NERVE REPAIR

NERVE REPAIR

Thomas M. Brushart, MD
PROFESSOR OF HAND SURGERY
JOHNS HOPKINS UNIVERSITY
VICE CHAIRMAN FOR RESEARCH, AND
CHIEF, DIVISION OF HAND SURGERY
DEPARTMENT OF ORTHOPAEDIC SURGERY
JOHN HOPKINS MEDICINE
BALTIMORE, MARYLAND

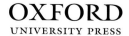

OXFORD
UNIVERSITY PRESS

Oxford University Press, Inc., publishes works that further Oxford University's objective of excellence
in research, scholarship, and education.

Oxford   New York
Auckland   Cape Town   Dar es Salaam   Hong Kong   Karachi   Kuala Lumpur   Madrid   Melbourne
Mexico City   Nairobi   New Delhi   Shanghai   Taipei   Toronto

With offices in
Argentina   Austria   Brazil   Chile   Czech Republic   France   Greece   Guatemala   Hungary   Italy
Japan   Poland   Portugal   Singapore   South Korea   Switzerland   Thailand   Turkey   Ukraine
Vietnam

Published by Oxford University Press, Inc.
198 Madison Avenue, New York, New York 10016

www.oup.com
Oxford is a registered trademark of Oxford University Press

Library of Congress Cataloging-in-Publication Data
Brushart, Thomas M.
  Nerve repair/Thomas M. Brushart.
      p.; cm.
  Includes bibliographical references.
  ISBN 978-0-19-516990-4 (hardcover)
ISBN-13 978-0-19-516990-4
1. Nervous system–Wounds and injuries. 2. Nervous system–Regeneration. 3. Nerves, Peripheral–Surgery. I. Title.
[DNLM: 1. Peripheral Nerves–surgery. 2. Nerve Regeneration. 3. Peripheral Nerves–physiology. 4. Treatment Outcome. WL 500]
RD593.B78 2011
617.4'81044–dc22   2010039082

9 8 7 6 5 4 3 2 1

Printed in China
on acid-free paper

Note to Readers

For my Family

PREFACE

The central objective of nerve repair is to assist regenerating axons to re-establish *useful* functional connections with the periphery.

Sir Sydney Sunderland

SURGICAL REUNION of proximal and distal nerve stumps has been the standard treatment of nerve transection injuries for over a century. Research carried out during this period has replaced empirical treatment of many diseases with novel therapies designed to combat specific molecular abnormalities. The twenty-first century has ushered in a genetic revolution that promises not only genetically engineered replacements for diseased or injured tissue, but ultimately the detection and treatment of genetic abnormalities before they result in disease. Unfortunately, today's peripheral nerve surgeon has not benefited from similar advances. We have made technical progress in the last 100 years—we operate with finer instruments and sutures, and view our work through the operating microscope—yet the repair of peripheral nerve remains an essentially mechanical undertaking.

Nerve Repair addresses a primary contributor to this therapeutic stasis, the progressive separation of surgical and scientific approaches to nerve injury. Today's surgeon, harried by a growing medical bureaucracy and dwindling resources, has little time for basic science research. In the operating room, the availability of prosthetic nerve tubes has actually decreased the emphasis placed on meticulous nerve repair. Ideally, the surgeon should approach each repair as an experiment in regeneration biology. The outcome will eventually manifest itself as the clinical result; the challenge is to identify the relevant variables and the degree to which they determine outcome in each case. The basic scientist, in contrast, can define variables and analyze their consequences at the molecular level. For this exercise to be relevant, however, it must be guided by clinical observation. Only by working together can the surgeon and scientist ask questions that will lead to molecular and genetic therapies for nerve injury.

This book was written to facilitate the dialog between surgeon and scientist by providing a translational review of the clinical and basic science relevant to nerve repair. It is designed to provide the clinician with an understanding of pertinent research, and the basic scientist with an overview of the clinical manifestations of nerve injury and regeneration. As clinical results are often published in summary form, they have been presented and analyzed to the extent possible with the information provided. Experimental results have been selected on the basis of their direct relevance to peripheral nerve regeneration in adult mammals. Most data are derived from experiments performed in living adult mammals or on adult mammalian neurons *in vitro*, and are presented in the context of the model system used in order to justify their inclusion.

Nerve Repair is grounded in the history of peripheral nerve surgery and biology so that modern concepts can be understood in the context of their origins. If there is a dominant theme, it is that neural organization is critical to function. In the periphery, axons must not only regenerate, they must also restore connections with functionally appropriate end organs. In the CNS, the normal organization of the systems used for motor control and sensory processing will determine the extent to which these systems can compensate for peripheral miswiring. Given the propensity for axonal misdirection at the site of nerve repair and the constrained flexibility of the CNS, enhancing the specificity of nerve regeneration is identified as a critical goal for future research.

ACKNOWLEDGMENTS

FROM INCEPTION to completion, this book has benefited from the contributions of many colleagues and friends. The project could not have been initiated without the support of the Thomas M. Brushart Chair in Hand Surgery, a generous gift from patients, family, and friends. Early funding was also provided by a grant from the National Library of Medicine. I am grateful to David Kline, Donald Price, Steve Scherer, Larry Schramm, Susan Standring, Giorgio Terengi, and James Urbaniak for writing in support of the grant application.

Nerve Repair would not be in its present form without the tireless enthusiasm of Kate Kiefe, whose graphics have done much to substantiate the text. I am also indebted to Tim Phelps for his meticulous artwork and to Norman Barker for his exceptional photography. As individual chapters were completed, I asked colleagues with particular expertise in the subject matter to review them. Art English, James Fawcett, Steven Hsiao, Richard Koerber, Goran Lundborg, Martijn Malessy, Beth Murinson, and Steve Scherer all responded with thoughtful suggestions, and I'm extremely grateful for their help. Thanks also to Pamela Talalay, who gently enforced the rules of English usage as she edited the text. I would especially like to acknowledge the generosity of Jack Griffin and Tessa Gordon, who read the entire manuscript and helped me recognize and correct many of its shortcomings.

Many others deserve thanks for more general contributions. Fiona Stevens and Craig Panner at Oxford University Press have been both supportive and patient in the face of what often seemed like glacial progress. My clinical partners, Dawn LaPorte, Gene Deune, and Heather Lochner kindly assumed my emergency call responsibilities when I was on sabbatical. Similarly, Kathy Cook in the office and Jennifer Kerr-Logan in the clinic protected my writing time; Jennifer also obtained the permissions for the book. Phil Kessens and several of my research fellows photocopied articles in the years before the Internet facilitated research. I owe a particular debt to my chairman, Frank Frassica, for allowing me the time to complete this project.

Finally, very special thanks go to my daughters Suzanne and Elizabeth and to my mother Ruthanna Weber for their patience in tolerating my all-too frequent absences, and to my wife Sandy, who steadfastly supported my dream for eight long years.

CONTENTS

NERVE REPAIR

The Adaxonal Membrane

The inner, adaxonal surface of the Schwann cell is enriched in myelin-associated glycoprotein (MAG) (Figure 1-2). MAG, a member of the immunoglobulin superfamily, is essential for signaling from Schwann cells to axons as part of normal myelin maintenance (reviewed in Quarles, 2002). MAG binds predominately to gangliosides on the axonal membrane (Yang et al., 1996). It may also bind to the Nogo-66 receptor (Domeniconi et al., 2002; Liu et al., 2002), and signal through a complex mechanism that involves the p75 (low affinity) neurotrophin receptor (Wang et al., 2002), though this mechanism has not been confirmed in the peripheral nervous system (PNS). MAG will be discussed further in the context of nerve regeneration (Chapter 9); it can inhibit axonal outgrowth (McKerracher et al., 1994), and it bears the HNK-1 carbohydrate, a specific marker of peripheral motor axons that may facilitate their selective reinnervation of previously motor pathways (Martini et al., 1994). Recently, nectin-like proteins (NECLs) have also been found to mediate adhesion between the adaxonal membrane and axon, both during myelination and in the mature nerve (Maurel et al., 2007; Spiegel et al., 2007). NECL-1 and NECL-2 on the axon both bind to NECL-4 on the adaxonal Schwann cell membrane (Figure 1-2).

Myelin

Myelin produced by the Schwann cell reduces the capacitance of the Schwann cell membrane, facilitating electrical conduction from one node of Ranvier to the next. The myelin sheath is a flattened extension of the Schwann cell that elongates and repeatedly encircles the axon (Figure 1-3). Once the layers formed by this process are compacted together, it is possible to distinguish the major dense line, a thin layer of cytoplasm bound by cell membranes, and the interperiod line, the extension of the extracellular space between these cellular components. Compact myelin is composed predominantly of cholesterol and sphingolipids, especially galactocerebroside and sulfatide (Suter, Snipes, 1995), but proteins also play a significant role in its structure. Po, the major protein of compact myelin, forms the interperiod line by linking its immunoglobulin G (IgG)-like extracellular domains to form a complex lattice (Shapiro et al., 1996). Myelin basic protein (MBP) is a cytoplasmic protein that constitutes

much of the major dense line of compact myelin (Lemke, Axel, 1985). An additional glycoprotein, PMP-22, has a major impact on myelin structure, as shown by the severe consequences of its under- or overexpression (reviewed in Quarles, 2002).

The interrelationship of the three primary structural characteristics of myelinated axons—axon diameter, myelin thickness, and internodal length—were clearly elucidated by extensive electronmicroscopic studies (discussed in Berthold, Rydmark, 1995). There is a nearly linear correlation between myelin cross-sectional area and the circumference of the axon, suggesting that myelin production is regulated by the contact area between axon and Schwann cell. Internodal length, in contrast, is proportional to the growth experienced by a given nerve. The adult internodal length is the product of the length of the Schwann cell at the time myelination begins (usually when the axon reaches a diameter of 1 μm; Murray, 1968) and the longitudinal growth that occurs subsequently. Since the axons that will become the largest are myelinated first, there is a positive correlation between internodal length and axon diameter (Berthold, Nilsson, 1983). As a general rule, internodal length is approximately 100x axon diameter (Hess, Young, 1952).

THE AXON

Structure

The myelinated axon is surrounded by the axon membrane, or axolemma. It contains a variety of organelles, including mitochondria, axoplasmic reticulum, and several types of vesicles and inclusions. It is supported by a dynamic cytoskeleton that consists of microtubules, neurofilaments, and the microtrabecular matrix. The axolemma interacts with its ensheathing Schwann cell across the periaxonal space (Figure 1-3). Throughout the internodal segment, the axolemma contains receptors that probably interact with MAG on the adjacent adaxonal Schwann cell membrane (see above: The Schwann Cell). This interaction results in maintenance of a constant gap between axon and Schwann cell.

The axolemma is specialized to facilitate conduction at both the node of Ranvier, the gap between adjacent Schwann cells, and the juxtaparanodal region, the transition between compact myelin and the paranode (Figure 1-1). Voltage-gated sodium channels are concentrated in the nodal axon membrane, primarily $Na_v 1.6$ (Caldwell et al., 2000), but also $Na_v 1.2$, $Na_v 1.8$, and $Na_v 1.9$ (reviewed in Scherer,

Arroyo, 2002). Channels of the Na$_v$1.x family are functionally similar, but differ significantly in their activation kinetics (Yu, Catterall, 2003). These channels are anchored to the cytoskeleton by two splice variants of ankyrin G (Kordeli et al., 1990, 1995), and are responsible for the initial rapid membrane depolarization of the action potential. Recently, the potassium channel KCNQ2 has also been identified in the nodes of PNS axons (Devaux et al., 2004), where it may serve to control membrane instability. In the mammal, unlike the amphibian, action potential repolarization is achieved without delayed activation of potassium channels (Chiu, 1993). Nonetheless, the delayed rectifying potassium channels K$_v$1.1 and K$_v$1.2 are present in the juxtaparanodal area, where they may dampen the excitability of myelinated fibers (reviewed in Scherer, Arroyo, 2002).

Impulse Conduction

The physiology of impulse conduction has been reviewed extensively (Ritchie, 1995; Koester, Siegelbaum, 2000). The axonal membrane functions as a capacitor, separating a positive external charge from a negative internal charge. The result of this charge separation, designated the resting membrane potential, is normally between −60 and −70 millivolts, and is determined by the relative concentrations of intra- and extracellular ions. Na+ and Cl⁻ are more concentrated outside the cell, while K+ and organic ions are more concentrated inside. These concentrations are regulated by Na+/K+ ATPase, the relative density and nature of ion channels, and the inability of organic ions to diffuse through the cell membrane.

Electrical conduction is initiated by opening voltage-gated sodium channels, which allows Na+ to move down its concentration gradient into the axon. The resulting decrease in membrane potential produces the rising phase of the action potential. In lower animals, voltage-gated potassium channels are then opened to allow potassium to leave the cell, returning the membrane potential to its resting value. These channels are not found in normal mammalian peripheral nerve, although they may contribute to repolarization in immature, regenerating, or demyelinated mammalian axons (Chiu, 1993). Instead, the activation of sodium channels is linked directly to their inactivation, briskly limiting the influx of ions, and passive K+ leakage returns the membrane potential to its resting value. The action potential generated in one segment of membrane supplies the depolarizing current to the adjacent segment, activating the voltage-gated channels and depolarizing the membrane in sequential fashion down the axon.

Were the axon not myelinated, conduction velocity would be slowed by the electrical resistance of the axon. Addition of myelin decreases the capacitance of the membrane, making it easier for a small amount of current to discharge the membrane and propagate the action potential passively along the axon. Myelin also limits the flux of ions across the cell membrane, however, interfering with the normal mechanism of action potential propagation. Membrane specializations at the node of Ranvier mitigate this problem. Voltage-gated sodium channels concentrated in the node of Ranvier amplify the signal by generating a strong inward Na+ current when stimulated by the more passive spread of depolarization from within the myelinated segment. The brief slowing of conduction during this amplification process at the node of Ranvier results in a relative jumping of the impulse from node to node, termed *saltatory conduction*.

The economies of myelination are considerable: a 10-μm myelinated fiber and a 500-μm unmyelinated fiber will both conduct at about 20 m/s (Ritchie, 1995). Myelin thickness is closely linked to axon diameter. Rushton (1951) calculated that the ideal relationship was achieved when the g ratio (axon diameter: total fiber diameter) was 0.6. In fact, most myelinated PNS axons have a g ratio between 0.47 and 0.74. Rushton's theory predicts that the conduction speed of myelinated fibers is roughly proportional to axon diameter, an observation borne out by findings in the cat (discussed in Ritchie, 1995). Rushton (1951) also calculated that conduction in axons smaller than 0.6 μm in diameter would not be improved by myelination.

Axoplasmic Transport

Neurons, by far the longest cells in the body, have also been adapted for the transport of materials. Transport may proceed in the anterograde direction, from the neuron to the periphery, or in the retrograde direction, from periphery back to neuron. Although transport may progress at a variety of speeds, it is usually characterized as fast or slow. Fast transport covers up to 400 mm/day in the anterograde direction and up to 300 mm/day in the retrograde direction (Grafstein, Forman, 1980). Slow transport, in contrast, proceeds at 0.1–4 mm/day (reviewed in Grafstein, 1995).

Fast transport conveys mitochondria, vesicles containing neurotransmitters, lysosomes and prelysosomal organelles, tubovesicular organelles that resemble smooth endoplasmic reticulum, membrane proteins such as sodium channels and transmitter receptors, and a variety of other molecular species including the calmodulin-binding protein GAP-43, agrin, and trophic factors (reviewed in Grafstein, 1995). The neurotrophin nerve growth factor (NGF) undergoes retrograde transport within endosomes, accompanied by its tyrosine kinase receptor, TrkA (Delcroix et al., 2003).

Fast transport proceeds along axonal microtubules. These unbranched tubulin polymers are 25 nm thick and may vary from 100 μm to 800 μm in length. Microtubules are polarized, with rapidly elongating "plus" ends and slowly elongating "minus" ends (Desai, Mitchison, 1997); the plus end is directed away from the cell body (Burton, Paige, 1981). Their density within an axon decreases with increasing axon size, from about $100/\mu m^2$ of cross-sectional area in small axons to $10/\mu m^2$ in large ones (Berthold, Rydmark, 1995). Microtubule density also varies along the course of the axon, and between afferent and efferent axons (summarized in Berthold,Rydmark, 1995). Organelles undergoing fast anterograde transport are linked to microtubules through the ATPase kinesin (Vallee, Shpetner, 1990). The selectivity of transport is controlled by the use of adaptor or scaffolding proteins to recognize and bind specific cargoes to the kinesin (reviewed in Hirokawa, Takemura, 2005). While bound to adenosine triphosphate (ATP), kinesin is tightly anchored to tubulin; when ATP is converted to adenosine diphosphate (ADP), the kinesin releases its hold, and transport occurs as the molecule changes configuration (Romberg, Vale, 1993). Fast retrograde transport also proceeds along microtubules, but is motored by the ATPase dynein (Vallee, Shpetner, 1990).

Slow transport was initially divided into two components, slow component a (SCa), the slowest, and slow component b (SCb). Microtubules and neurofilaments of the cytoskeleton were found to travel at the speed of SCa (Hoffman, Lasek, 1975), whereas SCb conveyed enzymes of intermediary metabolism as well as clathrin, calpain, actin and actin-binding proteins of the microfilament network, heat shock proteins, calmodulin, and synapsin I (reviewed in Grafstein, 1995). As the velocity of SCb corresponds to the speed of axon regeneration, manipulation of slow transport will play a crucial role in attempts to enhance regeneration.

The nature of slow transport continued to vex investigators long after the mechanism of fast transport had been clarified. Significant crossover was found between the two compartments, blurring the distinction between them (Vallee, Bloom, 1991). There was even debate as to whether the cytoskeleton was stationary or moving, depending on which techniques were used for analysis (summarized in Baas, 2002). This issue was resolved only recently through observation of fluorescence-tagged neurofilaments. Neurofilament proteins, a major constituent of the axonal cytoskeketon, are polymers of three separate monomers, each existing in several forms depending on their degree of phosphorylation (Nixon, Sihag, 1991). Neurofilament density is a relative constant at about $100/\mu m^2$ of axon cross-section, and is thought to be a primary determinant of axon caliber (Hoffman et al., 1984). Assembled neurofilaments were found to move in an intermittent and highly asynchronous manner, at peak rates up to 2.3 μm/s, but with pauses for extended periods between bursts of activity (Roy et al., 2000; Wang et al., 2000). This motion could be powered by a clever reversal of the mechanism for fast retrograde transport. The motor protein dynein is normally anchored to microtubules, and moves its cargo of organelles retrogradely in reference to them. If the dynein cargo domain is anchored to the actin microfilament matrix instead of to a readily mobile organelle, however, dynein activation could lead to paradoxical movement of the microtubule at the other end of the molecule, and in the anterograde direction relative to the fixed cargo domain (Ahmad et al., 1998).

THE DIVERSITY OF MYELINATED AXONS

Peripheral axons may be classified generally according to their conduction velocity, or more specifically on the basis of their size and end organ (Table 1-1). Erlanger and Gasser, pioneering electrophysiologists, observed that "the peculiar conglomerations of the constituent fibers of a nerve which give to conducted action potentials their characteristic configurations... are the expression of a segregation of fibers into different functional systems" (Erlanger, Gasser,1968, p68). They subdivided axons into three groups on the basis of their conduction properties. Group A axons, the most rapidly conducting, consisted of myelinated somatic efferent and afferent fibers. This group was further subdivided into alpha (70–120 m/s), beta

Table 1-1 Receptors that Participate in Somatic Sensation.
Their fibers are classified both as to conduction velocity and according to their size and end organ characteristics.

Receptor Types Active in Somatic Sensation

Receptor Type	Conduction Properties	Morphology, Modality	Sensation
Cutaneous & subcutaneous mechanoreceptors			*Touch*
Meissner's corpuscle	Aα, β	RA	Stroking, fluttering
Merkel disk receptor	Aα, β	SAI	Pressure, texture
Pacinian corpuscle	Aα, β	PC	Vibration
Ruffini ending	Aα, β	SAII	Skin stretch
Thermal receptors			*Temperature*
Cool receptors	Aδ	III	Skin cooling (25° C)
Warm receptors	C	IV	Skin warming (41° C)
Heat nociceptors	Aδ	III	Hot temperatures (>45° C)
Cold nociceptors	C	IV	Cold temperatures (<5° C)
Nociceptors			*Pain*
Mechanical	Aδ	III	Sharp, pricking pain
Thermal-mechanical	Aδ	III	Burning pain
Thermal-mechanical	C	IV	Freezing pain
Polymodal	C	IV	Slow, burning pain
Muscle and skeletal mechanoreceptors			*Limb proprioception*
Muscle spindle primary	Aα	Ia	Muscle length & speed
Muscle spindle secondary	Aβ	II	Muscle stretch
Golgi tendon organ	Aα	Ib	Muscle contraction
Joint capsule mechanoreceptors	Aβ	II	Joint angle
Stretch-sensitive free endings	Aδ	III	Excess stretch or force

Modified from Kandel, Schwartz, and Jessell, Principles of Neuroscience, 2000.

(30–70 m/s), gamma (15–30 m/s), and delta (12–30 m/s) subpopulations. Group B was limited to preganglionic autonomic fibers, and Group C, the slowest, included unmyelinated postganglionic autonomic fibers and unmyelinated somatic afferent fibers. In an alternative classification system, the alpha, beta, and gamma designations of group A were limited to efferent fibers (1965 Stockholm conference proceedings cited in Boyd, Davey, 1968) and afferent fibers were classified according to their size: type I—large myelinated; type II—intermediate myelinated; type III—small myelinated; type IV—unmyelinated (Lloyd, 1943). This scheme has been expanded to include designations such as rapidly adapting (RA) to distinguish an Aα or Aβ fiber with particular receptor properties, and Ia and Ib to differentiate primary muscle spindle fibers from those serving Golgi tendon organs (see Chapters 2 and 3). Figure 1-4 shows these various fiber populations in nerves that supply four functionally distinct tissues in the cat (Boyd, Davey, 1968). Peripheral nerve trunks thus convey a complex spectrum of fiber

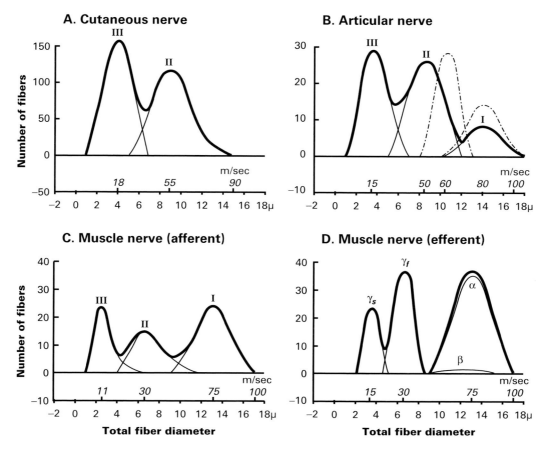

FIGURE 1-4 Distribution of axon diameters and conduction velocities in four functional classes of cat nerve. Fine lines define the distribution of axons within each subgroup; the thick line defines the entire population. The dotted line in B applies to the nerve to the interosseous membrane. The muscle efferents are classified as to conduction velocity, whereas the afferent axons are grouped by size. (Boyd and Davey, 1968, with permission).

types; even tributary branches destined for a single tissue contain a diverse axon population.

Axons may differ not only in their size and conduction velocity, but also in the molecular constituents present in their axoplasm and periaxonal environments. The enzyme acetylcholinesterase (AChE), a component of the cholinergic transmitter system, was one of the earliest factors found to differentiate myelinated motor from myelinated sensory axons (Adams et al., 1967). Histochemical demonstration of AChE on cross sections of nerve tissue was later used clinically to identify and selectively re-unite predominantly motor fascicles during peripheral nerve repair (Gruber, Zenker, 1973). Motor axons are also distinguished from myelinated afferent axons by selective binding of the ganglioside

antibody GD1a-1, consistent with the participation of anti-GD1a antibodies in acute motor axonal neuropathy (AMAN) (Gong et al., 2002). Myelinated sensory, but not motor axons contain carbonic anhydrase (Riley et al., 1982), an enzyme that catalyzes the breakdown of bicarbonate in a variety of tissues (Carter, 1972). Although these axonal constituents may be helpful in the identification of recently transected axons (Riley et al., 1988), a role in the selective guidance of regenerating axons seems unlikely; their clearance by Wallerian degeneration would limit their availability to only the most rapidly regenerating axons.

The periaxonal environment may also be modality-specific. The antibodies L2 and HNK-1 identify a carbohydrate epitope of several neural recognition molecules, including MAG and Po (Schachner, 1990). This epitope, now commonly referred to as HNK-1, is selectively expressed on the Schwann cells and Schwann cell basement membrane of motor axons, but is rarely found on those of sensory axons (Martini et al., 1988). HNK-1 is discussed further in Chapter 10 as a potential determinant of motor axon regeneration. Uninjured motor nerve is also characterized by selective expression of the extracellular matrix protein F-spondin. The uniform distribution of F-spondin after nerve injury suggests that it is unlikely to play a role in regeneration specificity (Burstyn-Cohen et al., 1998).

AXON/SCHWANN CELL INTERACTIONS

The axon and its Schwann cell partners engage in a dialog that regulates the form and function of the Schwann cell/axon complex throughout development and axon regeneration. Crucial interactions provide axons with the correct number of Schwann cells, match axon caliber with myelin of appropriate thickness, determine the structure of the internode, and provide myelinating Schwann cells with a modality-specific phenotype.

Several axon/Schwann cell interactions are mediated through the Neuregulin family of signaling molecules. Neuregulin-1 (NRG-1) is expressed by motor, sensory, and autonomic neurons (Corfas et al., 1995). NRG-1 modifies Schwann cell behavior by interacting with heterodimers of ErbB-2 and ErbB-3 tyrosine kinase receptors on the Schwann cell membrane (Figure 1-2) (reviewed in Citri et al., 2003). During early development, neuron-derived NRG-1 signaling promotes Schwann cell differentiation, proliferation, survival, and migration (reviewed in Falls, 2003). Later, axonal NRG-1 controls Schwann cell myelination to match axon caliber with myelin thickness. Experimentally, reduced NRG-1 expression results in hypomyelination and reduced nerve conduction velocity, while overexpression of NRG-1 induces hypermyelination (Michailov et al., 2004). The magnitude of axon-glial signaling through NRG-1 is thought to be a reflection of axon caliber that can be sensed by the Schwann cell and translated into appropriate myelin thickness.

Direct signaling between axon and Schwann cell also sculpts the node of Ranvier. As discussed above, sodium channels in the axonal membrane are tightly clustered at the node, potassium channels are localized to the juxtaparanode, and the two areas are separated by the firm anchoring of paranodal myelin loops to the axon (Figure 1-1). Soon after myelination is initiated, sodium channels cluster near Schwann cell processes (Vabnick et al., 1996). As the space between Schwann cells becomes narrowed, adjacent sodium channel clusters are packed together within the node of Ranvier (Pedraza et al., 2001). Studies in vitro confirm that physical contact with Schwann cells is necessary for this localization (Ching et al., 1999). The individual steps in this process are reviewed in Corfas et al., 2004.

The modulation of axon caliber by myelin was first elucidated by the classic nerve grafting experiments of Aguayo and coworkers (1979). In the Trembler mouse mutant, peripheral nerve is poorly myelinated. Segments of this nerve were grafted from Trembler mice into wild-type mice, so that wild-type axons would leave their normal environment, grow through hypomyelinating Trembler Schwann cells, then regain the company of normal Schwann cells. Once reinnervation had occurred, axon caliber was reduced within the graft, but not proximally or distally; the degree of myelination, dictated by the type of Schwann cell in a given area, determined the caliber of the normal axons passing through. The influence of myelin can also be inferred by examining the small unmyelinated segments of healthy myelinated axons, such as the node of Ranvier (Berthold, 1978) and the stem process of dorsal root ganglion (DRG) neurons (Hsieh et al., 1994), both of which are of reduced caliber. At the ultrastructural level, axon caliber correlates with the number of neurofilaments within the axon (Friede, Samorajski, 1970) and more specifically with the packing of these neurofilaments (Hoffman et al., 1984). Neurofilament is a structural protein formed by the aggregation of three distinct subunits, NF-L, NF-M, and NF-H (Schlaepfer, Freeman, 1978). The carboxyl-terminals on NF-M and NF-H bear varying numbers of lysine-serine-proline repeats and are associated with sidearms that extend from the neurofilament core (Geisler et al., 1983; Hisanga and Hirokawa, 1988).

The Aguayo experiments were repeated to examine neurofilament parameters within the narrowed axonal segments of the graft (DeWaegh et al., 1992). Neurofilaments in this region were less phosphorylated and more densely packed than their proximal and distal counterparts within axons of normal caliber. These observations led to the hypothesis that neurofilament phosphorylation results from a balance of kinase and phosphatase activities (summarized in Witt, Brady, 2000); the more phosphorylated the neurofilaments, the more their charges repel one another and the more widely they are spaced. Examination of the node of Ranvier and the DRG stem process, sites of normal axonal narrowing, appeared to confirm this hypothesis (Hsieh et al., 1994). However, removing the charged sites from the NF-H subunit of the neurofilament triplet did not alter neurofilament spacing or axon caliber (Rao et al., 2002), eliminating charge repulsion as the primary mechanism of spacing. An alternative explanation is that phosphorylation exerts its effect by stiffening the sidearm of the NF-M neurofilament subunit (Garcia et al., 2003), thus forcing the assembled neurofilaments farther apart. Similarly, phosphorylation of NF-H could slow the transport of neurofilament proteins (Ackerly et al., 2003), explaining the larger absolute volume of neurofilament proteins in areas of myelination. Most recently, however, preventing phosphorylation of NF-M has been shown to have no effect on axon caliber, opening the field to new alternative hypotheses (Garcia et al., 2009).

Signaling from Schwann cell myelination to neurofilament phosphorylation is thought to be initiated by the myelin-associated glycoprotein (MAG). MAG on the adaxonal Schwann cell membrane binds to gangliosides on the underlying axon (Yang et al., 1996) (Figure 1-2). Although MAG also engages the Nogo-66 receptor (Domeniconi et al., 2002; Liu et al., 2002) to signal through a complex mechanism that involves the p75 (low affinity) neurotrophin receptor (Wang et al., 2002), this mechanism has not been observed in the PNS. The subsequent events are complex, and may involve activation of the extracellular signal-related protein kinase 1/2 (ERK1/2) with a feedback loop involving cdk-5, a member of the cyclin-dependent protein kinase family (discussed in Griffin, Hoke, 2005).

Mature Schwann cells are traditionally viewed as expressing one of two possible phenotypes, myelinating or nonmyelinating (Jessen, Mirsky, 2002). Recent evidence, however, demonstrates that myelinating Schwann cells acquire secondary characteristics from their axonal partners, characteristics that persist after the original axon/Schwann cell partnership has ended. Initial evidence for this persisting identity was produced by experiments on the expression of the HNK-1 carbohydrate, an epitope of several neural adhesion molecules (Martini et al., 1994). HNK-1 is expressed normally by Schwann cells associated with motor axons, but not by those associated with cutaneous afferents. During regeneration, motor axons stimulate HNK-1 expression when they encounter previously motor Schwann cells, but not when they are paired with Schwann cells that previously served cutaneous afferents. Schwann cells thus derive a motor identity from their initial Schwann cell/axon pairing, and this identity persists after denervation and informs their subsequent behavior.

Ongoing exploration of the differences between cutaneous and muscle nerve has revealed that each is characterized by a unique pattern of trophic factor expression (Brushart et al., 2005; Hoke et al., 2006). Cutaneous nerve, denervated or reinnervated by cutaneous axons, dramatically upregulates nerve growth factor (NGF) and brain-derived neurotrophic factor (BDNF) but expresses little glial-derived neurotrophic factor (GDNF) or pleiotrophin (PT). Under similar conditions, ventral root upregulates GDNF and pleiotrophin 20- to 40-fold while expressing virtually no NGF or BDNF. Cutaneous and motor Schwann cells thus express growth factors appropriate to their axonal partners, and when challenged by axons with differing requirements do not change their expression patterns. Again, they acquire an identity from their initial axonal partners that influences their subsequent interactions. These observations have obvious consequences for both nerve regeneration and grafting.

THE UNMYELINATED AXON

Unmyelinated axons, or C fibers, account for 75% of the total axon number in cutaneous nerve and dorsal root and about 50% of the total in muscle nerve (Ochoa, 1976). They range in size from 0.1 to 2 μm in diameter; the diameter of a single axon may change by a factor of 3 or 4 over a distance of only 5 μm (Greenberg et al., 1990). In contrast to the one-to-one relationship between Schwann cell and myelinated axon, multiple unmyelinated axons can be ensheathed by a single Schwann cell (Figure 1-5). This assembly is termed a Remak bundle to honor the scientist who described it. The juxtaposition of axons without interposed myelin within the Remak bundle suggested to early observers that electrical signals might pass from one axon to another. This possibility stimulated the electrophysiologist Gasser

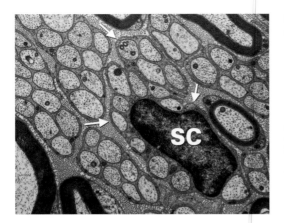

FIGURE 1-5   Fourteen unmyelinated axons are encompassed by the basement membrane (arrows) of a single Schwann cell to form a Remak bundle. Portions of myelinated axons are seen at the periphery. Electron micrograph, 4,000x.

to serially reconstruct the course of 54 axons through a 500 μm segment of cat saphenous nerve (Gasser, 1955). He found that axons were continuously exchanged from bundle to bundle, minimizing the possibility of intercommunication. Subsequent studies by Aguayo and coworkers confirmed the plexiform interactions of Remak bundles as they coursed distally, and established the variability in their size (Aguayo et al., 1976). As many as 100 axons may be served by a single Schwann cell in the dorsal root, while one-to-one relationships may be found in peripheral nerve. Recent immunohistochemical studies have demonstrated that a single Schwann cell may support diverse axon types with different growth factor dependencies (Murinson et al., 2005), further establishing the heterogeneous nature of the Remak bundle.

The majority of C fibers in peripheral nerve respond to both mechanical stimuli and heat, the so-called polymodal nociceptors that mediate a slow, burning pain (Bessou, Perl, 1969). Additional classes of C fiber respond individually to cold and heat (Table 1-1). Recent studies have also identified C fibers that respond to histamine to produce itch (Schmetz et al., 1997), and that respond to slow stroking of the skin to produce a sensation of pleasant touch (Olausson et al., 2002). As a group, C-fibers thus contribute to protective sensibility, but not to functional touch or the control of motion. In spite of these secondary functions, however, C fibers may compromise the recovery from nerve injury by contributing to the spontaneous generation of pain.

CONNECTIVE TISSUE LAYERS

Epineurium

Epineurium is the connective tissue that ensheaths peripheral nerve (Figure 1-6). It has been subdivided into outer epineurium, the superficial covering of nerve, and internal epineurium, the tissue that surrounds individual fascicles (Millesi, Terzis, 1983). Epineurium may comprise between 30 and 75% of the cross-sectional area of a nerve, with greater quantities found where fascicles are more numerous (Sunderland, 1965). Human epineurium is constructed largely of types I and III collagen (Salonen et al., 1985; Lorimier et al., 1992), with type I predominating (Seyer et al., 1977). Human collagen fibers range between 60 and 110 nm in diameter (Gamble, Eames, 1964). The equivalent fibers are 70–85 nm in diameter in the rabbit (Thomas, 1963) and 50–80 nm in the rat (Junqueira et al., 1979). The orientation of epineurial collagen was initially described as being predominantly longitudinal on the basis of transmission electron microscopy (TEM) of rabbit and human epineurium (Thomas, 1963; Gamble, Eames, 1964). More recent work with the scanning electron microscope (SEM) (Ushiki, Ide, 1990) and Nomarsky optics (Stolinski, 1995), however, has shown epineurial collagen to be gathered into bundles, 10–20 μm in width, that are arrayed around the circumference of the nerve in waves with a period of 39 μm (Figure 1-7). These bundles are more densely packed adjacent to the perineurium, and are interlaced throughout by a meshwork of fine collagen. This arrangement suggests that the epineurium is designed to accommodate stretch. Epineurium remains intact after nerve has been elongated to failure (stretched to the point that its elastic properties are lost) (Rydevik et al., 1990), indicating that epineurium does indeed stretch, so much so that it does not contribute significantly to the tensile strength of the nerve.

The epineurium contains elastin fibers that, like collagen, are more concentrated adjacent to the perineurium (Thomas, 1963). The cellular population includes fibroblasts, varying numbers of mast cells, and fat cells. The abundance of epineurial fat within the sciatic nerve in the buttock and thigh led Sunderland to suggest that epineurium might serve to cushion and protect the fascicles within its envelope (Sunderland, 1945b).

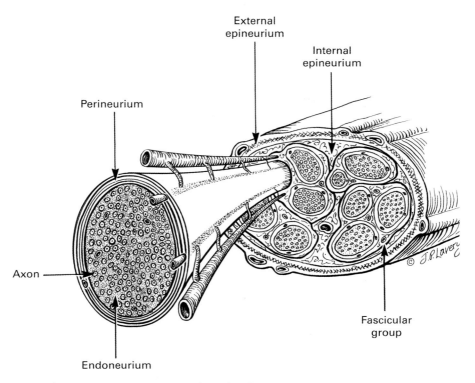

FIGURE 1-6   The macroscopic organization of peripheral nerve.

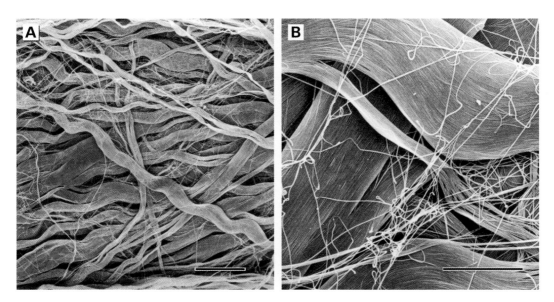

FIGURE 1-7   Scanning electron micrographs of epineurium that has been treated with NaOH. The proximo-distal axis of the nerve is horizontal. A: crimped collagen bundles run obliquely to the nerve axis, crossing each other at acute angles. Bar: 50 μm. B: At higher magnification, thick bundles are seen to give off smaller bundles (upper left). These are enmeshed with a loose network of fine collagen. Bar: 10 μm. (Ushiki, Ide, 1990, with permission).

Perineurium

The perineurium is the cellular layer that contains and thus defines the individual nerve fascicle. It is characterized by lamellae of flattened cells separated by thin layers of collagen that range from 40–80 nm in diameter in human nerve (Thomas, 1963; Gamble, Eames, 1964) (Figure 1-8). These fibers are predominantly fabricated of type III collagen, though some type I may be present (Lorimier et al., 1992). They are arranged in a wavy pattern similar to that of the epineurium, but with a shorter period of 6–9 μm (Stolinski, 1995). Additionally, the innermost perineurial cell layer adheres to a distinct boundary layer of densely woven collagen fibers and subperineurial fibroblasts that mechanically links the perineurium to its endoneurial contents (Ushiki, Ide, 1990).

Perineurial lamellae are more numerous in larger fascicles, and decrease in number peripherally until single axons are served by only a single cell layer (Lehman, 1957; Shanthaveerappa, Bourne, 1966; Burkel, 1967). The flattened, polygonal cells that constitute each lamella are specialized to function as a diffusion barrier (Shanthaveerappa, Bourne, 1966). Each cell is bounded on both inner and outer surfaces by basal lamina, and they are joined to one another by tight junctions. The basal lamina is composed of collagens IV and V (Shellswell et al., 1979; Timpl et al., 1981), heparin sulfate proteoglycan (Eldridge et al., 1986), fibronectin (Yamada, 1981), and laminin, which is found only on the innermost cell surface between perineurium and endoneurium (Schiff, Rosenbluth, 1986). The cells themselves are metabolically equipped to act as a diffusion barrier, with high levels of ATPase and creatine kinase activity (Shanthaveerappa, Bourne, 1962). Breakdown and recovery of barrier function are associated with changes in the expression of the intercellular junction proteins claudin-1, claudin-5, occludin, VE-cadherin, and connexin 43 (Hirakawa et al., 2003).

As could be predicted from the tightly adherent cellular structure and more longitudinally oriented collagen, the perineurium is less tolerant of elongation than is the adjacent epineurium. In the rabbit tibial nerve, mechanical failure during elongation coincides with disruption of the perineurium while the epineurium remains intact (Rydevik et al., 1990). The integrity of the diffusion barrier is maintained after 2 hours of 15% elongation (Lundborg, Rydevik, 1973); 27% elongation causes acute perineurial

disruption (Rydevik et al., 1990). The apparent strength of the bond between the innermost perineurial cell layer and the underlying sub-perineurial collagen is borne out by the observation that traction on the endoneurium results in shear through the innermost perineurial cell layer rather than between perineurium and endoneurium (Tillett et al., 2004).

Formation of the perineurium is controlled by Schwann cells (Mirsky et al., 1999). The signaling molecule Desert hedgehog is expressed by Schwann cell precursors and by Schwann cells up to postnatal day 10. The receptor for this molecule, patched, is expressed in mesenchymal cells that surround the developing nerve. In Desert hedgehog knockout mice, the perineurium develops poorly, forming mini-fascicles strongly reminiscent of those in the distal stump after nerve repair. In humans, mutation of the Desert hedgehog gene results in a similar picture in uninjured nerve (Umehara et al., 2002).

Endoneurium

The endoneurium is the collagenous matrix that surrounds individual axons within the perineurium (Figure 1-8). Endoneurial collagen fibers are smaller than those found in the epineurium, with ranges in diameter of 50–60 nm in rabbits (Thomas, 1963), 20–40 nm in rats (Junqueira et al., 1979), and 30–65 nm in humans (Gamble, Eames, 1964). These fibers are fabricated from types I and III collagen (Salonen et al., 1985; Lorimier et al., 1992). Endoneurial collagen in the surround of larger rat and rabbit axons can be divided into two layers (Thomas, 1963; Ushiki, Ide, 1990). An inner meshwork of fine collagen fibers adheres to the Schwann cell basal lamina, while a loosely arranged, more densely packed layer fills the space between axons. This arrangement has not been demonstrated in human nerve (Gamble, Eames, 1964). The endoneurium is populated by fibroblasts (Ochoa, Mair, 1969), many of which are concentrated superficially, adjacent to the perineurium (Ushiki, Ide, 1990). Between 2% and 9% of endoneurial cells are resident macrophages, the primary antigen-presenting cells of peripheral nerve (Griffin et al., 1993). These cells vigorously scavenge extracellular proteins and present them to T cells emerging from the circulation.

The interstices of the endoneurial collagen are packed with an extracellular matrix rich in glycoproteins, glycosaminoglycans, and proteoglycans

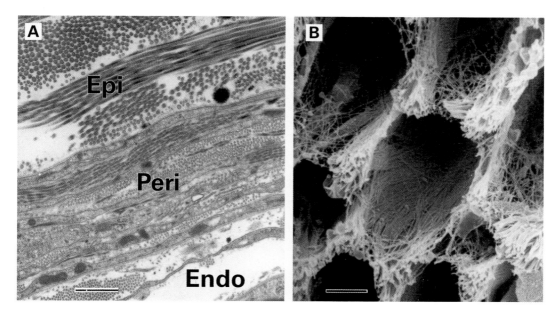

FIGURE 1-8   A. Transmission electron micrograph of the connective tissue layers that ensheath peripheral nerve. Layered collagen bundles with occasional elastin fibers (large black dots) characterize the epineurium. The perineurium contains finer collagen fibers sandwiched between cellular layers. The transition between perineurium and endoneurium is marked by fine collagen fibers (around scale bar) and endoneurial fibroblasts (right of scale bar). Bar: 1 μm. (Ushiki, Ide, 1990, with permission). B. Scanning electron micrograph of an endoneurial tube from which axon and Schwann cell have been removed. The inner layer of the tube is composed of a meshwork of thin collagen fibrils, while the outer one consists of longitudinally arranged collagen bundles. Bar: 2 μm. (Ushiki, Ide, 1990, with permission).

(Rutka et al., 1988; Chernousov, Carey, 2000; Dubovy et al, 2002). The best-characterized of these include the glycoproteins fibronectin, tenascin-C, and thrombospondin, and the Chondroitin sulfate proteoglycans (CSPGs) versican and decorin. The expression of these factors changes after nerve injury, so they are potentially relevant to the process of regeneration. In uninjured nerve, immuno-electron microscopy indicates that fibronectin co-localizes with endoneurial collagens types I and III, where it anchors cells to basal lamina and to one another (Lorimier et al., 1992). Tenascin-C is a boundary molecule the expression of which is confined to the node of Ranvier in normal nerve (Martini, 1994). Thrombospondin, ubiquitous during neural development, is restricted in the adult to areas capable of plasticity (Hoffman et al., 1994). It binds readily to both laminin and fibronectin (Lahav et al., 1984; Mumby et al., 1984). Two CSPGs immunologically related to decorin and versican bind to fibronectin in vitro, but do not bind to laminin or collagen (Braunewell et al., 1995). The tendency for axons to regenerate along the inner surface of the Schwann cell basal lamina, rather than through the endoneurium (Ide et al., 1983), characterizes the endoneurial environment as relatively nonpermissive when compared to that within the Schwann cell tube.

When viewed through the operating microscope, peripheral nerve appears to have alternating light and dark circumferential stripes, the so-called bands of Fontana. These are the optical consequence of axon organization within the epineurium (reviewed by Clarke, Bearn, 1972). When nerve is relaxed, axons take an undulating course; light reflecting from these undulations is responsible for the observed bands. When the nerve is stretched, the axons become straight and the bands disappear. The amount of stretch required to straighten the axons can thus be tolerated without axonal damage.

Vascular supply

Neurovascular anatomy has been reviewed by Adams (1942), Lundborg (1988), and Best and Mackinnon (1994). Peripheral nerve is supplied by segmental nutrient vessels that travel through the mesoneurium, the thin connective tissue layer that loosely anchors the nerve to its bed. These vessels join a longitudinally-oriented vascular network that extends throughout the epineurium, giving off lateral branches to the perineurium of each fascicle. The perineurium, in turn, is characterized by a second predominantly longitudinal vascular plexus. Transperineurial arterioles 10–25 μm in diameter pass from the epineurium to the endoneurium through sleeves of perineurial tissue (Beggs et al., 1991). These arterioles are often associated with clusters of unmyelinated fibers, suggesting that they may participate in the control of endoneurial blood flow. Their course through the perineurium is quite oblique, rendering them potentially susceptible to changes in intra- or extrafascicular pressure (Lundborg, 1988). The endoneurial microvessels are similar to capillaries histochemically (Bell, Weddell, 1984b), yet they are larger (Bell, Weddell, 1984a) and their extensive investment of pericytes is more consistent with a postcapillary venule (reviewed in Best, Mackinnon, 1994). This size may contribute to the unusually high baseline blood flow to nerve, which has been measured as twice that to spinal cord under comparable circumstances (Smith et al., 1977). The density of endoneurial microvessels varies significantly throughout the PNS, and these variations correlate with susceptibility to ischemic neuropathy (Kozu et al., 1992).

The outstanding characteristic of the peripheral neurovascular system is its flexibility. Peripheral nerve may be surgically mobilized, severing its nutrient vessels, to a surprising degree. The rabbit sciatic nerve can be mobilized to a 1:41 diameter: length ratio without interrupting blood flow (Maki et al., 1997), and the monkey sciatic nerve tolerates mobilization over 12 cm without compromising the outcome of subsequent transection and repair (Kline et al., 1972). Furthermore, the distribution of circulation within the endoneurium is exquisitely sensitive to physical and chemical manipulations (Lundborg, 1988). The vascular status of transected peripheral nerve will thus rarely be a significant variable in regeneration experiments, and should minimally influence the recovery from isolated nerve lacerations in humans.

THE INTRANEURAL ORGANIZATION OF AXONS

Dissection

The intraneural architecture of peripheral nerve was first described by Prochaska (1779) (Figure 1-9). He dissected human nerves into their fascicular subunits, recognizing that fascicles do not remain separate throughout the nerve but form an intraneural plexus. Intraneural anatomy was then neglected until a flurry of interest in the early twentieth century. Dissection, Wallerian degeneration, and electrical stimulation techniques were used, along with clinical observation, to study the location of functionally related axons within peripheral nerve (reviewed in Brushart, 1991). The results of these investigations varied widely. On the one hand, Sherren (1908) described no loss of function after transection of one-third of a proximal nerve trunk. On the other, stimulation around the circumference of intact human nerve defined a reproducible localization of fibers destined for specific muscles even at proximal levels (Marie et al., 1915; Kraus, Ingham, 1920). It was during this period that surgical repair of individual fascicles was first discussed (Langley, Hashimoto, 1917), though the necessary surgical techniques were not yet available.

More recent studies of intraneural organization with dissection and degeneration techniques have refined earlier observations. The most detailed anatomic and histologic explorations of intraneural organization were performed by Sunderland and his coworkers (Sunderland, 1945a; Sunderland, Ray, 1948; Sunderland et al., 1959). They determined that, despite the changing plexiform nature of the fascicular pattern, axons of peripheral branches are well localized to individual fascicles or fascicular groups for variable, but often considerable distances proximal to their exit from the nerve. Sunderland's findings were confirmed by Tamura's (1969) less extensive analysis of peripheral nerves in Japanese and by Perotto and Delagi's (1979) clinical study of partial median nerve lacerations at the wrist level. More recently, Jabaley et al. (1980) and Chow et al. (1986) have documented distal axon localization over distances somewhat greater than those found by Sunderland. However, intraneural plexus formation continues to defeat purely anatomical attempts to determine the proximal location of axons identified at the periphery (Figure 1-10). The dissector functionally identifies a fascicle by its distal

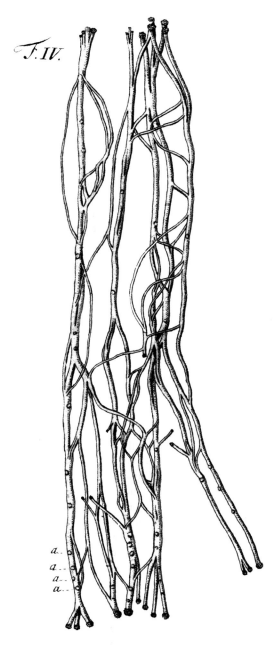

F. IV.

a--
a--
a--
a--

FIGURE 1-9   The internal architecture of the human median nerve. The connective tissues of the epineurium have been chemically digested to expose the fascicles within. The fascicles contributing to the thenar motor branch are at the lower right. Numerous interconnections among fascicles are present. Although this work was published by Prochaska in 1779, it had no practical significance until the development of microsurgery in the second half of the twentieth century.

termination, then works proximally, separating the fascicle from its neighbors. When an interfascicular plexus is encountered, it must be assumed that all proximal components contribute equally to the single fascicle being traced. As fascicular interconnections are repeatedly encountered, a progressively large number of fascicles are traced, most of which do not contribute significantly to the fascicle under study. Maps based on dissection thus represent the sum of all potential axon sources; they are maps of possibility rather than of fact, and cannot be used to argue against proximal localization of axons contributing to discrete distal functions.

Retrograde tracing

An entirely new perspective has been introduced through the use of axon tracing techniques based on axonal transport. The enzyme horseradish peroxidase (HRP) can be taken up by axons to which it is applied, carried back to the parent neurons by retrograde axonal transport, and demonstrated histochemically within the cell body (Mesulam, 1982). Although early techniques were not sufficiently sensitive to demonstrate HRP en route within axons, conjugation of HRP with the lectin wheat germ agglutinin increased uptake sufficiently to permit continuous labeling of axons from periphery to CNS (Brushart, Mesulam, 1980). With this new technique it was possible to trace the proximal course of primate digital nerve axons (Brushart, 1991), including their projections to the spinal cord (Brown et al., 1989) and brainstem (Culberson, Brushart, 1989). The location within the median nerve of axons contributing to the radial digital nerves of the thumb, index, and middle fingers was studied in six specimens (Brushart, 1991) (Figures 1-11 and 1-12). The axons of a single digital nerve were well-localized in the forearm, and were confined to 1/3 to 1/6 of the nerve cross section at the entrance to the brachial plexus. The territories occupied by axons of the three digital nerves were widely separated at the wrist level, whereas at proximal levels there was some intermingling of axons from adjacent digits. The location of axons serving each nerve was strikingly similar from right to left and from animal to animal. The long-accepted picture of intraneural chaos, reflecting the limitations of dissection technique, was thus replaced by a view of partial localization of distal function at proximal levels.

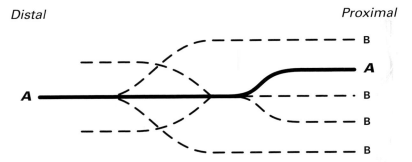

Distal   Proximal

FIGURE 1-10   Theoretical diagram of a nerve dissected into its fascicular elements to illustrate the limitations of dissection in determining axon location within a nerve trunk. Beginning with an identified branch A on the left, distal end of the nerve and dissecting proximally (to the right), one encounters interconnections with multiple fascicles (B) that could contribute axons to A, and would be labeled by Sunderland as doing so. The actual course of the axons, the solid line from A to A, can only be identified by axon tracing or neurographic techniques. Dissection thus provides an inappropriately negative view of axon localization at proximal levels.

Microneurography

Microneurography and intraneural microstimulation techniques have also circumvented the limitations imposed on anatomical dissection by intraneural plexus formation. Electrodes are placed within the nerves of awake humans and used to characterize the current arising from manipulation of peripheral receptive fields (microneurography), or are stimulated while the resulting sensory experience is characterized. Using a tungsten electrode to stimulate intact human median nerve axons, Schady et al. (1983) found that 42% of fascicles stimulated in the upper arm projected only to skin, and within these 67% of sensations elicited were confined to a single digital interspace. Axons with adjacent or overlapping cutaneous projections did not appear to be adjacent within the fascicle when this technique was used. However, Hallin (1990) was able to demonstrate topographic organization of axons within a fascicle by using a smaller concentric electrode. Further studies with the concentric electrode have demonstrated clustering of both Pacinian (Wu et al., 1998) and slowly adapting type II (Wu et al., 1999) afferents within nerve trunks. This clustering may have implications for nerve repair, in that it may increase the chances that an axon regenerating from the proximal end of a cluster will reinnervate an end organ of appropriate modality (Hallin, Wu, 2001).

CONCLUSIONS

Peripheral nerve is often described as a cable, connecting central neurons to peripheral end organs. Like a cable, its performance depends on uniting the structures at either end in a functionally and topographically appropriate manner. To achieve this goal with maximum efficiency, the axonal "wires" assume a variety of anatomic and physiologic properties that are matched to their individual tasks. Additionally, some axons carry information outward from neuron to end organ, while others work in the opposite direction, bringing information from end organ to neuron. The cable analogy breaks down, however, when one considers that wires maintain the same organization throughout a cable, whereas axons undergo dramatic rearrangement as they course through major peripheral nerves. In effect, nerve resembles an elongated plexus with distinct cross-sectional anatomy at each level. The details of this anatomy vary from person to person, so intraneural roadmaps will be only moderately predictive in a given patient. Peripheral nerve is thus a structure of great organizational complexity. When a nerve is injured, this complexity will increase the difficulty of matching axons in proximal and distal stumps, and will thus pose a major deterrant to reestablishing functional connections between neurons and their end organs.

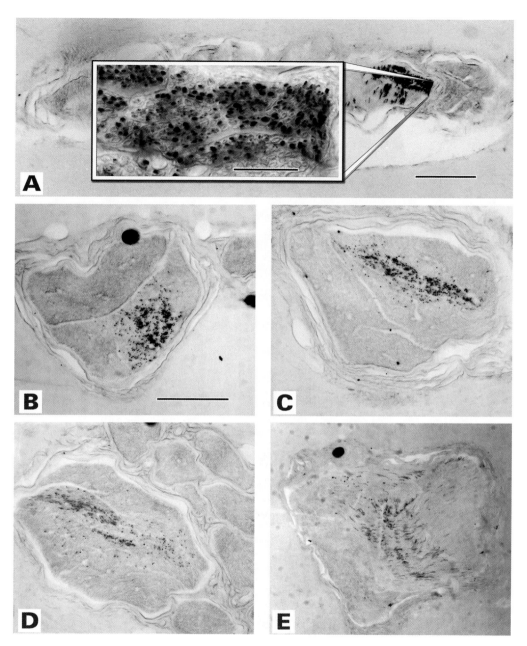

FIGURE 1-11   Photomicrographs of uncounterstained 80-μm cross sections of the monkey median nerve. The radial digital nerve of the middle finger has been exposed to HRP-WGA. The volar surface of the nerve is superior and the radial edge is on the left. A: The nerve is flattened as it passes through the carpal tunnel. Labeled axons are grouped within a single fascicle (Bar: 0.25 mm). This fascicle is enlarged to show individual labeled axons (Bar: 50 μm). B. Midforearm. Labeled axons are clustered within the dorso-ulnar aspect of the nerve. (Bar: 0.25 mm.) C: Proximal forearm. The digital nerve territory is now an elongated strip oriented from radio-volar to dorso-ulnar. D: proximal elbow, with several daughter fascicles destined to become forearm motor branches and the communicating branch to the ulnar nerve. Labeled axons within the core of the digital nerve territory are less densely packed, and there is a large area of sparse labeling about the periphery. E: The entrance to the brachial plexus. Still more axonal dispersion has occurred, yet the digital nerve territory remains well-defined. (Brushart, 1991).

RADIAL DIGITAL NERVES

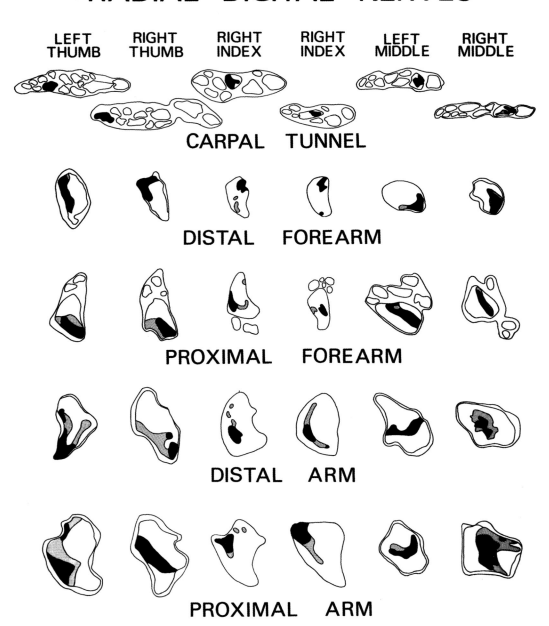

FIGURE 1-12 The location within the monkey median nerve of axons serving the radial aspect of the thumb, index finger, and middle finger. Images from the left arm have been reversed to facilitate comparison; same orientation as Figure 1-11. Solid black areas represent dense labeling, where labeled axons are separated from one another by no more than three unlabeled axons. There is a clear progression of digital nerve territories from the radial (thumb) to the ulnar (middle finger) aspects of the nerve. These territories are tightly localized within the wrist and forearm, then overlap progressively at proximal levels. In spite of this gradual dispersion, digital nerve axons are still clearly localized at the entrance to the brachial plexus. (Brushart, 1991).

REFERENCES

Ackerley S, Thornhill P, Grierson AJ, Brownlees J, Anderton BH, Leigh PN, Shaw CE, Miller CCJ (2003) Neurofilament heavy chain side arm phosphorylation regulates axonal transport of neurofilaments. J Cell Biol 161: 489–495.

Adams CW, Grant RT, Bayliss O (1967) Cholinesterases in peripheral nervous system I. Mixed, motor and sensory trunks. Brain Res 5: 366–376.

Adams WE (1942) The blood supply of nerves. J Anat 76: 323–341.

Aguayo A, Bray GM, Terry LC, Sweezey E (1976) Three dimensional analysis of unmyelinated fibers in normal and pathologic autonomic nerves. J Neuropathol Exp Neurol 35: 136–151.

Aguayo AJ, Bray GM, Perkins CS (1979) Axon-Schwann cell relationships in neuropathies of mutant mice. Ann NY Acad Sci 317: 512–531.

Ahmad FJ, Echeverri CJ, Vallee RB, Bass PW (1998) Cytoplasmic dynein and dynactin are required for microtubule transport into the axon. J Cell Biol 140: 391–402.

Arroyo EJ, Scherer SS (2000) On the molecular architecture of myelinated fibers. Histochem Cell Biol 113: 1–18.

Aumailley M, Bruckner-Tuderman L, Carter WG, Deutzmann R, Edgar D, Ekblom P, Engel J, Engvall E, Hohenester E, Jones JCR, Kleinman HK, Marinkovich MP, Martin GR, Mayer U, Meneguzzi G, Miner JH, Miyazaki K, Patarroyo M, Paulsson M, Quaranta V, Sanes JR, Sasaki T, Sekiguchi K, Sorokin LM (2005) A simplified laminin nomenclature. Matrix Biol 24: 326–332.

Baas PW (2002) Microtubule transport in the axon. Int Rev Cytol 212: 41–62.

Beggs J, Johnson PC, Olafsen A, Watkins CJ, Cleary C (1991) Transperineurial arterioles in human sural nerve. J Neuropathol Exp Neurol 50: 704–718.

Bell MA, Weddell AG (1984a) A morphometric study of intrafascicular vessels of mammalian sciatic nerve. Muscle & Nerve 7: 524–534.

Bell MA, Weddell AG (1984b) A descriptive study of the blood vessels of the sciatic nerve in the rat, man, and other mammals. Brain 107: 871–898.

Berthold, C.-H. (1978) Morphology of normal peripheral axons. In: Physiology and Pathobiology of Axons, S. Waxman, ed., pp. 3–63, New York: Raven.

Berthold C-H, Nilsson I (1983) Axon diameter and myelin sheath thickness in nerve fibers of the ventral spinal root of the seventh lumbar nerve of the adult and developing cat. J Anat 136: 483–508.

Berthold, C.-H. and M. Rydmark (1995) Morphology of normal peripheral axons. In: The Axon, S.G. Waxman, J.D. Kocsis and P.K. Stys, eds., pp. 13–48, New York: Oxford University Press.

Bessou P, Perl ER (1969) Responses of cutaneous sensory units with unmyelinated fibers to noxious stimuli. J Neurophysiol 32: 1025–1043.

Best TJ, Mackinnon SE (1994) Peripheral nerve revascularization: a current literature review. J Recon Micro 10: 193–204.

Bonneh-Barkay D, Shlissel M, Berman B, Shaoul E, Admon A, Vlodavsky I, Carey DJ, Asundi VK, Reich-Slotky R, Ron D (1997) Identification of glypican as a dual modulator of the biological activity of fibroblast growth factors. J Biol Chem 272: 12415–12421.

Boyd, I.A. and M.R. Davey (1968) Composition of Peripheral Nerves, Edinburgh: E & S Livingston.

Braunewell K-H, Pesheva P, McCarthy JB, Furcht LT, Schmitz B, Schachner M (1995) Functional involvement of sciatic nerve-derived versican- and decorin-like molecules and other chondroitin sulfate proteoglycans in ECM-mediated cell adhesion and neurite outgrowth. Eur J Neurosci 7: 805–814.

Brown PB, Brushart TM, Ritz LA (1989) Somatotopy of digital nerve projections to the dorsal horn in the monkey. Somatosens Motor Res 6(3): 309–317.

Brushart TM, Mesulam MM (1980) Transganglionic demonstration of central sensory projections from skin and muscle with HRP-lectin conjugates. Neurosci Lett 17: 1–6.

Brushart TM (1991) The central course of digital axons within the median nerve of macaca mulatta. J Comp Neurol 311: 197–209.

Brushart TM, Redett R, Hameed H, Li Z, Jari R, Zhou C, Hoke A (2005) Schwann cells express sensory and motor phenotypes that control axon regeneration. Soc Neurosci Abst 29.7.

Bunge MB, Williams AK, Wood PM (1982) Neuron-Schwann cell interaction in basal lamina formation. Dev Biol 92: 449–460.

Bunge RP, Bunge MB, Bates M (1989) Movements of the Schwann cell nucleus implicate progression of the inner (axon-related) Schwann cell process during myelination. J Cell Biol 109: 273–284.

Burkel WE (1967) The histological fine structure of perineurium. Anat Rec 158: 177–190.

Burstyn-Cohen T, Frumkin A, Xu Y-T, Scherer S, Klar A (1998) Accumulation of F-spondin in injured peripheral nerve promotes the outgrowth of sensory axons. J Neurosci 18: 8875–8885.

Burton PR, Paige JL (1981) Polarity of axoplasmic microtubules in the olfactory nerve of the frog. Proc Natl Acad Sci USA 78: 3269–3273.

Caldwell JH, Schaller KL, Lasher RS, Levinson SR (2000). Sodium channel Nav1.6 is localized at nodes of Ranvier, dendrites, and synapses. PNAS 97: 5616–5620.

Carey DJ, Evans DM, Stahl RC, Asundi VK, Conner KJ, Garbes P, Cizmeci-Smith G (1992) Molecular cloning and characterization of N-syndecan, a novel transmembrane heparin sulfate proteoglycan. J Cell Biol 117: 191–201.

Carey DJ, Stahl RC, Asundi V, Tucker B (1993) Processing and subcellular distribution of the Schwann cell-lipid anchored heparin sulfate proteoglycan and identification as glypican. Exp Cell Res 208: 10–18.

Carey DJ (1997) Syndecans: multifunctional cell-surface co-receptors. Biochem J 327: 1–16.

Carter MJ (1972) Carbonic anhydrase: Isoenzymes, properties, distribution, and functional significance. Biol Rev 47: 465–513.

Chernousov MA, Carey DJ (2000) Schwann cell extracellular matrix molecules and their receptors. Histol Histopath 15: 593–601.

Ching W, Zanazzi G, Levinson R, Salzer J (1999) Clustering of neuronal sodium channels requires contact with myelinating Schwann cells. J Neurocytol 28: 295–301.

Chiu, S.Y. (1993) Channel function in mammalian axons and support cells. In: *Peripheral Neuropathy*, Vol. 3, P.J. Dyck and P.K. Thomas, eds., pp. 94–108, Philadelphia: Saunders.

Chow JA, Van Beek AL, Bilos ZJ, Meyer DL, Johnson MC (1986) Anatomical basis for repair of ulnar and median nerves in the distal part of the forearm by group fascicular suture and nerve-grafting. J Bone Joint Surg 68-A: 273–280.

Citri A, Kochupurakkal B, Yarden Y (2003) The deaf and the dumb: the biology of ErbB-2 and ErbB-3. Exp Cell Res 284: 54–65.

Clarke E, Bearn JG (1972) The spiral nerve bands of Fontana. Brain 95: 1–20.

Colognato H, Yurchenco PD (2000) Form and function: the laminin family of heterotrimers. Dev Dyn 218: 213–234.

Corfas G, Rosen K, Aratake H, Krauss R, Fishbach G (1995) Differential expression of ARIA isoforms in the rat brain. Neuron 14: 103–115.

Corfas G, Velardez MO, Ko C-P, Ratner N, Peles E (2004) Mechanisms and roles of axon-Schwann cell interactions. J Neurosci 24: 9250–9260.

Culberson JL, Brushart TM (1989) Somatotopy of digital nerve projections to the cuneate nucleus in the monkey. Somatosens Motor Res 6(3): 319–330.

De Waegh SM, Lee V, Brady S (1992) Local modulation of neurofilament phosphorylation, axonal caliber, and slow axonal transport by myelinating Schwann cells. Cell 68: 451–463.

Delcroix JD, Valletta JS, Wu CB, Hunt SJ, Kowal AS, Mobley WC (2003) NGF signaling in sensory neurons: Evidence that early endosomes carry NGF retrograde signals. Neuron 39: 69–84.

Desai A, Mitchison TJ (1997) Microtubule polymerization dynamics. Ann Rev Cell Dev Biol 13: 83–117.

Devaux JJ, Kleopa KA, Cooper EC, Scherer SS (2004) KCNQ2 is a nodal K+ channel. J Neurosci 24: 1236–1244.

Domeniconi M, Cao ZU, Spencer T, Sivasankaran R, Wang KC, Nikulina E, Kimura N, Cai H, Deng KW, Gao Y, He ZG, Filbin MT (2002) Myelin-associated glycoprotein interacts with the Nogo66 receptor to inhibit neurite outgrowth. Neuron 35: 283–290.

Dubovy P, Klusakova I, Svizenska I (2002) A quantitative immunohistochemical study of the endoneurium in the rat dorsal and ventral spinal roots. Histochem Cell Biol 117: 473–480.

Einheber S, Milner TA, Giancotti F, Salzer JL (1993) Axonal regulation of Schwann cell integrin expression suggests a role for a6B4 in myelination. J Cell Biol 123: 1223–1236.

Eldridge CF, Sanes JR, Chiu AY (1986) Basal lamina-associated heparin sulfate proteoglycan in the rat PNS: characterization and localization using monoclonal antibodies. J Neurocytol 15: 37.

Eldridge CF, Bunge MB, Bunge RP (1989) Differentiation of axon-related Schwann cells in vitro. II. Control of myelin formation by basal lamina. J Neurosci 9: 625–638.

Erlanger, J. and H.S. Gasser (1968) *Electrical Signs of Nervous Activity*, Philadelphia: University of Pennsylvania Press.

Falls DL (2003) Neuregulins and the neuromuscular system: 10 years of answers and questions. J Neurocytol 32: 619–647.

Feltri ML, Scherer SS, Nemi R, Kamholz J, Vogelbacker H, Scott MO, Canal N, Quaranta V, Wrabetz L. (1994) ß4 integrin expression in myelinating Schwann cells is polarized, developmentally regulated and axonally dependent. Development 120: 1287–1301.

Feltri ML, Wrabetz L (2005) Laminins and their receptors in Schwann cells and hereditary neuropathies. JPNS 10: 128–143.

Friede RL, Samorajski T (1970) Axon caliber related to neurofilaments and microtubules in sciatic nerve fibers of rats and mice. Anat Rec 167: 379–388.

Gamble HJ, Eames RA (1964) An electron microscope study of the connective tissues of human peripheral nerve. J Anat 98: 655–663.

Garcia ML, Lobsiger CS, Shah SB, Deerinck TJ, Crum J, Young D, Ward CM, Crawford TO, Gotow T, Uchiyama Y, Ellisman MH, Calcutt NA, Cleveland DW (2003) NF-M is an essential target for the myelin-directed "outside-in" signaling cascade that mediates radial axonal growth. J Cell Biol 163: 1011–1020.

Gasser HS (1955) Properties of dorsal root unmedullated fibers on the two sides of the ganglion. J Gen Physiol 38: 709–728.

Geisler N, Kaufmann E, Fischer S, Plessman U, Weber K (1983) Neurofilament architecture combines structural principles of intermediate filaments with carboxy-terminal extensions increasing in size between triplet proteins. EMBO J 2: 1295–1302.

Garcia ML, Rao MV, Fujimoto J, Garcia VB, Shah SB, Crum J, Gotow T, Uchiyama Y, Ellisman M, Calcutt NA, Cleveland DW (2009) Phosphorylation of highly conserved neurofilament medium KSP repeats is not required for myelin-dependent radial axonal growth. J Neurosci 29: 1277–1284.

Gong Y, Tagawa Y, Lunn MPT, Laroy W, Heffer-Lauc M, Li CY, Griffin JW, Schnaar RL, Sheikh KA (2002) Localization of major gangliosides in the PNS: implications for immune neuropathies. Brain 125: 2491–2506.

Grafstein B, Forman DS (1980) Intracellular transport in neurons. Physiol Rev 60: 1167–1283.

Grafstein, B. (1995) Axonal transport: Function and mechanisms. In: The Axon, S. Waxman, J.D. Kocsis and P.K. Stys, eds., pp. 185–199, New York: Oxford University Press.

Greenberg MM, Leitao C, Trogadis J, Stevens JK (1990) Irregular geometries in normal unmyelinated axons: A 3D serial EM analysis. J Neurocytol 20: 978–988.

Griffin, J. and A. Hoke (2005) The control of axonal caliber. In: Peripheral Neuropathy, Philadelphia: Saunders.

Griffin JW, George R, Ho T (1993) Macrophage systems in peripheral nerves. A review. J Neuropathol Exp Neurol 52: 553–560.

Gruber H, Zenker W (1973) Acetylcholinesterase: histochemical differentiation between motor and sensory fibers. Brain Res 51: 207–214.

Hallin RG (1990) Microneurography in relation to intraneural topography: somatotopic organisation of median nerve fascicles in humans. Neurol Neurosurg Psychiatry 9: 736–744.

Hallin RG, Wu G (2001) Fitting pieces in the peripheral nerve puzzle. ExpNeurol 172: 482–492.

Hartmann U, Maurer P (2001) Proteoglycans in the nervous system: the quest for functional roles in vivo. Matrix Biology 20: 23–35.

Hess A, Young JZ (1952) The nodes of Ranvier. Proc R Soc Lond [Biol] 140: 301–319.

Hirakawa H, Okajima S, Nagaoka T, Takamatsu T, Oyamada M (2003) Loss and recovery of the blood-nerve barrier in the rat sciatic nerve after crush injury are associated with expression of intercellular junctional proteins. Exp Cell Res 284: 196–210.

Hirokawa N,Takemura R (2005). Molecular motors and mechanisms of directional transport in neurons. Nat Rev Neurosci 6(3): 201–214.

Hisanaga S-I, Hirokawa N (1988) Structure of the peripheral domains of neurofilaments revealed by low angle rotary shadowing. J Mol Biol 202: 297–305.

Hoffman JR, Dixit VM, O'Shea KS (1994) Expression of thrombospondin in the adult nervous system. J Comp Neurol 340: 126–139.

Hoffman P, Lasek RJ (1975) The slow component of axonal transport: Identification of major structural peptides and their generality among mammalian neurons. J Cell Biol 66: 351–366.

Hoffman PN, Griffin JW, Price DL (1984) Control of axon caliber by neurofilament transport. J Cell Biol 99: 705–714.

Hoke A, Redett R, Hameed H, Jari R, Li Z-B, Griffin J, Brushart TM (2006) Schwann cells express motor and sensory phenotypes that regulate axon regeneration. J Neurosci 26: 9646–9655.

Hsieh S-T, Kidd GJ, Crawford TO, Xu Z, Lin W-M, Trapp BD, Cleveland DW, Griffin JW (1994) Regional modulation of neurofilament organization by myelination in normal axons. J Neurosci 14: 6392–6401.

Ide C, Tohyama K, Yokota R, Nitatori T, Onodepa H (1983) Schwann Cell basal lamina and nerve regeneration. Brain Res 288: 61–65.

Jabaley ME, Wallace WH, Heckler FR (1980) Internal topography of major nerves of the forearm and hand. J Hand Surg 5: 1–18.

Jessen KR, Mirsky R (2002) Signals that determine Schwann cell identity. J Anat 200: 367–375.

Junqueira LC, Montes GS, Kristzan RM (1979) The collagen of the vertebrate peripheral nervous system. Cell Tissue Res 202: 453–460.

Kandel ER, Schwartz JH, and Jessell TM (2000) Principles of Neural Science, ed 4. New York, McGraw-Hill.

Kline DG, Hackett ER, Davis GD, Myers MB (1972) Effect of mobilization on the blood supply and regeneration of injured nerves. J Surg Res 12: 254–266.

Koester J, Siegelbaum SA (2000). Propagated signaling: The action potential. *Principles of Neural Science*. New York, McGraw-Hill: Chapter 9. (pages 150–170 if you also need pages, and editors are Kandel ER, Schwartz JH, and Jessell TM)

Kordeli E, Davis J, Trapp B, Bennett V (1990) An isoform of ankyrin is localized at nodes of Ranvier in myelinated axons of central and peripheral nerves. J Cell Biol 110: 1341–1352.

Kordeli E, Lambert S, Bennett V (1995) Ankyrin G: a new ankyrin gene with neural-specific isoforms localized at the axonal initial segment and node of Ranvier. J Biol Chem 270: 2352–2359.

Kozu H, Tamura E, Parry G (1992) Endoneurial blood supply to peripheral nerves is not uniform. J Neurol Sci 111: 204–208.

Kraus WM, Ingham SD (1920) Electrical stimulation of peripheral nerves exposed at operation. JAMA 74: 586–589.

Lahav J, Lawler J, Gimbrone MA (1984) Thrombospondin interactions with fibronectin and fibrinogen: Mutual inhibition in binding. Eur J Biochem 145: 151–156.

Langley JN, Hashimoto M (1917) On the suture of separate nerve bundles in a nerve trunk and on internal nerve plexuses. J Physiol 51: 318–345.

Lehman HJ (1957) Uber struktur und funktion der perineuralen diffusionsbarriere. Z Zellforsch Mikrosk Anat 46: 232–241.

Lemke G, Axel R (1985) Isolation and sequence of a cDNA encoding the major structural protein of peripheral myelin. Cell 40: 501–508.

Liu BP, Fournier A, Grand Pré T, Strittmatter SM (2002) Myelin-associated glycoprotein as a functional ligand for the Nogo-66 receptor. Science 297: 1190–1193.

Lloyd DP (1943) Neuron patterns controlling transmission of ipsilateral hind limb reflexes in cat. J Neurophysiol 6: 293–315.

Lorimier P, Mezin P, Labat Moleur F, Pinel N, Peyrol S, Stoebner P (1992) Ultrastructural localization of the major components of the extracellular matrix in normal rat nerve. J Histochem Cytochem 40: 859–868.

Lundborg G, Rydevik B (1973) Effects of stretching the tibial nerve of the rabbit: a preliminary study of the intraneural circulation and the barrier function of the perineurium. JBJS 5B: 390–401.

Lundborg G (1988) Intraneural microcirculation. OCNA 19: 1–12.

Maki Y, Firrell JC, Breidenbach WC (1997) Blood flow in mobilized nerves: results in a rabbit sciatic nerve model. Plast Reconstr Surg 100: 627–633.

Malave C, Villegas GM, Hernandez M, Martinez JC, Castillo C, Suarez de Mata Z, Villegas R (2003) Role of the glypican-1 in the trophic activity on PC12 cells induced by cultured sciatic nerve conditioned medium: identification of a glypican-1-neuregulin complex. Brain Res 983: 74–83.

Marie MP, Meige H, Gosset A (1915) Les localisations motrices dans les nerfs peripheriques. Bull Acad Med 74: 798–810.

Martini R, Bollensen E, Schachner M (1988) Immunocytological localization of the major peripheral nervous system glycoprotein Po and the L2/HNK-1 and L3 carbohydrate structures in developing and adult mouse sciatic nerve. Dev Biol 129: 330–338.

Martini R (1994) Expression and functional roles of neural cell surface molecules and extracellular matrix components during development and regeneration of peripheral nerves. J Neurocytol 23: 1–28.

Martini R, Schachner M, Brushart TM (1994) The L2/HNK-1 carbohydrate is preferentially expressed by previously motor axon-associated Schwann cells in reinnervated peripheral nerves. J Neurosci 14: 7180–7191.

Maurel P, Einheber S, Galinska J, Thaker P, Lam I, Rubin M, Scherer SS, Murakami Y, Gutmann DH, Salzer JL (2007) Nectin-like proteins mediate axon-Schwann cell interactions along the internode and are essential for myelination. J Cell Biol 178: 861–874.

McKerracher L, David S, Jackson DL, Kottis V, Dunn RJ, Braun PE (1994) Identification of myelin-associated glycoprotein as a major myelin-derived inhibitor of neurite growth. Neuron 13: 805–811.

Mesulam, M.-M. (1982) *Tracing Neural Connections with Horseradish Peroxidase*, New York: Wiley.

Michailov GV, Sereda MW, Brinkmann BG, Fischer TM, Haug B, Birchmeier C, Role L, Lai C, Schwab MH, Nave K-A (2004) Axonal neuregulin-1 regulates myelin sheath thickness. Science 304: 700–703.

Millesi H, Terzis JK (1983) Problems of terminology in peripheral nerve surgery: committee report of the International Society of Reconstructive Microsurgery. Microsurgery 4: 51–56.

Mirsky R, Parmantier E, McMahon AP, Jessen KR (1999) Schwann cell-derived desert hedgehog signals nerve sheath formation. Ann NY Acad Sci 883: 196–202.

Mumby SM, Raugi GJ, Bornstein P (1984) Interactions of thrombospondin and extracellular matrix proteins: selective binding to type V collagen. J Cell Biol 98: 1603–1611.

Murinson BB, Hoffman PN, Banihashemi MR, Meyer RA, Griffin JW (2005) C-Fiber (Remak) bundles contain both isolectin B4-binding and calcitonin gene-related peptide-positive axons. J Comp Neurol 484: 392–402.

Murray MA (1968) An electron microscopic study of the relationship between axon diameter and the initiation of myelin production in the peripheral nervous system. Anat Rec 161: 337–352.

Nixon RA, Sihag RK (1991) Neurofilament phosphorylation: a new look at regulation and function. TINS 14: 501–506.

Ochoa J, Mair W (1969) The normal sural nerve in man. I. Ultrastructure and numbers of fibers and cells. Acta Neuropath 13: 197.

Ochoa, J. (1976) The unmyelinated nerve fiber. In: The Peripheral Nerve, D.N. Landon, ed., pp. 106–158, London: Chapman and Hall.

Olausson H, Lamarre Y, Backlund H, Morin C, Wallin BG, Starck G, Ekholm S, Strigo I, Worsley K, Vallbo AB, Bushnell MC (2002) Unmyelinated tactile afferents signal touch and project to insular cortex. Nature Neuroscience 5: 900–904.

Patton BL (2000) Laminins of the neuromuscular system. Microsc Res Tech 51: 247–261.

Pedraza L, Huang JK, Colman DR (2001) Organizing principles of the axoglial apparatus. Neuron 30: 335–344.

Perotto AO, Delagi EF (1979) Funicular localization in partial median nerve injury at the wrist. Arch Phys Med Rehab 60: 165–169.

Poliak S, Peles E (2003) The local differentiation of myelinated axons at nodes of Ranvier. Nat Rev Neurosci 4: 968–980.

Prochaska, G. (1779) De Structura Nervorum, Vienna: R. Graeffer.

Quarles RH (2002) Myelin sheaths: glycoproteins involved in their formation, maintenance and degeneration. Cell Mol Life Sci 59: 1851–1871.

Rao MV, Garcia ML, Miyazaki Y, Gotow T, Yuan A, Mattina S, Ward CM, Calcutt NA, Uchiyama Y, Nixon RA, Cleveland DW (2002) Gene replacement in mice reveals that the heavily phosphorylated tail of neurofilament heavy subunit does not affect axonal caliber or the transit of cargoes in slow axonal transport. J Cell Biol 158: 681–693.

Riley DA, Ellis S, Bain J (1982) Carbonic anhydrase activity in skeletal muscle fiber types, axons, spindles, and capillaries of rat soleus and extensor digitorum longus muscles. J Histochem Cytochem 30: 1275–1288.

Riley DA, Sanger JR, Matloub HS, Yousif NJ, Bain JL, Moore GH (1988) Identifying motor and sensory myelinated axons in rabbit peripheral nerves by histochemical staining for carbonic anhydrase and cholinesterase activities. Brain Res 453: 79–88.

Ritchie, M. (1995) Physiology of axons. In: The Axon, S. Waxman, J.D. Kocsis and P.K. Stys, eds., pp. 68–96, New York: Oxford University Press.

Romberg L, Vale RD (1993) Chemomechanical cycle of kinesin differs from that of myosin. Nature 361: 168–170.

Rothblum K, Stahl RC, Carey DJ (2004) Constitutive release of a4 type V collagen n-terminal domain by Schwann cells and binding to cell surface and extracellular matrix heparin sulfate proteoglycans. J Biol Chem 279: 51282–51288.

Roy S, Coffee P, Smith G, Liem RK, Brady S, Black S (2000) Neurofilaments are transported rapidly but intermittently in axons: implications for slow axonal transport. J Neurosci 20: 6849–6861.

Rushton WA (1951) A theory of the effects of fibre size in medullated nerve. J Physiol (Lond) 115: 101–122.

Rutka JT, Apodaca G, Stern R, Rosenblum M (1988) The extracellular matrix of the central and peripheral nervous systems: structure and function. J Neurosurg 69: 155–170.

Rydevik BL, Kwan MK, Myers R, Brown RA, Triggs KJ, Woo S, Garfin SR (1990) An in vivo mechanical and histological study of acute stretching on rabbit tibial nerve. J Orthop Res 8: 694–701.

Salonen V, Lehto M, Vaheri A, Aro H, Pelonten J (1985) Endoneurial fibrosis following nerve transection. Acta Neuropathol (Berl) 67: 315–321.

Salzer JL (2003) Polarized domains of myelinated axons. Neuron 40: 297–318.

Schachner M (1990) Functional implications of glial cell recognition molecules. Seminars Neurosci 2: 497–507.

Schady W, Ochoa JL, Torebjork HE, Chen LS (1983) Peripheral projections of fascicles in the human median nerve. Brain 106: 745–760.

Scherer SS (1996) Molecular specializations at nodes and paranodes in peripheral nerve. Microsc Res Tech 34: 452–461.

Scherer SS, Arroyo EJ (2002) Recent progress on the molecular organization of myelinated axons. JPNS 7: 1–12.

Scherer, S., E.J. Arroyo, and E. Peles (2004) Functional organization of the nodes of Ranvier. In: *Myelin Biology and Disorders*, R.A. Lazzarini, ed., Chapter 4, pp. 89–116. San Diego: Elsevier.

Schiff R, Rosenbluth J (1986) Ultrastructural localization of laminin in rat sensory ganglia. J Histochem Cytochem 34: 1691–1699.

Schlaepfer WW, Freeman LA (1978) Neurofilament proteins of rat peripheral nerve and spinal cord. J Cell Biol 78: 653–662.

Schmelz M, Schmidt R, Bickel A, Handwerker HO, Torebjork HE (1997) Specific C-receptors for itch in human skin. J Neurosci 17: 8003–8008.

Seyer JM, Kang AH, Whitaker N (1977) The characterization of type I and type III collagens from human peripheral nerve. Biochim Biophys Acta 492: 415–425.

Shanthaveerappa TR, Bourne GH (1962) The "perineurial epithelium," a metabolically active, continuous, protoplasmic cell barrier surrounding peripheral nerve fasciculi. JAnat 96: 527.

Shanthaveerappa T, Bourne G (1966) Perineural epithelium: a new concept of its role in the Integrity of the peripheral nervous system. Science 154: 1464–1467.

Shapiro L, Doyle J, Hensley P, Colman D, Hendrickson W (1996) Crystal structure of the extracellular domain from Po, the major structural protein of peripheral nerve myelin. Neuron 17: 435–449.

Shellswell GB, Restall DJ, Duance VC, Bailey AJ (1979) Identification and differential distribution of collagen types in the central and peripheral nervous systems. FEBS Lett 106: 305–308.

Sherman DL, Fabrizi C, Gillespie CS, Brophy PJ (2001) Specific disruption of a Schwann cell dystrophin-related protein complex in a demyelinating neuropathy. Neuron 30: 677–687.

Sherren, J. (1908) *Injuries of Nerves and Their Treatment*, London: James Nisbit.

Smith DR, Kobrine AI, Rizzoli HV (1977) Blood flow in peripheral nerves. J Neurol Sci 33: 341–346.

Spiegel I, Adamsky K, Eshed Y, Milo R, Sabanay H, Sarig-Nadir O, Horresh I, Scherer SS, Rasband MN, Peles E (2007) A central role for Necl4 (SynCAM4) in Schwann cell-axon interaction and myelination. Nat Neurosci 10: 861–869.

Stolinski C (1995) Structure and composition of the outer connective tissue sheaths of peripheral nerve. J Anat 186: 123–130.

Sunderland S (1945a) The internal topography of the radial, median and ulnar nerves. Brain 68: 243–298.

Sunderland S (1945b) The adipose tissue of peripheral nerves. Brain 68: 118–122.

Sunderland S, Ray LJ (1948) The internal topography of the sciatic nerve and its popliteal divisions in man. Brain 71: 242–273.

Sunderland S, Marshall RD, Swaney WE (1959) The intraneural topography of the circumflex, musculocutaneous, and obturator nerves. Brain 82: 116–129.

Sunderland S (1965) The connective tissue of peripheral nerves. Brain 88: 841–854.

Suter U, Snipes GJ (1995) Biology and genetics of hereditory motor and sensory neuropathies. Annu Rev Neurosci 18: 45–75.

Tamura K (1969) The funicular pattern of Japanese peripheral nerves. Arch Jap Surg 38: 35–57.

Thomas PK (1963) The connective tissue of peripheral nerve: an electron microscope study. J Anat 97: 35–44.

Tillett RL, Afoke A, Hall SM, Brown R, Phillips JB (2004) Investigating mechanical behaviour at a core-sheath interface in peripheral nerve. JPNS 9: 255–262.

Timpl R, Wiedemann H, Van Delden V, Furthmayr H, Kuhn K (1981) A network model for the organization of type IV collagen molecules in basement membranes. Eur Neurol 41 (Suppl. 1): 35–43.

Timpl R, Brown JC (1996) Supramolecular assembly of basement membranes. Bio Essays 18: 123–132.

Tumova S, Woods A, Couchman JR (2000) Heparin sulfate proteoglycans on the cell surface: versatile coordinators of cellular functions. Int J Biochem Cell Biol 32: 269–288.

Umehara F, Tate G, Itoh K, Osame M (2002) Minifascicular neuropathy: A new concept of the human disease caused by *Desert hedgehog* gene mutation. Cell Mol Biol 48: 187–189.

Ushiki T, Ide C (1990) Three-dimensional organization of the collagen fibrils in the rat sciatic nerve as revealed by transmission- and scanning electron microscopy. Cell Tissue Res 260: 175–184.

Uziyel Y, Hall S, Cohen J (2000) Influence of laminin-2 on Schwann cell-axon interactions. Glia 32: 109–121.

Vabnick I, Novakovic SD, Levinson SR, Schachner M, Shrager P (1996) The clustering of axonal sodium channels during development of the peripheral nervous system. J Neurosci 16: 4914–4922.

Vallee RB, Shpetner HS (1990) Motor proteins of cytoplasmic microtubules. Ann Rev Biochem 59: 909–932.

Vallee RB, Bloom GS (1991) Mechanisms of fast and slow axonal transport. Ann Rev Neurosci 14: 59–92.

Vogelezang MG, Scherer SS, Fawcett JW, French-Constant C (1999) Regulation of fibronectin alternative splicing during peripheral nerve repair. J Neurosci Res 56: 323–333.

Wang KC, Kim JA, Sivasankaran R, Segal R, He ZG (2002) p75 interacts with the Nogo receptor as a co-receptor for Nogo, MAG and OMgp. Nature 420: 74–78.

Wang L, Ho C-L, Sun D, Liem RK, Brown A (2000) Rapid movement of axonal neurofilaments interrupted by prolonged pauses. Nat Cell Biol 2: 137–141.

Witt A, Brady ST (2000) Unwrapping new layers of complexity in axon/glial relationships. Glia 29: 112–117.

Wu G, Ekedahl R, Hallin RG (1998) Clustering of slowly adapting type II mechanoreceptors in human peripheral nerve and skin. Brain 121: 265–279.

Wu G, Ekedahl R, Stark B, Carlstedt T, Nilsson B, Hallin RG (1999) Clustering of Pacinian corpuscle

afferent fibres in the human median nerve. Exp Brain Res 126: 399–409.

Yamada H, Denzer AJ, Hori H, Tanaka T, Anderson L, Fujita S, Fukuta-Ohi H, Shimizu T, Ruegg MA, Matsumura K (1996) Dystroglycan is a dual receptor for agrin and laminin-2 in Schwann cell membrane. J Biol Chem 271: 23418–23423.

Yamada, K.M. (1981) Fibronectin and other structural proteins. In: *Cell Biology of the Extracellular Matrix*, E.D. Hay, ed., p. 95, New York: Plenum Press.

Yang L, Zeller C, Shaper NL, Kiso M, Hasegawa A, Shapiro RE, Schnaar RL (1996) Gangliosides are neuronal ligands for myelin-associated glycoprotein. PNAS 93: 814–818.

Yu FH, Catterall WA (2003) Overview of the voltage-gated sodium channel family. Genome Biol 4: 207–1–207–7.

Yurchenco PD, O'Rear JJ (1994) Basal lamina assembly. Curr Opin Cell Biol 6: 674–681.

Zhang F, Ronca F, Linhardt RJ, Margolis RU (2004) Structural determinants of heparin sulfate interactions with Slit proteins. Biochem Biophys Res Commun 317: 352–357.

2

TOUCH

CUTANEOUS SENSATION may be characterized by its modality, location, intensity, and timing. The mechanoreceptors that respond to cutaneous stimulation are classified by their adaptive properties: slowly adapting receptors (SA) continue to fire as long as the stimulus is present, while rapidly adapting receptors (RA) fire only at the onset and termination of the stimulus. Four types of cutaneous mechanoreceptor contribute to touch: (1) The Merkel cell, the SA I receptor, is superficial in the skin, sensitive to skin stress, and signals information about form and texture; (2) The Ruffini organ, the SA II receptor, is placed deeply, is sensitive to skin stretch, and signals hand conformation; (3) The Meissner corpuscle, the RA I receptor, is closest to the skin surface, senses flutter and low frequency vibration, and signals the slippage of objects across the skin; and (4) The Pacinian corpuscle, the RA II receptor (often designated as the PC receptor), lies deep, is sensitive to high frequency vibration, and signals information applied either directly to the skin or indirectly through a tool.

The output of these receptors is transmitted by primary neurons in the dorsal root ganglion through relay neurons in the cuneate nucleus and thalamus to the primary somatosensory cortex (SI). A secondary pathway to cortex is based on collateral projections to the dorsal horn of the spinal cord. The organization of ascending mechanosensitive information by both modality and topographic location is preserved throughout this relay process, although both ascending and descending pathways may influence its passage at each relay nucleus. Brodmann's area 3b is the portion of SI devoted to cutaneous mechanoreceptive stimuli. It is organized topographically, with further subdivision by sensory modality. Individual sensory channels for SA I, RA, and PC activity thus extend from skin to cortex, where they terminate in modality-specific cortical columns. Initial processing in area 3b is performed by receptive fields with complex geometries, after which information is relayed to other areas of SI, then to secondary somatosensory cortex (SII) and to higher association cortex to be used in conjunction with sensory inputs from other modalities and with motor outputs.

GENERAL PROPERTIES OF SENSATION

The multiplicity of sensations we experience can all be classified as to modality, location, intensity, and timing (discussed in Gardner and Martin, 2000). In sensory systems, modality represents the pairing of a specialized peripheral receptor with a neuron whose central projections are appropriate to the information conveyed. This constant relationship is formalized as the "labeled line" code. In the glabrous skin, each type of mechanoreceptor is activated by a specific pattern of skin deformation or by stimuli of a limited frequency range. Mechanoreceptors thus serve as spatiotemporal filters, responding selectively to specific qualities of stimuli while minimizing others.

The energy imparted to the skin is translated by cutaneous receptors into the electrical energy of the action potential, a signaling mechanism used by all sensory modalities. A specific sensation results from this generalized signal because it is directed to cortical centers that, when activated, are programmed to produce that sensation. The result is the same regardless of whether the impulse is generated through receptor activation, or by direct stimulation of the peripheral axon along its course. This fundamental property of sensation was formulated by Muller as the "law of specific nerve energies." He stated "sensation is not the conduction of a quality or state of external bodies to consciousness, but a conduction of a quality or a state of our nerves to consciousness, excited by an external cause" (cited in Clarke and O'Malley, 1968, p206).

Cutaneous mechanoreceptors convey reliable information about the location of surface stimuli because of the fixed anatomic relationship between individual receptors and their projection to the central nervous system (CNS). The area of skin within which a stimulus causes a change in the firing rate of a neuron is termed the *receptive field* of that neuron. In the absence of disease or injury, stimulation of the same receptive field will always activate the same primary neuron in the dorsal root ganglion. In a given area of skin, the density of receptors and the size of their receptive fields will determine the spatial acuity of the system. Receptor density varies both within a given receptor type and among different receptors, with high concentrations of mechanoreceptors on the tongue, lips, and fingertips and low concentrations on the back and thigh.

The response to cutaneous stimuli of varying intensity was an object of early scientific scrutiny, as both the magnitude of the stimulus and the resulting sensation could be determined without the need for specialized equipment. Ernst Weber, best known to those who treat patients with nerve injuries for his two-point discrimination test (see Chapter 4), was a pioneering student of psychophysics. He came to appreciate that a just noticeable difference in the pressure of a stimulus is a constant function of the force applied, a relationship now formalized as "Weber's law" (Weber, 1846; Finger, 1994). In practical terms, if adding 1 gram provides the just noticeable difference for a 20-gram weight, then 2 gm will provide the just noticeable difference for a 40-gram weight. Weber's law was subsequently modified by Fechner, who hypothesized that the magnitude of sensation would increase linearly as the magnitude of stimulus increased geometrically (Mountcastle, 2006a). Additional analysis by Stevens (1961) revealed that stimulus intensity was best described by a power function. Although further advances in psychophysics have yielded multiple refinements of Weber's law to deal with especially weak or strong stimuli (reviewed in Gardner and Martin, 2000), the basic principle roughly describes behavior in the midrange for many stimuli. The lowest stimulus intensity that can be perceived is termed the *sensory threshold*, usually defined as the minimum stimulus amplitude that can be detected with a frequency midway between chance and 100% correct. The way in which stimulus intensity is signaled to the neuron was revealed by the pioneering electophysiologic experiments of Adrian, who demonstrated that the frequency of action potentials from a given receptor increased as more intense stimulation was applied (Adrian, Zotterman, 1926). Intensity may also be signaled, however, by any measure of neural activity that increases with the intensity of the stimulus, such as the total number of receptors stimulated or the total number of action potentials evoked.

Mechanoreceptors vary in their response to duration of stimulus. All four types of cutaneous mechanoreceptor afferent fire both at the onset and termination of stimulation (Table 2-1). Their ongoing activity, however, varies according to their

Table 2-1 Properties of the Cutaneous Mechanoreceptors that Contribute to Touch

	Merkel	Meissner	Pacinian	(Ruffini)
Adaptation				
Receptors/ RF	~100	30 - 80	1	1
RF Diameter	2 – 3mm	3 – 5mm	Finger/ hand	10 – 30mm
Primary Frequency		40 – 60 Hz	100 – 300 Hz	
Location	Superficial	Superficial	Deep	Deep
Detects	Strain energy density	Skin motion	Distant vibration	Deep tissue strain
1° Sensation	Pressure	Flutter	Vibration	None
Function	Form and texture	Grip control, motion detection	Tool manipulation	Hand conformation, forces acting on hand

adaptation to the stimulus. The Meissner and Pacinian corpuscles are rapidly adapting (RA); they fire a burst at the onset of stimulation, then become silent as long as the stimulus remains constant. They are thus ideally suited to detect and signal change. The Merkel cell and Ruffini ending, in contrast, continue to fire as long as the stimulus is applied, and are thus slowly adapting (SA).

A *sensory channel* consists of a specific receptor type and the pathways that convey its information to the cerebral cortex. In the glabrous skin of the palm and fingers, the Merkel cell is the receptor for the SA I channel, the Meissner corpuscle is the receptor for the RA (RA I) channel, and the Pacinian corpuscle is the receptor for the PC (RA II) channel. The receptor for the SA II channel, initially thought to be the Ruffini ending, is currently unknown (Paré et al., 2003). Each of the channels is exquisitely sensitive to appropriate stimulation; during normal activity, they are all activated simultaneously (Johnson, 2001; Jenmalm et al., 2003). Isolated movement of the hand, such as making a fist, activates 57% of RA, 66% of SA I, 94% of SA II, and 100% of PC afferents (Hulliger et al., 1979). It is thus important to resist the temptation, obvious in many clinical publications, to oversimplify the relationship between individual tests of sensation and specific fiber systems.

CUTANEOUS MECHANORECEPTORS

This discussion will be confined to the four cutaneous mechanoreceptors that are capable of contributing to discriminative touch: the Merkel cell, Meissner corpuscle, Pacinian corpuscle, and Ruffini ending (Figure 2-1, Table 2-1).

The Merkel Cell-Neurite Complex

The Merkel cell-neurite complex, or Merkel disc, is the cellular unit of the SA I (slowly adapting type I) receptor of glabrous skin (Figure 2-1). It was described by Merkel as a *tastzellen*, or touch receptor (Merkel, 1875). Individual Merkel cells are 9–16 μm

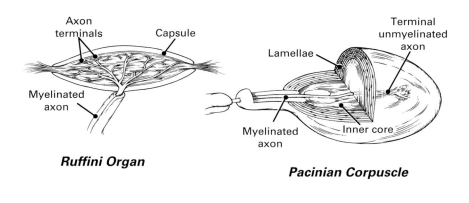

Ruffini Organ

Pacinian Corpuscle

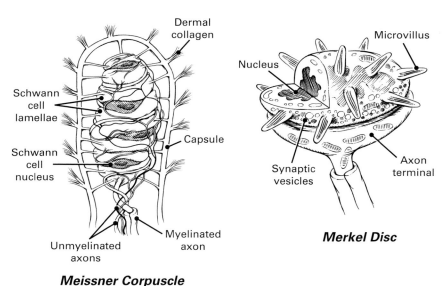

Meissner Corpuscle

Merkel Disc

FIGURE 2-1   The four cutaneous mechanoreceptors that contribute to touch.

in diameter, and are embedded along the basal lamina of the intermediate epidermal ridges, the inner structures that mirror the ridges of the finger-prints (Figure 2-2) (Smith, 1970). Merkel cells and their axons form a complex web. A single parent axon may innervate several small grape-like clusters of Merkel cells, or may give off a series of lateral branches, each with clusters, to extend a chain of receptors for up to 300 μm (Paré et al., 2002). Clusters served by an individual axon may be spread out over 5 mm² (Iggo and Andres, 1982). Although each Merkel cell is contacted by only one axon branch, each cluster or chain of Merkel cells receives the interdigitated terminals of several axons. The SA I receptive field is 2–3 mm in diameter, is contributed

to by roughly 100 Merkel cells, and has "hot spots" that correspond to individual branches of the affer-ent axon (Figure 2-3). When small stimuli are pre-sented, a single hot spot may become dominant, permitting the resolution of spatial detail smaller than the receptive field diameter (Phillips, Johnson, 1981; Johnson, 2001). The density of SA I receptive fields has been estimated at 70 per cm² in the human fingertip (Johansson, Vallbo, 1980), corresponding to a spacing between receptive field centers of 1 mm (Johnson et al., 2000).

Whether the Merkel cell actively transmits impulses to the axon, or merely supports and modulates its function, has long been the subject of debate (summa-rized in Tachibana, 1995; Lucarz and Brand, 2007).

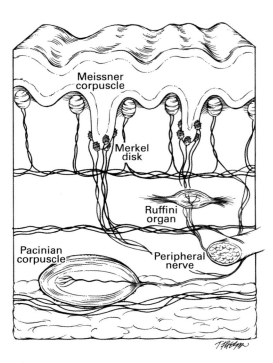

FIGURE 2-2   The location of cutaneous mechanoreceptors in the skin. Merkel cell/neurite complexes are arrayed along the intermediate ridge, the internal mirror image of the external fingerprint ridge. Merkel cells may be linked in receptor chains of up to 300 μm in length (not shown). Meissner corpuscles lie closer to the skin surface, between the lateral ridges. Pacinian corpuscles and Ruffini endings are deeper, within the subcutaneous tissues.

The junction between Merkel cell and axon resembles, but is not entirely structured like, a synapse (Hartschuh, Weihe, 1980). Merkel cells contain dense granules that package neuropeptides, ATP, and serotonin, each discussed as potential neurotransmitters (Tachibana, Nawa, 2002; Tachibana et al., 2005). Recently, neurotransmission through release of glutamate has emerged as a realistic possibility. Micro-array and protein expression studies have accounted for the molecular machinery needed for glutamate release (Haeberle et al., 2004; Hitchcock et al., 2004), and antagonism of glutamate receptors has been shown to cause dose-dependent reduction in the response of SA I receptors to stimulation (Fagan, 2001). Nonetheless, there is strong evidence that action potentials are initiated by mechanosensitive ion channels in the terminal portions of the nerve (Diamond et al., 1988), isolated Merkel cells are not mechanosensitive (Yamashita et al., 1992),

and numbers and response properties of SA I receptors are well maintained in mice that lack most of their Merkel cells (Kinkelin et al., 1999). The true function of the Merkel cell thus remains enigmatic.

The role of neurotrophins in the development and maintenance of the Merkel cell-neurite complex has also challenged investigators. During development, Merkel cells colonize the skin before their neural partners have arrived (English et al., 1980). Initial observations in knockout mice revealed that Merkel innervation initially requires both the TrkA (tyrosine kinase receptor for NGF) and TrkC (tyrosine kinase receptor for NT-3) receptors, but becomes solely dependent on TrkC postnatally (Margolis, Margolis, 1997). Neurotrophin 3 (NT-3), the TrkC ligand, thus emerged as the primary neurotrophin regulating the Merkel cell-neurite complex in adults. The importance of NT-3 was emphasized further by the observation of increased numbers of Merkel cells in mice overexpressing NT-3 (Albers et al., 1996), and decreased numbers in NT-3 knockout animals (Airaksinen et al., 1996). Physiologically, NT-3 overexpression was found to increase the magnitude of the SA I response to stimulation and to enhance the speed of SA I fiber conduction (McIlwrath et al., 2007). As additional subtleties have emerged, however, the apparent role of NT-3 has been modified. The truncated (nonkinase) form of the TrkC receptor, $TrkC_t$, has proven to be the most important regulator of early Merkel cell development (Cronk et al., 2002), and NT-3 has been shown to mediate Merkel cell number indirectly through neural effects rather than directly as a survival factor (Krimm et al., 2004).

The Merkel cell-neurite complex is slowly adapting, and its rate of discharge increases linearly with the depth of skin indentation from 0 to at least 1500 μm (Mountcastle et al., 1966; Johnson et al., 2000). The receptor fires in response to local tissue distortion, or strain. Evaluation of biomechanical models of the fingertip revealed that observable behavior was best explained by an SA I response to a specific aspect of strain such as the strain energy density (Srinivasan, Dandekar, 1996) or maximum compressive strain (Phillips, Johnson, 1981). These measures of tissue distortion are scalar quantities that do not depend on the direction of measurement. A consequence of this pattern of end organ sensitivity is *surround suppression* (Vega-Bermudez, Johnson, 1999b); the SA I response to structures within a receptive field is decreased by stimuli in the surrounding area, as these peripheral stimuli reduce

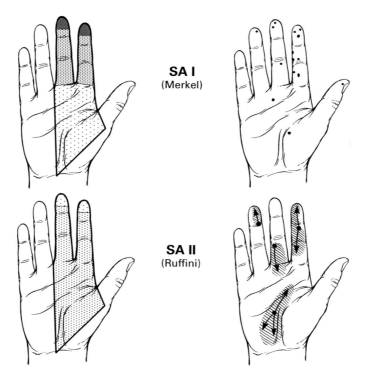

FIGURE 2-3   The relative density of the slowly adapting receptors (left), and the size of their individual receptive fields (right). For SAII units, the arrows indicate directions of skin stretch that gave rise to increased discharge. Redrawn with permission from Vallbo and Johansson, 1978, and Johansson and Vallbo, 1983.

the strain at the receptor. As a result, SA I receptors respond most briskly to stimuli that are completely isolated, such as a point, or partially isolated, such as an edge or curve. Experimentally, SA I afferents provide an accurate representation of Braille dot patterns (Phillips et al., 1990), and an edge elicits 20 times as much SA I response as does a smooth surface (Philips, Johnson, 1981). Electrical stimulation of individual, identified SA I fibers in human peripheral nerve elicits the primary sensation of pressure (Ochoa, Torebjork, 1983). The perceptions arising from stimulation of groups of SA I fibers will be discussed below.

The Meissner Corpuscle

The Meissner corpuscle, described by Wagner and Meissner in 1852, is the cellular transducer for rapidly adapting (RA) cutaneous mechanotransduction. Meissner corpuscles in adult human skin measure 20–40 μm in diameter and 80–150 μm in length. They are embedded in the dermal papillae,

between the intermediate and limiting ridges (Figure 2-2), and are arrayed in parallel rows that follow the contours of the overlying fingerprint (Bolanowski, Pawson, 2003) (Figure 2-4, 2-5). This places them as close as possible to the skin surface (Quilliam, 1978). The pattern of Meissner corpuscle innervation by RA afferent fibers is highly complex. Each corpuscle is innervated by between two and nine RA afferents (Cauna, 1956; Paré et al., 2002). A single afferent fiber supplies approximately 80 corpuscles in the young, decreasing with age-related loss to 30 in the aged (Bolton et al., 1964; Johnson et al., 2000). An individual corpuscle may be innervated by axons with distinct anatomical patterns of arborization, suggesting that it participates in an overlapping continuum of afferents with varying resolutions (Paré et al., 2002). The average RA receptive field is 3–5 mm in diameter, provides a uniform response to stimuli throughout its area, and is most sensitive to vibratory stimuli between 40 and 60 Hz (Figure 2-4) (Johnson et al., 2000).

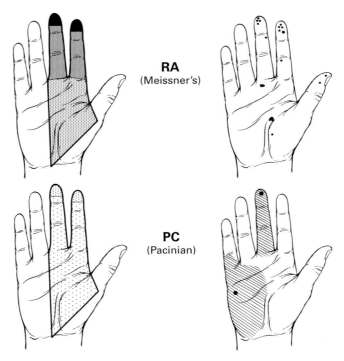

FIGURE 2-4   The relative density of the rapidly adapting receptors (left), and the size of their individual receptive fields (right). For PC units, the zone of maximum sensitivity is indicated by black dots. Redrawn with permission from Vallbo and Johansson, 1978, and Johansson and Vallbo, 1983.

The individual Meissner corpuscle is an ovoid structure that, on closer inspection, is a stack of flattened, plate-like lamellae of Schwann cell lineage (Figure 2-1) (Cauna, 1956; Ide, 1988). The terminals of RA axons are sandwiched between these lamellae to form the mechanosensitive transducer (Munger, Ide, 1988). The Meissner corpuscle is also innervated by both peptidergic and nonpeptidergic C-fibers, suggesting a role in nociception (Paré et al., 2001). A connective tissue capsule links the Meissner corpuscle to the surrounding tissues. Externally, dermal collagen fibers bind the capsule to the epidermis; internally, collagen trabeculae anchor it to projections from the discoid Schwann cells (Takahashi-Iwanaga, Shimoda, 2003). The contrast of peripheral stimulation with central damping is

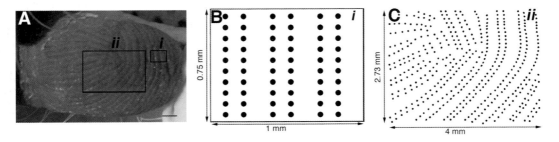

FIGURE 2-5   A. Photograph of the glabrous skin of the index finger of a Macaque monkey. B,C. Maps of Meissner corpuscle distribution corresponding to the areas outlined in A. The association between rows of Meissner corpuscles and the fingerprint ridge is striking. Reprinted with permission from Bolanowski and Pawson, 2003.

thought to maximize bending, and thus stimulation, of the RA axon tip. A strong role for BDNF signaling in the support of Meissner corpuscles is suggested by: (1) a developmental requirement for TrkB, the tyrosine kinase receptor for BDNF, but not for TrkA or TrkC, the other high-affinity neurotrophin receptors (LeMaster et al., 1999; González-Martínez et al., 2004; Perez-Pinera, et al., 2008); and (2) the presence of enlarged, densely innervated Meissner corpuscles in animals overexpressing BDNF (LeMaster et al., 1999).

The Meissner corpuscle responds to low frequency vibration, the skin movement perceived as flutter (Mountcastle, 1975; Ochoa and Torebjork, 1983). In contrast to the SA I receptor, it is insensitive to static skin deformation, is four times more sensitive to skin motion, and resolves spatial detail poorly (Johnson, 2001). Signaling by populations of Meissner corpuscles to control grip is discussed below.

The Pacinian Corpuscle

The Pacinian corpuscle is the only cutaneous mechanoreceptor large enough to be visible to the naked eye, appearing at surgery as a small, lustrous grain of rice. In humans it can reach sizes up to 1–2 mm in width and 4 mm in length. Although discovered by Vater and first described in a thesis in 1741, the corpuscle became more widely known as a result of Pacini's publication of 1835 (Hamann, 1995). Pacinian corpuscles are embedded singly or in clusters within the deep dermis or subcutaneous fat (Figure 2-2). Unlike the receptors described previously, they have a strictly one-to-one relationship with their innervating axons. There are approximately 2,500 Pacinian corpuscles in the hand, with 300–400 in each finger and 800 in the palm (Brisben et al., 1999). The Pacinian receptive field is vast compared to those considered previously, including an entire finger or even the whole hand (Figure 2-4) (Johannson, Vallbo, 1979).

The Pacinian corpuscle encapsulates a terminal axon within an onion-like structure that is differentiated into inner core, intermediate cell layer, and capsule (Figure 2-1). The axon, myelinated as it enters the capsule, terminates within the inner core as an unmyelinated shaft several hundred micrometers long. This shaft bristles with up to 1600 lateral spines that penetrate the inner core (Munger and Ide, 1988). A membrane specialization at the base of the spines, the subaxolemmal lamina, is thought to

participate in signal transduction (Spencer and Schaumberg, 1973). The inner core is assembled from hemilaminae, stacked on either side of the axon like concentric gutter tiles and separated by opposing radial clefts (Munger and Ide, 1988). These hemilamellar cells of Schwann cell origin (Pease, Quilliam, 1957; Nava, 1974) enclose the terminal axon except at its tip, where it contacts the intermediate layer (Spencer, Schaumberg, 1973). The intermediate cell layer, separated from the core by a free space containing collagen, is two to three cell layers thick (Munger, Ide, 1988). It is surrounded by the capsule, 30–60 thin concentric layers of perineurial origin (Pease, Quilliam, 1957; Nava, 1974) that are invested with basal laminae and separated by fluid-filled spaces (Halata, 1975). Development of the Pacinian corpuscle appears to involve multiple neurotrophin signaling pathways, most prominently through NT-3, probably as a result of their action on DRG neurons (Gonzalez-Martinez et al., 2004; Sedy et al., 2004).

The Pacinian corpuscle is exquisitely sensitive to vibration, so much so that early electrophysiologic experiments were confounded by ambient vibrations in the laboratory (Hunt, 1961). It responds to displacement amplitudes as fine as 3 nm at the capsule surface (Bolanowski, Zwislocki, 1984) and 10 nm at the skin (Brisben et al., 1999) within its tuning frequency of 80–300 Hz. As a by-product of this sensitivity, however, the Pacinian corpuscle has little if any spatial resolution (Johnson et al., 2000). At low frequencies, the multilayered capsule is a highly effective filter that minimizes the impact of the high-amplitude, low-frequency vibrations produced by the working hand (Lowenstein, Skalak, 1966); as the frequency of stimulation is decreased from 150 to 20 Hz, the Pacinian vibration threshold rises from 0.03 μm to 5.6 μm (Brisben et al., 1999). A further consequence of its sensitivity and filtering properties is that the Pacinian corpuscle is especially suited to provide a high-fidelity neural image of vibratory stimuli transmitted to the hand through a tool (Brisben et al., 1999; Johnson et al., 2000). The surgeon may grasp a scalpel firmly, yet still appreciate the textural nuances of the tissue being cut.

(The Ruffini Organ)

The Ruffini organ, or Ruffini corpuscle, is the receptor traditionally associated with slowly adapting type II (SA II) afferent activity. Described by Ruffini in 1894 (Ruffini, 1894), the receptor is quite large, measuring up to 200 x 1,000 μm, and is located in the deep dermis (Figure 2-2). Each receptor is innervated by a single axon, though one axon may serve several corpuscles. A fusiform capsule contains a fluid-filled subcapsular space that surrounds the core of the receptor, where axon processes are surrounded by Schwann cells and mechanically linked to the surrounding connective tissue through collagen fibrils (Willis and Coggeshall, 2004b). The role of the Ruffini organ in mechanotransduction is the subject of ongoing debate. Ruffini corpuscles are not found in the glabrous skin of monkeys (Paré et al., 2002), nor are SA II responses obtained from stimulating monkey skin (Johnson et al., 2000). As SA II responses can be obtained readily from the glabrous skin of humans (Johannson and Vallbo, 1979), the assumption was made that a lack of Ruffini corpuscles in monkeys was responsible for the difference between species. More recently, however, histologic evaluation of human fingerpad skin from three individuals revealed only a single Ruffini corpuscle, leading the investigators to conclude that human SA II activity must rely on structures other than the Ruffini ending (Paré et al., 2003). The complex innervation pattern of the Merkel cell (Paré et al., 2002) and its ability to respond to skin stretch under some circumstances (Bisley et al., 2000) suggest that it may contribute to SA II activity, although definitive proof is lacking.

The SA II receptor, whatever it may be, is sensitive to vertical displacement over an area of 2.5 cm^2; it responds to skin stretch over an area as great as 25 cm^2 (Figure 2-3) (Chambers et al., 1972). Stimulation of identified SA II fibers in awake humans results in no consistent sensory experience (Ochoa and Torebjork, 1983). SA II afferents can be differentiated from SA I afferents by several criteria (summarized in Johnson et al., 2000): (1) Their receptive fields are 5 times larger and less distinct (Johannson, Vallbo, 1980); (2) they are 6 times less sensitive to skin indentation (Johannson, Vallbo, 1979); (3) they are 2–4 times more sensitive to skin stretch (Edin, 1992); and (4) their discharges are more uniform (Edin, 1992).

CENTRAL PROCESSING OF MECHANOSENSITIVE INPUT

The pathways that communicate information from individual cutaneous receptors to the cerebral cortex are remarkable for their functional and somatotopic organization as they convey impulses from one relay to the next. After nerve injury and regeneration, with many axons reinnervating receptors of incorrect modality and/or in an incorrect somatotopic location, the information arriving in the spinal cord and brain will be disordered. Both the modality and location of a stimulus may be misrepresented. It is thus important to understand both the normal wiring diagram and the tools applied by the CNS to normal sensory input, as these will be the same tools used to translate the "new language spoken by the hand to the brain" after nerve repair (Lundborg, 2000).

The Dorsal Root Ganglion

The neurons that innervate cutaneous mechanoreceptors are located in the dorsal root ganglion (DRG), adjacent to the spinal cord. These neurons are described as pseudo-unipolar: a single process, the initial axon segment, leaves the cell before bifurcating into a peripheral process that brings information from the end organ, and a central process that penetrates the dorsal root entry zone of the spinal cord. Once within the cord, the central process sends branches medially to laminae III and IV of the dorsal horn of the spinal cord and centrally to the cuneate and gracile nuclei within the medulla. DRG neurons exhibit a dizzying array of often overlapping chemical phenotypes that emphasize the great diversity of functions represented within each ganglion (reviewed in Willis and Coggeshall, 2004a; Lawson, 2005). This diversity, in turn, suggests the potential for many categories of functional mismatch as regenerating axons contact inappropriate targets distally.

NEURONAL PHENOTYPE

Within the diversity of the DRG it is possible to characterize the neurons of cutaneous mechanoreceptors on a broad basis. Histograms of DRG neuron size are usually bimodal, allowing separation of large and small cell populations (Lieberman, 1976; Lawson, 1979). Furthermore, the staining properties of these populations are generally different, leading to division of DRG neurons into large light neurons (L) and small dark neurons (SD) (Lieberman, 1976). The cytoplasm of L cells is less dark because it contains high concentrations of microtubules and neurofilaments, neuronal constituents that stain lightly with routine basic aniline dyes. An antibody to a phosphorylated neurofilament subunit, RT97, binds exclusively to L neurons and has been used to identify them immunohistochemically (Lawson, 1992). Human cutaneous mechanoreceptors are served by large axons that conduct rapidly at speeds of 45–60 m/sec (Knibestol, 1973, 1975). As conduction velocity and cell size are strongly correlated (Yoshida, Matsuda, 1979; Harper, Lawson, 1985), one would expect the neurons of cutaneous mechanoreceptors to be L cells, an hypothesis confirmed by combined electrophysiologic and labeling studies (discussed in Lawson, 2005).

The variability in molecular phenotype of large DRG neurons is less complex than that of their smaller, often nociceptive counterparts. Growth factors and their receptors are among the best-studied of these phenotypic markers. The neurotrophin NT-3 is required for survival and function of approximately 20% of DRG neurons, and may be supplied to these neurons by either muscle or skin (Botchkarev et al., 1999). L neurons participate in proprioception and mechanotransduction, especially that mediated by the Merkel cell-neurite complex (Enfors et al., 1994; Zhou et al., 1998). Ninety-four percent of DRG neurons immunoreactive for NT-3 express TrkC, the high-affinity NT-3 receptor (Chen et al., 1996), and these are among the largest neurons in the ganglion (Mu et al., 1993). Several members of the interleukin family of cytokines also influence large DRG neurons. The receptor for ciliary neuronotrophic factor (CNTF) is expressed by all DRG neurons, consistent with a significant role for CNTF in both development and adulthood (MacLennan et al., 1996). Interleukin 1β is expressed in most medium and large neurons, where it may function as an auto/paracrine signaling molecule in sensory transmission (Copray et al., 2001). IL-6, in contrast, is expressed in medium and large neurons only after axotomy (Murphy et al., 2000).

L neurons are also characterized by a variety of other molecular components. The ganglioside GM-1, a neural receptor that binds the subunit of cholera toxin, is present on most RT97-positive L neurons (Robertson et al., 1991). Other surface markers of large DRG neurons include antibodies to embryonic antigens (SSEA3, SSEA4) and the lectins *Griffonia simplicifolia* agglutinin II (GSAII), *Pisum sativum* antigen (PSA), and *Lens culinaris* antigen (LCA) (Lawson, 2005). Functionally, L neurons express high levels of the enzymes cytochrome oxidase and carbonic anhydrase, and the calcium-binding proteins parvalbumin and calbindin D28k

(Carr, Nagy, 1993). Cytochrome oxidase activity is correlated with cellular oxygen consumption, carbonic anhydrase regulates intraneuronal CO_2 levels, and the calcium-binding proteins control intracellular calcium concentrations during neuronal activity (discussed in Carr, Nagy, 1993).

SOMATOTOPY

In addition to their functional and molecular attributes, DRG neurons may be characterized by their somatotopic organization. On the rostrocaudal axis of the body, there are two DRGs per spinal segment, one for each side of the median sagittal plane. The peripheral axons emanating from each DRG define a dermatome, or strip of skin innervated by the DRG neurons of that spinal level. The central processes define a somatotopically organized territory within the dorsal horn of the spinal cord and brainstem. This strict organization of peripheral and central projections might suggest that DRG neurons should be similarly organized within the DRG. In reality, their organization is more difficult to discern. Axonal tracing studies in rat and cat have determined that discrete patches of skin project to longitudinal columns within a ganglion (Kaus, Rethelyi, 1985), that projections of major limb nerves tend to occupy the rostral or caudal half of multiple ganglia (Wessels et al., 1994), and that muscle afferent neurons are organized in a manner that suggests grouping by muscle compartment (Peyronnard et al, 1990). In the primate, individual digital nerves project to longitudinal columns that are bilaterally symmetrical, but that do not occupy a consistent rostrocaudal position (Figure 2-6).

The Dorsal Column–Lemniscal System

Mechanosensitive DRG neurons serving the hand extend their primary axons centrally through the ipsilateral dorsal column of the spinal cord to form synapses in the nucleus cuneatus of the medulla (Mountcastle, 1984). By the time information leaves this first relay, it has been transformed from the dermatomal organization of the roots to a somatotopic format (Figure 2-7) (Culberson, Brushart, 1989; Florence et al., 1991). This reorganization may occur both within dorsal column pathways approaching the nucleus (Culberson, Albright, 1984) and within the nucleus itself (summarized in Mountcastle, 2006b). Afferent mechanosensitive

Radial Digital Thumb

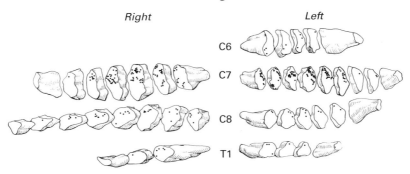

Right   *Left*

C6

C7

C8

T1

Radial Digital Index

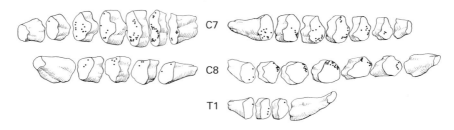

C7

C8

T1

Radial Digital Middle

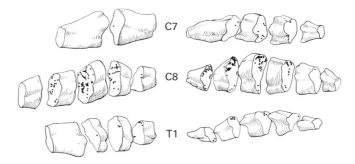

C7

C8

T1

FIGURE 2-6   The location of neurons serving median digital nerves in the Macaque. The radial digital nerves of the thumb, index, and middle finger have been exposed to HRP-WGA to label proximal axons and their neurons. The ganglia are viewed from the ventral surface. The radial digital nerve of the thumb projects to the rostral portions of both C7 and C8, the radial digital index to caudal C7 and rostral C8, and the radial digital middle to rostral and mid-C8. Neurons are usually distributed throughout the length of the ganglion, and there is moderate correspondence from side to side. Drawing by Suzanne Merrick, MA.

information is also reordered on the basis of modality; axons serving a specific function are grouped together in small bundles, each corresponding to a modality-specific column within the cuneate nucleus (Florence et al., 1988, 1989). Axons emanating from cuneate relay neurons then cross the midline of the body and course proximally in the medial lemniscus to terminate in the ventral posterior lateral nucleus of the thalamus (VPL) (Mountcastle, Henneman, 1952). This secondary relay nucleus is also organized somatotopically by modality (Mountcastle, Henneman, 1952; Dykes

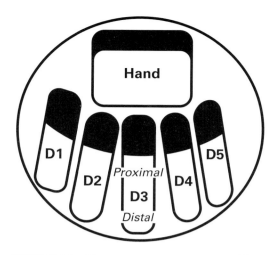

FIGURE 2-7   The somatotopic organization of the hand representation in the cuneate nucleus of the macaque. Dorsal above, medial to the right. Reprinted with permission from Florence et al., 1991.

et al., 1981; Jones et al., 1982). The image is reversed, however, as axons have crossed from one side of the body to the other.

The input resulting from stimulation of individual cutaneous mechanoreceptors is subject to many influences as it passes through relay nuclei on its path from skin to cortex (summarized in Gardner and Martin, 2000). Brainstem and thalamic relay neurons have receptive fields that are progressively larger than those of individual primary neurons. The DRG receptive field is determined by the distribution of a single peripheral axon, whereas that of a relay neuron is defined by the entire population of more peripheral neurons that interact with it through synaptic connections. This *convergence* of peripheral inputs onto a relay neuron is mirrored by *divergence* of outputs from this neuron onto several more central neurons. Convergence and divergence allow relay nuclei to interpret the output of an individual receptor in the context of surrounding activity. The activity of relay neurons is also modified by the action of inhibitory interneurons (Figure 2-8). The most active afferents can suppress the firing of neighboring relay neurons, thus sharpening the signal through afferent or *feed-forward* inhibition; the most active relay neurons can accomplish the same through *feed-back* inhibition. Additional influences are provided by descending cortical signals that modify transmission based on behavioral context, and input from secondary afferent pathways that

project through the dorsal horn of the spinal cord (Mountcastle, 2006b).

The abundance of influences poised to modify the central transmission of mechanosensitive information suggests that it could be altered substantially by the time it reaches the cortex. If all convergent and divergent connections were active, the signal from a single peripheral receptor would be delivered to a large cortical area, limiting its usefulness. This is not, however, the case; the receptive field of a cortical neuron is only 2–3 times larger than that of a primary neuron (DiCarlo & Johnson, 2000). As Mountcastle has emphasized, "The dynamic characteristics of the lemniscal somatic afferent systems are determined by a strong synaptic security up to and through the initial stages of intracortical processing, a throughput function that belies the anatomical divergence and convergence within them" (Mountcastle, 2006c, p239).

The Dorsal Horn of the Spinal Cord

In addition to their primary central projections through the dorsal column–lemniscal system, mechanosensitive afferents from the hand also distribute collaterals to the dorsal horn of the spinal cord. These collaterals terminate somatotopically in the primate, with individual digital nerves projecting to narrow strips that penetrate from the surface to the depths of the dorsal horn (Figure 2-9). The digits are represented sequentially along the medial two-thirds of the dorsal horn, with the skin of the hand itself represented laterally, and that of the forearm both proximal and distal to the hand and digits (Brown et al., 1989; Florence et al., 1991) (Figure 2-10). The dorsal horn terminations of identified mechanoreceptors have been mapped individually with combined intracellular recording and labeling techniques (Brown et al., 1978; Brown et al., 1980; Brown et al., 1981). Each of the four cutaneous mechanoreceptors has a morphologically distinct projection pattern, although all send collaterals both rostrally and caudally for at least several millimeters. Interneurons in the area of these mechanosensitive projections are involved in a variety of interactions. Some project through the dorsal columns to the cuneate nucleus (Gordon, Grant, 1982), some project directly to the thalamus (Willis et al., 2001), and others presumably mediate cutaneous reflexes.

Dorsal horn collaterals of primary mechanoreceptive neurons also interact with neurons involved

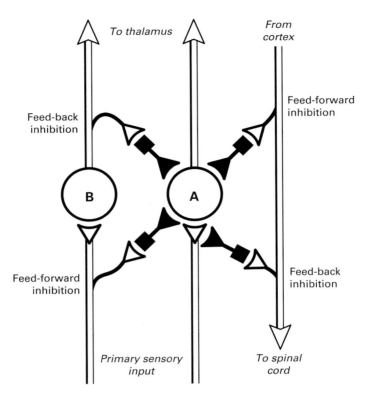

To thalamus

From cortex

Feed-forward inhibition

Feed-back inhibition

B

A

Feed-forward inhibition

Feed-back inhibition

Primary sensory input

To spinal cord

FIGURE 2-8   Schematic summary of the potential inhibitory influences within the cuneate nucleus. A and B are relay neurons, and the small dark neurons are inhibitory interneurons. Excitatory synapses are indicated by open triangles, and inhibitory synapses by closed triangles. Neuron A displays the variety of inhibitory influences that can be exerted by neighboring relay neurons (B) and descending cortical pathways.

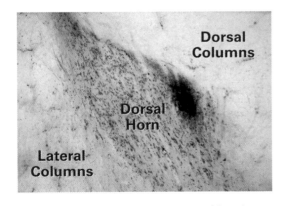

Dorsal Columns

Dorsal Horn

Lateral Columns

FIGURE 2-9   Somatotopic projection of digital nerve to the dorsal horn of the spinal cord in the macaque. HRP-WGA has been applied to the radial digital nerve of the index finger, and labels a discrete strip of medial dorsal horn with black reaction product. Same animal as Figure 2-6. This and similar photos were used to map the dorsal horn projections of the medial digital nerves. Reprinted from Brown et al., 1989.

in the transmission of pain. Vibration of the skin temporarily relieves pain of neural origin (Bini et al., 1984), while electrical stimulation of large caliber afferents may provide lasting pain relief (Melzack, 1975). These interactions are consistent with the gate theory of pain proposed by Melzack and Wall (1965); practically, they allow us to apply vibration to lessen the pain of cutaneous injection, or to reduce chronic pain with transcutaneous electrical nerve stimulation (TENS) of large caliber afferents.

In the absence of clear DRG somatotopy, the sharply circumscribed projections to the dorsal horn provide the first spatial representation of mechano-receptive activity along the neural axis. This map of cutaneous projections will be redrawn after periph-eral nerve injury and regeneration (Brushart et al., 1981). Although the technology is not yet available to obtain such a map in humans, one would expect the degree of distortion after reinnervation to

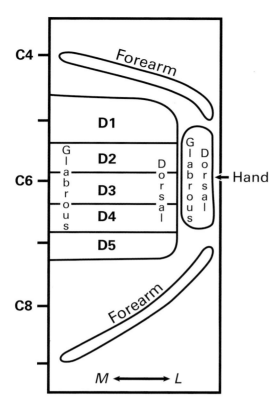

C4

Forearm

D1

G
l
a
b
r
o
u
s

D2

D
o
r
s
a
l

G
l
a
b
r
o
u
s

D
o
r
s
a
l

C6

D3

D4

D5

Forearm

C8

M ⟷ L

← Hand

FIGURE 2-10 The somatotopic organization of the hand representation in the dorsal horn of the spinal cord in squirrel monkeys, determined physiologically. M—medial, L—lateral. The representation of each digit is more circumscribed on the rostrocaudal axis than that suggested by the distribution of labeled neurons in the DRG (Figure 2-6). Reprinted with permission from Florence et al., 1991.

correlate with the degree to which sensory stimuli are inappropriately localized by the patient.

Primary Somatosensory Cortex

SOMATOTOPY

Mechanosensitive neurons in the VPL nucleus of the thalamus project to the primary somatosensory cortex (SI), located in the postcentral gyrus of the parietal lobe (Figure 2-11). A century ago Brodmann subdivided this region on the basis of cellular architecture into areas 1, 2, and 3 (Brodmann, 1903). Area 3 was later subdivided into areas 3a and 3b (Vogt, Vogt, 1919). The connections linking the thalamus to each area, and the areas one to another, have been studied extensively. Of the four subdivisions of SI, area 3b

has been found to receive the most abundant cutaneous mechanoreceptive input from the thalamus (Jones et al., 1982). Additional evidence confirms the dominant role of area 3b in cutaneous sensation: (1) It devotes the largest cortical surface to the digits (Sur, 1980); (2) It contains the highest proportion of cells receptive to light touch (Powell, Mountcastle, 1959b) and static skin indentation (Paul et al., 1972); and (3) neurons in area 3b have the smallest receptive fields, exhibiting less convergence of signals from multiple receptors than other areas (Paul et al., 1972; Iwamura et al., 1993).

Each of the four Brodmann areas in SI contains a somatotopic map of the body surface (Kaas et al., 1979; Nelson et al., 1980) (Figure 2-11). This statement summarizes nearly a century of work on one of the core problems of neuroscience, the organization and function of the cerebral cortex (history reviewed in Kaas et al., 1981 and Mountcastle, 2006d). Progress was saltatory, with flurries of activity as new techniques were introduced. Observation of the consequences of cortical wounds by Head and Holmes (1911) and intraoperative cortical stimulation by Harvey Cushing (1909) identified the presence of a somatotopic sensory map in the human postcentral gyrus. Charting the cortical potentials evoked by peripheral stimulation in the monkey, a technique introduced in the 1930s and employed extensively by Woolsey (1942), extended the sensory map to include Brodmann's areas 3, 1, and 2, and established that each half of the body, divided through the midsagittal plane, is mapped along the contralateral postcentral gyrus. The body surface is represented along its rostrocaudal axis, with the tail medially and the head laterally (Figure 2-11). Additionally, the area of cortex apportioned to an area of skin was found to be proportional to tactile acuity. The scale of this relationship was later refined by showing that a unit of glabrous digital skin commands 100x the cortical area of an equivalent area of skin on the trunk (Sur et al., 1980).

The 1950s saw great progress: the intraoperative studies of Penfield defined human cortical localization (Penfield and Jasper, 1954), and the introduction of single-cell recording techniques ushered in the modern era of cortical mapping in the primate. Mountcastle used this new tool to reveal that most neurons in area 2 responded to stimulation of deep tissues (joint, fascia, periosteum), most in area 3 (now 3b) responded to stimulation of skin, and those in area 1 represented a gradient between the

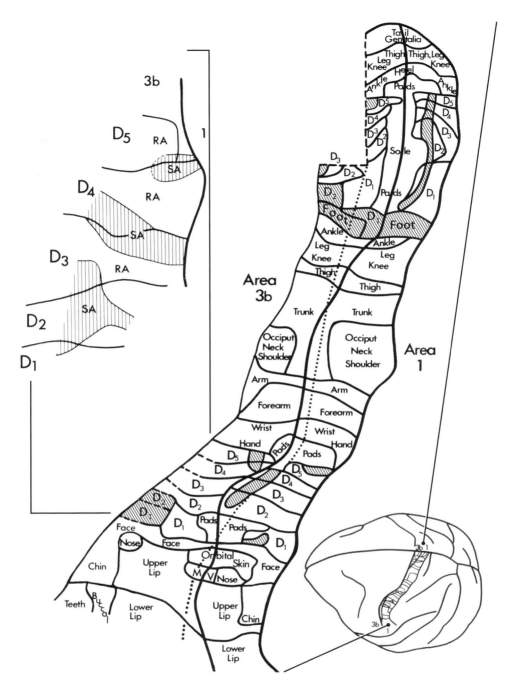

FIGURE 2-11   The somatotopic and modality-specific mapping of cutaneous projections to cortex in the monkey. Lower right—The location of areas 3b and 1 in the postcentral gyrus of the brain as seen in a dorso-lateral view. Center—Detailed mapping of cutaneous projections to areas 3b and 1. The heavy vertical line separates areas 3b and 1; the dotted line indicates the location of the central sulcus; shaded areas correspond to hairy skin on the dorsum of the fingers and toes. The digits are labeled D1–D5, beginning with the thumb and numbering ulnarward. Reprinted with permission from Nelson et al., 1980. Upper left—The distribution of RA and SA regions within the cortical representation of the digits. There is considerable overlap from one digit to the next. Reprinted with permission from Sur et al., 1984.

other two. He also found that stimulation of a single body area could elicit responses in more than one Brodmann area (Powell, Mountcastle, 1959a). These observations ruled out the possibility of a single somatotopic map spread over the four Brodmann areas in SI. The coexistence of two somatotopic maps, one in area 3b and the other in area I, was confirmed by Paul, Merzenich, and Goodman (1972), and the full picture of four separate maps was defined soon thereafter (Kaas et al.,1981; Pons et al., 1992). It is now known that areas 3b and 1 receive the output of cutaneous mechanoreceptors (Powell, Mountcastle, 1959a, Phillips et al., 1971, Kaas et al., 1981). In the awake animal, some of these neurons also respond to input from deep tissues (Iwamura et al., 1993), and their responses may be altered by motor activity (Nelson, 1996). Neurons of area 2 respond to both proprioceptive and tactile stimulation (Hyvarinen, Poranen, 1978; Iwamura et al., 1993) and manifest complex receptive fields with direction sensitivity and multimodal input (Whitsel et al., 1972; Hyvarinen, Poranen, 1978; Iwamura et al., 1985). Area 3a neurons receive proprioceptive and deep tissue inputs, although a small number have cutaneous receptive fields (Jones, Porter, 1980; Iwamura et al., 1993). The newest technique of cortical analysis, functional MRI (fMRI), is further advancing our knowledge of human cortical organization, allowing confirmation of the somatotopic principles established in nonhuman primates (McGlone et al., 2002; Blankenburg et al., 2003). The ability to image the human cortical response to peripheral stimuli will prove especially useful in the analysis of cortical reorganization after nerve repair (Chapter 11).

Topographically distinct areas of SI cortex are further subdivided by sensory modality. This additional level of complexity was suggested by the differing response of cortical neurons to uniform stimuli applied during routine topographic mapping. It was confirmed by detailed remapping of the digital territories in area 3b, probing the skin for one second to allow differentiation of RA and SA responses (Sur et al., 1984) (Figure 2-11). This technique revealed separate bands of RA and SA neurons, in the same general orientation of the bands representing each digit, but of variable conformation and often overlapping the territories of adjacent digits (Figure 2-11). When modality-specific stimuli are applied, it is possible to refine this mapping even further, identifying separate areas of termination for SA I, RA, and PC channels within each topographic area (Chen et al., 2001).

Similar localization has also been found when modality-specific probes are applied to area 1 (Friedman et al., 2004).

The Cortical Column

The cortical column is the unit of modality-specific cortical function. Histologic studies a century ago led to the realization that the entire cerebral cortex can be divided into six distinct cellular layers, and that these layers differ in their relative thickness based on the function of the region in which they are observed (Brodmann, 1909). The cells of specific cortical layers were found to connect stereotypically within the brain: layers II and III project to other cortical regions, layer IV receives input from the thalamus, layer V projects to subcortical structures, and layer VI projects to the thalamus (Gardner and Kandell, 2000). It was not until the pioneering electrophysiologic work of Mountcastle, however, that the functional consequences of this pattern were fully appreciated (summarized in Mountcastle, 1997). He determined that the smallest unit of cortical function is the "minicolumn," a narrow chain of 80–100 interconnected cells that span cortical layers II–VI perpendicular to the cortical surface. Approximately 80 minicolumns associate to become a column, or module, a hexagonal structure 300–400 μm wide that is surrounded by 6 similar columns (Favorov and Diamond, 1990). Layer II, just below the cortical surface, can thus be viewed as a pavement fashioned of hexagonal tiles. Each tile is the uppermost layer of a six-layered hexagonal column that projects inward, perpendicular to the cortical surface. In SI, each column is modality-specific, yet relates to other areas of the brain through a stereotypical pattern of connections. The modality-specific cortical column is thus the termination of the sensory channel, defined by its peripheral receptor and preserved faithfully throughout its course from skin to brain. The identity of the cortical column as a basic building block of the brain is emphasized further by its evolutionary history; cortical size is expanded not by increasing cortical thickness or the size of cortical columns, but by adding more columnar units to the structure as evolution proceeds (Rakic, 1995).

The discussion so far has emphasized the anatomy and function of individual sensory channels. Stimulation of single, identified human peripheral axons activates a single channel and results in a specific primary sensation. Activity in the RA channel is interpreted as flutter, activity in the SA I channel as pressure, and activity in the PC channel as vibration (Ochoa, Torebjork, 1983). Stimulation of identified SA II fibers does not elicit a consistent sensory experience. With the exception of the SA II channel, one can visualize the core elements of the pathway from peripheral receptor to cortical column with little difficulty. Superimposed on this relative simplicity, however, is wide variability in both the receptive fields of 3b neurons and in their response to complex stimuli. The direct, isomorphic representation of form in the periphery is thus modified in area 3b to produce neural responses that signal specific stimulus features (Hsiao et al., 2002)

Corticoneuronal Receptive Field

The ability to define the receptive field of a cortical neuron is highly dependent on the nature of the stimulus applied to the skin.In early studies, application of a single point to the skin resulted in the impression that most neurons had homogeneous, excitatory receptive fields (Mountcastle, Powell, 1959; Sur, 1980). The observation of more varied responses in some neurons (summarized in DiCarlo et al., 1998)—excitatory summation, surround inhibition, directional selectivity, and orientation selectivity—suggested that cortical receptive fields in area 3b were more complex than was initially thought. DiCarlo and colleagues set out to define this complexity by presenting the finger with a random pattern of dot stimuli, an approach designed to eliminate spatial cues by making the number of stimuli and alternative responses so high that performance is based only on appreciation of the spatial structure (Johnson et al., 1994).

In initial studies, DiCarlo and his coworkers found that most receptive fields contained a single, central region of excitation with areas of inhibition on one, two, three, or all sides of the excitatory center (DiCarlo et al., 1998). The images formed were independent of scanning velocity over a wide range, consistent with our ability to perceive texture and form under a wide variety of tactile conditions (DiCarlo, Johnson, 1999). These observations also support the observation that motion does not affect the accuracy of a robust clinical test of sensory acuity. The relationship between excitatory and inhibitory regions was explored further by scanning a single receptive field from several directions (DiCarlo, Johnson, 2000). This revealed: (1) a single, central excitatory region of short duration; (2) one or more

brief inhibitory regions adjacent to and nearly synchronous with the excitation; and (3) an area of inhibition that overlapped the excitatory region to varying degrees, but that was temporally delayed (Figure 2-12). The location of the excitatory and initial inhibitory areas were fixed and independent of the direction of stimulus movement, while the delayed inhibitory component always trailed the center of the receptive field.

The function of each component of the receptive field has been summarized by Hsiao et al. (2002). The fixed inhibitory component interacts with the area of central excitation to enhance detection of specific stimulus features, such as edges or corners, irrespective of scanning direction or speed. The delayed inhibitory component has three functions: (1) It emphasizes changes in the character of the stimulus along the axis of scanning, enhancing pattern and feature recognition. (2) When the area of delayed inhibition is centered on the area of excitation, it increases the discharge rate in parallel with scanning velocity. This mechanism permits uniform pattern recognition as scanning velocity is increased; progressively shorter contact times are compensated for by a progressive increase in signaling frequency, keeping the signaling per unit of skin relatively constant (Vega-Bermudez et al., 1991). (3) It provides directional sensitivity when the area of delayed inhibition is displaced from the center of excitation.

COMPLEX SENSIBILITY

The perception of form is attributed to the activity of groups of SA I afferents (Johnson et al., 2000). Of the four cutaneous mechanoreceptors, Pacinian and Ruffini endings are too sparse and too far from the surface of the skin to resolve spatial detail. SA I and RA receptors are both spaced appropriately in the fingertip to provide detailed information (see above). The crucial difference between them lies in receptive field geometry; SA I receptive fields are smaller than their RA counterparts, and thus are able to produce information at higher resolution (Vega-Bermudez, Johnson, 1999a). Additionally, SA I receptors signal increased intensity of stimulation by firing the same receptors more rapidly (Mountcastle et al., 1966). The pivotal role of SA I afferents is borne out by experiments in which they outperformed the other receptor types in detecting gradients as fine as 0.5 mm (Johnson, Lamb, 1981; Phillips, Johnson, 1981).

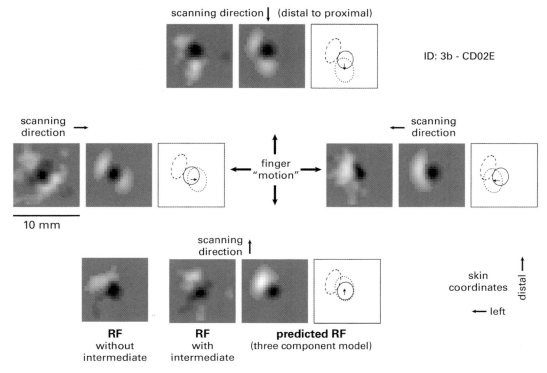

scanning direction ↓ (distal to proximal)

ID: 3b - CD02E

scanning direction →

← scanning direction

finger "motion"

10 mm

scanning direction ↑

skin coordinates

distal ↑

← left

RF without intermediate

RF with intermediate

predicted RF (three component model)

FIGURE 2-12   Receptive fields in area 3b in four scanning directions. The excitatory component is shown by the solid ellipse, the fixed inhibitory component by the dashed ellipse, and the lagged inhibitory component by the dotted ellipse. The left-hand square in each group represents the raw data, the middle square represents the receptive field predicted by the three component model, and the right-hand square diagrams the middle square. The relative location of the excitatory and fixed inhibitory components are unaffected by scanning direction, while the lagged inhibitory component always trails behind. Reprinted with permission from DiCarlo and Johnson, 2000.

Populations of SA I afferents also contribute to the perception of roughness, curvature, and orientation. The majority of texture judgments are made along the axes of rough/smooth and soft/hard (Hollins et al., 1993); of these, roughness has received the most attention. Perception of roughness is unidimensional, depends on element height, diameter, shape, and density, and is minimally affected by scanning velocity, contact force, and friction (discussed in Hsiao et al., 2002). A complex series of psychophysical studies has led to the conclusion that roughness is signaled by the differences in firing rates among closely spaced SA I afferents (summarized in Johnson, 2000). Interestingly, the receptive field architecture characterized by DiCarlo and Johnson (see above) is appropriate for this function (discussed in Hsiao et al., 2002). The SA I response to the curvature and orientation of

cylinders has also been studied in monkeys, leading to predictions of population responses that code for both variables (Wheat et al., 1995; Dodson et al., 1998). The minimum orientation difference that is signaled by the neural population response in monkeys was found to be 20 degrees, similar to the threshold demonstrated by humans during perceptual testing (Bensmaia et al., 2008a,b).

RA activity has been implicated in the identification of slippage between objects and the hand, a function crucial to the control of grip (summarized in Johnson et al., 2000). Within the first 0.1 second of grasping an object, the hand is able to assay its slipperiness, or coefficient of friction, and adjust the force of grip accordingly (Johansson, Westling, 1987). The response to sudden changes in load force is similar (Macefield et al., 1996). The Meissner (RA) system is implicated as the mediator of these functions for several reasons, as summarized by Johnson (2001): (1) RA afferents are 4x more sensitive to skin motion than are SA I afferents (Johannson, Vallbo, 1979), and are the only receptors able to detect slippage within the first 100 ms of contact (Johannson, Westling, 1987). (2) The RA system is exquisitely sensitive to small surface imperfections, as fine as 2 μm, whereas the threshold for the SA I system is at least 8 μm (LaMotte, Whitehouse, 1986). (3) Unlike SA I afferents, RA afferents are uniformly sensitive throughout their receptive fields, enhancing response to broad-based stimuli like slippage at the expense of spatial acuity (Phillips, Johnson, 1981; Vega-Bermudez, Johnson, 1999a). (4) The fluid-filled corpuscle is likely to have a damping effect on static force and very low frequency vibration, by-products of grasping activity that could interfere with sensation (Johnson et al., 2000).

Groups of SA II afferents provide information about skin stretch while minimizing interference from the skin indentation caused by holding an object in the hand, thereby optimizing perception of the direction of object motion (Olausson et al., 2000). The SA II afferent system also has a role in sensing hand conformation. The perception of joint angle was initially attributed to joint receptors (Goodwin et al., 1972), then to muscle spindles (Matthews, 1982). Recently, however, cutaneous receptors have also been implicated (Johnson, 2004). Stretching the skin near an anesthetized joint produces the sensation of joint movement, while movement of the anaesthetized joint in the absence of skin stretch is not perceived (Edin, Johansson, 1995). Furthermore, skin stretch can modify the response to muscle spindle activation, indicating that the two systems work together to signal joint position (Collins, 2000).

SECONDARY CORTICAL PROJECTIONS

As mechanosensitive information passes from area 3b to area 1 and beyond, its organizational framework changes dramatically (summarized in Gardner and Kandell 2000). In higher centers, neurons respond to combinations of stimuli or stimulus patterns; their inputs are selected from larger collections of primary receptive fields to emphasize features such as the orientation and direction of stimuli.

The process of tactile object recognition has been the focus of recent work that illustrates the interaction of area 3b with the other areas of SI and with SII

(reviewed in Hsiao, 2008). Area 3b provides the dominant input to area 1 (Garraghty et al., 1990), where receptive fields are larger, often spanning more than 1 digit. Area 1 neurons are able to extract information about more complex features than those in area 3b, and play a key role in processing tactile motion (Hsiao, 2008). Area 2, the next processor in the sequence, receives cutaneous inputs from areas 3b and 1, and proprioceptive inputs from the thalamus and area 3a (Jones, 1986). In humans, fMRI studies confirm that this area is activated by both cutaneous and proprioceptive inputs (Moore et al., 2000). Receptive fields in area 2 are even larger than those in area 1, often spanning the entire hand. Area 2 neurons modify their sensitivity to cutaneous stimuli on the basis of hand conformation and contribute to object recognition; they are not sensitive to motion (Hsiao, 2008).

The final step in shape perception occurs in SII, which receives inputs from all four areas of SI. Although some evidence suggests that SI and SII process information in parallel, the bulk of available data suggests that serial processing predominates (discussed in Hsiao et al., 2002). The anterior and posterior portions of SII receive both proprioceptive and cutaneous input, while the central portion processes primarily cutaneous information (Fitzgerald et al., 2004). The receptive fields of SII neurons vary widely in size, with the majority receiving input from both hands (Fitzgerald et al., 2004). In many instances, all the digits that are included in the field have the same orientation selectivity, suggesting that they integrate information about objects that touch multiple fingers, and are the neurons responsible for tactile object recognition (Fitzgerald et al., 2006a,b).

CONCLUSIONS

The experimental work of the last century has provided us with a topographic map of the primate brain, and is beginning to reveal the techniques used by the brain to process sensory information. Many challenges remain, such as determining how a stimulus property not seen in the responses of a single fiber is encoded in a population response, and how information about multiple properties—texture, form, orientation—can be encoded in the same population discharge, yet discriminated separately (Mountcastle, 2006e).

The normal functioning of the cutaneous sensory system is predicated on the correspondence between a receiver in the skin and its projection to the SI cortex. Although afferent signals may be modified in relay nuclei, their transmission is controlled so rigidly that a single cutaneous receptor may activate a single cortical neuron. That neuron is programmed to interpret the incoming signal as coming from a specific receptor type in a specific location as codified by the "labeled line" hypothesis. After nerve injury and regeneration, misrouting of regenerating axons will alter the correspondence between peripheral receptors and neurons in SI; a cortical neuron could potentially receive information from a novel receptor type that is located far from the receptor it originally responded to. The way in which this information is handled will determine the quality of the resulting sensation. The sensory experience arising from stimulation of reinnervated human skin (Chapter 5), the specificity with which receptor types and topographic areas are reinnervated (Chapter 10), and the electrophysiologic responses to peripheral miswiring (Chapter 11) will all shed light on this process.

REFERENCES

Adrian ED, Zotterman Y (1926) The impulses produced by sensory nerve-endings. Part 2. The response of a single end-organ. J Physiol (Lond) 61: 151–171.

Airaksinen MS, Koltzenburg M, Lewin GR, Masu Y, Helbig C, Wolf E, Brem G, Toyka KV, Thoenen H, Meyer M (1996) Specific subtypes of cutaneous mechanoreceptors require neurotrophin-3 following peripheral target innervation. Neuron 16: 287–295.

Albers KM, Perrone TN, Goodness TP, Jones ME, Green MA, Davis BM (1996) Cutaneous overexpression of NT-3 increases sensory and sympathetic neuron number and enhances touch dome and hair follicle innervation. J Cell Biol 134: 487–497.

Bensmaia SJ, Denchev PV, Dammann JF 3rd, Craig JC, Hsiao SS (2008a) The representation of stimulus orientation in the early stages of somatosensory processing. J Neurosci 28(3): 776–786.

Bensmaia SJ, Hsiao SS, Denchev PV, Killebrew JH, Craig JC (2008b) The tactile perception of stimulus orientation. Somatosens Mot Res 25(1): 49–59.

Bini G, Cruccu G, Hagbarth K-E, Shady W, Torebjörk E (1984) Analgesic effect of vibration and cooling on pain induced by intraneural electrical stimulation. Pain 18: 239–248.

Bisley JW, Goodwin AW, Wheat HE (2000) Slowly adapting type I afferents from the sides and ends of the finger respond to stimuli on the center of the fingerpad. J Neurophysiol 84: 57–64.

Blankenburg F, Ruben J, Meyer R, Schwiemann J, Villringer A (2003) Cerebral Cortex 13: 987–993.

Bolanowski SJ, Zwislocki JJ (1984) Intensity and frequency characteristics of Pacinian corpuscles. I. Action potentials. J Neurophysiol 51: 793–811.

Bolanowski SJ, Pawson L (2003) Organization of Meissner corpuscles in the glabrous skin of monkey and cat. Somatosens Mot Res 20: 223–231.

Bolton CF, Winkelmann RK, Dyck PJ (1964) A quantitative study of Meissner's corpuscles in man. Trans Am Neurol Assn 89: 190–192.

Botchkarev VA, Metz M, Botchkaerva NV, Welker P, Lommatzsch M, Renz H, Paus R (1999) Brain-derived neurotrophic factor, neurotrophin-3, and neurotrophin-4 act as "epitheliotrophins" in murine skin. Lab Invest 79: 557–572.

Brisben AJ, Hsiao SS, Johnson KO (1999) Detection of vibration transmitted through an object grasped in the hand. J Neurophysiol 81: 1548–1558.

Brodmann K (1903) Beitrage zur histologischen Lokalisation der Grosshirnrinde. Dritte Mitteilung: Die Rindenfelder der niederen Affen. J Psychol Neurol 4: 177–226.

Brodmann, K. (1909) *Vergleichende Lokalisationslehre der Grosshirnrinde in ihren Prinzipien dargestellt auf Grund des Zellenbaues*, Leipzig: Barth.

Brown AG, Rose PK, Snow PJ (1978) Morphology and organization of axon collaterals from afferent fibers of slowly adapting Type I units in cat spinal cord. J Physiol 277: 15–27.

Brown AG, Fyffe RE, Noble R (1980) Projections from Pacinian corpuscles and rapidly adapting mechanoreceptors of glabrous skin to the cat's spinal cord. J Physiol 307: 385–400.

Brown AG, Fyffe RE, Rose PK, Snow PJ (1981) Spinal cord collaterals from axons of type II slowly adapting units in the cat. J Physiol 316: 469–480.

Brown PB, Brushart TM, Ritz LA (1989) Somatotopy of digital nerve projections to the dorsal horn in the monkey. Somatosens Motor Res 6(3): 309–317.

Brushart TM, Henry EW, Mesulam M-M (1981) Reorganization of muscle afferent projections accompanies peripheral nerve regeneration. Neuroscience 6: 2053–2061.

Carr PA, Nagy JI (1993) Emerging relationships between cytochemical properties and sensory modality transmission in primary sensory neurons. Brain Res Bull 30: 209–219.

Cauna N (1956) Nerve supply and nerve endings in Meissner's corpuscles. Am J Anat 99: 315–350.

Chambers MR, Andres KH, Duering M, Iggo A (1972) The structure and function of the slowly adapting type II mechanoreceptor in hairy skin. Quart J Exp Physiol 57: 417–445.

Chen C, Zhou XF, Rush RA (1996) Neurotrophin-3 and TrkC-immunoreactive neurons in rat dorsal root ganglia correlate by distribution and morphology. Neurochem Res 21: 809–814.

Chen LM, Friedman RM, Ramsden BM, LaMotte RH, Roe AW (2001) Fine-scale organization of SI (area 3b) in the squirrel monkey revealed with intrinsic optical imaging. J.Neurophysiol. 86: 3011–3029.

Clarke, E. and C.D. O'Malley (1968) *The Human Brain and Spinal Cord*, Berkeley: University of California Press.

Collins DF (2000) Sensory integration in the perception of movements at the human metacarpophalyngeal joint. J Physiol 529: 505–515.

Copray JC, Mantingh I, Brouwer N, Biber K, Kust BM, Liem RS, Huitinga I, Tilders FJ, Van Dam A-M, Boddeke HW (2001) Expression of interleukin-1 beta in rat dorsal root ganglia. J Neuroimmunol 118: 203–211.

Cronk KM, Wilkinson GA, Grimes R, Wheeler EF, Jhaveri S, Fundin BT, Silos-Santiago I, Tessarollo L, Reichardt LF, Rice FL (2002) Diverse dependencies of developing Merkel innervation on the trkA and both full-length and truncated isoforms of trkC. Development 129: 3739–3750.

Culberson JL, Albright BC (1984) Morphological evidence for fiber sorting in the fasciculus cuneatus. Exp Neurol 85: 358–370.

Culberson JL, Brushart TM (1989) Somatotopy of digital nerve projections to the cuneate nucleus in the monkey. Somatosens Motor Res 6(3): 319–330.

Cushing H (1909) A note on the faradic stimulation of the postcentral gyrus in a conscious patient. Brain 32: 44–53.

Diamond J, Mills LR, Mearow KM (1988) Evidence that the Merkel cell is not the transducer in the mechanosensory Merkel cell-neurite complex. Prog Br Res 74: 51–56.

DiCarlo JJ, Johnson K, Hsiao SS (1998) Structure of receptive fields in area 3b of primary somatosensory cortex in the alert monkey. J Neurosci 18: 2626–2645.

DiCarlo JJ, Johnson KO (1999) Velocity invariance of receptive field structure in somatosensory cortical area 3b of the alert monkey. J Neurosci 19: 401–419.

DiCarlo JJ, Johnson KO (2000) Spatial and temporal structure of receptive fields in primate somatosensory area 3b: effects of stimulus scanning direction and orientation. J Neurosci 20: 495–510.

Dodson MJ, Goodwin AW, Browning AS, Gehring HM (1998) Peripheral neural mechanisms determining the orientation of cylinders grasped by the digits. J Neurosci 18: 521–530.

Dykes RW, Sur M, Merzenich MM, Kaas JH, Nelson RJ (1981) Regional segregation of neurons responding to quickly adapting, slowly adapting, deep and Pacinian receptors within thalamic ventroposterior lateral and venteroposterior inferior nuclei in the squirrel monkey (Saimiri sciureus). Neuroscience 6: 1687–1981.

Edin BB (1992) Quantitative analysis of static strain sensitivity in human mechanoreceptors from hairy skin. J Neurophysiol 67: 1105–1113.

Edin BB, Johansson N (1995) Skin strain patterns provide kinaesthetic information to the human central nervous system. J Physiol (Lond) 487: 243–251.

English KB, Burgess PR, Kavka-Van Norman D (1980) Development of rat Merkel cells. J Comp Neurol 194: 475–496.

Ernfors P, Lee K-F, Kucera J, Jaenisch R (1994) Lack of neurotrophin-3 leads to deficiencies in the peripheral nervous system and loss of proprioceptive afferents. Cell 77: 503–512.

Fagan BM (2001) Evidence for glutamate receptor mediated transmission at mechanoreceptors in the skin. Neuroreport 12: 341–347.

Favorov OV, Diamond ME (1990) Demonstration of discrete place-defined columns-segregates-in the cat SI. J Comp Neurol 298: 97–112.

Finger, S. (1994) *Origins of Neuroscience: A History of Explorations into Brain Function*, New York: Oxford University Press.

Fitzgerald PJ, Lane JW, Thakur PH, Hsiao SS (2004) Receptive field properties of the macaque second somatosensory cortex: evidence for multiple functional representations. J Neurosci 24: 11193–11204.

Fitzgerald PJ, Lane JW, Thakur PH, Hsiao SS (2006a) Receptive field (RF) properties of the macaque second somatosensory cortex: RF size, shape, and somatotopic organization. J Neurosci 26: 6485–6495.

Fitzgerald PJ, Lane JW, Thakur PH, Hsiao SS (2006b) Receptive field properties of the macaque second somatosensory cortex: representation of orientation on different finger pads. J Neurosci 26: 6473–6484.

Florence SL, Wall JT, Kaas JH. (1988) The somatotopic pattern of afferent projections from the digits to the spinal cord and cuneate nucleus in macaque monkeys. Brain Res 452: 388–392.

Florence SL, Wall JT, Kaas JH. (1989) Somatotopic organization of inputs from the hand to the spinal gray and cuneate nucleus of monkeys with observation on the cuneate nucleus of humans. J Comp Neurol 286: 48–79.

Florence SL, Wall JT, Kaas JH (1991) Central projections from the skin of the hand in squirrel monkeys. J Comp Neurol 311: 563–578.

Friedman RM, Chen LM, Roe AW (2004) Modality maps within primate somatosensory cortex. PNAS 101: 12724–12729.

Gardner, E.P. and E.R. Kandel (2000) Touch. In: *Principles of Neural Science*, Vol. 4, E.R. Kandel, J.H. Schwartz and T.M. Jessell, eds., pp. 451–471, New York: McGraw-Hill.

Gardner, E.P. and J.H. Martin (2000) Coding of sensory information. In: *Principles of Neural Science*, Vol. 4, E.R. Kandel, J.H. Schwartz and T.M. Jessell, eds., pp. 411–429, New York: McGraw-Hill.

Garraghty PE, Florence SL, Kaas JH (1990) Ablations of areas 3a and 3b of monkey somatosensory cortex abolish cutaneous responsivity in area 1. Brain Res 528: 165–169.

González-Martínez T, Germaná GP, Monjil DF, Silos-Santiago I, De Carlos F, Germanà G, Cobo J, Vega JA (2004) Absence of Meissner corpuscles in the digital pads of mice lacking functional TrkB. Brain Res 1002: 120–128.

Goodwin GM, McCloskey DI, Matthews PB (1972) The contribution of muscle afferents to kinaesthesia shown by vibration induced illusions of movement and by the effects of paralyzing joint afferents. Brain 95: 705–748.

Gordon G, Grant G (1982) Dorsolateral spinal afferents to some medullary sensory nuclei: an anatomical study in the cat. Exp Brain Res 46: 12–23.

Haeberle H, Fujiwara M, Chuang J, Medina MM, Panditrao MV, Bechstedt S, Howard J, Lumpkin EA (2004) Molecular profiling reveals synaptic release machinery in Merkel cells. Neuroscience 101: 14503–14508.

Halata Z (1975) The mechanoreceptors of the mammalian skin: ultrastructure and morphological classification. Adv Anat Embryol Cell Biol 50: 1–77.

Hamann W (1995) Mammalian cutaneous mechanoreceptors. Prog Biophys Mol Biol 64: 81–104.

Harper AA, Lawson SN (1985) Conduction velocity is related to morphological cell type in rat dorsal root ganglion neurons. J Physiol 359: 31–46.

Hartschuh W, Weihe E (1980) Fine structural analysis of the synaptic junction of Merkel cell-axon complexes. J Invest Dermatol 75: 159–165.

Head H, Holmes G (1911) Sensory disturbances from cerebral lesions. Brain 34: 102–254.

Hitchcock IS, Genever PG, Cahusac PM (2004) Essential components for a glutamatergic synapse between Merkel cell and nerve terminal in rats. Neurosci Lett 362: 196–199.

Hollins M, Faldowski R, Rao S, Young F (1993) Perceptual dimensions of tactile surface texture: a multidimensional-scaling analysis. Percept Psychophysiol 54: 697–705.

Hsiao, S., K. Johnson, and T. Yoshioka (2002) Processing of tactile information in the primate brain. In: *Handbook of Psychology, Vol. 3, Biological Psychology*, M. Gallagher and R.J. Nelson, eds., pp. 211–236. New York: Wiley.

Hsiao S (2008) Central mechanisms of tactile shape perception. Curr Opin Neurobiol 18: 418–424.

Hulliger M, Nordh E, Thelin AE, Vallbo AB (1979) The responses of afferent fibers from the glabrous skin of the hand during voluntary finger movements in man. J Physiol (Lond) 291: 233–249.

Hyvarinen J, Poranen A (1978) Movement-sensitive and direction and orientation-selective cutaneous receptive fields in the hand area of the post-central gyrus in monkeys. J. Physiol (Lond) 283: 523–527.

Hunt CC (1961) On the nature of vibration receptors in the hind limb of the cat. J Physiol (Lond) 155: 175–186.

Ide C (1988) The development of the Meissner corpuscle of mouse toe pad. Anat Rec 188: 49–67.

Iggo A, Andres KH (1982) Morphology of cutaneous receptors. Ann Rev Neurosci 5: 1–31.

Iwamura Y, Tanaka M, Sakamoto M, Hikosaka O (1985) Vertical neuronal arrays in the postcentral gyrus signaling active touch: a receptive field study in the conscious monkey. Exp Brain Res 58: 412–420.

Iwamura Y, Tanaka M, Sakamoto M, Hikosaka O (1993) Rostrocaudal gradients in the neuronal receptive field complexity in the finger region of the alert monkey's postcentral gyrus. Exp Brain Res 92: 360–368.

Jenmalm P, Birznieks I, Goodwin AW, Johansson RS (2003) Influence of object shape on responses of human tactile afferents under conditions characteristic of manipulation. Eur J Neurosci 18: 164–176.

Johannson RS, Vallbo AB (1979) Tactile sensibility in the human hand: relative and absolute densities of four types of mechanoreceptive units in glabrous skin. J Physiol (Lond) 286: 283–300.

Johansson RS, Vallbo AB (1980) Spatial properties of the population of mechanoreceptive units in the glabrous skin of the human hand. Brain Res 184: 353–366.

Johansson RS, Westling G (1987) Signals in tactile afferents from the fingers eliciting adaptive motor responses during precision grip. Exp Brain Res 66: 141–154.

Johnson K (2004) Closing in on the neural mechanisms of finger joint angle sense. Focus on "Quantitative analysis of dynamic strain sensitivity in human skin mechanoreceptors." J Neurophysiol 92: 3167–3168.

Johnson KO, Lamb GD (1981) Neural mechanisms of spatial tactile discrimination: neural patterns evoked by Braille-like dot patterns in the monkey. J Physiol (Lond) 310: 117–144.

Johnson, K.O., R.W. VanBoven, and S.S. Hsiao (1994) The perception of two points is not the spatial resolution threshold. In: Progress in Pain Research and Management, J. Boivie, P. Hansson and U. Lindblom, eds., pp. 389–404, Seattle: ISAP Press.

Johnson KO, Yoshioka T, Vega-Bermudez F (2000) Tactile functions of mechanoreceptive afferents innervating the hand. J Clin Neurophys 17: 539–558.

Johnson KO (2001) The roles and functions of cutaneous mechanoreceptors. Curr Opin Neurobiol 11: 455–461.

Jones EG, Porter R (1980) What is area 3a? Brain Res Rev 2: 1–43.

Jones EG, Friedman DP, Hendry SH (1982) Thalamic basis of place- and modality-specific columns in monkey somatosensory cortex: A correlative anatomical and physiological study. J Neurophysiol 48: 545–568.

Jones, E.G. (1986) Connectivity of the primate sensory-motor cortex. In: Cerebral Cortex, 5th Edition, E.G. Jones and A. Peters, eds., pp. 113–184. New York: Plenum Press.

Kaas, J.H., R.J. Nelson, M. Sur, and M.M. Merzenich (1981) Organization of somatosensory cortex in primates. In: The Organization of the Cerebral Cortex: Proceedings of a Neurosciences Research Program Colloquium, F.O. Schmitt, F.G. Worden, G. Adelman and S.G. Dennis, eds., pp. 237–261, Cambridge, MA: MIT Press.

Kaas JH, Nelson RJ, Sur M, Lin C-S, Merzenich MM (1979) Multiple representations of the body within the primary somatosensory cortex of primates. Science 204: 521–523.

Kausz M, Rethelyi M (1985) Lamellar arrangement of neuronal somata in the dorsal root ganglion of the cat. Somatosens Res 2(3): 193–204.

Kinkelin I, Stuckey CL, Koltzenburg M (1999) Postnatal loss of Merkel cells, but not of slowly adapting mechanoreceptors in mice lacking the neurotrophin receptor p75. Eur J Neurosci 11: 3963–3969.

Knibestol M (1973) Stimulus-response functions of rapidly adapting mechanoreceptors in the human glabrous skin area. J Physiol 232: 427–452.

Knibestol M (1975) Stimulus-response functions of slowly adapting mechanoreceptors in the human glabrous skin area. J Physiol 245: 63–80.

Krimm RF, Davis BM, Woodbury J, Albers K (2004) NT3 expressed in skin causes enhancement of SA1 sensory neurons that leads to postnatal enhancement of Merkel cells. J Comp Neurol 471: 352–360.

LaMotte RH, Whitehouse JM (1986) Tactile detection of a dot on a smooth surface: peripheral neural events. J Neurophysiol 56: 1109–1128.

Lawson, S. (2005) The peripheral sensory nervous system: Dorsal root ganglion neurons. In: Peripheral Neuropathy, Vol. 4, P.J. Dyck and P.K. Thomas, eds., pp. 163–202, Philadelphia: Elsevier/Saunders.

Lawson SN (1979) The postnatal development of large light and small dark neurons in the mouse dorsal root ganglion: A statistical analysis of cell numbers and size. J Neurocytol 8: 275–294.

Lawson, S.N. (1992) Morphological and biochemical cell types of sensory neurons. In: Sensory Neurons: Diversity, Development, and Plasticity, S.A. Scott, ed., pp. 27–59, New York: Oxford.

LeMaster AM, Krimm RF, Davis BM, Noel T, Forbes ME, Johnson JE, Albers KM (1999) Overexpression of brain-derived neurotrophic factor enhances sensory innervation and selectively increases neuron number. J Neurosci 19: 5919–5931.

Lieberman, A.R. (1976) Sensory ganglia. In: The Peripheral Nerve, D.N. Landon, ed., pp. 188–278, London: Chapman & Hall.

Lowenstein WR, Skalak R (1966) Mechanical transmission in a Pacinian corpuscle: an analysis and a theory. J Physiol (Lond) 182: 346–378.

Lucarz A, Brand G (2007) Current considerations about Merkel cells. Eur J Cell Biol 86: 243–251.

Lundborg G (2000) Brain plasticity and hand surgery: an overview. J Hand Surg [BrEur] 25B: 242–252.

Macefield VG, Hager-Ross C, Johansson RS (1996) Control of grip force during restraint of an object held between finger and thumb: responses of cutaneous afferents from the digits. Exp Brain Res 108: 155–171.

MacLennan AJ, Vinson EN, Marks L, McLaurin DL, Pfeifer M, Lee N (1996) Immunohistochemical localization of ciliary neurotrophic factor receptor alpha expression in the rat nervous system. J Neurosci 15: 621–630.

Margolis RU, Margolis RK (1997) Chondroitin sulfate proteoglycans as mediators of axon growth and pathfinding. Cell Tissue Res 290: 343–348.

Matthews PB (1982) Where does Sherrington's "muscular sense" originate? Muscles, joints, corollary discharges? Ann Rev Neurosci 5: 189–218.

McGlonne F, Kelly EF, Trulsson M, Francis ST, Westling G, Bowtell R (2002) Functional neuroimaging studies of human somatosensory cortex. Behav Brain Res 135: 147–158.

McIlwrath SL, Lawson JJ, Anderson CE, Albers KM, Koerber HR (2007) Overexpression of neurotrophin-3 enhances the mechanical response properties of slowly adapting type 1 afferents and myelinated nociceptors. Eur J Neurosci 26: 1801–1812.

Melzack R, Wall PD (1965) Pain mechanisms: a new theory. Science 150: 971–979.

Melzack R (1975) Prolonged relief of pain by brief transcutaneous somatic stimulation. Pain 1:357–373.

Merkel F (1875) Tastzellen und Tastkorperchen bei den Hausthieren und beim Menschen. Arch Mikrosk Anat 11: 636–652.

Moore CI, Stern CE, Corkin S, Fischl B, Gray AC, Rosen BR, Dale AM (2000) Segregation of somatosensory activation in the human rolandic cortex using fMRI. J Neurophysiol 84: 558–569.

Mountcastle VB, Henneman E (1952) The representation of tactile sensibility in the thalamus of the monkey. J Comp Neurol 97: 409.

Mountcastle VB, Powell TP (1959) Neural mechanisms subserving cutaneous sensibility, with special reference to the role of afferent inhibition in sensory perception and discrimination. Bull Johns Hopkins Hosp 105: 201–232.

Mountcastle, V.B., W.H. Talbot, and H.H. Kornhuber (1966) Touch, Heat, Pain, and Itch, London: Churchill.

Mountcastle VB (1975) The view from within: pathways to the study of perception. Johns Hopkins Med Jnl 136: 109–131.

Mountcastle, V.B. (1984) Central nervous system mechanisms in mechanoreceptive sensibility. In: Handbook of Physiology, S.R. Geiger, I. Darian-Smith, J.M. Brookhart and V.B. Mountcastle, eds., pp. 789–878, Baltimore: Waverly.

Mountcastle VB (1997) The columnar organization of the neocortex. Brain 120: 701–722.

Mountcastle, V.B. (2006a) The Sensory Hand. Chap. 1, pp. 1–26. Perception and the World of Somesthesis. Cambridge, MA: Harvard University Press.

Ibid (2006b) Chap. 6, pp. 136–165. Dorsal Systems and the Dorsal Column Nuclear Complex.

Ibid (2006c) Chap. 9, pp. 214–259. Dual Functions of the Dorsal Thalamus.

Ibid (2006d) Chap. 10, pp. 260–300. Postcentral Somatic Sensory Cortical Areas in Primates.

Ibid (2006e) Chap. 11, pp. 301–340. Parietal Lateral System and Somatic Sensibility.

Mu X, Silos-Santiago I, Carroll SL, Snider W (1993) Neurotrophin receptor genes are expressed in distinct patterns in developing dorsal root ganglia. J Neurosci 13: 4029–4041.

Munger BL, Ide C (1988) The structure and function of cutaneous sensory receptors. Arch Histol Cytol 51: 1–34.

Murphy PG, Borthwick LA, Altares M, Gauldie J, Kaplan D, Richardson PM (2000) Reciprocal actions of interleukin-6 and brain-derived neurotrophic factor on rat and mouse primary sensory neurons. Eur J Neurosci 12: 1891–1899.

Nava PB (1974) The development and fine structure of Pacinian corpuscles. Anat Rec 178: 424P–425P.

Nelson RJ, Sur M, Felleman DJ, Kaas JH (1980) Representations of the body surface in postcentral parietal cortex of Macaca fascicularis. J Comp Neurol 192: 611–643.

Nelson RJ (1996) Interactions between motor commands and somatic perception in sensorimotor cortex. Curr Opin Neurobiol 6: 801–810.

Ochoa J, Torebjork E (1983) Sensations evoked by intraneural microstimulation of single mechanoreceptor units innervating the human hand. J Physiol Lond 342: 633–654.

Olausson H, Wessberg J, Kakuda N (2000) Tactile directional sensibility: peripheral neural mechanisms in man. Brain Res 866: 178–187.

Paré M, Smith AM, Rice FL (2002) Distribution and terminal arborizations of cutaneous mechanoreceptors in the glabrous finger pads of the monkey. J Comp Neurol 445: 347–359.

Paré M, Behets C, Cornu O (2003) Paucity of presumptive Ruffini corpuscles in the index finger pad of humans. J Comp Neurol 456: 260–266.

Paré M, Elde R, Mazurkiewicz JE, Smith AM, Rice FL (2001) The Meissner corpuscle revised: a multiafferented mechanoreceptor with nociceptor immunochemical properties. J Neurosci 21: 7236–7246.

Paul RL, Merzenich MM, Goodman H (1972) Representation of slowly and rapidly adapting cutaneous mechanoreceptors of the hand in Brodmann's areas 3 and 1 of Macaca mulatta. Brain Res 36: 229–249.

Pease DC, Quilliam TA (1957) Electron microscopy of the Pacinian corpuscle. J Biophys Biochem Cytol 3: 331–342.

Penfield, W. and H.H. Jasper (1954) *Epilepsy and the Functional Anatomy of the Human Brain*, Boston: Little Brown.

Perez-Pinera P, Garcia-Suarez O, Germana A, Diaz-Esnal B, de Carlos F, Silos-Santiago I, del Valle ME, Cobo J, Vega JA (2008) Characterization of sensory deficits in TrkB knockout mice Neurosci Lett 433(1): 43–47.

Peyronnard J-M, Messier J-P, Dubreuil M, Charron L, Lebel F (1990) Three-dimensional computer-aided analysis of the intraganglionic topography of primary muscle afferent neurons in the rat. Anat Rec 227: 405–417.

Phillips CG, Powell TP, Wiesendanger M (1971) Projection from low-threshold muscle afferents of hand and forearm to area 3a of baboon's cortex. J Physiol Lond 217: 419–446.

Phillips JR, Johnson KO (1981) Tactile spatial resolution II. Neural representation of bars, edges, and gratings in monkey primary afferents. J Neurophysiol 46: 1192–1203.

Phillips JR, Johansson RS, Johnson KO (1990) Representation of Braille characters in human nerve fibers. Exp Brain Res 81: 589–592.

Pons TP, Garraghty PE, Mishkin M (1992) Serial and parallel processing of tactual information in somatosensory cortex of rhesus monkeys. J Neurophysiol 68(2): 518–527.

Powell TP, Mountcastle VB (1959a) Some aspects of the functional organization of the cortex of the postcentral gyrus of the monkey. Bull Johns Hopkins Hosp 105: 133–162.

Powell TP, Mountcastle VB (1959b) The cytoarchitecture of the post-central gyrus of the monkey Macaca mulatta. Bull Johns Hopkins Hosp 105: 108–131.

Quilliam, T.A. (1978) The structure of finger print skin. In: *Active Touch*, G. Gordon, ed., pp. 1–18, Oxford: Pergamon Press.

Rakic P (1995) Radial versus tangential migration of neuronal clones in the developing cerebral cortex (comments). PNAS 92: 11323–11327.

Robertson B, Perry MJ, Lawson SN (1991) Populations of rat spinal primary afferent neurons with choleragenoid binding compared with those labelled by markers for neurofilament and carbohydrate groups: a quantitative immunocytochemical study. J Neurocytol 20: 387–395.

Ruffini A (1894) Sur un nouvel organe nerveux terminal et sur la présence des corpuscules Golgi-Mazzoni dans le conjonctif sous-cutané de la pulpe des doigts de l'homme. Arch Ital Biol 21: 249–265.

Sedy J, Szeder V, Walro JM, Ren ZG, Nanka O, Tessarollo L, Sieber-Blum M, Grim M, Kucera J (2004) Pacinian corpuscle development involves multiple Trk signaling pathways. Dev Dynamics 231: 551–563.

Smith KR (1970) The ultrastructure of human "Haarscheibe" and Merkel cell. J Invest Dermatol 54: 150–159.

Spencer PS, Schaumburg HH (1973) An ultrastructural study of the inner core of the Pacinian corpuscle. J Neurocytol 2: 217–235.

Srinivasan MA, Dandekar K (1996) An investigation of the mechanics of tactile sense using two-dimensional models of the primate fingertip. J Biomed Eng 118: 48–55.

Stevens SS (1961) To honor Fechner and repeal his law Science 133:80–86.

Sur M (1980) Receptive fields of neurons in areas 3b and 1 of somatosensory cortex in monkeys. Brain Res 198: 465–471.

Sur M, Merzenich MM, Kaas JH (1980) Magnification, receptive-field area, and "hypercolumn" size in areas 3b and 1 of somatosensory cortex in owl monkeys. J Neurophysiol 44: 295–311.

Sur M, Wall JT, Kaas JH (1984) Modular distribution of neurons with slowly adapting and rapidly adapting responses in area 3b of somatosensory cortex in monkeys. J Neurophysiol 51: 724–744.

Tachibana T (1995) The Merkel cell: recent findings and unresolved problems. Arch Histol Cytol 58: 379–396.

Tachibana T, Nawa T (2002) Recent progress in studies on Merkel cell biology. Anat Sci Intl 77: 26–33.

Tachibana T, Endoh M, Fujiwara N, Nawa T (2005) Receptors and transporter for serotonin in Merkel cell-nerve endings in the rat sinus hair follicle: an immunohistochemical study. Arch Histol Cytol 68: 19–28.

Takahashi-Iwanaga H, Shimoda H (2003) The three-dimensional microanatomy of Meissner corpuscles in monkey palmar skin. J Neurocytol 32: 363–371.

Johansson RS, Vallbo AB (1983) Tactile sensory coding in the glabrous skin of the human hand. TINS. 6: 27–35.

Vega-Bermudez F, Johnson KO, Hsiao SS (1991) Human tactile pattern recognition: active versus passive touch, velocity effects, and patterns of confusion. J Neurophysiol 65: 531–546.

Vega-Bermudez F, Johnson KO (1999a) SAI and RA receptive fields, response variability, and population responses mapped with a probe array. J Neurophysiol 81: 2701–2710.

Vega-Bermudez F, Johnson KO (1999b) Surround suppression in the responses of primate SA-I and RA mechanoreceptive afferents mapped with a probe array. J Neurophysiol 81: 2711–2719.

Vogt O, Vogt C (1919) Allgemeine Ergebnisse unserer hirnforschung. J Psych Neuro 25: 273–462.

Wagner R, Meissner G (1852) Über das Vorhandensein bisher unbekannter eigentümlicher Tastkörperchen (corpuscula tacus) in den Gefühlswärzchen der menschlichen Haut und über die Endausbreitung sensitiver Nerven. Unikonigl Ges Wiss Gottingen 2: 17–30.

Wang GY, Scott SA (2002) Development of "normal" dermatomes and somatotopic maps by "abnormal" populations of cutaneous neurons. Dev Biol 251: 424–433.

Weber, E.H. (1846) Handworterbuch der Physiologie, Braunschweig: Vieweg.

Wessels WJT, Feirabend HKP, Marani E (1994) The rostrocaudal organization in the dorsal root ganglia of the rat: a consequence of plexus formation? Anat Embryol (Berl) 190: 1–11.

Wheat HE, Goodwin AW, Browning AS (1995) Tactile resolution: peripheral neural mechanisms underlying the human capacity to determine positions of objects contacting the fingerpad. J Neurosci 15: 5582–5595.

Whitsel BL, Roppolo JR, Werner G (1972) Cortical information processing of motion on primate skin. J Neurophysiol 35: 691–717.

Willis WD, Zhang X, Honda CN, Geisler GJ Jr. (2001) Projections from the marginal zone and deep dorsal horn to the ventrobasal nuclei of the primate thalamus. Pain 92: 267–276.

Willis, W.D. and R.E. Coggeshall (2004a) Dorsal root ganglion cells and their processes. In: Sensory Mechanisms of the Spinal Cord, Ed 3, pp. 103–154, New York: Kluwer/Plenum.

Willis, W.D. and R.E. Coggeshall (2004b) Sensory receptors and peripheral nerves. In: Sensory Mechanisms of the Spinal Cord, pp 19–101, New York: Kluwer/Plenum.

Woolsey CN, Marshall WH, Bard P (1942) Representation of cutaneous tactile sensibility in the cerebral cortex of the monkey as indicated by evoked potentials. Bull Johns Hopkins Hosp 70: 399–441.

Yamashita Y, Akaita N, Wakamori W, Ikeda Z, Ogawa H. (1992) Voltage dependent currents in isolated single Merkel cells in rats. J Physiol Lond 450: 143–162.

Yoshida S, Matsuda Y (1979) Studies on sensory neurons of the mouse with intracellular recording and horseradish peroxidase injection techniques. J Neurophysiol 42: 1134–1146.

Zhou X-F, Cameron D, Rush RA (1998) Endogenous neurotrophin-3 supports the survival of a subpopulation of sensory neurons in neonatal rat. Neuroscience 86: 1155–1164.

3

MOTION

THE SARCOMERE, the basic structural unit of muscle, is powered by the interaction of overlapping myosin and actin filaments. Muscle contraction is initiated at the motor endplate, where acetylcholine released from axon terminals interacts with receptors on the muscle surface. Specialization of muscle fibers has resulted in a spectrum of fiber types. These may be ordered on a physiologic continuum from the fastest, most glycolytic, type IIb, to the slowest, most oxidative, type I. Muscle activity is monitored by proprioceptors; the Golgi tendon organ responds to stretch, while the muscle spindle signals muscle length. The motor unit, the elemental circuit of motor control, consists of a motoneuron and the muscle fibers it serves. Motor units are classified as fast-twitch, fatigable (FF), fast-twitch, intermediate (Fint), fast-twitch, fatigue-resistant (FR), and slow (S). Motor unit size is proportional to the speed with which its fibers contract, with type S units the smallest and type FF the largest. During a progressively forceful muscle contraction, motor units are recruited according to their size, beginning with small type S units and ending with large type FF units. Motoneurons serving individual muscles are grouped together within pools in the anterior horn of the spinal cord. Regulation of motor function is a complex process involving a hierarchical system of controls centered in spinal cord, brainstem, and cortex, each with afferent input and output to the motoneuron pool. Of potential interest in the context of regeneration are the patterns of direct input to the motoneuron through Ia afferents, cortico-motoneuronal neurons, Ia inhibitory interneurons, and Ib interneurons.

THE SARCOMERE

The sarcomere is the structural and functional unit of muscle (Figure 3-1). Sarcomeres vary in length between 1.5 and 3.5 μm, depending on their state of contraction. Several thousand sarcomeres are attached in series to form a myofibril; hundreds or thousands of myofibrils are linked in parallel to form a multinucleate muscle cell. The sarcomere consists

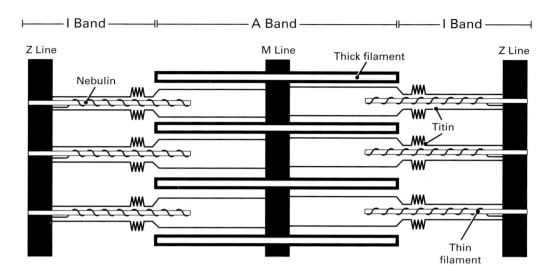

FIGURE 3-1   Diagram of the sarcomere. Myosin thick filaments are anchored to the M line, and actin thin filaments are anchored to the Z line. They interdigitate in an arrangement organized by the giant molecule titin. Nebulin spans the length of the thin filament, controlling its dimensions. The interaction of myosin and actin draws the thick and thin filaments into greater overlap, resulting in muscle contraction.

primarily of interdigitating thick myosin filaments and thin actin filaments that slide past one another to produce muscle contraction (Huxley and Hanson, 1954). The activation of these contractile proteins is modulated by the regulatory proteins troponin and tropomyosin, and their three-dimensional structure is maintained by structural proteins.

The myosin molecule is a protein hexamer with two "heads" that enzymatically hydrolyze ATP, and a long structural "tail." Its shape resembles that of a golf club with two adjacent heads at one end. The thick filament of the sarcomere is assembled from several hundred myosin molecules, arranged in a longitudinal bundle with tails parallel and partially overlapping, and heads protruding outward from the bundle at regular intervals (Hudson et al., 1997). This configuration is stabilized by myosin binding proteins, the most prevalent of which is C protein (Squire et al., 2003). Thick filaments of myosin are anchored at one end to the M line (it appears as a line when the sarcomere is cut longitudinally as in Figure 3-1, but is actually a plate that defines the circumference of the myofibril when seen end-on) and arrayed in parallel at regular intervals, like the bristles protruding from a brush. The M line contains a lattice of M protein and myomesin that anchors myosin filaments, and creatine kinase that

recharges ADP to power the sarcomere (Wallimann, Eppenberger, 1985; Furst et al., 1999).

Thin filaments consist largely of actin, a globular protein that aggregates to form a longitudinally oriented helical polymer, F-actin (Sheterline et al., 1995). The F-actin filament is decorated at regular intervals with the regulatory proteins tropomyosin and troponin, and is accompanied throughout its length by the giant protein nebulin, which is thought to limit overall filament length (Horowits et al., 1996; Gordon et al., 2000). Just as thick filaments are anchored in the M line at the center of the sarcomere, thin filaments are anchored in the Z lines at the ends of the sarcomere (Yamaguchi et al., 1985). In effect, two brush-like structures are stacked together with their respective thick and thin filaments overlapping, aligned parallel to one another in a regular double hexagonal array. The giant protein titin bridges thick and thin filaments, running from Z line to M line (Labeit, Kolmerer, 1995). During development titin serves as a blueprint for sarcomere assembly; in the adult, it maintains filament order and its elastic components provide the resting tension of the muscle.

Muscle contraction is produced by a change in configuration of the myosin head (reviewed in Craig, Padron, 2004). At rest, the head is in a "cocked" position, is bound to ADP, and is prevented from interacting with actin by troponin-tropomyosin complexes that cover binding sites on the thin actin filaments. Muscle contraction is initiated by release of calcium, which binds to tropomyosin, changing its configuration and exposing binding sites on actin that now attach to myosin. The myosin head then changes configuration, advancing the thin filament and drawing the M and Z lines closer together by increasing the overlap between thick and thin filaments. At the completion of this cycle the myosin-bound ADP is replaced by ATP, which is dephosphorylated to provide the energy for "recocking" the myosin head.

MUSCLE FIBER TYPES

The human central nervous system, with its complex circuits for the gathering and analysis of sensory input, can interact with the world in only one way: by contracting muscle. As a result, muscle has been adapted to perform a wide variety of functions. It has responded to diverse job requirements by developing specialized muscle fiber types, several of which may be present in a single muscle. Fiber types may be distinguished by their ATPase activity (Barany, 1967), their particular isoforms of contractile and regulatory proteins such as the myosin heavy chain (MyHC) (Arndt, Pepe, 1975) or troponin (TnT) (Lees-Miller, Helfman, 1991), or by their physiologic properties (Burke et al. 1973) (Figures 3-2, 3-3).

Myosin ATPase activity determines the speed of muscle contraction. Brooke and Kaiser (1970),

building on earlier work by Guth and Samaha (1969), defined three fiber types based on ATPase staining: Type I, slow fibers, and Types IIa and IIb, fast fibers with differing responses depending on the pH (Figures 3-2, 3-3). Classification by ATPase activity is limited, however, as new myosin heavy chain isoforms have been identified that cannot be distinguished with this technique. For instance, type IIx (also called IId) fibers have ATPase activity similar to that of type IIb fibers (Schiaffino et al. 1989). At least 10 myosin heavy chains have been identified in adult extrafusal muscle fibers (Pette, Staron, 2000). Fiber types I, IIa, IIb, and IIx each contain a single MyHC isoform. Additionally, however, different isoforms may be combined to generate hybrid fiber types with intermediate properties, so that a continuum of function is present from Type I at one extreme to type IIb at the other. Sequential interconversion is possible through the series MHCIß<>MHCIIa<>MHCIId<> MHCIIb (Pette, Staron, 2000). This sequence can be driven in the fast-to-slow direction by increased neuronal activity, mechanical loading, or hypothyroidism, and in the reverse direction by reduced neuronal activity, mechanical unloading, or hyperthyroidism. These transitions are thought to relate to changes in the energy cost of force production (Bottinelli et al., 1994).

The troponin gene provides for even more variability than does the MyHC gene. Differential splicing can generate up to 64 fast troponin isoforms (Breibart, Nadal-Ginard, 1987) in addition to the slow isoforms.

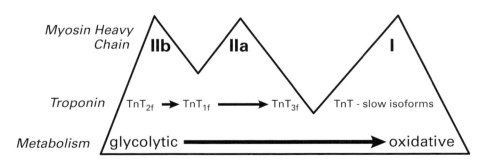

FIGURE 3-2   Three related properties of muscle fiber types. Fiber type is determined by the identity of the myosin heavy chain (MyHC), at the top of each pyramid, which is completely distinct from one fiber type to another. Type IIb is found in FF fibers, type IIa in FR fibers, and type I in S fibers. Correspondence of troponin (TnT) isoforms with MyHC types is less rigid, so that there is overlap between types IIb and IIa, but none with the slow isoforms in type I. Metabolic capabilities, at the base of the pyramid, span the continuum from glycolytic to oxidative, and are the characteristic least able to clearly differentiate one fiber class from another. From Rubinstein and Kelly, 2004, with permission.

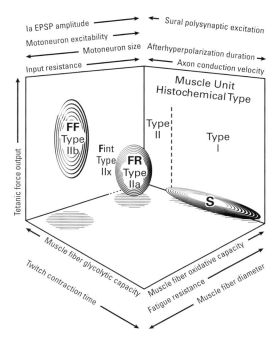

Ia EPSP amplitude ⟶   ⟵ Sural polysynaptic excitation

Motoneuron excitability ⟶

⟵ Motoneuron size   Afterhyperpolarization duration →

Input resistance ⟶   Axon conduction velocity →

Muscle Unit Histochemical Type

Type II

FF Type IIb

Fint Type IIx

FR Type IIa

Type I

S

Tetanic force output

Muscle fiber glycolytic capacity

Twitch contraction time

Muscle fiber oxidative capacity

Fatigue resistance

Muscle fiber diameter

FIGURE 3-3   The interrelationship of motor unit physiology and muscle fiber histochemistry. From Burke, 2006, with permission.

Specific combinations of troponin, tropomyosin, and actin isoforms often occur together in so-called *canonical programs* (Schachat et al. 1990) (Figure 3-2). These are identified by their troponin isoforms as 1f, 2f, and 3f. The 2f program is the most calcium-responsive, while the 3f program allows the most graded response to calcium (Rubinstein, Kelly, 2004). Expression of canonical programs may be correlated, in turn, with MyHC expression (Schmitt, Pette, 1990). TnT-2f is co-expressed with MyHCIIb, TnT-3f with MyHCIIa, and TnT-4f with MyHCIIx (Figure 3-2). There are myriad possible combinations of the protein isoforms expressed in muscle; that relatively few, predictable patterns are encountered suggests that the expression of muscle proteins is well coordinated.

THE MOTOR UNIT

Physiologic Classification

Sherrington introduced the term "motor unit" to emphasize that the motoneuron and the muscle fibers it serves are the irreducible unit of motor control (Liddell, Sherrington, 1925; Burke, 1999). When a motoneuron discharges an action potential, all the muscle fibers in the motor unit contract. Since

these all have the same properties (Burke at al. 1973), physiologic analysis has been performed on motor units rather than on individual muscle fibers.

Burke and coworkers (1973) characterized cat gastrocnemius motor units on the basis of their resistance to fatigue and their ability to maintain force output during low-frequency tetanic stimulation (Figure 3-3). They defined three distinct motor unit types: fast-twitch, fatigable (FF) units fatigued rapidly; fast-twitch, fatigue-resistant (FR) units were more resistant to fatigue; and slow (S) units were extremely resistant to fatigue. Subsequent investigations added a fourth category, fast-intermediate (Fint) (McDonagh et al. 1980), with properties intermediate between FF and FR. Smaller, distal muscles are less easily categorized because they present a continuum of physiologic properties (Appelberg, Emont-Denand, 1967; Gates et al. 1991). When motor unit types were analyzed in the context of myosin ATPase activity, it was found that FF motor units were type IIB, FR muscles were type IIA, and S units were type I (Burke et al. 1973; Dum, Kennedy, 1980a) (Figure 3-3).

Burke (2006) has summarized the more general physiologic properties of the various motor unit types (Figure 3-3). The type IIB fibers of FF motor units are characterized by high glycogen content, few mitochondria, low levels of oxidative enzymes and myoglobin, large fiber diameter, and few capillaries. They are thus specialized to run anaerobically for as long as their glycogen stores hold out. At the opposite extreme, type I fibers of S motor units are well supplied with mitochondria, oxidative enzymes, myoglobin, and capillaries, but store little glycogen. They continue to function as long as their circulation is maintained. Type IIA fibers of FR units contain both aerobic and anaerobic enzyme systems and store glycogen, and are thus equipped to contract rapidly but also to resist fatigue during longer periods of activation.

Distribution and Innervation Ratio

The distribution and size of motor units have been defined relatively well in animals. Much of the experimental evidence has been obtained by stimulating single motor axons to deplete muscle glycogen stores within the motor unit, then mapping the distribution of depleted muscle fibers. This approach has revealed that motor units are not dispersed throughout an entire muscle (Burke et al., 1973). In the cat tibialis anterior they may occupy from 8 to

22% of the muscle cross section, while in the soleus they are spread over 41–76% of the cross-sectional area (Bodine-Fowler et al., 1990). An individual motor unit overlaps with from 15 to 30 other motor units when viewed on muscle cross-section (Burke et al., 1973; Roy et al., 1995). On the longitudinal axis, muscle fibers, and as a consequence motor units, may not extend from one end of a muscle to the other (Ounjian et al., 1991). Some muscles are compartmentalized, with each compartment served by a different terminal nerve branch and capable of discrete function (English, Ledbetter, 1982; English, Weeks, 1987). Within these muscles, motor units are usually restricted to a single compartment (English, 1984).

The *innervation ratio*, the number of muscle fibers innervated by a single motoneuron, can be determined with reasonable precision using the glycogen depletion technique. It has been found to increase progressively in large limb muscles from the smallest motor units containing type S muscle, to larger units composed of type F muscle, to the largest units with type FF muscle (Bodine et al., 1987; Kanda, Hashizume, 1992; Totosy de Zepetnek et al., 1992). Representative innervation ratios for the tibialis anterior of the cat are 93 for type S motor units, 197 for type FR units, and 255 for type FF units (Bodine et al., 1987). The maximal force generated by a given motor unit is determined by several factors (summarized in Enoka, 1995). It can be calculated as the product of the number of muscle fibers in the motor unit (innervation ratio) and the force that can be generated by an individual fiber; this force, in turn, depends on the cross-sectional area of the muscle fiber and its force-generating capacity, or *specific force*. Of these variables, the innervation ratio has been found to have the most significant influence on motor unit force (Totosy de Zepetnek et al., 1992).

In humans, the mean innervation ratio has traditionally been calculated using estimates of the number of fibers in the muscle and the number of motor axons in a muscle nerve, approximately 60% of the large myelinated fiber population (Christensen, 1959; summarized in Enoka, 1995). This technique has produced innervation ratios ranging from 5 for the lateral rectus muscle of the eye to 595 for the opponens pollicis and 1,900 for the medial gastrocnemius. In general, smaller muscles have lower innervation ratios and are capable of more precise control of muscle force. More recently, a variety of electrophysiologic techniques for motor unit number estimation (MUNE) have been devised (Daube, 1995; Doherty et al., 1995). There is good correlation between morphologic and physiologic estimates for small muscles of the hand, but considerable variability in the estimates for limb muscles (Enoka, 1995). The relative ratios from muscle to muscle, however, appear to be more accurate.

Recruitment

Sherrington's discovery of the motor unit posed a new question for neurophysiologists: How are motor units recruited in an orderly fashion to produce smooth increments of force? Denny-Brown, a pupil of Sherrington's, observed that motor units were enlisted in a fairly reproducible order during voluntary movement, and that this order proceeded from small to large (Denny-Brown, 1929; Denny-Brown, Pennybacker, 1939). Henneman subsequently proposed that recruitment order was determined by motoneuron size, from smallest to largest (reviewed in Mendell, 2005). This robust predictor of recruitment order became known as the "size principle." Henneman initially considered input resistance to be the important physiological concomitant of size: smaller neurons with less surface area would have higher input resistance, and would respond to a given synaptic input with a greater voltage change than would a larger neuron (Mendell, 2005). Further research has indicated that there are actually several motoneuron properties that are size-related and may influence recruitment order (Munson, 1990; Heckman, Minder, 1993). As discussed below, recruitment will also be influenced by the relative intensity of various inputs to the motoneuron and the resting membrane potential.

Burke (2006) (Figure 3-3) has summarized the relationships among motor neuron and motor unit properties. Most strikingly, motoneuron size, like motor unit size, increases from small type S motoneurons through intermediate type FR to large type FF motoneurons (Burke et al., 1982), linking muscle fiber type to the size principle. Several physiological properties also correlate with motoneuron size and muscle fiber type. Input resistance, as noted by Sherrington, as well as motoneuron excitability, increase as motoneurons become smaller (Fleshman et al., 1981). The duration of afterhyperpolarization, the main factor limiting the firing rate of a motoneuron, is greater in type I (S) muscles than in type II (FR, FF) muscle, placing intrinsic limits on the firing rate of type S muscle (Powers, Binder, 2001).

Afferent input to motoneurons also varies by motor unit fiber type. Monosynaptic Ia input is strongest to type S muscle and weakest to type FF muscle (Burke et al., 1976b), consistent with the relative ease of activating type S muscle through the stretch reflex (Burke, 1968). Conversely, polysynaptic inputs from cutaneous withdrawal reflexes are strongest to fast, type II motoneurons (Burke et al., 1970).

Further exploration of the size principle revealed that motor unit force is perhaps the best predictor of recruitment order (Zajac, Fadden, 1985), and can vary by up to 100-fold in a given muscle (Burke, 1981). Recruitment begins with type S units, proceeds to type FR, and only includes FF when high force is required (Walmsey et al., 1978) (Figure 3-4). The first motor units recruited generate the least force; when half the motoneurons serving the cat peroneus longus are firing, the muscle is only at 10% of maximum output (Kernell et al., 1983). As a consequence, fine gradations of relatively weak force can be produced. This force is being generated by oxidative type S muscle, so it can be sustained for long periods. At the opposite extreme, recruiting FF units adds larger increments of force that cannot be sustained. Although this sequence applies to the majority of situations, there are special circumstances in which large motor units may be brought into play earlier than normal (Enoka, 1995).

Firing Rate

The force developed by a muscle depends not only on the identity of the motor units firing, but also on the frequency of their discharge. In the small muscles of the hand, voluntary recruitment of all motor units results in only 50% of maximum force generation; the remaining force is produced by increasing the firing rate of motor units that have already been recruited (Milner-Brown et al., 1973a). Human motor units fire in two fundamentally different patterns; one to produce force that is constant or changing slowly, and the other to generate explosive bursts of strength (Burke, 2006). To exert low forces, motoneurons begin firing at 5–10 Hz (Hertz, or contractions per second), and respond to incremental demands by raising their firing rate to a maximum of 20–40 Hz (Enoka, Fuglevand, 2001). In some human distal extremity muscles, fast and slow motor units have similar minimum and maximum firing rates (Milner-Brown et al., 1973b; Monster, Chan, 1977), but this is not always the case (DeLuca et al., 1996). Instantaneous production of high forces, in contrast,

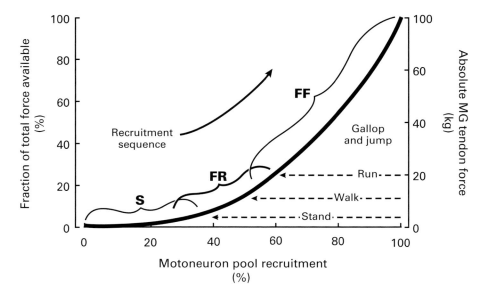

FIGURE 3-4   Hypothetical graph of force generation during cat locomotion, assuming that motor units are recruited on the basis of their force output. The relationship is not linear, with small increments from addition of type S units, slightly larger increments from addition of type FR units, and substantial increments from addition of type FF units. As force increments increase with addition of progressively larger motor units the potential for fine control of force gradation decreases. From Burke, 2006, with permission.

begins with a brief period of contraction at 50–60 Hz, followed by a rapid decline in discharge frequency (Desmedt, Godaux, 1977). When muscle is activated repetitively, force production does not increase as a linear function of firing rate (Burke et al., 1976a; discussed in Burke, 2006). For instance, when activating an FR motor unit in the cat, advancing the second pulse from 65 ms to 10 ms after the initial pulse will double force production. This "doublet" effect also occurs in humans (Thomas et al., 1999), where it may serve to diminish the consequences of fatigue (Bigland-Ritchie et al., 2000). During repeated activation, force generation is most efficient when the interval between stimuli approximates the twitch contraction time (Burke et al., 1976a).

MOTONEURON-MUSCLE INTERACTIONS

As suggested by the above discussion, the properties of muscle and motoneuron are shaped by an ongoing dialogue. Motoneurons were initially thought to determine the properties of developing muscle, potentially through their firing pattern (Hennig, Lomo, 1985; Vrbova et al., 1985). Several lines of evidence indicate, however, that fiber types may be determined without innervation, or even with incorrect innervation (summarized in Rubinstein, Kelly, 2004). Motoneuron control of muscle properties is more straightforward in the adult. Cross-reinnervation of predominantly fast and slow muscles provokes variable degrees of muscle plasticity, so that muscles are more closely matched to their reinnervating neurons (Buller et al., 1960). The details of this conversion will be discussed in the context of muscle reinnervation after nerve repair (Chapter 11). Modification of neuronal firing rates with electrical stimulation can also transform muscle type, both from fast to slow (Pette, Vrbova, 1999) and from slow to fast (Vrbova, 1963), clearly implicating motoneuronal activity as a determinant of MyHC gene expression. The motoneuron, in turn, is subject to modification in response to input from muscle. Blockade of transmission in the cat soleus nerve with tetrodotoxin (TTX) is normally accompanied by a decrease in the duration of motoneuron afterhyperpolarization, an alteration that can be prevented by stimulating muscle contraction distal to the cuff (Czeh et al., 1977). Similarly, changes in muscle properties are accompanied by synaptic changes on the innervating motoneurons (Mendell, Munson, 1999). Retrograde

signaling from muscle to motoneuron depends on acetylcholine receptor activation for its normal operation (Nakanishi et al., 2005), and may involve the transport of NT-4 (Funakoshi et al., 1995). Motoneuron and muscle are thus truly interdependent, each undergoing modifications in response to signals from the other.

THE MOTONEURON POOL

Sherrington (1892) discovered that motoneurons serving a given muscle are grouped together in the anterior horn of the spinal cord. The first extensive maps of human motoneuron "pools" were made by correlating motoneuron loss in the spinal cords of patients who had been stricken by poliomyelitis with the distribution of their muscle atrophy (Sharrard, 1955). Similar information was obtained experimentally by injuring muscle nerves, then mapping the distribution of chromatolytic motoneurons (Goering, 1928; Romanes, 1951). It became clear that motoneurons serving axial muscles were placed medially, while those to the extremities were more lateral. The lateral extremity group could be subdivided further into a medial flexor group and a lateral extensor group (Figure 3-5). Overall, however, the topography of motoneuron pools was difficult to map onto that of the muscles they served.

The use of retrograde motoneuron labeling with HRP to study the neurons within a pool (Burke et al., 1977) and the topographic relationship of flexor and extensor motoneurons (Brushart, Mesulam, 1980) introduced a new level of precision to spinal cord mapping. Motoneuron organization was investigated in a variety of species (e.g., Fritz et al., 1986a; Fritz et al., 1986b; Swett et al., 1991), and it was found that a muscle's embryonic origin, rather than its position in the mature animal, correlated best with the location of its motoneuron pool (Gutman et al., 1993). Motoneuron pools serving individual compartments of compartmentalized muscles were found to overlap extensively, yet maintain characteristic topography and neuron size distributions (Weeks, English, 1985). The clear definition of motoneuron pools has served as a basis for the study of connections formed by regenerating peripheral nerves (Brushart, Mesulam, 1980), has guided numerous physiological experiments, and will become increasingly important to the surgeon as techniques of direct reinnervation from the spinal cord are developed (Carlstedt et al., 2000).

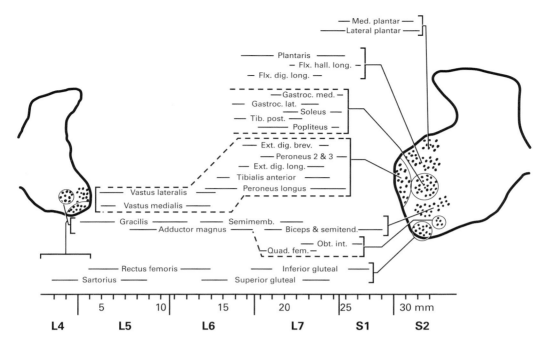

FIGURE 3-5 The longitudinal extent and topographic arrangement of motoneuron pools in the cat. Individual muscle nerves were crushed repeatedly, causing chromatolytic changes in the parent motoneurons. The distribution of these chromatolytic motoneurons was then mapped on spinal cord cross sections. From Romanes, 1951, with permission.

THE MOTOR ENDPLATE

The motor endplate converts the electrical activity of the axon into muscle contraction. It has three cellular components: the axon terminal, the muscle fiber, and the perisynaptic Schwann cell. The accessibility and relatively large size of the motor endplate made it the primary model for the study of synaptic transmission for many years. The vast literature that resulted from these efforts has been summarized recently in reviews that serve as the basis for this brief summary (Vincent, 2001; Kandel, Siegelbaum, 2000; Engel, 2004).

The axon terminal occupies a shallow depression in the muscle fiber (Figure 3-6). It contains numerous clear synaptic vesicles that are 50–60 nm in diameter and are concentrated near the presynaptic membrane. These vesicles package the neurotransmitter acetylcholine (ACh) (Whittaker, 1984). The cytoplasm also contains giant synaptic vesicles, thought to arise from fusion of smaller vesicles, coated vesicles that participate in endocytosis, and dense core vesicles that contain calcitonin gene-related peptide (CGRP)

and other neuroactive substances (Hall and Sanes, 1993). The presynaptic membrane is studded with active zones, areas rich in voltage-gated calcium channels that are positioned opposite clefts in the postsynaptic membrane. The active zones are the focus of a cytoskeletal framework that anchors synaptic vesicles through synapsin-I and draws them to the presynaptic membrane for release using kinesin motors (reviewed in Vincent, 2001).

The pre- and postsynaptic membranes are separated by a layer of specialized basal lamina (Patton, 2003) that contains acetylcholinesterase (AChE) (Rotundo, 2003), a unique form of laminin with ß2 subunits (originally called s-laminin), agrin, type IV collagen, entactin, neuregulin, and perlecan. It is folded into the synaptic clefts, and is continuous with the basal lamina of both muscle and perisynaptic Schwann cell. The postsynaptic membrane includes the primary synaptic cleft, the space where the pre- and postsynaptic membranes directly oppose one another, and the secondary synaptic cleft, or synaptic fold, an invagination of the postsynaptic membrane into the muscle surface. The primary synaptic

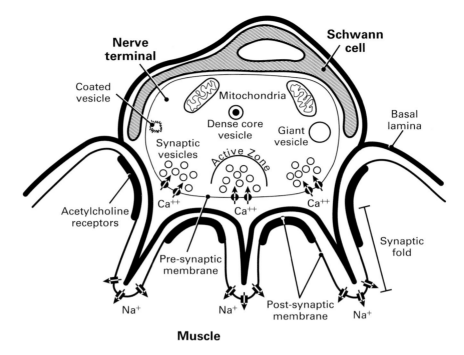

FIGURE 3-6 Diagram of the motor end plate. In addition to the labeled components, acetylcholinesterase is concentrated in the basal lamina of the synaptic cleft.

cleft is rich in acetylcholine receptors that are anchored through a complex interaction with the protein RAPsyn (receptor aggregating protein at the synapse) (Sanes et al. 1998; Vincent, 2001). The depths of the synaptic folds, in contrast, are rich in voltage-gated sodium channels (Caldwell, 2000).

Perisynaptic Schwann cells, their unique relationship with the neuromuscular junction long neglected, have recently been recognized as functionally significant (summarized in Feng et al. 2005). These cells express several ion channels and receptors for neurotransmitters, and are able to respond to synaptic activity by increasing intracellular calcium; whether they can then modulate this synaptic activity remains to be seen. A role in maintenance of the neuromuscular junction is suggested by experiments in which perisynaptic Schwann cells were either ablated (Reddy et al. 2003), resulting in progressive structural and functional deterioration, or caused to migrate (Trachtenberg, Thompson, 1997), resulting in axon retraction from the endplate.

The phenomenon of neuromuscular transmission is a generalized process that is restored after nerve injury and regeneration, and has been reviewed extensively (Vincent, 2001; Engel, 2004). When the nerve action potential reaches the nerve terminal, it opens voltage-gated calcium channels that permit a brief, focal increase in intracellular calcium concentration. This calcium, in turn, triggers exocytosis of ACh-containing vesicles in the active zone by interacting with the vesicular protein synaptotagmin. The exocytotic process is thought to involve binding of a V-SNARE protein on the vesicle to a T-SNARE protein on the nerve terminal membrane (Sudhof, 2004). Once released, ACh travels across the synaptic cleft to interact with ACh receptors (AChR) that are localized to the adjoining portion of the postsynaptic membrane. The acetylcholine receptor is a transmembrane protein that is assembled from 5 subunits (Miyazawa et al., 1999). When ACh binds to the extracellular domain of the receptor, the subunits rotate in such a way as to open a pore through the receptor, permitting sodium to enter the cell and depolarize the membrane (reviewed in Vincent, 2001). This depolarization spreads into the synaptic folds, where it opens numerous voltage-gated sodium channels that greatly amplify the effects of the AChR. The brevity of response to ACh release is ensured by a high concentration of acetylcholinesterase (AChE) in the basal lamina within the synaptic cleft.

MUSCLE RECEPTORS

Proprioception—from *proprius* (L., one's own) and *recipere* (L., to sense)—is the process of obtaining information not about the outside world, but about oneself. Proprioceptive information about muscle tension and length that is needed to control posture and movement is provided by Golgi tendon organs and muscle spindles. In the late nineteenth century, it was known that tapping on a tendon could stimulate muscle contraction, yet the receptor for the tap had not been identified. Golgi attacked the problem with a systematic histological evaluation of tendon and its junction with muscle (Mazzarello, 1999), describing the "musculo-tendinous end-organ" that bears his name in 1878 (Golgi, 1878) and correctly inferring that it responded to muscle tension. He also provided an early description of the muscle spindle (Golgi, 1880), more complete than those of Kolliker, Weismann, and Kuhne (Mazzarello, 1999), yet still lacking the crucial recognition of its sensory function. Golgi thus made an early and substantial contribution to our knowledge of the anatomic basis of proprioception.

Golgi Tendon Organ

The Golgi receptor, which resembles the Ruffini organ (Chapter 2), is an encapsulated corpuscle interposed, in series, between muscle and its insertion (structure reviewed in Jami, 1992) (Figure 3-7). Within the capsule, collagen bundles extend from individual muscle fibers, interconnect and divide in a complex process during which their number is reduced, then attach to muscle tendon or aponeurosis. Several motor units contribute muscle fibers to a single tendon organ (Houck, Henneman, 1967), and the fibers of a single motor unit may activate several receptors (Jami, Petit, 1976), allowing a relatively small number of receptors to sense the activity of a large muscle. Many, but not all, collagen bundles in a Golgi organ are innervated by a single Ib afferent axon (Chapter 1, Table 1-1); the function of bundles lacking innervation remains unclear. The receptor may also be influenced by adjacent muscle fibers that insert directly on tendon or bone and are thus in parallel with the receptor, and can "unload" it by contracting (Houck, Henneman, 1967).

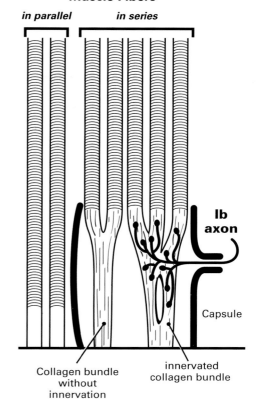

Muscle Fibers

in parallel   *in series*

Ib
axon

Capsule

Collagen bundle without innervation

innervated collagen bundle

FIGURE 3-7   Diagram of the Golgi tendon organ. Not all collagen bundles within the capsule are innervated. The forces transmitted to innervated collagen bundles may be influenced by adjacent parallel fibers that unload the end organ through their contraction.

The Golgi organ was initially thought to be a low threshold receptor for passive muscle stretch (Matthews, 1933). Subsequent studies, however, revealed that it responds primarily to stretch resulting from active muscle contraction (Houck, Henneman, 1967; Houck et al., 1970). Each receptor signals only the changes occurring in the muscle fibers to which it is attached (Proske, Gregory, 2002). The Golgi organ responds to tetanic contraction of an activating motor unit with an initial high frequency burst, decreasing to a steady rate of discharge as tension is maintained (Petit et al., 1994). Unlike the motor unit, which contains only one type of muscle fiber, a single Golgi organ may serve motor units representing several fiber types (Reinking et al., 1975). This heterogeneity results in different firing patterns from the same Golgi organ in response to contraction of each of its constituent fiber types (Gregory, Proske, 1979), and is one of the factors confounding efforts to derive a consistent relationship between applied force and the output of Golgi tendon organs (discussed in Jami, 1992; Prochazka, 1996; Scott, 2005).

The contribution of Ib afferent input to function is highly dependent on context. In the cat, Ib afferent volleys inhibit motoneuron firing in the resting preparation, but are excitatory during gait (Conway et al., 1987). During the stance phase, the output from Golgi tendon organs can double the contractile activity of extensor muscles (Gorassini et al., 1994; Stein et al., 2000; Pearson et al., 1993). Muscle stretch increases Ib firing, which in turn increases the force of muscle contraction, tending to return the muscle to its previous length and stabilize the joint it crosses. Activation of Ib afferents may also regulate the duration of the stance phase by signaling the progressive unloading of extensor muscles, a prerequisite for the initiation of the swing phase (Conway et al., 1987; Pearson et al., 1992).

The Muscle Spindle

The muscle spindle, the most complex extracranial sensory receptor, signals muscle length. It contains three types of intrafusal (inside the spindle) muscle fiber, and is innervated by two classes of sensory axon and up to four types of motoneuron (Figure 3-6) (reviewed in Banks, Barker, 2004). Mammalian spindles are typically 7–10 mm long and are aligned in parallel with adjacent extrafusal muscle fibers. The central portion of the spindle, where innervating axons terminate, is enclosed within a fluid-filled capsule. Spindles tend to be concentrated near points of muscle innervation, and are usually found in deeper, more oxidative portions of the muscle. They are much more abundant than Golgi tendon organs; the human abductor pollicis has nearly 100 spindles, while the quadriceps femoris contains 1350 (Voss, 1971). Spindle density in human muscle has been found to vary as the square root of muscle mass (Banks, Stacey, 1998). When viewed in this context, the small muscles of the hand once thought to have unusually rich spindle innervation and thus exceptional control actually fall within the normal continuum (Banks, Barker, 2004). In a recent reanalysis of the topic, Banks (2006) found that muscle spindles are most abundant in axial muscles and least abundant in muscles of the shoulder girdle;

no differences were found between large and small muscles that functioned synergistically.

The three types of intrafusal muscle fiber found in the muscle spindle are differentiated on the basis of histochemical properties, and on the configuration and location of the nucleus (reviewed in Banks, Barker, 2004). Bag fibers are characterized by clumping of their nuclei in a "bag" at the longitudinal midpoint, or equator, of the muscle fiber. Chain fibers are smaller in diameter and have a single, longitudinal row of nuclei that resembles a chain. Analysis of myosin heavy chains and the appearance of the sarcomere M line permit further differentiation of type 1 and 2 bag fibers, both from one another and from chain fibers. The spindle is innervated at the equator by a primary Ia afferent axon that is distributed predominantly to the bag 1 fiber (Banks, 1986) (Figure 3-8). One or more type II secondary afferent axons may be distributed in more peripheral locations within the capsule, with the majority of their terminations on chain fibers (Banks et al., 1982). The terminal branches of these axons often spiral around the fiber they are innervating. Intrafusal muscle fibers are most commonly powered by gamma motoneurons that can be of either the dynamic or static type (Matthews, 1962). Contraction of intrafusal muscle in response to gamma motoneuron firing will modify the forces applied to afferent axons at the center of the spindle. Dynamic gamma motoneurons are distributed exclusively to bag 1 intrafusal muscle fibers, whereas static gamma motoneurons serve both bag 2 and chain fibers. In many instances muscle spindles are also innervated by ß or skeletofusimotor neurons (Bessou et al., 1963). Slow dynamic ß terminals are found almost exclusively on bag 1 fibers within the spindle; their extrafusal collaterals are confined to type I (S) muscle (Barker et al., 1977). Fast ß motoneurons, in contrast, insert on long chain fibers in the spindle (Figure 3-8) (Harker et al., 1977) and innervate extrafusal type IIa (FR) fibers (Jami et al., 1982).

Muscle spindles signal muscle length (Vallbo, 1974). They are extremely sensitive to their environment; some even respond to breathing or arterial pulsations (Hagbarth et al., 1975; McKeon, Burke, 1981). Within their own muscle, they can respond to the activity of a single motor unit (McKeon, Burke, 1983). When muscle lacking gamma innervation is stretched, the muscle spindle fires with increasing speed, adapting and leveling off when a new constant length is reached. The relationship between muscle length and the rate of firing at that

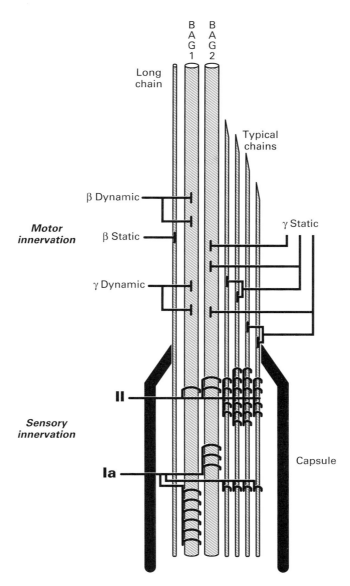

FIGURE 3-8   Schematic of one half of a muscle spindle, omitting the bottom half in this orientation. The Ia afferent axon defines the equator, or longitudinal midpoint, of the structure. Intrafusal muscle fibers are described as bag or chain, depending on their nuclear morphology. Both gamma and beta dynamic innervation are shown, though only one is present in a given spindle. Examples of motor innervation patterns are depicted without reference to their frequency of occurrence; sensory innervation of each class of intrafusal fiber is depicted on a proportional basis based on information from Banks (1986, 1994, 2006) and Banks et al., 1982.

length, after adaptation, is approximately linear (Lennerstrand, 1968; Banks, Barker, 2004). The addition of gamma motoneuron function results in predictable modifications of spindle activity. Firing of dynamic gamma motoneurons activates bag 1 fibers, resulting in little change in spindle discharge when muscle length is kept static, but magnifying the response to length change, or the dynamic sensitivity of the spindle. Firing of static gamma motoneurons, in contrast, activates bag 2 or chain fibers. The spindle discharge rate at a fixed muscle length is increased, thus increasing the sensitivity of the system to muscle length, but the dynamic response is not altered significantly (Proske, Gregory, 2002; Banks, Barker, 2004). If alpha motoneurons fire alone, only extrafusal muscle fibers will contract; the muscle spindle will be shortened passively, and Ia output will cease (Hunt, Kuffler, 1951). The resulting gap in sensory feedback can be prevented by the coactivation of alpha and gamma motoneurons, allowing the spindle to keep pace with changing muscle length (Rothwell et al., 1990; Hagbarth, 1993). This ability is constrained, however, as muscle spindle fibers contain only the slower MHC isoforms, and are thus unable to keep pace with fast extrafusal contraction (McWhorter et al., 1995; Walro, Kucera, 1999). Alpha-gamma linkage is not absolute, as the effects of motion on Ia output usually predominate over those of linkage (Al-Falahe et al., 1990). In addition to partial control by alpha motoneurons, gamma motoneurons may be influenced by a variety of CNS centers including the brainstem and cerebellum (summarized in Prochazka, 1996).

In the decerebrate cat, Ia afferent activity influences both the strength and timing of muscle activity. Ia afferent volleys, resulting from muscle spindle stimulation, strengthen the inciting contraction through monosynaptic Ia contacts on motoneurons (Pearson, Collins, 1993). During fictive locomotion, Ia input from ankle extensors can reset the locomotor rhythm (Guertin et al., 1995). Similarly, the transition from stance to swing may be initiated by the Ia activity of hip muscles when the joint is extended (Andersson, Grillner, 1983; Kriellaars et al., 1994).

NT-3, a member of the neurotrophin family of growth factors, plays a pivotal role in the development and maintenance of the muscle spindle. Mice lacking NT-3 or its receptor TrkC fail to develop muscle spindles altogether (Enfors et al., 1994; Klein et al., 1994). NT-3 produced by developing muscle supports the survival of TrkC-positive Ia neurons as their axons reach the periphery; the number of neurons that survive depends on the supply of available NT-3 (summarized in Chen, Frank, 1999). Ia axons, in turn, express neuregulin 1 that interacts with the ErbB2 receptor on muscle to initiate the differentiation of the muscle spindle (discussed in Chen et al., 2003). As the spindle develops, the bag fibers themselves become a source of NT-3, and continue to produce it into adulthood (Copray, Brouwer, 1994). This supply is crucial for the contribution of the Ia neuron to the reflex arc (Mendell et al., 2001). The large DRG neurons that supply afferent axons to muscle spindles and Golgi tendon organs have been characterized broadly as to their gene expression and biochemical markers as described in Chapter 2.

THE FUNCTIONAL ANATOMY OF MOTOR CONTROL

The control of motor function is a complex process that has been explored from the perspective of systems function at one end and the physiology of isolated circuits at the other; the process of melding these perspectives to form a unified model is incomplete. This brief overview of functional neuroanatomy, guided by several reviews (Orlovsky et al., 1999; Bizzi et al., 2000; Ghez, Krakauer, 2000; Drew et al., 2004), will provide a conceptual framework for the more detailed discussion of inputs to the motoneuron pool that follows. Motoneuronal activity is regulated by a hierarchical system of controls involving the spinal cord, brainstem, and cortex, with afferent input and output to the motoneuron pool at each level (Figure 3-9). Three features of this hierarchy are particularly important (Ghez, Krakauer, 2000): (1) The information that enters and leaves each processing level is organized somatotopically; (2) each level receives peripheral sensory information that may be used to shape motor output, and in turn provides information back to sensory centers; and (3) motor programs are shaped by learning on an ongoing basis. Inherent in this multitiered pattern of organization is also the potential for substantial plasticity in response to a focal lesion.

The primary motor cortex (M1) lies across the central sulcus from the sensory cortex, in the precentral gyrus (Brodman area 4). It projects to the spinal cord directly through the corticospinal tract, and indirectly through the brainstem. Trans-synaptic transport of rabies virus from individual primate muscles has been used to define two subdivisions of M1 (Rathelot and Strick, 2009). The rostral, "old" M1, found in many mammals, has no direct corticomotoneuronal (CM) projections, whereas the "new," caudal M1, present in some higher primates and humans, bypasses intermediate nuclei to communicate directly from cortex to motoneuron. Cortical motor cells represent either specific muscle activity or specific motions, irrespective of the muscles used to generate them (Kakei et al., 1999). These neurons thus lack the strict somatotopic organization that is characteristic of sensory cortex (Chapter 2).

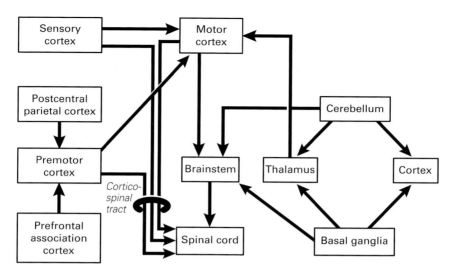

FIGURE 3-9 Schematic summary of the major projections that contribute to motor control. Multiple discrete projections from one area to another have been combined for simplicity. The hierarchical system of cortex/ brainstem/ spinal cord is influenced strongly by both cerebellum and basal ganglia.

The response of M1 to motor learning suggests that it stores the internal representation of skilled sequential movements (Matsuzaka et al., 2007). Neighboring cortical motor cells with common target muscles form functional groups that activate similar combinations of muscles (Cheney, Fetz, 1985). M1 receives direct input from the sensory cortex, and from the premotor cortex in Brodman area 6. Premotor cortex is responsible for the planning and coordination of complex motor functions, and is influenced by postcentral parietal cortex and prefrontal association cortex, which contributes working memory to the planning process. Primary sensory cortex (Chapter 2) projects directly to M1 as noted, but also contributes fibers to the corticospinal tract that modulate afferent input to the dorsal horn of the spinal cord. The brainstem receives input from motor cortex, and projects to the spinal cord through medial pathways that control postural muscles and lateral pathways that contribute to target-specific limb placement.

The spinal cord is the seat of a variety of reflexes as exemplified by the monosynaptic stretch reflex (Figure 3-10). Spinal interneurons also generate patterns of rhythmic motion for stereotyped, fundamental behaviors such as locomotion or scratching. Circuits known as "central pattern generators" are thought to control a small number of synergistic muscles that act at a single joint (Grillner, 1985).

Coordinated motion thus results from the sequential recruitment of appropriate units. The actual mechanism of central pattern generation is still under debate (reviewed in McCrea and Rybak, 2008). A necessary concomitant of spinal autonomy is reliance on proprioceptive feedback. In the cat, feedback from muscle proprioceptors is now known to alter the timing of phase transitions during gait, to contribute to the activation of central pattern generators, to generate some aspects of the motor program, and to alter gait in response to changes in leg mechanics (Pearson, 2004).

Transmission within the hierarchical system of cortex/brainstem/spinal cord is influenced strongly by the cerebellum and basal ganglia. Both of these structures receive cortical input, project directly to the brainstem, and project to M1 through the thalamus (Figure 3-9). The cerebellum participates in the timing and coordination of ongoing movement as well as in the learning of motor skills; the basal ganglia represent the interface of motivation with movement, and influence the choice of motor sequences needed to produce a specified outcome.

INPUTS TO THE MOTONEURON POOL

Discussions of motor control usually focus on the organization and function of the controlling circuitry,

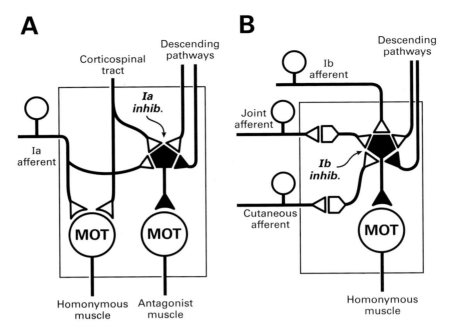

FIGURE 3-10   A. Ia muscle spindle afferents and cortical neurons excite homonymous motoneurons monosynaptically. They reciprocally inhibit antagonistic motoneurons through their contacts with Ia inhibitory interneurons. The firing of these interneurons is also modulated by descending control from other sources. A single Ia or cortical impulse can thus simultaneously contract one muscle and relax its antagonist. B. Ib Golgi tendon afferents inhibit motoneuron firing disynaptically through the Ib inhibitory interneuron. This class of interneuron may be influenced by several types of input, and functions to coordinate muscle force at several joints.

mentioning the motoneuron or motoneuron pool as an effector only. This approach is appropriate to studies of normal CNS function and its alteration by disease. It does little, however, to help one evaluate the possible consequences of peripheral nerve injury and regeneration. Motoneurons may reinnervate incorrect muscles; sensory neurons may err both as to receptor type and location. Both types of neuron, at least initially, will maintain their normal relationships with higher centers in spite of their new distal connections. Motoneuron firing is an all-or-nothing event, Sherrington's "final common pathway" (Sherrington, 1906), determined by the summation of excitatory and inhibitory inputs in the context of persistent inward currents that alter membrane potential (Binder et al., 1993; Heckman et al., 2005). It is thus important to focus on the organization of these inputs to set the stage for later analysis of misdirected reinnervation and its consequences. This section will discuss four of the most significant classes of neuron that synapse on the motoneuron: excitatory Ia afferents, cortical neurons, Ia inhibitory

interneurons, and Ib interneurons. The degree to which these projections are generalized to the entire motoneuron pool or are capable of postinjury plasticity might determine their role, positive or negative, after the connections between end organs and their central neurons have been rewired by regeneration.

IA Afferent Projections

The monosynaptic stretch reflex, based on direct synapses between Ia muscle spindle afferents and motoneurons (Figure 3-10), was among the first forms of motor control to be identified (Sherrington, 1906). Nonetheless, details of the relationship between afferent and efferent neurons remained inaccessible until techniques of intracellular recording and HRP labeling were perfected. The central projections of individual Ia neurons have been mapped in great detail by injecting horseradish peroxidase (HRP) into axons that have first been identified by functional criteria (Brown, Fyffe, 1978;

Ishizuka et al., 1979). These axons bifurcate as they enter the dorsal columns, sending ascending and descending branches at least several millimeters. Collaterals arise from both branches at approximately 1-mm intervals, and support terminal arborizations in Rexed lamina VI (Rexed, 1962) (the intermediate region), lamina VII (Ia inhibitory interneurons), and lamina IX (motoneuron pools) (Figure 3-11). The intracellular HRP technique can be extended by injecting both neurons of a reflex arc to identify the contacts between them (Brown, Fyffe, 1981). This combined approach revealed that motoneurons receive between 2 and 6 contacts from an individual Ia afferent (mean 2.05), and that these are localized to the neuronal soma and the proximal 30 μm of the proximal dendrite. In spite of the arborization of the motoneuron dendritic tree for 2–3 mm in all directions, each motoneuron interacts with only one collateral from a given Ia afferent, suggesting some form of selectivity in establishing the Ia-motoneuron relationship (Brown, Fyffe, 1981).

HRP technique provides magnificent anatomical detail of structures that have been filled with the enzyme (Figure 3-11). Injected HRP may not fill more distant portions of an extensive arbor, however, and cannot be relied on to demonstrate the full extent of a neuron's projections. Purely electrophysiologic techniques, such as spike-triggered averaging, give a better picture of the overall organization of afferent projections. In the study that introduced this technique, Mendell and Henneman (1968) found that single Ia gastrocnemius afferents projected to nearly all (94%) of the motoneurons in the gastrocnemius (homonymous) motoneuron pool, a finding that has been confirmed repeatedly (Munson et al., 1984; Munson, 1990). In addition to their homonymous projections, Ia afferents also project to the motoneuron pools of neighboring synergistic (heteronymous) muscles. These connections follow a "neighborhood principle," being more frequent to the motoneurons of adjacent than to those of more distant muscles (Fritz et al., 1989; Illert, 1996). Similarly, Ia afferent fibers give off more functional synaptic endings to motoneurons close to their spinal cord entry level than to those farther away (Luscher et al., 1984). In multicompartment muscles, Ia afferents are distributed preferentially to motoneurons from the compartment containing the receptor (Lucas, Binder, 1984). The presence or absence of shared Ia afferent input has been correlated with the functional independence of muscle. For instance, the shared Ia input of

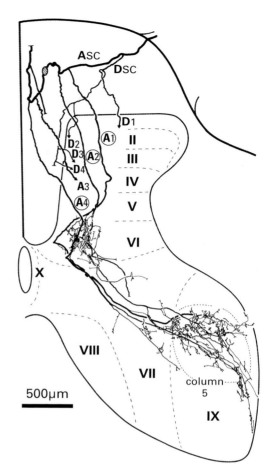

FIGURE 3-11   The trajectory of a Ia afferent fiber within the spinal cord, demonstrating terminations in Rexed laminae VI, VII, and IX. Asc—ascending branch; Dsc—descending branch; A1, A2, A4—collaterals completely traced; A3, D1, D2, D3, D4—collaterals leaving the plane for proximal and distal levels; I–X—Rexed laminae. Reproduced with permission from Brown and Fyffe, 1979.

muscles above and below the elbow in cats, but not in humans, has been attributed to the respective demands of quadripedal and bipedal locomotion, the latter freeing up the forearm for more independent motion (Illert, Kummel, 1999).

In addition to conforming to these topographic principles, Ia afferents have stronger inputs to low-threshold than to high-threshold neurons (Burke, 1968; Heckman, Binder, 1988), magnifying the inherent differences in motoneuron recruitment thresholds that underlie the size principle.

Direct Cortico-Motoneuronal Projections

Motor control in the primate is uniquely characterized by direct projections from motor cortex to the motoneurons that control the hand (Lemon, 1993; Figure 3-9). These cortico-motoneuronal neurons (CM neurons) are located primarily in M1, but have also been found in supplementary motor areas (Maier et al., 2002). Approximately 80% of CM neurons project to muscles within the hand; the other 20% of the neurons project to more proximal portions of the limb (Lemon, 1993). The electrical activity evoked in motoneurons serving proximal muscles by CM firing is relatively weak, whereas that evoked in the motoneurons of intrinsic hand muscles is strong enough to fire the motoneuron without other inputs (Porter, Lemon, 1993). Within the human intrinsic muscles, CM neurons project most strongly to the 1st dorsal interosseous muscle, and less strongly to the abductor pollicis brevis and adductor digiti quinti muscles (Ziemann et al., 2004).

The processes of individual CM neurons contact many motoneurons, and each motoneuron is influenced by input from several CM neurons. HRP studies reveal extensive branching of CM processes within Rexed lamina IX, which contains the motoneuron pools (Lawrence et al., 1985). Electrophysiologically, single CM cells project to most low-threshold motor units within a target muscle activated during precision grip (Mantel, Lemon, 1987). CM neurons may also project more widely. In a sample of 80 CM neurons, Lemon found that each projected to a mean of 1.9 muscles (Lemon, 1993). Nineteen of these facilitated the firing of only one muscle, most often an intrinsic hand muscle. The term "muscle field" was coined to describe the group of muscles innervated by a single CM cell (Fetz, Cheney, 1980). A single motoneuron, in turn, receives input from an entire "colony" of CM neurons (discussed in Lemon, 1993). In general, the organization of CM neurons mirrors that of the motor cortex as a whole. There is no 1:1 mapping of CM neurons to muscles, and CM neurons do not represent individual muscle functions. Instead, they appear to represent groups of muscles that are activated for discrete components of a motion, or the motion itself, without reference to the muscles used to produce it (Lemon, 1993; Kakei et al., 1999). CM neurons with common target muscles tend to fire synchronously, while inhibitory mechanisms act between neurons with opposing effects (Jackson et al., 2003).

Several features of the CM projection are consistent with relatively independent functioning of this pathway. Presynaptic inhibition is absent (Nielsen, Petersen, 1994), and there is a high proportion of beta innervation with little direct control from muscle spindles (Marsden et al., 1972; Buller et al., 1980). Lemon (1993) has summarized additional evidence that these projections are at least equipped to control independent finger movement: CM connections have a purely excitatory effect on motoneurons, destruction of CM projections in primates eliminates independent finger movement without harming general motor behavior, the development of CM projections parallels the acquisition of skilled hand control, and species with the greatest dexterity have the largest CM projections. This evidence is supported by recordings made from primate CM neurons during voluntary manual activity that show CM cell firing to be appropriately timed and distributed to facilitate the motor performance observed (summarized in Lemon et al., 2004).

The role of the CM projection can be appreciated further through analysis of its possible evolutionary role. Fine coordination of digital motion may not be possible using the spinal circuitry evolved for control of posture and gait (Sherrington, 1906). A monosynaptic cortico-motoneuronal connection, in contrast, shifts control to areas that receive direct input from visual and somatosensory cortex. Lemon has hypothesized that the CM system provides an "executive pathway" for the integration of innate spinal motor patterns to produce complex activities. The direct availability of cognitive and sensory input from nearby cortex could allow motion to be controlled through a progressively "feed-forward," or anticipatory, fashion, rather than relying on muscle proprioceptors for more time-consuming and imprecise "feedback" control.

IA Inhibitory Interneurons

Ia inhibitory interneurons are interposed between the collaterals of Ia muscle spindle afferents and motoneurons (Figure 3-10). The muscles that receive this inhibitory input are antagonistic to those in which the Ia impulse arose. Muscle stretch thus provokes simultaneous contraction of the stretched muscle through monosynaptic excitatory Ia activity, and relaxation of antagonistic muscles through the action of Ia inhibitory interneurons, a process termed *reciprocal inhibition*.

Ia inhibitory interneurons are so named because they are strongly influenced by the activity of Ia afferent impulses (Hultborn et al., 1971a). As was shown for excitatory Ia effects (see above), the amplitudes of inhibitory postsynaptic potentials (IPSPs) vary systematically by motoneuron type: S > FR > Fint > FF (Burke et al., 1976b; Dum, Kennedy, 1980b). The gradient of Ia inhibition across the motoneuron pool is less steep than that of Ia excitation (Heckman, Binder, 1991), however, a differential that may favor orderly recruitment in accordance with the size principle.

In addition to their primary input from muscle spindles, Ia inhibitory interneurons receive input from several other sources. They are influenced by interneurons that relay a variety of peripheral inputs (Eccles, Lindberg, 1959: Bruggencate et al., 1969; Hultborn et al., 1971a), as well as by those that contribute to the generation of locomotor patterns (discussed in Jankowska, 1992), although they themselves do not generate motion (Pratt, Jordan, 1987). Input is also received from descending systems; in primates, Ia inhibitory interneurons interact with collaterals of CM neurons (see above) in a pattern similar to that described for Ia afferents (summarized in Jankowska, 1992) (Figure 3-10). A CM neuron may thus, with a single impulse, facilitate contraction of some muscles and relaxation of their antagonists. The activity of Ia inhibitory interneurons may be depressed, in turn, by input from other neurons, most prominently Renshaw cells (Hultborn et al., 1971a; 1971b). These unique inhibitory interneurons are interposed between motor axon collaterals and the motoneurons themselves. By modulating the activity of Renshaw cells, higher motor centers adjust co-contraction of flexors and extensors (Hultborn, Lundberg, 1972). The Ia interneuron is thus subject to a wide variety of influences that support its role in the fine tuning of motoneuron excitability (Jankowska, 1992).

Individual Ia inhibitory interneurons are situated in Rexed lamina VII (Figure 3-11), adjacent to motor nuclei that receive the same Ia input (Hultborn et al., 1971a; Rastad et al., 1990). Their dendritic trees extend in a predominantly dorso-volar orientation; there is relatively little dendritic branching, yet the combined length of dendritic elements may reach 7 mm (Rastad et al., 1990). Each neuron is excited by input from a few synergistic muscles (Hultborn et al., 1971a). The axons of Ia interneurons enter the white matter, laterally or ventrally depending on their orientation (Jankowska,

Lindstrom, 1972), and travel to the motoneuron pools of antagonistic muscles. In the cat, in which Ia projections have been studied most extensively, individual quadriceps Ia inhibitory axons project extensively to the four antagonistic motor nuclei that have been examined (Jankowska, Roberts, 1972; Rastad, 1981; Brink et al., 1983), making contact with up to 20% of the motoneurons within each pool (Jankowska, Roberts, 1972). It seems likely, therefore, that the Ia inhibitory interneuron generalizes input from a single or small number of muscles to a larger pool of antagonists.

IB Interneurons

Type Ib interneurons were defined initially by their response to input from Golgi tendon organs: disynaptic inhibition of homonymous and synergistic motoneurons, coupled with excitation of their antagonists (LaPorte, Lloyd, 1952) (Figure 3-10). It soon became apparent, however, that these interneurons receive input from a variety of sources, can be inhibitory or excitatory depending on context, and can discharge their output through any one of a variety of channels under the control of descending motor commands (Jami, 1992). In light of these findings, their function is now described more inclusively as *Ia* or *Group I nonreciprocal inhibition*, although the neurons themselves are still referred to as Ib interneurons (Jankowska et al., 1981b).

The distribution of Golgi tendon organ (Ib) afferents, the dominant source of input to Ib interneurons (Jankowska, 1992), has been mapped in the cat by injection of HRP into functionally identified neurons (Hongo et al., 1978; Brown, Fyffe, 1979). Ib axons bifurcate upon entering the spinal cord, sending rostral and caudal processes that have been filled with HRP for up to 1 cm and probably extend even farther. Collaterals arise from these processes approximately every 1 mm, penetrate the dorsal horn of the spinal cord, and form fan-like projections within Rexed lamina VI and the dorsal portion of lamina VII, where they interact with interneurons. Ib afferent input is stronger from extensor muscles than it is from flexors (Jankowska et al., 1981a), consistent with the observation of stronger reflex activity from extensor muscles (Eccles et al., 1957a; 1957b). Input from several muscles converges on each interneuron; no single input is of sufficient strength to fire the Ib interneuron, so that strong input from one muscle or input from several muscles is required (Jankowska, 1992).

Ib interneurons are subject to a host of influences beyond their dominant Ib input. Ia afferents synapse on 30–50% of Ib interneurons, each of which may be influenced by several muscles (Czarkowska et al., 1981). Ia input could allow adjustments of Ib reflex actions based on changes in muscle length, and modulations of these adjustments by gamma and beta fusimotor activity (Jankowska, McCrea, 1983; Jankowska, 1992). Cutaneous and joint afferents project to Ib interneurons through one or two additional synapses (Harrison, Jankowska, 1985b), and may be important for restricting movement when an obstacle is encountered (Lundberg et al., 1975). More distant excitatory influences include long propriospinal neurons and cortico- and rubrospinal descending tracts (discussed in Jankowska, 1992). Inhibitory input is received from other Ib interneurons, from presynaptic modification of peripheral input, and from descending inhibitory pathways (Jankowska, 1992). There appears to be little specialization of Ib interneurons by type of afferent input, as all modalities appear to be distributed evenly (Harrison, Jankowska, 1985a; Jankowska, 1992).

Synergistic motoneurons, predominantly extensors, are the principal target of Ia inhibitory interneurons; antagonistic motoneurons, predominantly flexors, are the principal target of Ib excitatory motoneurons. Nonetheless, the effect of Ia afferent activity on any motoneuron may be reversed by using alternative interneuronal pathways (summarized in Jankowska, 1992). Individual Ib interneurons project to several motoneuron pools (Czarkowska et al., 1981; Jankowska et al., 1981a), yet make contact with few motoneurons within each (Harrison, Riddell, 1989). They influence not only alpha motoneurons, but probably gamma motoneurons as well (Fetz et al., 1979). Ib interneurons also send extensive projections to other interneurons in the intermediate zone (Czarkowska et al., 1981), and may project to the cerebellum (Lundberg, 1971). Jankowska (1992) has summarized the probable role of Ib interneurons in the control of movement. Because of their widespread connections, they are ideally suited to coordinate the muscle activity around multiple joints. Subpopulations of Ib interneurons may be activated selectively to contribute to specific motor synergies (Hongo et al., 1969), a function that has been observed in man (Fournier, Pierrot-Deseilligny, 1989). They have also been shown to contribute specifically to the control of

walking, modulating the yield of extensors during stance, and adjusting muscle tension according to the speed of gait (Eccles, Lundberg, 1959; Hongo et al., 1969).

CONCLUSIONS

The principles that govern motor function are fundamentally different from those that regulate the processing of sensory information (Chapter 2). The cutaneous afferent system is tightly organized, with precise correspondence between receptors and cortical neurons, and cannot function without cortical participation. The motor system, in contrast, does not provide a cortical neuron for each motor unit or muscle. Instead, MI cortical neurons are programmed more generally to produce specific motions or joint positions, and their organization does not rigidly mirror the topography of the limb. The relative role of the cortex is also different, as a panel of basic motions such as reaching can result from activation of pattern generators in the spinal cord, relying on cortical input for overall control rather than step-by-step instructions. Additionally, normal motor function requires the activation of both efferent and afferent axons, whereas sensory communication is unidirectional.

Regenerating peripheral axons are imprecise in their targeting, and may reinnervate end organs that are functionally and/or topographically inappropriate (Chapter 10). It is possible, based on the structure of the motor system, to anticipate potential consequences of this imprecision and to identify the circuits that might be used to compensate for it. On the efferent side, regenerating motor axons may reinnervate inappropriate muscles (Chapter 10). Motoneurons that initially controlled one muscle can reinnervate several, potentially antagonistic muscles. Conversely, a single muscle could be reinnervated by motoneurons from several pools. As a consequence, a signal that normally stimulated contraction of one muscle would fire several muscles, and each muscle could receive potentially conflicting commands from several motoneuron pools.

Compensation for mismatch between motoneuron pools and muscles would, at the very least, require rerouting of signals through existing circuits. To be capable of performing this task, a circuit would need to address motoneurons individually. It is clear from the outset that motor system organization central to the motoneuron pool varies substantially between most mammals on the one hand

and higher primates and man on the other. In the former, spinal cord pattern generators have a relatively dominant role; a spinal cat suspended on a treadmill can generate a fairly normal gait in response to movement of the surface beneath it. In higher primates and man, many cortical neurons synapse directly on motoneurons (CM neurons). CM projections have been described in the context of cortical "executive function," allowing feed-forward, or anticipatory control of motor activities. These unique circuits could potentially facilitate compensation for peripheral miswiring. They are highly independent, and lack most of the inhibitory controls that influence indirect projections. A motoneuron may be contacted by several cortical neurons, and can thus be accessed in a variety of functional contexts. It is important to note, however, that most CM neurons fire one or more motoneuron pools as units. Whereas these neurons might facilitate adjustment to altering the function of an entire motoneuron pool, such as in nerve transfer, they provide no circuitry capable of electrically coupling selected motoneurons from several motoneuron pools. The projections of individual neurons within the afferent portion of the motor system are also distributed widely. Ia afferents project to all motoneurons within a pool, and to a lesser degree to synergistic motoneuron pools. Ia inhibitory neurons generalize from a single or small number of motoneuron pools to a larger number of antagonistic motoneuron pools, and Ib inhibitory neurons project even more extensively.

Although the motor unit clearly represents the quantum of motor function, the preceding analysis of efferent and afferent spinal cord circuitry suggests that the motoneuron pool is the most discrete unit that can be addressed individually. There are no projections from more centrally located neurons to individual motoneurons, and thus no circuitry through which signals could be rerouted to compensate for the reinnervation of several muscles by a single motoneuron pool. The degree to which normal function can be restored in these circumstances is thus likely to depend on the plasticity of existing synapses, allowing some circuits to be strengthened at the expense of others, or the potential for the formation of entirely new connections (Chapter 11).

REFERENCES

Al-Falahe NA, Nagaoka M, Vallbo AB (1990) Response profiles of human muscle afferents during active finger movements. Brain 113: 325–346.

Andersson O, Grillner S (1983) Peripheral control of the cat's step cycle. II. Entrainment of the central pattern generators for locomotion by sinusoidal hip movements during fictive locomotion. Acta Physiol Scand 118: 229–239.

Appelberg B, Emonet-Denand F (1967) Motor units of the first superficial lumbrical muscle of the cat. J Neurophysiol 30: 154–160.

Arndt I, Pepe FA (1975) Antigenic specificity of red and white muscle myosin. J Histochem Cytochem 23: 159–168.

Banks RW, Barker D, Stacey MJ (1982) Form and distribution of sensory terminals in cat hindlimb muscle spindles. Philos Trans R Soc Lond [Biol] 299: 329–364.

Banks RW (1986) Observations on the primary sensory ending of tenuissimus muscle spindles in the cat. Cell Tissue Res 246: 309–319.

Banks RW (1994) The motor innervation of mammalian muscle spindles. Prog Neurobiol 43: 323–362.

Banks RW, Stacey M (1998) On the number of spindles in mammalian muscles. J Physiol 511: 69P.

Banks, R.W. and D. Barker (2004) The muscle spindle. In: *Myology*, Vol. 3, A.G. Engel and C. Franzini-Armstrong, eds., pp. 489–509, New York: McGraw Hill.

Banks RW (2006) An allometric analysis of the number of muscle spindles in mammalian skeletal muscles. J Anat 208: 753–768.

Barany M (1967) ATPase activity of myosin correlated with speed of muscle shortening. J Gen Physiol 50 (suppl): 197–218.

Barker D, Emonet-Denand F, Harker DW, Jami L, Laporte Y (1977) Types of intra- and extrafusal muscle fibre innervated by dynamic skeletofusimotor axons in cat peroneus brevis and tenuissimus muscles, as determined by the glycogen-depletion method. J Physiol Lond 266: 713–726.

Bessou P, Emonet-Denand F, Laporte Y (1963) Occurrence of intrafusal muscle fibers innervated by branches of slow a motor fibers in the cat. Nature 198: 594–595.

Bigland-Ritchie B, Zijdewind I, Thomas CK (2000) Muscle fatigue induced by stimulation with and without doublets. Muscle Nerve 23: 1348–1355.

Binder MD, Heckman CJ, Powers RK (1993) How different afferent inputs control motoneuron discharge and the output of the motoneuron pool. Current Biology 3: 1028–1034.

Bizzi E, Tresch MC, Saltiel P, d'Avella A (2000) New perspectives on spinal motor systems. Nat. Rev. Neurosci. 1: 101–108.

Bodine SC, Roy RR, Eldred E, Edgerton VR (1987) Maximal force as a function of anatomical features of motor units in the cat tibialis anterior. J Neurophysiol 57: 1730–1745.

Bodine-Fowler SC, Garfinkel A, Roy RR, Edgerton VR (1990) Spatial distribution of muscle fibers within the territory of a motor unit. Muscle Nerve 13: 1133–1145.

Bottinelli R, Canepari M, Reggiani C, Stienen GJ (1994) Myofibrillar ATPase activity during isometric contraction and isomyosin composition in rat single skinned muscle fibers. J. Physiol (Lond.) 481: 663–675.

Breitbart RE, Nadal-Ginard B (1987) Developmentally induced, muscle-specific trans factors control the differential splicing of alternative and constitutive troponin T exons. Cell 49: 793–803.

Brink E, Harrison PJ, Jankowska E, McCrea D, Skoog B (1983) Postsynaptic potentials in a population of motoneurones following activity of single interneurones in the cat. J Physiol 343: 341–359.

Brooke MH, Kaiser KK (1970) Three "myosin adenosine triphosphate" systems: the nature of their pH lability and sulfhydral dependence. J Histochem Cytochem 18: 670–672.

Brown AG, Fyffe RE (1978) The morphology of group Ia afferent fibre collaterals in the spinal cord of the cat. J Physiol 274: 111–127.

Brown AG, Fyffe RE (1979) The morphology of group Ib afferent fibre collaterals in the spinal cord of the cat. J Physiol 296: 215–228.

Brown AG, Fyffe REW (1981) Direct observations on the contacts made between Ia afferent fibers and alpha motoneurones in the cat's lumbosacral spinal cord. JPhysiol 313: 121–140.

Bruggencate G, Burke RE, Lundberg A, Udo M (1969) Interactions between the vestibulospinal tract, contralateral flexor reflex afferents and Ia afferents. Brain Res 14: 529–532.

Brushart TM, Mesulam M-M (1980) Alteration in connections between muscle and anterior horn motoneurons after peripheral nerve repair. Science 208: 603–605.

Buller AJ, Eccles JC, Eccles RM (1960) Interactions between motoneurons and muscles in respect of the characteristic speeds of their responses. J Physiol 150: 417–439.

Buller NP, Garnett R, Stephens JA (1980) The reflex responses of single motor units in human hand muscles following muscle afferent stimulation. J Physiol 303: 337–349.

Burke, R.E. (2006) The structure and function of motor units. In: *Myology*, Vol. 3, A.G. Engel and C. Franzini-Armstrong, eds., pp. 104–118, New York: McGraw Hill.

Burke RE (1968) Firing patterns of gastrocnemius motor units in the decerebrate cat. J Physiol (Lond) 196: 631–645.

Burke RE, Jankowska E, ten Bruggencate G (1970) A comparison of peripheral and rubrospinal synaptic input to slow and fast twitch motor units of the triceps surae. J Physiol (Lond) 207: 709–732.

Burke RE, Levine DN, Tsairis P, Zajac FE (1973) Physiological types and histochemical profiles in motor units of the cat gastrocnemius. J Physiol 234: 723–748.

Burke RE, Rudomin P, Zajac FE (1976a) The effect of activation history on tension production by individual muscle units. Brain Res 109: 515–529.

Burke RE, Rymer WZ, Walsh JV (1976b) Relative strength of synaptic input from short latency pathways to motor units of defined type in cat medial gastrocnemius. J Neurophysiol 39: 447–458.

Burke RE, Strick PL, Kanda K, Kim CC, Walmsley B (1977) Anatomy of medial gastrocnemius and soleus motor nuclei in cat spinal cord. J Neurophysiol 40: 667–680.

Burke, R.E. (1981) Motor units: anatomy, physiology, and functional organization. In: *Handbook of Physiology*, V.B. Brooks, ed., pp. 345–422, Washington, DC: American Physiological Society.

Burke RE, Dum RP, Fleshman JW, Glenn LL, Lev TA, O'Donovan MJ, Pinter MJ (1982) A HRP study of the relation between cell size and motor unit type in cat ankle extensor motoneurons. J Comp Neurol 209: 17–28.

Burke RE (1999) Revisiting the notion of "motor unit types." Prog Brain Res 123: 167–175.

Caldwell JH (2000) Clustering of sodium channels at the neuromuscular junction. Microsc Res Tech 49: 84–89.

Carlstedt T, Anand P, Hallin R, Misra PV, Norén G, Seferlis T (2000) Spinal nerve root repair and reimplantation of avulsed ventral roots into the spinal cord after brachial plexus injury. J Neurosurg 93 Suppl.: 237–247.

Chen H-H, Hippenmeyer S, Arber S, Frank E (2003) Development of the monosynaptic stretch reflex circuit. Curr Opin Neurobiol 13: 96–102.

Chen HH, Frank E (1999) Development and specification of muscle sensory neurons. Curr Opin Neurobiol 9: 405–409.

Cheney PD, Fetz EE (1985) Comparable patterns of muscle facilitation evoked by individual corticomotoneuronal (CM) cells and by single intracortical microstimuli in primates: evidence for functional groups of CM cells. J Neurophysiol 53: 786–804.

Christensen E (1959) Topography of terminal motor innervation in striated muscles from stillborn infants. Am J Phys Med 38: 65–78.

Conway BA, Hultborn H, Kiehn O (1987) Proprioceptive input resets central locomotor rhythm in the spinal cat. Exp Brain Res 68: 643–656.

Copray JCVM, Brouwer N (1994) Selective expression of neurotrophin-3 messenger RNA in muscle spindles of the rat. Neuroscience 63: 1125–1135.

Craig, RW. and R. Padron (2004) Muscle contraction. In: *Myology*, Vol. 3, A.G. Engel and C. Franzini-Armstrong, eds., pp. 129–166, New York: McGraw-Hill.

Czeh, G (1977) Ventral root elicited depression of the dorsal root evoked response in frog motoneurons. Exp Brain Res 27(3–4): 441–449.

Czarkowska J, Jankowska E, Sybirska E (1981) Common interneurones in reflex pathways from group Ia and Ib afferents of knee flexors and extensors in the cat. J Physiol 310: 367–380.

Daube JR (1995) Estimating the number of motor units in a muscle. J Clin Neurophys 12: 585–594.

De Luca CJ, Foley PJ, Erim Z (1996) Motor unit control properties in constant-force isometric contractions. J Neurophysiol 76: 1503–1516.

Denny-Brown D (1929) On the nature of postural reflexes. Proc Roy Soc, Ser B 104: 252–301.

Denny-Brown D, Pennybacker JB (1939) Fibrillation and fasciculation in voluntary muscle. Brain 61: 311–334.

Desmedt JE, Godaux E (1977) Ballistic contractions in man: Characteristic recruitment pattern of single motor units of the tibialis anterior muscle. J Physiol (Lond) 264: 673–694.

Doherty T, Simmons Z, O'Connell B, Felice KJ, Conwit R, Chan M, Komori T, Brown T, Stashuk DW, Brown W (1995) Methods for estimating the numbers of motor units in human muscles. J Clin Neurophys 12: 565–584.

Drew T, Prentice S, Schepens B (2004) Cortical and brainstem control of locomotion. Prog Brain Res 143: 251–261.

Dum RP, Kennedy T (1980a) Physiological and histochemical characteristics of motor units in cat tibialis anterior and extensor digitorum longus muscles. J Neurophysiol 43: 1615–1630.

Dum RP, Kennedy TT (1980b) Synaptic organization of defined motor-unit types in cat tibialis anterior. J Neurophysiol 43: 1631–1644.

Eccles JC, Eccles RM, Lundberg A (1957a) Synaptic actions in motoneurones caused by impulses in Golgi tendon afferents. J Physiol 138: 227–252.

Eccles JC, Eccles RM, Lundberg A (1957b) Synaptic actions on motoneurones in relation to the two components of the group I muscle afferent volley. J Physiol 136: 527–546.

Eccles RM, Lundberg A (1959) Synaptic actions in motoneurones by afferents which may evoke the flexion reflex. Arch Ital Biol 97: 199–221.

Enfors P, Lee KF, Kucera J, Jaenisch R (1994) Lack of neurotrophin-3 leads to deficiencies in the peripheral nervous system and loss of limb proprioceptive afferents. Cell 77: 503–512.

Engel, A.G. (2004) Neuromuscular transmission. In: *Myology*, Vol. 3, A.G. Engel and C. Franzini-Armstrong, eds., pp. 325–372, New York: McGraw Hill.

English AW, Ledbetter WD (1982) Anatomy and innervation patterns of cat lateral gastrocnemius and plantaris muscles. Am J Anat 164: 67–77.

English AW (1984) Compartmentalization of single muscle units in cat lateral gastrocnemius. Exp Brain Res 56: 361–368.

English AW, Weeks OI (1987) An anatomical and functional analysis of cat biceps femoris and semitendinosus muscles. J Morphol 191: 161–175.

Enoka R (1995) Morphological features and activation patterns of motor units. J Clin Neurophys 12: 538–559.

Enoka RM, Fuglevand AJ (2001) Motor unit physiology: Some unresolved issues. Muscle & Nerve 24: 4–17.

Feng Z, Koirala S, Ko C-P (2005) Synapse-glia interactions at the vertebrate neuromuscular junction. The Neuroscientist 11: 503–513.

Fetz EE, Jankowska E, Johannisson T, Lipski J (1979) Autogenic inhibition of motoneurones by impulses in group Ia muscle spindle afferents. J Physiol 293: 173–195.

Fetz EE, Cheney PD (1980) Postspike facilitation of forelimb muscle activity by primate corticomotoneuronal cells. J Neurophysiol 44: 751–772.

Fleshman JW, Munson JB, Sypert GW, Friedman WA (1981) Rheobase, input resistance, and motor-unit type in medial gastrocnemius motoneurons in the cat. J Neurophysiol 46: 1326–1338.

Fournier E, Pierrot-Deseilligny E (1989) Changes in transmission in some reflex pathways during movement in humans. New Physiol Sci 4: 29–32.

Fritz N, Illert M, Reeh P (1986a) Location of motoneurones projecting to the cat distal forelimb. II. Median and ulnar motornuclei. J Comp Neurol 244: 302–312.

Fritz N, Illert M, Saggau P (1986b) Location of motoneurons projecting to the cat distal forelimb. I. Deep radial motornuclei. J Comp Neurol 244: 286–301.

Fritz N, Illert M, de la Motte S, Reeh P, Saggau P (1989) Pattern of monosynaptic Ia connections in the cat forelimb. J Physiol 419: 321–351.

Funakoshi H, Belluardo N, Arenas E, Yamamoto Y, Casabona A, Persson H, Ibanez CF (1995) Muscle-derived neurotrophin-4 as an activity-dependent trophic signal for adult motor neurons. Science 268: 1495–1499.

Furst DO, Obermann WM, van der Ven PF (1999) Structure and assembly of the sarcomeric M band. Rev Physiol Biochem Pharmacol 138: 163–202.

Gates HJ, Ridge RM, Rowlerson A (1991) Motor units of the fourth deep lumbrical muscle of the adult rat: isometric contractions and fibre type compositions. J Physiol (Lond) 443: 193–215.

Ghez, C. and J. Krakauer (2000) The organization of movement. In: *Principles of Neural Science*, Vol. 4, E.R. Kandel, J.H. Schwartz and T.M. Jessell, eds., pp. 653–673, New York: McGraw-Hill.

Goering JH (1928) An experimental analysis of the motor-cell columns in the cervical enlargement of the spinal cord in the albino rat. J Comp Neurol 46: 125–151.

Golgi C (1878) Intorno alla distribuzione e terminazione dei nervi nei tendini dell'uomo e di altri vertebrati. Rend Rist Lomb Sci Lett B11: 445–453.

Golgi C (1880) Sui nervi dei tendini dell'uomo e di altri vertebrati e di un nuovo organo nervoso terminale muscolo-tendineo. Memorie della R Acad della Scienze di Torino Serie 2, 32: 359–386.

Gorassini M, Prochazka A, Hiebert GW, Gauthier MJA (1994) Corrective responses to loss of ground support during walking. I. Intact cats. J Neurophysiol 71: 603–610.

Gordon AM, Homsher E, Regnier M (2000) Regulation of contraction in striated muscle. Physiol Rev 80: 853–924.

Gregory JE, Proske U (1979) The responses of Golgi tendon organs to stimulation of different combinations of motor units. J Physiol Lond 295: 251–262.

Grillner S (1985) Neurobiological bases of rhythmic motor acts in vertebrates. Science 228: 143–149.

Guertin P, Angel M, Perreault M-C, McCrea DA (1995) Ankle extensor group I afferents excite extensors throughout the hindlimb during fictive locomotion in the cat. J Physiol (Lond) 487: 197–209.

Guth L, Samaha FJ (1969) Qualitative differences between actomyosin ATPase of slow and fast mammalian muscle. Exp Neurol 25: 138–152.

Gutman CR, Ajmera MK, Hollyday M (1993) Organization of motor pools supplying axial muscles in the chicken. Brain Res 609: 129–136.

Hagbarth K-E, Wallin BG, Burke D, Lofstedt L (1975) Effect of the Jendrassik manoeuver on muscle spindle activity in man. J Neurol Neurosurg Psychiatry 38: 1143–1153.

Hagbarth K-E (1993) Microneurography and applications to issues of motor control: fifth annual Stuart Reiner Memorial Lecture. Muscle Nerve 16: 693–705.

Hall ZW, Sanes JR (1993) Synaptic structure and development: the neuromuscular junction. Cell 72 Suppl: 99–121.

Harker DW, Jami L, Laporte Y, Petit J (1977) Fast conducting skeletofusimotor axons supplying intrafusal chain fibers in the cat peroneus tertius muscle. J Neurophysiol 40: 791–799.

Harrison PJ, Jankowska E (1985a) Organization of input to the interneurones mediating group I non-reciprocal inhibition of motoneurones in the cat. J Physiol 361: 403–418.

Harrison PJ, Jankowska E (1985b) Sources of input to interneurones mediating group I non-reciprocal inhibition of motoneurones in the cat. J Physiol 361: 379–401.

Harrison PJ, Riddell JS (1989) Estimation of the projection frequencies of single inhibitory interneurones to motoneurones in the cat spinal cord. J Q exp Physiol 74: 79–82.

Heckman CJ, Binder MD (1988) Analysis of effective synaptic currents generated by homonymous Ia afferent fibers in motoneurons of the cat. J Neurophysiol 60: 1946–1966.

Heckman CJ, Binder MD (1991) Analysis of Ia-inhibitory synaptic input to cat spinal motoneurons evoked by vibration of antagonistic muscles. J Neurophysiol 66: 1888–1893.

Heckman CJ, Binder MD (1993) Computer simulations of the effects of different synaptic input systems on motor unit recruitment. J Neurophysiol 70: 1827–1840.

Heckman CJ, Gorassini MA, Bennett DJ (2005) Persistent inward currents in motoneuron dendrites: implications for motor output. Muscle Nerve 31: 135–156.

Hennig R, Lomo T (1985) Firing patterns of motor units in normal rats. Nature 314: 164–166.

Hongo T, Jankowska E, Lundberg A (1969) The rubrospinal tract. II. Facilitation of interneuronal transmission in reflex paths to motoneurons. Exp Brain Res 7: 365–391.

Hongo T, Ishizuka N, Mannen H, Sasaki S (1978) Axonal trajectory of single group Ia and Ib fibers in the cat spinal cord. Neurosci Lett 8: 321–328.

Horowits R, Luo G, Zhang JQ, Herrera AH (1996) Nebulin and nebulin-related proteins in striated muscle. Adv Biophys 33: 143–150.

Houck JC, Henneman E (1967) Responses of Golgi tendon organs to active contraction of the soleus muscle of the cat. J Neurophysiol 30: 466–481.

Houck JC, Singer JJ, Goldman MR (1970) An evaluation of length and force feedback to soleus muscle of decerebrate cats. J Neurophysiol 33: 784–811.

Hudson L, Harford JJ, Denny RC, Squire JM (1997) Myosin head configuration in relaxed fish muscle: resting state myosin heads must swing axially by up to 150 A or turn upside down to reach rigor. J Mol Biol 273: 440–455.

Hultborn H, Jankowska E, Lindstrom S (1971a) Recurrent inhibition of interneurones monosynaptically activated from group Ia afferents. J Physiol 215: 613–636.

Hultborn H, Jankowska E, Lindstrom S (1971b) Recurrent inhibition from motor axon collaterals of transmission in the Ia inhibitory pathway to motoneurons. J Physiol 215: 591–612.

Hultborn H, Lundberg A (1972) Reciprocal inhibition during the stretch reflex. Acta Physiol Scand 85: 136–138.

Hunt CC, Kuffler SW (1951) Stretch receptor discharges during muscle contraction. J Physiol (Lond) 113: 298–315.

Huxley H, Hanson J (1954) Changes in the cross-striations of muscle during contraction and stretch and their structural interpretation. Nature 173: 973–976.

Illert M (1996) Monosynaptic Ia pathways and motor behaviour of the cat distal forelimb. Acta Neurobiol Exp (Warsz) 56: 423–433.

Illert M, Kümmel H (1999) Reflex pathways from large muscle spindle afferents and recurrent axon collaterals to motoneurones of wrist and digit muscles: a comparison in cats, monkeys, and humans. Exp Brain Res 128: 13–19.

Ishizuka N, Mannen H, Hongo T, Sasaki S (1979) Trajectory of group Ia afferent fibers stained with horseradish peroxidase in the lumbosacral spinal cord of the cat: three dimensional reconstructions from serial sections. J Comp Neurol 186: 189–212.

Jackson A, Gee VJ, Baker SN, Lemon RN (2003) Synchrony between neurons with similar muscle fields in monkey motor cortex. Neuron 38: 115–125.

Jami L, Petit J (1976) Heterogeneity of motor units activating single Golgi tendon organs in cat leg muscles. Exp Brain Res 24: 485–493.

Jami L, Murthy KSK, Petit J (1982) A quantitative study of skeletofusimotor innervation in the cat peroneus tertius muscle. J Physiol 325: 125–144.

Jami L (1992) Golgi tendon organs in mammalian skeletal muscle: functional properties and central actions. Physiol Rev 72: 623–666.

Jankowska E, Lindstrom S (1972) Morphology of interneurones mediating Ia reciprocal inhibition of motoneurons in the spinal cord of the cat. J Physiol 226: 805–823.

Jankowska E, Roberts WJ (1972) An electrophysiological demonstration of the axonal projections of single spinal interneurones in the cat. J Physiol 222: 597–622.

Jankowska E, Johannisson T, Lipski J (1981a) Common interneurones in reflex pathways from group Ia and Ib afferents of ankle extensors in the cat. J Physiol 310: 381–402.

Jankowska E, McCrea D, Mackel R (1981b) Pattern of "nonreciprocal" inhibition of motoneurones by impulses in group Ia muscle spindle afferents. J Physiol 316: 393–409.

Jankowska E, McCrea D (1983) Shared reflex pathways from Ib tendon organ afferents and Ia muscle spindle afferents in the cat. J Physiol 338: 99–111.

Jankowska E (1992) Interneuronal relay in spinal pathways from proprioceptors. Prog Neurobiol 38: 335–378.

Kakei S, Hoffman DS, Strick PL (1999) Muscle and movement representations in the primary motor cortex. Science 285: 2136–2139.

Kanda K, Hashizume K (1992) Factors causing difference in force output among motor units in the rat medial gastrocnemius muscle. JPhysiol(Lond) 448: 677–695.

Kandel, E.R. and S.A. Siegelbaum (2000) Signaling at the nerve-muscle synapse: directly gated transmission. In: Principles of Neural Science, Vol. 4, E.R. Kandel, J.H. Schwartz and T.M. Jessell, eds., pp. 187–206, New York: McGraw Hill.

Kernell D, Eerbeek O, Verhey BA (1983) Motor unit categorization on the basis of contractile properties: an experimental analysis of the composition of the cat's m. peroneus longus. Exp Brain Res 50: 211–219.

Klein R, Silos-Santiago I, Smeyne RJ, Lira SA, Brambilla R, Bryant S, Zhang L, Snider W, Barbacid M (1994) Disruption of the neurotrophin-3 receptor gene trkC eliminated Ia muscle afferents and results in abnormal movements. Nature 368: 249–251.

Kriellaars DJ, Broenstone RM, Noga BR, Jordan LM (1994) Mechanical entrainment of fictive locomotion in the decerebrate cat. J Neurophysiol 71: 2074–2086.

Labeit S, Kolmerer B (1995) Titins: giant proteins in charge of muscle ultrastructure and elasticity. Science 270: 293–296.

Laporte Y, Lloyd DPC (1952) Nature and significance of the reflex connections established by large afferent fibers of muscular origin. Am J Physiol 169: 609–621.

Lawrence DG, Porter R, Redman SJ (1985) Corticomotoneuronal synapses in the monkey: light microscopic localization upon motoneurons of intrinsic muscles of the hand. J Comp Neurol 232: 499–510.

Lees-Miller JP, Helfman JP (1991) The molecular basis for tropomyosin isoform diversity. Bio Essays 13: 429–436.

Lemon RN (1993) Cortical control of the primate hand. Exp Physiol 78: 263–301.

Lemon RN, Kirkwood PA, Maier MA, Nakajima K, Nathan P (2004) Direct and indirect pathways for corticospinal control of upper limb motoneurons in the primate. Prog Brain Res 143: 263–279.

Lennerstrand G (1968) Position and velocity sensitivity of muscle spindles in the cat I. Primary and secondary endings deprived of fusimotor activation. Acta Physiol Scand 73: 281–299.

Liddell EGT, Sherrington CS (1925) Recruitment and some other factors of reflex inhibition. Proc Roy Soc, SerB 97: 488–518.

Lucas SM, Binder MD (1984) Topographic factors in distribution of homonymous group Ia-afferent input to cat medial gastrocnemius motoneurons. J Neurophysiol 51: 50–63.

Lundberg A (1971) Function of the ventral spinocerebellar tract. A new hypothesis. Exp Brain Res 12: 317–330.

Lundberg A, Malgrem K, Schomburg ED (1975) Convergence from Ib, cutaneous and joint afferents in reflex pathways to motoneurons. Brain Res 87: 81–84.

Luscher H-R, Mathis J, Henneman E (1984) Wiring diagrams of functional connectivity in monosynaptic reflex arcs of the spinal cord. Neurosci Lett 45: 217–222.

Maier MA, Armand J, Kirkwood PA, Yang H-W, Davis JN, Lemon RN (2002) Differences in the corticospinal projection from primary motor cortex and supplementary motor area to macaque upper limb motoneurons: an anatomical and electrophysiological study. Cerebral Cortex 12: 281–296.

Mantel GW, Lemon RN (1987) Cross-correlation reveals facilitation of single motor units in thenar muscles by single corticospinal neurones in the conscious monkey. Neurosci Lett 77: 113–118.

Marsden CD, Merton PA, Morton HB (1972) Servo action in human voluntary movement. Nature 238: 140–143.

Matsuzaka Y, Picard N, Strick PL (2007) Skill representation in the primary motor cortex after long-term practice. J Neurophysiol 97: 1819–1832.

Matthews BHC (1933) Nerve endings in mammalian muscle. J Physiol Lond 78: 1–33.

Matthews PBC (1962) The differentiation of two types of fusimotor fiber by their effects on the dynamic response of muscle spindle primary endings. Q J Exp Physiol 47: 324–333.

Mazzarello, P. (1999) Professor at Pavia. In: The Hidden Structure: A Scientific Biography of Camillo Golgi, H. Buchtel and A. Badiani, eds., pp. 101–117, Oxford: Oxford University Press.

McCrea DA, Rybak IA (2008) Organization of mammalian locomotor rhythm and pattern generation. Brain Res Rev 57: 134–146.

McDonagh JC, Binder M, Reinking RM, Stuart DG (1980) Tetrapartite classification of motor units of cat tibialis posterior. J Neurophysiol 44: 696–712.

McKeon B, Burke D (1981) Component of muscle spindle discharge related to arterial pulse. J Neurophysiol 46: 788–796.

McKeon B, Burke D (1983) Muscle spindle discharge in response to contraction of single motor units. J Neurophysiol 49: 291–302.

McWhorter DL, Walro JM, Signs SA, Wang J (1995) Expression of alpha-cardiac myosin heavy chain in normal and denervated rat muscle spindles. Neurosci Lett 200: 2–4.

Mendell LM, Henneman E (1968) Terminals of single Ia fibers: distribution within a pool of 300 homonymous motor neurons. Science 160: 96–98.

Mendell LM, Munson JB (1999) Retrograde effects on synaptic transmission at the Ia/motoneuron connection. J Physiol Paris 93: 297–304.

Mendell LM, Munson JB, Arvanian VL (2001) Neurotrophins and synaptic plasticity in the mammalian spinal cord. J Physiol (Lond) 533: 91–97.

Mendell LM (2005) The size principle: a rule describing the recruitment of motoneurons. J Neurophysiol 93: 3024–3026.

Milner-Brown HS, Stein RB, Yemm R (1973a) The contractile properties of human motor units during voluntary isometric contractions. J Physiol(Lond) 228: 285–306.

Milner-Brown HS, Stein RB, Yemm R (1973b) Changes in firing rate of human motor units during linearly changing voluntary contractions. J Physiol(Lond) 230: 371–390.

Miyazawa A, Fujiyoshi Y, Stowell M, Unwin N (1999) Nicotinic acetylcholine receptor at 4.6 A resolution: transverse tunnels in the channel wall. J Mol Biol 288: 765–786.

Monster AW, Chan H (1977) Isometric force production by motor units of extensor digitorum communis muscle in man. J Neurophysiol 40: 1432–1443.

Munson JB, Fleshman JW, Zengel JE, Sypert GW (1984) Synaptic and mechanical coupling between type-identified motor units and individual spindle afferents of medial gastrocnemius muscle of the cat. J Neurophysiol 51: 1268–1283.

Munson, J.B. (1990) Synaptic inputs to type-identified motor units. In: The Segmental Motor System, M.D. Binder and L.M. Mendell, eds., pp. 291–307, New York: Oxford University Press.

Nakanishi ST, Cope T, Rich M, Carrasco DI, Pinter MJ (2005) Regulation of motoneuron excitability via motor endplate acetylcholine receptor activation. J Neurosci 25: 2226–2232.

Nielsen J, Petersen N (1994) Is presynaptic inhibition distributed to corticospinal fibers in man? J Physiol (Lond) 477: 47–58.

Orlovsky, G.N., T.G. Deliagina, and S. Grillner (1999) Neuronal Control of Locomotion: From Mollusc to Man, Oxford: Oxford University Press.

Ounjian M, Roy RR, Eldred E, Garfinkel A, Payne JR, Armstrong A, Toga AW, Edgerton VR (1991) Physiological and developmental implications of motor unit anatomy. J Neurobiol 22: 547–559.

Patton B (2003) Basal lamina and the organization of neuromuscular synapses. J Neurocytol 32: 883–903.

Pearson KG, Ramirez JM, Jiang W (1992) Entrainment of the locomotor rhythm by group Ib afferents from ankle extensor muscles in spinal cats. Exp Brain Res 90: 557–566.

Pearson KG, Collins DF (1993) Reversal of the influence of group Ib afferents from plantaris on activity in medial gastrocnemius muscle during locomotor activity. J Neurophysiol 70: 1009–1017.

Pearson KG (2004) Generating the walking gait: role of sensory feedback. Prog Brain Res 143: 123–129.

Petit J, Davies P, Scott JJ (1994) Static sensitivity of tendon organs to tetanic contraction of in-series motor units in feline peroneus tertius muscle. J Physiol (Lond) 481: 177–184.

Pette D, Vrbova G (1999) What does chronic electrical stimulation teach us about muscle plasticity? Muscle Nerve 22(6): 666–677.

Pette D, Staron RS (2000) Myosin isoforms, muscle fiber types, and transitions. Mic Res Tech 50: 500–509.

Porter, R. and R.N. Lemon (1993) Corticospinal Function and Voluntary Movement: Physiological Society Monograph, Oxford: Oxford University Press.

Powers RK, Binder MD (2001) Input-output functions of mammalian motoneurons. Rev Physiol Biochem Pharmacol 143: 137–263.

Pratt C, Jordan L (1987) Ia inhibitory interneurons and Renshaw cells as contributors to the spinal mechanisms of fictive locomotion. J Neurophysiol 57: 56–71.

Prochazka, A. (1996) Proprioceptive feedback and movement regulation. In: Handbook of Physiology: Regulation and Integration of Multiple Systems, L. Rowell and J.T. Sheperd, eds., pp. 89–127, New York: Am. Physiol. Soc.

Proske U, Gregory JE (2002) Signaling properties of muscle spindles and tendon organs. Adv Exp Med Biol 508: 5–12.

Rastad J (1981) Ultrastructural morphology of axon terminals of an inhibitory spinal interneurone in the cat. Brain Res 223: 397–401.

Rastad J, Gad P, Jankowska E, McCrea D, Westman J (1990) Light microscopical study of dendrites and perikarya of interneurones mediating Ia reciprocal inhibition of cat lumbar alpha-motoneurones. Anat Embryol 181: 381–388.

Rathelot JA, Strick PL (2009) Subdivisions of primary motor cortex based on cortico-motoneuronal cells. Proc Natl Acad Sci U S A 106: 918–923.

Reddy LV, Koirala S, Sugiura Y, Herrera AA, Ko C-P (2003) Glial cells maintain synaptic structure and function and promote development of the neuromuscular junction in vivo. Neuron 40: 563–580.

Reinking RM, Stephens JA, Stuart DG (1975) The tendon organs of cat medial gastrocnemius: significance of motor unit type and size for the activation of Ib afferents. J Physiol Lond 250: 491–512.

Rexed BR (1962) The cytoarchitectonic organisation of the spinal cord of the cat. J Comp Neurol 96: 415–496.

Romanes GJ (1951) The motor cell columns of the lumbo-sacral spinal cord of the cat. J Comp Neurol 94: 313–364.

Rothwell JC, Gandevia SC, Burke D (1990) Activation of fusimotor neurons by motor cortical stimulation in human subjects. J Physiol (Lond) 431: 743–756.

Rotundo RL (2003) Expression and localization of acetylcholinesterase at the neuromuscular junction. J Neurocytol 32: 743–766.

Roy RR, Garfinkel A, Ounjian M, Payne J, Hirahara A, Hsu E, Edgerton VR (1995) Three-dimensional structure of cat tibialis anterior motor units. Muscle Nerve 18: 1187–1195.

Rubinstein, N.A., and A.M. Kelly (2004) The diversity of muscle fiber types and its origin during development. In: *Myology*, Vol. 3, A.G. Engel and C. Franzini-Armstrong, eds., pp. 87–103, New York: McGraw Hill.

Sanes JR, Apel E, Burgess RW, Emerson RB, Feng G, Gautam M, Glass D, Grady M, Krejci E, Lichtman J, Lu JT, Massoulie J, Miner J, Moscoso LM, Nguyen Q, Nichol M, Noakes PG, Patton B, Son Y-J, Yancopoulos GD, Zhou H (1998) Development of the neuromuscular junction: genetic analysis in mice. J Physiol Paris 92: 167–172.

Schachat, R., M. Briggs, and E. Williamson (1990) Expression of fast thin filament proteins: Defining their archetypes in a molecular continuum. In: *The Dynamic State of Muscle Fibers*, D. Pette, ed., pp. 279–292, Berlin: de Gruyter.

Schiaffino S, Gorza L, Sartore S, Saggin L, Ausoni S, Vianello M, Gundersen K, Lomo T (1989) Three myosin heavy chain isoforms in type 2 skeletal muscle fibers. J Muscle Res Cell Motil 10: 197–205.

Schmitt, T.L. and D. Pette (1990) Correlations between troponin-T and myosin heavy chain isoforms in normal and transformed rabbit muscle fibers. In: *The Dynamic State of Muscle Fibers*, D. Pette, ed., pp. 293–302, Berlin: de Gruyter.

Scott, J.A. (2005) The Golgi tendon organ. In: *Peripheral Neuropathy*, Vol. 4, P.J. Dyck and P.K. Thomas, eds., pp. 151–161, Philadelphia: Elsevier.

Sharrard WJW (1955) The distribution of the permanent paralysis in the lower limb in poliomyelitis. JBJS 37B: 540–558.

Sherrington CS (1892) Notes on the arrangement of some motor fibers in the lumbosacral plexus. J Physiol (Lond) 13: 621–772.

Sherrington, C.S. (1906) *Integrative Actions of the Nervous System*, New Haven, CT: Yale University Press.

Sheterline P, Clayton J, Sparrow J (1995) Actin. Protein Profile 2: 1–103.

Squire JM, Luther PK, Knupp C (2003) Structural evidence for the interaction of C-protein (MyBP-C) with actin and sequence identification of a possible actin-binding domain. J Mol Biol 331: 713–724.

Stein RB, Misiaszek JE, Pearson KG (2000) Functional role of muscle reflexes for force generation in the decerebrate walking cat. J. Physiol (Lond) 525: 781–791.

Sudhof TC (2004) The synaptic vesicle cycle. Annu Rev Neurosci 27: 509–547.

Swett JE, Hong C-Z, Miller PG (1991) All peroneal motoneurons of the rat survive crush injury but some fail to reinnervate their original targets. J Comp Neurol 304: 234–252.

Thomas CK, Johansson RS, Bigland-Ritchie B (1999) Pattern of pulses that maximize force output from single human thenar motor units. J Neurophysiol 82: 3188–3195.

Totosy de Zepetnek J, Zung H, Erdebil S, Gordon T (1992) Innervation ratio is an important determinant of force in normal and reinnervated rat tibialis anterior muscle. J Neurophysiol 67: 1385–1403.

Trachtenberg JT, Thompson WJ (1997) Nerve terminal withdrawal from rat neuromuscular junctions induced by neuregulin and Schwann cells. J Neurosci 17: 6243–6255.

Vallbo AB (1974) Afferent discharge from human muscle spindles in non-contracting muscles: steady state impulse frequency as a function of joint angle. Acta Physiol Scand 90: 303–318.

Vincent, A. (2001) The neuromuscular junction and neuromuscular transmission. In: *Disorders of Voluntary Muscle*, Vol. 7, G. Karpati, D. Hilton-Jones and R.C. Griggs, eds., pp. 142–167, Cambridge: Cambridge University Press.

Voss VH (1971) Tabelle der absoluten und relativen Muskelspindelzahlen der menschlichen Skelettmuskulatur. Anat Anz Bd 129: 562–572.

Vrbova G (1963) Changes in the motor reflexes produced by tenotomy. J Physiol 166: 241–250.

Vrbova G, Navarrete R, Lowrie M (1985) Matching of muscle properties and motoneurone firing patterns during early stages of development. J Exp Biol 115: 113–123.

Wallimann T, Eppenberger HM (1985) Localization and function of M-line-bound creatine kinase. M-band model and creatine phosphate shuttle. Cell Muscle Motil 6: 239–285.

Walmsey B, Hodgson JA, Burke RE (1978) Forces produced by medial gastrocnemius and soleus muscles during locomotion in freely moving cats. J Neurophysiol 41: 1203–1216.

Walro JM, Kucera J (1999) Why adult mammalian intrafusal and extrafusal fibers contain different myosin heavy-chain isoforms. TINS 22: 180–184.

Weeks OI, English AW (1985) Compartmentalization of the cat lateral gastrocnemius motor nucleus. J Comp Neurol 235: 255–267.

Whittaker VP (1984) The structure and function of cholinergic synaptic vesicles. The Third Thudichum Lecture. Biochem Soc Trans 12: 561–576.

Yamaguchi M, Izumimoto M, Robson RM, Stromer MH (1985) Fine structure of wide and narrow vertebrate muscle Z-lines. A proposed model and computer simulation of Z-line architecture. J Mol Biol 184: 621–643.

Zajac FE, Faden JS (1985) Relationship among recruitment order, axonal conduction velocity, and muscle-unit properties of type-identified motor units in cat plantaris muscle. J Neurophysiol 53: 1303–1322.

Ziemann U, Ilic TV, Alle H, Meintzschel F (2004) Cortico-motoneuronal excitation of three hand muscles determined by a novel penta-stimulation technique. Brain 127: 1887–1898.

4

DETERMINING CLINICAL OUTCOMES

CUTANEOUS SENSATION is evaluated at three levels: detection of threshold stimuli, integration of stimuli for spatial discrimination, and object recognition. Touch threshold is measured by Semmes-Weinstein monofilament testing (SWMT), a thoroughly validated procedure that predicts function moderately well. Vibration threshold is not determined routinely, as it does not predict function. Spatial discrimination is evaluated most often by measuring two-point discrimination (2-PD). This convenient but critically flawed procedure presents nonspatial cues that can be learned to improve performance without physiologic change. The grating orientation test has been designed to eliminate these problems, but has not been evaluated in the setting of peripheral nerve injury. Tests of localization also depend on spatial discrimination and often predict function, but have not been standardized. Until recently object recognition was tested with a variety of "pick-up" tests, but now the validated shape texture identification (STI) test is available. Manual muscle testing, a mainstay of physical examination, is

imprecise. Use of a hand-held dynamometer improves accuracy, as does measurement of grip and pinch strength with purpose-built devices. The results of electrodiagnostic testing correlate poorly with functional outcome. Frameworks for reporting the results of nerve repair have diverged widely from their World War II (WWII) origin in the Medical Research Council. The first outcome instrument validated specifically for peripheral nerve has been introduced recently by Rosén and Lundborg (2000). In accordance with current outcomes standards, reports of nerve repair are also graded according to the level of evidence they present.

RATIONALE AND ORGANIZATION OF SENSORY TESTING

Sensory testing was first undertaken to answer questions about human sensory physiology and neuro-anatomy (von Frey, 1895). It was not until the mid twentieth century, however, that objective sensory testing was used to evaluate the outcome of nerve repair (Moberg, 1958; Onne, 1962). The WWII experience raised questions that required more precise measures of outcome than those available, such as: How much could a nerve be shortened by excising damaged tissue before end-to-end repair is no longer possible? Did the timing of nerve repair matter? Was age a factor in outcome? Reproducible criteria were required that could be used to compare outcomes from center to center. Within a given center, it was necessary to establish criteria for satisfactory progress in the months and years after surgery. Poor progress was recognized as the harbinger of poor outcome and the potential need for reoperation.

Tests of sensory function were initially organized by the cutaneous end organ they were thought to stimulate (Frey, 1895; Finger, 1994; Norrsell et al., 1999). More recently, Dellon proposed a similar classification based on current understanding of the four types of receptor found in glabrous skin (Dellon, 1981). Although conceptually useful, this simplification breaks down when one considers that moving stimuli may excite not only rapidly adapting receptors, but slowly adapting receptors as well. In fact, most stimuli excite all four receptor populations to some degree (Chapter 2). Jerosch-Herold has modified an organizational scheme initially proposed by Fess to organize sensory tests hierarchically by the complexity of what is tested (Fess, 1995; Jerosch-Herold, 2005). The most basic tests are for the detection of threshold, most commonly light touch and vibration. The next level requires the integration of stimuli for spatial discrimination to determine two-point discrimination, grating orientation, or localization of stimuli in the hand. The third and most complex level is that of object recognition, which requires both movement and the temporal summation of acquired information. This hierarchical scheme will be used in this chapter because it satisfies both mechanistic and practical criteria.

SENSORY TESTING: THRESHOLD

Touch

MONOFILAMENTS

The study of sensory thresholds was initiated by Max von Frey (1895). He assigned specific functions to the cutaneous sensory receptors known at the time, and developed an instrument to test cutaneous pressure thresholds. A chuck similar to that used to hold drill

bits was modified to grasp hairs of various diameters by one end so that their opposite ends could be pressed against the skin. Each hair was modified to standardize the area contacting the skin, and the force produced by each had to be calibrated by pressing it on a balance. Half a century later, Weinstein standardized and simplified this cumbersome procedure by permanently mounting nylon monofilaments of varying sizes in individual plastic handles (Weinstein, 1993; Figure 4-1). Each filament was identified by the logarithm of the force produced, expressed in milligrams. This counterintuitive labeling resulted from Weinstein's desire to simplify the statistical analysis of results (discussed in Weinstein, 1993).

Extensive use of the Semmes-Weinstein monofilament test (SWMT) in the military by von Prince and Butler (1967) and Werner and Omer (1970) led to the formulation of a relationship between specific filaments and the level of sensory function present when they could be recognized. This relationship was strikingly similar to that later formalized by Bell-Krotoski (1990) (Table 4-1). Nonetheless, citing the lack of "unequivocal evidence that touch threshold is predictive of function," Jerosch-Herold (2005, p260) recommends that results be reported as the force of the smallest detectable filament rather than by descriptors of function. In addition to their counterintuitive labeling, the Semmes-Weinstein filaments have several potential shortcomings; testing with the full range of filaments is time-consuming, the smaller filaments are fragile and inaccurate once bent (Weinstein, 1993), the force applied may vary by as much as a factor of 8 depending on the angle of application (Levin et al., 1978), the geometry of filament tips is not uniform (Levin et al., 1978), and detected threshold varies with the duration of contact between filament and skin (Van Vliet et al., 1993) and the rate of application (Bell-Krotoski, Buford, 1997). Nonetheless, if filaments are in their intended structural configuration and are applied appropriately, the forces they generate are reproducible within a predictable range (Bell-Krotoski, Tomanicik, 1987).

In response to several of these problems, Weinstein developed the Weinstein Enhanced Sensory Test (WEST) (Weinstein, 1993). The five filaments in this hand-held device have oval tips to diminish the change in contact area during buckling, resulting in more consistent appreciation of applied force, and textured contact areas to minimize skidding of the filament along the skin. They are calibrated as to the force applied to facilitate the understanding of test results. Others chose the route of computerized,

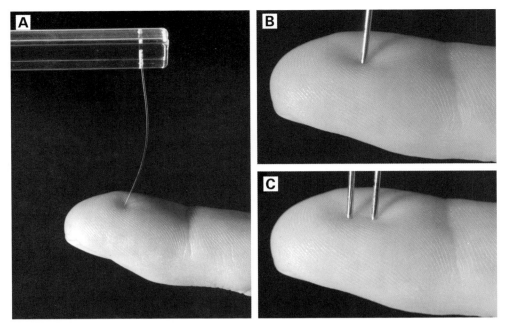

FIGURE 4-1   A. Application of a Semmes-Weinstein monofilament to the fingertip. The filament is perpendicular to the skin surface, and has just buckled. B,C. Testing two-point discrimination. The contact area of two points is always greater than that of one point, providing nonspatial cues that can be learned to improve performance without physiologic change.

Table 4-1 Interpretation of Semmes-Weinstein Monofilaments. The markings used to identify each filament are grouped with the corresponding forces produced by filament application. These have been divided, by consensus, into functional groupings, each of which is represented by a distinct color.

Color	Function	Filament markings	Calculated force (g)
Green	Normal	1.65 – 2.83	0.0045 – 0.068
Blue	Diminished light touch	3.22 – 3.61	0.166 – 0.408
Purple	Diminished protective sensation	3.84 – 4.31	0.697 – 2.06
Red	Loss of protective sensation	4.56 – 6.65	3.63 – 447
Red-lined	Untestable	> 6.65	> 447

Modified from Bell-Krotosky, 1990.

automated devices to evaluate sensibility (Dyck et al., 1978, 1993; Cohen, Dellon, 2001; Siao, Cros, 2003). These devices use a single probe, eliminating the variable of filament tip size, the rate and force of tip application may be controlled precisely, and testing algorithms have been chosen with great care. Although automated testing devices are applied most often to patients with peripheral neuropathy, they may also be useful in the evaluation of patients with nerve injuries (Cohen, Dellon, 2001).

A STATISTICAL DIGRESSION

Meaningful evaluation of the responsiveness, reliability, and validity of any sensory test requires the choice and application of appropriate statistical methods. These will be summarized briefly to facilitate understanding of the material that follows. *Effect size* can be used to measure the relevance of a change in health status over time, and is defined as the mean change in a variable divided by the standard deviation of that variable (Kazis et al., 1989). An effect size of > 0.2 is small, one of > 0.5 is moderate, and one of > 0.8 is large (Cohen, 1977). The *Pearson* and *Spearman* tests are used to evaluate the association between two continuous variables (Altman, 1994). The Pearson is a parametric test (it makes assumptions about the distribution of data) that evaluates the degree of straight-line association between two variables. The Spearman, in contrast, is a nonparametric test (it makes no assumptions about a linear distribution) that evaluates more general association; it is essentially a Pearson test performed on the ranks of the observations rather than the observations themselves. The results of both are reported as an *r* value, a measure of the scatter around an underlying linear trend, ranging from 0 for no association to 1 or –1 for a straight line. Confidence limits can be calculated for r values derived from either Pearson or Spearman tests. Although these tests are often used to compare the results of two testing methods, or the degree of intra- or interobserver reliability of a test, it is important to realize that they both assess only the association between two groups of data.

To measure the actual agreement between two sets of observations, one must calculate the kappa value, a chance-corrected measure of proportional agreement (Altman, 1994). The kappa value is often weighted to take into account the magnitude of disagreement between measurements. Alternatively, an intraclass correlation coefficient (ICC) may be used. Kappa values range from 0 for no agreement to 1 for

absolute agreement (< 0.2, poor; 0.21–0.40, fair; 0.41–0.60, moderate; 0.61–0.80, good; 0.81–1.00, very good (Altman, 1994). It is not unusual for a high r value to indicate a clear association between groups of measurements when the kappa value for the same data is low, indicating little agreement among individual measurements (Altman, 1994; Jerosch-Herold, 2005), and therefore limited ability of one test to predict the results of the other. Often, test results will be influenced by more than one variable. By removing the effects of one or more of these, one may assess the interaction of those that remain. Various techniques of regression analysis are useful for this purpose. The simplest, linear regression, allows one to predict one continuous variable from another. More commonly, multiple regression is used to evaluate the interaction of several variables. If the relation among the variables is not linear, a polynomial regression is required. If one variable is categorical, logistic regression is the appropriate technique.

EFFECTIVENESS OF THRESHOLD TESTING

The effectiveness of Semmes-Weinstein monofilaments has been subjected to repeated scrutiny. The responsiveness of both the SWMT (Rosén et al., 2000) and WEST (Jerosch-Herold, 2003) to changes over time has been confirmed, with substantial size effects of 1.5 between 3 and 48 months after surgery for SWMT and 1.2 between 6 and 18 months after surgery for WEST. The interrater reliability was found to be high, with an ICC of 0.965 (95% confidence limit 0.934) in a diverse group of patients including many with nerve injury (Novak et al., 1993b). In normal individuals, however, inter- and intra-observer reliability are were found to be only fair in one study (kappa = 0.40, median nerve), suggesting that comparison of normal and abnormal values may be unreliable (Rozental et al., 2000). SWMT has been validated as a predictor of function by correlation of threshold and object identification scores. In the study mentioned above (Novak et al., 1993b), the Spearman rank correlation coefficients relating pressure thresholds to the number of objects identified for each of two observers were r = –0.69 and r = –0.67 (95% confidence intervals –0.507 and –0.478, respectively), similar to the correlations found between two-point discrimination (2-PD) and object recognition (r = –0.73, r = –0.754). A polynomial regression analysis on the data from a second study of 18 patients (12 after median nerve repair, 6 with carpal tunnel syndrome) found that pressure threshold correlated strongly with time to object recognition ($p < 0.002$), but less so with number of objects identified ($p = 0.12$) (Dellon, Kallman, 1983). In contrast, after Marsh subjected Onne's published data to multiple regression analysis correcting for the effects of age, delay in repair, and follow-up time, the Spearman rank correlation coefficients were : 2-PD—$r = -0.22$, $p = 0.22$; threshold—$r = -0.66$, $p < 0.01$ (Onne, 1962; Marsh, 1990). Threshold tests, not 2-PD, emerged as the best predictors of function when patient age was removed from the equation. Tests of threshold have been proven to be fairly robust predictors of function. Nonetheless, significant questions remain unanswered: What does threshold mean in the context of regenerating nerve? Does the threshold for a given axon decline as it reinnervates progressively more receptors? Can bare axon tips fire, presumably at high threshold, before they contact end organs? Do increasing numbers of regenerating axons in the skin interact to lower threshold? Correlation of the physiology and microanatomy of individual regenerating fibers will be required to answer these questions.

Vibration

Traditionally, the ability to sense vibration has been evaluated by touching the skin with a vibrating tuning fork. This technique is fraught with inaccuracy, as application pressures vary from 2 to 25 g and vibration can be masked to varying degrees by the person holding the device (Bell-Krotosky, Buford, 1997). As patients are often asked to compare one hand to the other, any variation in application pressure would invalidate comparison of stimulus intensities (Novak, 2001). The development of mechanical vibrometers overcame many of these problems. In assessing a fixed frequency (120 Hz), variable amplitude vibrometer, Novak et al. (1993b) found a high interrater reliability with an ICC of 0.982 (95% confidence limit 0.967). Similarly, the results of evaluation with a multifrequency vibrometer correlated fairly well with those of SWMT (Spearman: $r = 0.56$, $p = 0.007$; Rosén, 1996). The results of vibratory testing have not, however, been found to correlate with hand function after nerve repair (Dellon, Kallman, 1983; Rosén, 1996). This technique has found its greatest applicability in the evaluation of patients with nerve

compression and peripheral neuropathy (Lundborg et al., 1986; Lundborg et al., 1992).

SENSORY TESTING: SPATIAL DISCRIMINATION

Two-point Discrimination (2-PD)

HISTORICAL PERSPECTIVE

The first detailed analysis of innervation density was performed in the nineteenth century by Weber, who applied the points of a compass to the skin to determine the distance at which they could be identified as two points rather than one (Weber, 1978). At a time when the modes of axon termination in the skin had not been defined, Weber believed "the skin is divided into small *sensory circles*, i.e., into small subdivisions each of which owes its sensitivity to a single elementary nerve-fiber" (Weber, 1978, p187). It followed that two points could be perceived as such when they contacted two separate sensory circles; the size and density of sensory circles in a given location would determine its discriminative capacity.

The validity of two-point testing as a measure of spatial discrimination was rapidly undermined by the discovery that results could be modified by both peripheral and central factors. Dresslar found that not only could the 2-PD in the forearm be reduced by repeated testing (21 mm to 4 mm in one individual, 33 mm to 3 mm in another), but this reduction could also be seen in the opposite, untested forearm (Dresslar, 1894); subjects could learn to interpret the test and improve results without a change in peripheral physiology. Results were often inconsistent, with two-point thresholds varying by as much as an order of magnitude in the same subject (Friedline, 1918). Alertness and attention were also found to play a role, so much so that 2-PD was applied to schoolchildren as a test of fatigue (Finger, 1994). The test fell from favor after wide criticism of a study purporting to show that Murray Island natives had more acute 2-PD than native Englishmen (discussed in Finger, 1994).

A fascinating anecdote recalled by Weinstein objectifies the role of central processing in two-point discrimination (Weinstein, 1993, p16). While working at Albert Einstein hospital in New York City he had the opportunity to test awake patients during craniotomy. He found that touch threshold as measured with Semmes-Weinstein monofilaments was not altered by stimulation of the cortex with electric current. Two-point discrimination, in contrast, was abolished on the contralateral side of the body by even weak cortical stimulation; removal of the stimulus restored normal 2-PD. From this experience he concluded that "pressure sensitivity is subsumed by subcortical structures . . . whereas spatial ability depends much more upon cortical integrity."

In the 1950s, Moberg evaluated the tests then available for assessing sensibility of the hand, as he had found them to be of little use in predicting the function of his patients. Not only did he reject the cotton wool and pinprick of the neurologist, he also noted that the Weber 2-PD test was "subjective," depending on the ability of the subject and examiner to concentrate, and was "apt to give a false impression" (Moberg, 1958, p456). Searching for alternatives, he initially proposed chemical tests of sweating as an objective measure of sensibility, but these were soon found to have little correlation with function (Onne, 1962). Moberg eventually settled on his "pick-up test" to evaluate what he termed tactile gnosis, "the complex sensibility that gives the hand sight" (Moberg, 1962). He then asked how tests of sensibility predicted function as measured by the pick-up test. The 10 patients he reviewed had index pulp touch thresholds between 0.5 and 2.5 g, and 2-PD between 8 mm and > 60 mm. The three patients who scored well on the pick-up test had the best three 2-PD scores—8 mm, 12 mm, and 15 mm. He concluded that "The determination of two-point discrimination with the Weber method is the only test, the results of which are scored in figures, which is reliable for testing the functional value of this sensibility" (Moberg, 1962, p19). Nonetheless, a touch threshold of 1 g or better was found in 4 patients, including all three who scored well on the pick-up test. His evaluation thus provides no sound basis for choosing one test over the other.

2-PD AND AGE

In 1962 Onne published a landmark study of sensory recovery after nerve repair, remarkable for its meticulous evaluation and documentation of results (Onne, 1962). Unlike others who reported on nerve repair at that time, (Nicholson, Seddon, 1957; Larsen, Posch, 1958; Sakellarides, 1962), Onne used statistics to evaluate relationships between some measures of outcome. After repair of the median or digital nerves, he found the results of 2-PD testing and tactile thresholds, measured with a modified von Frey device, to correlate significantly with one another. He did not attempt, however, to correlate the results of either test with function. Onne concluded, "it is not possible, however, to decide which of the two tests provides the more correct impression of the sensibility. From earlier work (the Moberg paper cited above) it is evident, however, that in general the 2 pd value is the more reliable" (Onne, 1962, p61). The recent resurgence of 2-PD as a test of sensory function thus rests on evidence that would not survive the level of scrutiny applied to studies published today.

Onne's paper is cited most often for its correlation of 2-PD and age. He noted that "Roughly speaking, the 2-PD value in millimeters corresponded to the patient's age up to 20 years" (Onne, 1962, p58). For the next two decades the assumption was that young age somehow allowed better recovery after nerve injury. This assumption was subsequently challenged by Marsh (1990), who, thanks to Onne's meticulous reporting, was able to subject his original data on 2-PD, touch thresholds, pick-up testing, and object recognition to multiple regression analysis. After correcting for age, 2-PD no longer predicted function, leading Marsh to conclude that "2-PD is not a valid index of sensory capacity underlying integrated hand function" (Marsh, 1990, p32). In other words, age did not act through 2-PD to influence outcome, but acted on 2-PD and outcome independently.

PSYCHOPHYSICS

Interpretation of the results of 2-PD testing is difficult because the process generates perceptions arrayed along a continuum of sensations, rather than two completely different sensations that correspond to one or two points (Tawney, 1895). These may include point, circle, dumbbell, and hourglass (Boring, 1921). In the clinic, patients may signal the ambiguous nature of two-point testing by responding "I can tell its not one" when asked if they are being touched with one or two points. The decrease in 2-PD seen with repeated testing is thought to result from increasing familiarity with this continuum, manifested as shifting criteria for one vs. two points (Johnson et al., 1994). The extreme is reached when patients are able to distinguish between one point and two points that are touching each other. Under these circumstances, they are clearly responding to nonspatial cues (Johnson, Phillips, 1981; Van Boven, Johnson, 1994b). This is possible because two points cover a greater area than one (Figure 4-1) and recruit more fibers to discharge, but at a lower peak impulse rate than that elicited by one point (Vega-Bermudez, Johnson, 1991). Drawing two points across the skin, the moving two-point discrimination test (Dellon, 1978), does nothing to alleviate this problem, as one and two points will always evoke different sensations regardless of the way in which they are presented (Johnson et al., 1994).

EFFECTIVENESS OF 2-PD TESTING

Testing of 2-PD has been evaluated thoroughly for responsiveness, reliability, and validity, often with a wide range of conclusions. The responsiveness of 2-PD testing—its ability to respond to progressive recovery over time—has been found wanting. A prospective, longitudinal study of 23 patients with nerve injury found 2-PD to have an effect size of 0.1 as compared with a value of 1.2 for evaluation of threshold by using the WEST device (Jerosch-Herold, 2003). A similar study that followed 14 patients for 4 years found an effect size of essentially 0, as there was no significant change in 2-PD over time (Rosén et al., 2000). Excellent interobserver reliability has been documented in nerve-injured patients by Dellon (linear regression analysis, $p < 0.0001$) (Dellon et al., 1987) and by Novak et al. (1993b; ICC = 0.991 for moving 2-PD, ICC = 0.989 for static 2-PD). The results of 2-PD testing vary dramatically, however, from center to center. At one extreme, Novak et al. documented 2-PD of 12 mm or less in 9/14 patients after median nerve graft (Novak et al., 1992). At the other, two experienced examiners found that only 1 of 40 patients with nerve repairs recovered 2-PD to 10 mm in one series (Jerosch-Herold, 2000), while 16 of 25 patients never regained 2-PD better than 16 mm in a second series (Rosén, 1996). As only the grafted patients received sensory reeducation with the two-point testing device, they had ample opportunity to adjust their perception of one and two points as discussed above. This could be an important factor distinguishing them from patients who had not had this opportunity.

The degree to which 2PD predicts function has varied according to the techniques of functional testing and data analysis. In two separate series Novak et al. found Spearman coefficients of 0.77 and 0.74 ($p < 0.005$ in both instances) (Novak et al., 1992, 1993a). After polynomial regression analysis of object recognition time and speed on four tests of sensibility, Dellon and Kallman (1983) reported that moving 2-PD correlated best with number of

objects identified ($p < 0.001$) while static 2-PD correlated best with the speed of identification ($p = 0.001$). The results are less consistent when regression analysis is used to correct for age. Marsh correlated combined pick-up and object recognition data with 2-PD results; he obtained an r of –0.79 ($p < 0.001$) on uncorrected data; this was reduced to only –0.18 ($p = 0.17$) after correcting the data for age (Marsh, 1990, p32). He concluded "2-PD is not a valid index of the sensory capacity underlying integrated hand function." In contrast, Chassard et al. (1993), evaluating patients with both median and ulnar nerve injury with an untimed object recognition test, found that 2-PD correlated significantly with function ($p < 0.005$), even after multiple regression analysis to correct for age.

Two-point discrimination thus has poor responsiveness, good intra-observer repeatability, but poor agreement among different centers, and a variable ability to predict function. In spite of these shortcomings, it is the test used most frequently to measure sensory function after nerve injury and repair (Chapter 5). This choice probably reflects the ease of patient testing and the need for only a single device to obtain results.

Grating Orientation Test

The physiologists K. Johnson, R. Van Boven, and J. Phillips, having rejected 2-PD as a meaningful test of spatial acuity (Johnson et al., 1994; Craig, Johnson, 2000), went on to design their own apparatus (Van Boven, Johnson, 1994a). This consists of a series of plastic domes, all 25 mm in diameter, that can be applied to the skin surface by a handle attached to their flat surface (Figure 4-2). The curved, testing surface of the domes is crossed by parallel rectangular ridges separated by grooves of equal width, ranging from 0.35 to 3.0 mm, and is applied to the skin in either transverse or longitudinal orientation. The closest spacing at which groove orientation can be detected in 75% of trials is the test result.

Whereas tests of threshold and 2-PD evolved through many years of trial and error, the grating orientation test was designed in accordance with current psychophysical principles (summarized in Van Boven, Johnson, 1994a). The skin surface area tested is always the same, eliminating the variability in contact area described above for 2-PD. The results of the grating orientation test are consistent with those of more complex tests that can only be resolved by spatial cues (Johnson, Phillips, 1981), and the

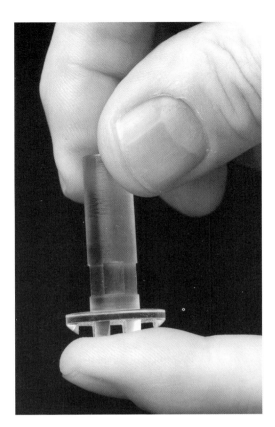

FIGURE 4-2   Application of the JVP grating dome to the fingertip. The device was designed for sensory testing on the face; it is difficult to bring the entire dome into contact with the fingertip.

test is known to evaluate primarily the function of the SA I (Merkel cell) population and provide reliable information throughout a wide range of application pressures (see discussion in Chapter 2). The grating orientation test has been evaluated in normal individuals and found to have excellent intra-observer reliability over time (Van Boven, Johnson, 1994a). When used in a battery of tests to evaluate sensibility after injury and repair of the trigeminal nerve, the test was the only measure of sensory function to correlate strongly with the patients' assessment of recovery (Van Boven, Johnson, 1994b). Although the grating test embodies current understanding of physiologic principles, it is difficult to apply to the fingers because of the relatively large size of the testing devices. It has not been evaluated formally in the context of peripheral nerve injury.

Stimulus Localization

Faulty sensory localization occurs when a stimulus applied to one area is perceived in another, distant location. This phenomenon was first described by John Mitchell in a 30-year follow-up of patients treated by his father, Silas Weir Mitchell, during the Civil War (Mitchell, 1895). More recently, Hallin et al. have mapped out areas of faulty localization after median nerve injury with great precision, and have shown that it persists in both adults and children for many years (Hallin et al., 1981). Individuals without nerve pathology can localize stimuli to within 1–2 mm on the fingertips and 5–6 mm in the palm (Weinstein, 1968; Nakada, 1993). Techniques of measuring locognosia, the ability to localize stimuli, involve dividing the hand into compartments and measuring the ability to identify the compartment within which the stimulus is delivered. The size of the compartments, the nature of the stimulus, and the scoring system have not been standardized (Marsh, 1990; Nakada, 1993; Rosén, 1996; Jerosch-Herold, 2003). Locognosia has been found to have a large effect size (0.9; Jerosch-Herold, 2003), excellent test-retest reliability (Jerosch-Herold et al., 2006), and a variable correlation with function. The ability to localize correlated with the ability to perform activities of daily living (ADL) (Pearson r = 0.57, p = 0.045; Jerosch-Herold, 1993), and to varying degrees with the pick-up test (Spearman r = 0.48, p = 0.001; Marsh, 1990; Spearman r = 0.29, p = 0.07; Jerosch-Herold, 2000). Standardization of the testing protocol and more uniform application of testing could well reveal a consistent relationship between the ability to localize and hand function.

SENSORY TESTING: OBJECT RECOGNITION

Moberg's primary goal in evaluating tests of sensibility was to see which ones correlated with hand function (Moberg, 1962). He divided function into "gross grips" and "precision grips," and devised the pick-up test to evaluate the latter. The patient was asked to pick up a series of small objects and place them in a small box as quickly as possible, initially with vision but then blindfolded. The outcome was scored simply as + or – based on a comparison of injured and uninjured hands. Soon thereafter Wynn Parry and Salter (1976) devised a test in which patients were asked to identify textures and objects while blindfolded. Performance was graded based on recognition time. These two approaches, timed manipulation and timed identification, were then combined by Dellon, who emphasized the role of motion in object identification (Dellon, 1981; Dellon, Kallman, 1983). Variations on this technique have been devised subsequently by several authors (Marsh, 1986; Jerosch-Herold, 1993; Novak et al., 1993b; Imai et al., 1996), pointing out both the usefulness of the concept and the lack of testing standardization—especially important, because these tests have been used repeatedly to validate tests of sensibility (see above).

Rosén and Lundborg have recently described a standardized object recognition test, the shape texture identification test (STI test) that has been subjected to rigorous evaluation (Rosén, Lundborg, 1998). Without the aid of vision, patients are presented with a series of objects (circle, cube, hexagon) of progressively smaller diameter (15, 8, or 5 mm) and a series of textures (1, 2, or 3 raised dots) of varying coarseness (dots separated by 15, 8, or 3 mm) (Figure 4-3). All 3 items in each category (shape, texture) at each level of difficulty (15, 8, 5, or 3 mm) must be identified correctly to score one point out of a possible 6 points. The test has a large size effect when evaluated in patients recovering from nerve injury over a 6-month period (ES = 0.73) (Rosén, Jerosch-Herold, 2000), and has been found to have good test-retest and interobserver reliability (weighted kappa 0.79–0.81 for the former (Rosén, Lundborg, 1998) and 0.66 for the latter (Rosén, 2003). Validity has been confirmed in the context of an overall evaluation of nerve repair outcomes (Rosén, Lundborg,

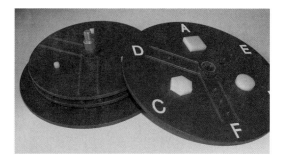

FIGURE 4-3   STI test. The device consists of three discs, each of which displays shapes and textures on a progressively larger scale. Each disc is placed on the platform at the left and rotated by the examiner to present a random sequence of shapes and textures to the patient, who identifies them without the aid of vision. Photograph courtesy of Ms. Brigitta Rosén.

2000). The STI test thus stands alone as a reproducible, validated test of object and texture recognition.

MUSCLE TESTING

Manual Muscle Testing

Manual muscle testing (MMT) has been used to quantify motor function in most studies of nerve repair. The results obtained with MMT are highly dependent on the technique used. Each muscle should be tested in a standard position with the extremity stabilized to prevent trick motions (Beasley, 1956; Sapega, 1990; Brandsma et al., 1995). In order to maximize force, one-joint muscles are tested near the end of the range of motion, while two-joint muscles are tested within the midrange of the overall length of the muscle (Kendall, 1991). Tests can be performed in either "make" or "break" fashion (Bohannon, 1992). In a make test, the examiner applies an isometric counterforce at the end of the range of motion and judges how much force is needed to offset the muscle being tested. In a break test, the examiner exerts enough force at the end of the range to overcome, or "break," the patient's contraction. The break test is usually preferred, as it maximizes the force exerted by the patient (Bohannon, 1992).

Strength of individual muscles is often graded using the ordinal scale established by the Medical Research Council (Medical Research Council, 1975) (Table 4-2): 0 = no contraction; 1 = trace, flicker or trace of contraction; 2 = poor, active movement with gravity eliminated; 3 = fair, active movement against gravity; 4 = good, active movement against gravity and resistance; and 5 = normal power. This scale has been expanded to include a variety of gradations between the integral scores (reviewed in Bohannon, 1992). The good, fair, and poor categories correspond roughly to 75%, 50%, and 25% of normal strength (Sapega, 1990). There is, however, great variability; patients with up to 50% loss of strength may be rated as normal (Beasley, 1956), those rated as fair may have anywhere from 6 to 32% of normal strength (Sapega, 1990), and experienced examiners have difficulty in identifying up to a 25% difference in strength between paired limbs (Beasley, 1956).

The reliability of MMT has been evaluated primarily in patients with neuromuscular disease and significant weakness. In this setting intra-examiner reliability can be excellent, with weighted kappa values of 0.65–0.93 for various muscles in patients

Table 4-2 Commonly Used Frameworks for Grading Sensory and Motor Recovery. Their evolution is described in the text.

Motor - Zachary and Holmes, 1946

Grade	Median Nerve	Ulnar Nerve
M0	No contraction in any muscles.	No contraction in any muscles.
M1	Contraction in the proximal (long flexor) muscles but they do not act against gravity.	Return of the voluntary power in the proximal (long flexor) muscles although they are not able to act against gravity.
M1+	The proximal muscles act against gravity but there is no return of power in the thenar muscles.	The proximal muscles act against gravity.
M2	The proximal muscles act against gravity and there is a flicker in the thenar muscles.	The proximal muscles are acting and there is a contraction in the hypothenar muscles at least, with either no action in the interossei or not more than a flicker.
M2+		The proximal muscles and the intrinsic muscles are acting, and the first dorsal interosseous muscle produces a definite movement but does not act against resistance.
M3	The thenar muscles act against resistance.	The long flexor muscles, the hypo-thenars and the first dorsal interosseous act against resistance.
M4	All muscles act against strong resistance and some independent action is possible.	As in grade 3 but some independent lateral movement of the fingers is possible.
M4+		Recovery to grade 4 but the independent movement is good although not perfect.
M5	Full recovery in all muscles.	Complete recovery.

Sensory - Mackinnon and Dellon, 1988

Grade	
S0	No recovery of sensibility in the autonomous zone of the nerve
S1	Recovery of deep cutaneous pain sensibility within the autonomous zone of the nerve
S1+	Recovery of superficial pain sensibility
S2	Recovery of superficial pain and some touch sensibility
S2+	As in S2, but with overresponse
S3	Recovery of pain and touch sensibility with disappearance of overresponse; 2pd >15mm
S3+	As in S3, but localization of the stimulus is good and there is imperfect recovery of two-point discrimination; 2pd 7–15mm
S4	Complete recovery; 2pd 2–6mm

Modified from Zachary, Holmes, 1946 and Mackinnon, Dellon, 1988.

with Duchenne muscular dystrophy (Florence et al., 1992), and 0.96 for testing of thumb abduction in patients with leprosy (Brandsma et al., 1995). Reliability was greatest for grades 1 and 2 (gravity eliminated). In a more diverse population in which muscle strength was graded as either normal or reduced, examination of intertester reliability resulted in a weighted kappa of only 0.54. When the results of MMT are compared to those of more quantitative tests of strength (see below), MMT is uniformly found to be less reliable (Aitkens et al., 1989; Schwartz et al., 1992; Escolar et al., 2001). Although MMT can discriminate reliably between injured and uninjured nerves (Aberg et al., 2007) the wide variability inherent in manual muscle testing has led experts to conclude "the results of manual muscle-testing are of little value except when there is a debilitating degree of muscular weakness" (Sapega, 1990, p1565).

Dynamometry

Frustrated with the vagaries of MMT, neurologists caring for patients with neuromuscular disease sought more reliable means of detecting modest changes in strength as disease progressed or was treated successfully (Drachman et al., 1974). Interposition of a hand-held dynamometer between examiner and patient provides quantitative information on a continuous scale, and is convenient enough for routine use. The technique may be compromised by excursion of the device with increasing application of force, leading to overestimation of strength and underestimation of weakness (Cook, Soutter, 1987); the examiner must also be strong enough to counter the patient's maximum force (Bohannon, 1997). The superiority of dynamometry in detecting changes not revealed by MMT was confirmed readily in patients with neuromuscular disease and spinal cord injury (Aitkens et al., 1989; Schwartz et al., 1992).

Dynamometry has been found to have high intrarater reliability in testing elbow flexion/extension in patients with ALS (Spearman r = 0.99; Beck et al., 1999) and spinal muscular atrophy (ICC = 0.98; Merlini et al., 2002). Testing thumb abduction in normals has both high intrarater (ICC = 0.92) and interrater (ICC = 0.89) reliability (Liu et al., 2000); extensive normative data are available (An et al., 1980; Boatright et al., 1997). In patients with nerve injury, testing thumb abduction with an industrial strain gauge yielded high correlation coefficients (intra-observer ICC = 0.96, interobserver ICC = 0.95), but the smallest detectable difference of 30–50% indicated that this technique was less reliable for detecting change in a given patient (Schreuders et al., 2000). Overall, hand-held dynamometry has high intrarater but only moderate interrater reliability (Bohannon, 1990). Recent approaches to improving the reliability of dynamometry include customization of the hand-held dynamometer for testing of specific muscles (e.g., Schreuders et al., 2004; ICC = 0.94–0.97, smallest detectable difference = 6.1 N) and the use of fixed devices that minimize tester variability (Escolar et al., 2001).

TESTING COMPOSITE STRENGTH

Tests of grip and pinch, actions that depend on the function of several muscle groups, have also been used to evaluate the outcome of nerve repair. The Jamar dynamometer (Figure 4-4), a test of grip strength, (Jamar; Smith and Nephew, Memphis TN) has been evaluated thoroughly by the hand therapy community. The device is highly accurate when tested against external standards with minimal variation among instruments (Harkonen et al., 1993; Mathiowetz, 2002). Recording the mean of three trials is recommended by the American Society of Hand Therapists (Fess, 1992) and has been found to produce the greatest test-retest reliability in normal individuals (Mathiowetz et al., 1984), though one trial may be adequate in those with pathology that results in pain with grasp (Coldham et al., 2006). In normals, intertester reliability is outstanding (Pearson r = 0.99; Mathiowetz

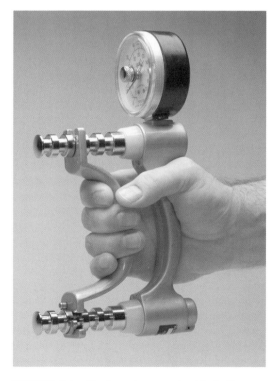

FIGURE 4-4   Testing grip strength with the Jamar dynamometer set in the third position.

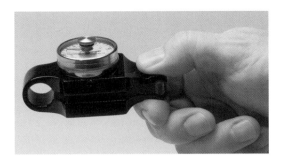

FIGURE 4-5   Testing key pinch strength with the Pinch Gauge (B & L Engineering).

et al., 1984; ICC = 0.98; Peolsson et al., 2001). Intratester reliability in normals is excellent but more variable (Pearson r = 0.883-0.929; Mathiowetz et al., 1984; ICC = 0.93; Nitschke et al., 1999) and is affected in women by hand shape; those with long hands produce consistent results (ICC = 0.92), whereas in those with square hands results are more likely to be variable (ICC = 0.476; Clerke et al., 2005). Intratester reliability is also excellent but somewhat variable in patients with upper extremity pathology: cervical radiculopathy, ICC = 0.90 (Peolsson et al., 2001); nonspecific regional pain syndrome, ICC = 0.95 (Nitschke et al., 1999); hand injury, ICC = 0.97 (Schreuders et al., 2004). Overall, the Jamar dynamometer is one of the most thoroughly scrutinized and reliable of devices.

Evaluation of pinch strength has been studied less extensively, but also appears to be reliable. Determination of key pinch in normals with the Pinch Gauge (B & L Engineering) (Figure 4-5) was found to have high intertester reliability (Pearson r = 0.98) and somewhat less intratester reliability (Pearson r = 0.832–0.870; Mathiowetz et al., 1984). In patients with nerve injury, intratester reliability was excellent (ICC = 0.97; Schreuders et al., 2004).

ELECTRODIAGNOSTIC TESTING

Intra-operative evaluation of conduction through damaged nerve has proven valuable in the diagnosis and management of incomplete nerve injuries (Kline, Hudson, 1995). Attempts to predict functional outcome on the basis of routine neurodiagnostic testing, in contrast, have been uniformly disappointing (Rosén, 1996). After nerve repair, the sensory nerve action potential (SNAP) may remain undetectable in up to 50% of patients (Tallis et al., 1978; Van der Kar et al., 2002). The signal is widely dispersed (Buchtal, Kuhl, 1979), reflecting both fiber heterogeneity and staggered regeneration (Chapter 9), and neither SNAP amplitude nor sensory conduction velocity correlate with restoration of sensory function (Almquist, Eeg-Olofsson, 1970; Tallis et al., 1978; Donoso et al., 1979). Parameters of motor conduction tend to increase more reliably with the passage of time (Donoso et al., 1979) and may be used to differentiate normal and injured nerve (Aberg et al., 2007), yet motor conduction velocity reaches a peak at 40–80% of normal (Tallis et al., 1978; Buchtal, Kuhl, 1979). A recent correlation of clinical motor function with a composite motor electrophysiologic score derived a weighted kappa value of 0.39, indicating only a fair correlation between the two measures (Van der Kar et al., 2002). Overall, these findings suggest that the recovery of electrical conduction is necessary but not sufficient to restore function, and that some other factor such as the specificity of regenerated connections plays a critical role.

Newer approaches to electrodiagnosis may yet provide functionally significant measurements. Techniques of motor unit number estimation (MUNE) have proven useful in the study of neuromuscular diseases (Scarfone et al., 1999; Doherty et al., 1995), and their successful application to the study of regeneration in nonhuman primates (Krarup et al., 2002) suggests the potential to quantify motor recovery after human nerve repair.

REPORTING FRAMEWORKS

The first published series to document the consequences of nerve injury and regeneration was not only the most detailed, but also provided the longest follow-up on record—30 years. Patients first described by Wier Mitchell during the Civil War (Mitchell et al., 1864) were reviewed by him in 1872 (Mitchell, 1872), and again by his son John Mitchell in 1895 (Mitchell, 1895). The Mitchell series was remarkable for the quality of observation and the precision of recording that formed the basis for detailed portrayal of individual patients. As war repeatedly focused attention on nerve injury and its consequences, however, the need for a systematic approach to reporting results became evident. This need was met initially by W. B. Highet, who devised general criteria for the grading of sensory and motor recovery (Highet, Holmes, 1943) (Table 4-2). The return of motor function was graded in five stages that accounted for both proximal and distal muscles, while sensory recovery was divided into four stages, the last of which included return of some two-point discrimination. Soon thereafter, Zachary and Holmes (1946) individualized the motor scale for specific peripheral nerves while adding intermediate grades of function. Unfortunately, they changed the nomenclature from "stages" to an M0–M5 scale that can be confused easily with the MRC scale for individual muscles. An "American" scale that included six grades of function was introduced at the same time, but has received little use (Woodhall, Beebe, 1956). The sensory scale was modified by Mackinnon and Dellon (1988) to include more specific 2-PD criteria (Table 4-2) as had been suggested by Moberg (1978).

The second half of the twentieth century witnessed a proliferation of scales for grading recovery. Some involved particular groupings of MRC/Zachary and Holmes ratings (Strickland et al., 1991), often with reassignment of 2-PD criteria (Birch, 1991). The Louisiana State University (LSU) scale, developed by Kline and Hudson (1995), reconfigured the MRC scale for grading individual muscles by shifting emphasis away from severe weakness. More gradations were introduced at the high end to better differentiate the wide range of patients formerly confined to grade 4, and the emphasis on 2-PD was removed from the sensory scale. A progression of sensory and motor recovery was then specified for each nerve. The greatest deviation from the MRC framework was undertaken by Millesi (1985), who generated a composite rating from the range of motion of all joints in the hand, the results of 2-PD testing and a pick-up test, and strength measurements; a normal hand rated 10,000. Although the LSU scale has been used extensively by Kline and his collaborators, none of the scales has been validated formally.

Recently, a validated instrument for the grading of outcomes after nerve repair has become available. Rosén and Lundborg developed a numerical scoring system based on the correlation between individual test results and outcome as judged by the patient (Rosén, 1996; Rosén, Lundborg, 2000). They sought out quantitative tests that had been validated individually, that changed during the process of nerve regeneration, that could be used to predict final outcome, and that were convenient and cost-effective enough to be clinically applicable. Patients were evaluated with a variety of tests, then a factor analysis was used to identify variables that were related to one another. This analysis identified a sensory domain, tested by SWMT, 2-PD, the STI

test, and selected elements of the Sollerman test (Sollerman, Ejeskar, 1995), a motor domain tested by MMT and grip strength, and a pain/discomfort domain evaluated by patient assessment of cold intolerance and hyperaesthesia (Table 4-3). The consistency within each domain was then confirmed using Cronbach alpha statistics. When this instrument was used to follow patients after nerve repair, recovery was documented by significant improvement in the outcome score (Rosén, Lundborg, 2000). Subsequent use by other observers has confirmed the effectiveness of this grading system (Vordemvenne et al., 2007).

Overall upper extremity status is often assessed with the disabilities of the arm, shoulder, and hand instrument (DASH). This rigorously validated, self-administered questionnaire evaluates disability and functional limitations in the context of activities of daily living (ADLs), work, and recreational activities (Hudak et al., 1996; Jester et al., 2005). The original 34-item questionnaire has recently been shortened to an 11-item version (QuickDash) (Beaton et al., 2005). In its frequent application to joint-specific problems, the DASH is equally responsive to proximal and distal complaints (Beaton et al., 2001); when used to evaluate a small number of patients with median nerve injuries, it was able to differentiate them from patients with other classes of problem. If validated more extensively in the specific context of nerve injury, the DASH may in turn prove useful in determining whether the results of a particular test truly reflect patient experience. In addition to the DASH, the Michigan Hand Outcomes Questionnaire (Chung et al., 1998, 1999; Kotsis and Chung, 2005; Shauver and Chung, 2009) and the Patient Outcomes of Surgery-Hand/Arm (Cano et al., 2004) instruments have been validated for use in the upper extremity, but have yet to be applied to the specific evaluation of nerve repair.

Reports of outcome after nerve repair must now be judged not only on the relevance of their findings to patient performance, but also on the design of the study that produced those findings. Within the last decade, the tenets of evidence-based medicine have been applied by many journals (Sackett et al., 1996; Spindler et al., 2005). Criteria have been established to grade the quality of evidence presented, so that clinicians may place appropriate weight on a paper's conclusions when making clinical decisions (Table 4-4). The majority of papers that describe the results of peripheral nerve repair fall into Level 4, or case series, and thus provide fairly weak evidence.

Table 4-3 The Rosén/Lundborg Instrument for Grading Recovery after Nerve Repair.

The vertical columns at the right are used to add up scores from successive time periods. The results are grouped into sensory, motor, and pain/discomfort domains.

Domain	Instrument & quantification		Month	Score*						
Sensory Innervation 	**Semmes–Weinstein Monofilament** 0 = not testable 1 = filament 6.65 2 = filament 4.56 3 = filament 4.31 4 = filament 3.61 5 = filament 2.83	Result: 0 – 15 Normal median: 15 Normal ulnar: 15								
Tactile gnosis	**s2PD** (digit II or V) 0 = ≥16 mm 1 = 11 – 15 mm 2 = 6 – 10 mm 3 = ≤5 mm	Result: 0 – 3 Normal ulnar: 15								
	STI–test (digit II or V)	Result: 0 – 6 Normal: 6								
Dexterity	**Sollerman test** (task 4, 8, 10)	Result: 0 – 12 Normal: 12								
	Mean sensory domain									
Motor Innervation	**Manual muscle test 0 – 5** Median: palmar abd Ulnar: abd dig II, V add dig V	Result median: 0 – 5 Result ulnar: 0 – 15 Normal median: 5 Normal ulnar: 15								
Grip strength	**Jamar dynamometer** Mean of 3 trials in 2nd position, right and left	Normal = Result uninjured hand								
	Mean motor domain									
Pain/ discomfort Cold intolerance	**Patient's estimation of problem** 0 = hinders function 1 = disturbing 2 = moderate 3 = none/ minor	Result: 0 – 3 Normal: 3								
Hyperesthesias	As for cold intolerance									
	Mean pain/ discomfort domain									
	Total score (sensory + motor + pain/ discomfort)									

*Scoring key: result/ normal

Reprinted with permission from Rosén, Lundborg, 2000.

Table 4-4 Levels of Evidence for Therapeutic Studies. The majority of follow-up studies of nerve repair fall into Level 4, and thus provide relatively weak evidence on which to base therapeutic decisions.

Level 1	• High-quality randomized controlled trial with statistically significant difference or no statistically significant difference but narrow confidence intervals
	• Systematic review[1] of **Level 1** randomized controlled trials (and study results were homogeneous[2])
Level 2	• Lesser-quality randomized controlled trial (e.g. <80% follow-up, no blinding, or improper randomization)
	• Prospective[3] comparative study[4]
	• Systematic review[1] of **Level 2** studies or **Level 1** studies with inconsistent results
Level 3	• Case-control study[5]
	• Retrospective[6] comparative study[4]
	• Systematic review[1] of **Level 3** studies
Level 4	• Case series[7]
Level 5	• Expert opinion

[1] A combination of results from two or more prior studies.

[2] Studies provided consistent results.

[3] Study was started before the first patient was enrolled.

[4] Patients treated one way (e.g. with cemented hip arthroplasty) compared with patients treated another way (e.g. with cementless hip arthroplasty) at the same institution.

[5] Patients identified for the study on the basis of their outcome (e.g. failed total hip arthroplasty), called "cases," are compared with those who did not have the outcome (e.g. had a successful total hip arthroplasty) called "controls."

[6] Study was started after the first patient was enrolled.

[7] Patients treated one way with no comparison group of patients treated another way.

Reprinted with permission from Spindler et al., 2005.

CONCLUSIONS

The clinical evaluation of sensation has progressed through the efforts of a small number of dedicated enthusiasts. Nonetheless, there remains a substantial gap between clinical practice, shaped by convenience, and the possibilities suggested by recent advances in sensory physiology. Inroads have been made, such as the design of the grating orientation test by physiologists in accordance with their experimental findings, yet this apparatus is difficult to apply to the hand. When evaluating spatial discrimination we still rely heavily on 2-PD testing, a convenient yet critically flawed procedure. Development of a convenient, physiologically sound testing device would thus be a substantial contribution. Similarly, the already promising tests of sensory localization could be standardized to facilitate comparison of results among clinical investigators. At the level of object recognition, the STI test is a standardized, validated procedure that can be recommended for widespread use.

Clinical evaluation of muscle function also relies heavily on an imprecise technique, manual muscle testing. The hand-held dynamometer, a more accurate yet still convenient tool, could help refine our ability to quantify muscle strength in the clinical setting. Purpose-built fixed dynamometers, though more cumbersome, could improve this accuracy even further. Ultimately, evaluation of dynamic muscle function, increasingly common in the sports medicine setting, could provide additional insights into the quality of muscle reinnervation after nerve injury.

The combined grading of sensory and motor outcomes, rooted in the consensus of the MRC system, has evolved along divergent paths. Only one nerve-specific outcomes instrument, however, that of Lundborg and Rosén, has been validated rigorously. It has set a new standard for clinical evaluation, and should enhance our ability to evaluate the utility of therapeutic interventions and to predict ultimate outcome from early progress.

REFERENCES

Aberg M, Ljunberg C, Edin E, Jenmalm P, Millquist H, Nordh E, Wiberg M (2007)t Considerations in evaluating new treatment alternatives following peripheral nerve injuries: A prospective clinical study of methods used to investigate sensory, motor, and functional recovery. J Plas Recon Aes Surg 60: 103–113.

Aitkens S, Lord J, Bernauer E, Fowler WM, Lieberman JS, Berck P (1989) Relationship of manual muscle testing to objective strength measurements. Muscle & Nerve 12: 173–177.

Almquist E, Eeg-Olofsson O (1970) Sensory-nerve-conduction velocity and two-point discrimination in sutured nerves. JBJS 52A: 791–796.

Altman, D.G. (1994) Practical Statistics for Medical Research, London: Chapman and Hall.

An K-N, Chao EY, Askew LJ (1980) Hand strength measurement instruments. Arch Phys Med Rehab 61: 366–368.

Beasley W (1956) Influence of method on estimates of normal knee extensor force among normal and postpolio children. Phys Ther Rev 36: 21–41.

Beaton DE, Katz JN, Fossel AH, Wright JG, Tarasuk V, Bombardier C (2001) Measuring the whole or the parts? Validity, reliability, and responsiveness of the Disabilities of the Arm, Shoulder and Hand outcome measure in different regions of the upper extremity. J Hand Ther 14: 128–146.

Beaton DE, Wright J, Katz JN, UECG (2005) Development of the QuickDASH: Comparison of three item-reduction approaches. JBJS 87: 1038–1046.

Beck M, Giess R, Wurffel W, Magnus T, Ochs G, Toyka KV (1999) Comparison of maximal voluntary isometric contraction and Drachman's hand-held dynamometry in evaluating patients with amyotrophic lateral sclerosis. Muscle & Nerve 22: 1265–1270.

Bell-Krotoski J, Tomanicik E (1987) The repeatability of testing with Semmes-Weinstein monofilaments. J Hand Surg 12A: 155–161.

Bell-Krotoski, J.A. (1990) Light touch-deep pressure testing using Semmes-Weinstein monofilaments. In: Rehabilitation of the Hand, Vol. 3, J.M. Hunter, L.H. Schneider, E.J. Mackin and A.D. Callahan, eds., pp. 585–593, St. Louis: Mosby.

Bell-Krotoski JA, Buford W (1997) The force/time relationship of clinically used sensory testing instruments. J Hand Ther 10: 297–309.

Birch R (1991) Repair of median and ulnar Nerves. JBJS 73B: 154–157.

Boatright JR, Kiebzak GM, O'Neil DM, Peindl RD (1997) Measurement of thumb abduction strength: Normative data and a comparison with grip and pinch strength. J Hand Surg 22A: 843–848.

Bohannon R (1997) Hand-held dynamometry: factors influencing reliability and validity. Clinical Rehab 11: 263–264.

Bohannon, R.W. (1990) Muscle strength testing with hand-held dynamometers. In: Muscle Strength Testing: Instrumented and Non-Instrumented Systems, L.R. Amundsen, ed., pp. 69–88, New York: Churchill Livingston.

Bohannon RW (1992) Manual muscle testing of the limbs: Considerations, limitations, and alternatives. Phys Ther Pract 2: 11–21.

Boring EG (1921) The stimulus error. Am J Psychol 32: 449–471.

Brandsma JW, Schreuders TA, Birke JA, Piefer A, Oostendorp R (1995) Manual muscle strength testing: intraobserver and interobserver reliabilities for intrinsic muscles of the hand. J Hand Ther 8: 185–190.

Buchtal F, Kuhl V (1979) Nerve conduction, tactile sensibility, and the electromyogram after suture or compression of peripheral nerve: a longitudinal study in man. J Neurol Neurosurg Psych 42: 436–451.

Cano SJ, Browne JP, Lamping DL, Roberts AH, McGrouther DA, Black NA (2004) The Patient Outcomes of Surgery-Hand/Arm

(POS-Hand/Arm): a new patient-based outcome measure. J Hand Surg Br 29: 477–485.

Chassard M, Pham E, Comtet JJ (1993) Two-point discrimination tests versus functional sensory recovery in both median and ulnar nerve complete transections. J Hand Surg 18B: 790–796.

Chung KC, Pillsbury MS, Walters MR, Hayward RA (1998) Reliability and validity testing of the Michigan Hand Outcomes Questionnaire. J Hand Surg Am 23: 575–587.

Chung KC, Hamill JB, Walters MR, Hayward RA (1999) The Michigan Hand Outcomes Questionnaire (MHQ): assessment of responsiveness to clinical change. Ann Plast Surg 42: 619–622.

Clerke AM, Clerke JP, Adams RD (2005) Effects of hand shape on maximal isometric grip strength and its reliability in teenagers. J Hand Ther 18: 19–29.

Cohen, J. (1977) *Statistical Power Analysis for the Behaviour Sciences*, New York: Academic Press,

Cohen MD, Dellon AL (2001) Computer-assisted sensorimotor testing documents neural regeneration after ulnar nerve repair at the wrist. PRS 107: 501–505.

Coldham F, Lewis J, Lee H (2006) The reliability of one vs. three grip trials in symptomatic and asymptomatic subjects. J Hand Ther 19: 318–326.

Cook DJ, Soutter DS (1987) Strength evaluation in neuromuscular disease. Neurol Clin 5: 101–123.

Craig JC, Johnson KO (2000) The two-point threshold: not a measure of tactile spatial resolution. Curr Dir Psych Sci 9: 29–32.

Dellon AL (1978) The moving two-point discrimination test: clinical evaluation of the quickly adapting fiber receptor system. J Hand Surg 3: 474–481.

Dellon, A.L. (1981) *Evaluation of Sensibility and Re-education of Sensation in the Hand*, Baltimore: Williams and Wilkins.

Dellon AL, Kallman CH (1983) Evaluation of functional sensation in the hand. J Hand Surg 8: 865–870.

Dellon AL, Mackinnon SE, Crosby PM (1987) Reliability of two-point discrimination measurements. J Hand Surg 12A: 693–696.

Doherty T, Simmons Z, O'Connell B, Felice KJ, Conwit R, Chan M, Komori T, Brown T, Stashuk DW, Brown W (1995) Methods for estimating the numbers of motor units in human muscles. J Clin Neurophys 12: 565–584.

Donoso R, Ballantyne JP, Hansen S (1979) Regeneration of sutured human peripheral nerves: an electrophysiological study. J Neurol Neurosurg Psych 42: 97–106.

Drachman DB, Toyka KV, Myer E (1974) Prednisone in Duchenne muscular dystrophy. Lancet 2(7894): 1409–1412.

Dresslar FB (1894) Studies in the psychology of touch. Am J Psych 6: 313–368.

Dyck PJ, Zimmerman IR, O'Brien PC, Ness A, Caskey PE, Karnes J, Bushek W (1978) Introduction of automated systems to evaluate touch-pressure, vibration, and thermal cutaneous sensation in man. Ann Neurol 4: 502–510.

Dyck PJ, O'Brien PC, Kosanke JL, Gillen DA, Karnes JL (1993) A 4, 2, and 1 stepping algorithm for quick and accurate estimation of cutaneous sensation threshold. Neurology 43: 1508–1512.

Escolar DM, Henricson EK, Mayhew J, Florence J, Leshner R, Patel KM, Clemens PR (2001) Clinical evaluator reliability for quantitative and manual muscle testing measures of strength in children. Muscle & Nerve 24: 787–793.

Fess, E.E. (1992) Grip strength. In: *Clinical Assessment Recommendations*, Vol. 2, J.S. Casanova, ed., pp. 41–45, Chicago: ASHT.

Fess, E.E. (1995) Documentation: Essential elements of an upper extremity assessment battery. In: *Rehabilitation of the Hand*, J. Hunter, L. Schneider, E. Mackin and A. Callahan, eds., pp. 185–214, St. Louis: CV Mosby.

Finger, S. (1994) *Origins of Neuroscience: A History of Explorations into Brain Function*, New York: Oxford University Press.

Florence JM, Pandya S, King WM, Robinson JD, Baty J, Miller JP, Schierbecker J, Signore LC (1992) Intrarater reliability of manual muscle test (Medical Research Council Scale) grades in Duchenne's muscular dystrophy. Phys Ther 72: 115–122.

Frey M von (1895) Beitrage sur sinnesphysiologie der haut. Sachsischen Akademie der Wissenschaften zu Leipzig Math-Phy Cl 47: 166–184.

Friedline CL (1918) Discrimination of cutaneous patterns below the two-point limen. Am J Psych 29: 400–419.

Hallin RG, Wiesenfeld Z, Lindblom U (1981) Neurophysiological studies on patients with sutured median nerves: faulty sensory localization after nerve regeneration and its physiological correlates. Exp Neurol 73: 90–106.

Harkonen R, Harju R, Alaranta H (1993) Accuracy of the Jamar dynamometer. J Hand Ther 6: 259–262.

Highet WB, Holmes W (1943) Traction injuries to the lateral popliteal nerve and traction injuries to peripheral nerves after suture. Br J Surg 30: 212–233.

Hudak PL, Amadio P, Bombardier C, UECG (1996) Development of an upper extremity outcome measure: The DASH (disabilities of the arm, shoulder, and hand). Am J Ind Med 29: 602–608.

Imai H, Tajima T, Natsumi Y (1996) Successful reeducation of functional sensibility after median nerve repair at the wrist. J Hand Surg 16A: 60–65.

Jerosch-Herold C (1993) Measuring outcome in median nerve injuries. J Hand Surg 18B: 624–628.

Jerosch-Herold C (2000) Should sensory function after median nerve injury and repair be quantified using two-point discrimination as the critical measure? Scand J Plast Reconstr Surg Hand Surg 34: 339–343.

Jerosch-Herold C (2003) Study of the relative responsiveness of five sensibility tests for assessment of recovery after median nerve injury and repair. J Hand Surg 28B: 255–260.

Jerosch-Herold C (2005) Assessment of sensibility after nerve injury and repair: a systematic review of evidence for validity, reliability and responsiveness of tests. J Hand Surg 30B: 252–264.

Jerosch-Herold C, Rosén B, Shepstone L (2006) The reliability and validity of the locognosia test after injuries to peripheral nerves in the hand. JBJS 88B: 1048–1052.

Jester A, Harth A, Wind G, German G, Sauerbier M (2005) Disabilities of the arm, shoulder and hand (DASH) questionnaire: determining functional activity profiles in patients with upper extremity disorders. J Hand Surg 30B: 23–28.

Johnson KO, Phillips JR (1981) Tactile spatial resolution: I. Two-point discrimination, gap detection, grating resolution, and letter recognition. J Neurophysiol 46: 1177–1191.

Johnson, K.O., R.W. Van Boven, and S.S. Hsiao (1994) The perception of two points is not the spatial resolution threshold. In: Progress in Pain Research and Management, J. Boivie, P. Hansson and U. Lindblom, eds., pp. 389–404, Seattle: ISAP Press.

Kazis LE, Anderson JJ, Meenan RF (1989) Effect sizes for interpreting changes in health status. Medical Care 27: S178–S189.

Kendall FP (1991) Manual muscle testing: there is no substitute. J Hand Ther 4: 159–161.

Kline, D.G. and A.R. Hudson. (1995) Nerve Injuries, Philadelphia: W.B. Saunders Company.

Kotsis SV, Chung KC (2005) Responsiveness of the Michigan Hand Outcomes Questionnaire and the Disabilities of the Arm, Shoulder and Hand questionnaire in carpal tunnel surgery. J Hand Surg Am 30: 81–86.

Krarup C, Archibald SJ, Madison RD (2002) Factors that influence peripheral nerve regeneration: An electrophysiological study of the monkey median nerve. Ann Neurol 51: 69–81.

Larsen RD, Posch JL (1958) Nerve injuries in the upper extremity. Arch Surg 77: 469–482.

Levin S, Pearsall G, Ruderman RJ (1978) von Frey's method of measuring pressure sensibility in the hand: an engineering analysis of the Weinstein-Semmes pressure aesthesiometer. J Hand Surg 3: 211–216.

Liu F, Carlson L, Watson HK (2000) Quantitative abductor pollicis brevis strength testing: Reliability and normative values. J Hand Surg 25A: 752–759.

Lundborg G, Lie-Stenstrom A, Stromberg T, Pyykko I (1986) Digital vibrogram: a new diagnostic tool for sensory testing in compression neuropathy. J Hand Surg 11A: 693–699.

Lundborg G, Dahlin LB, Lundström R, Necking LE, Strömberg T (1992) Vibrotactile function of the hand in compression and vibration-induced neuropathy. Sensibility index—A new measure. Scand J Plast Reconstr Surg Hand Surg 26: 275–279.

Mackinnon, S.E. and A.L. Dellon. (1988) Surgery of the Peripheral Nerve, New York: Thieme.

Marsh D (1986) Timed functional tests to evaluate sensory recovery in sutured nerves. Brit J Occup Ther 49: 79–82.

Marsh D (1990) The validation of measures of outcome following suture of divided peripheral nerves supplying the hand. J Hand Surg 15–B: 25–34.

Mathiowetz V, Weber K, Volland G, Kashman N (1984) Reliability and validity of grip and pinch strength evaluations. J Hand Surg 9A: 222–226.

Mathiowetz V (2002) Comparison of Roylan and Jamar dynamometers for measuring grip strength. Occ Ther Intl 9: 201–209.

Medical Research Council (1975) Aids to the Examination of the Peripheral Nervous System, London: Her Majesty's Stationary Office,

Merlini L, Mazzone ES, Solari A, Morandi L (2002) Reliability of hand-held dynamometry in spinal muscular atrophy. Muscle Nerve 26: 64–70.

Millesi, H. (1985) Microsurgical restoration of nerves and evaluation of results. In: Clinical neurophysiology in peripheral neuropathies, P.J. Delwaid and A. Gorio, eds., pp. 67–90, Amsterdam: Elsevier.

Mitchell, J.K. (1895) Remote Consequences of Injuries of Nerves, and Their Treatment. An Examination of the *Present Condition of Wounds Received 1863–5, with Additional Illustrative Cases*, Philadelphia: Lea Brothers.

Mitchell, S.W., G.R. Morehouse, and W.W. Keen (1864) *Gunshot Wounds and Other Injuries of Nerves*, Philadelphia: Lippincott.

Mitchell, S.W. (1872) *Injuries of Nerves*, Philadelphia: Lippincott.

Moberg E (1958) Objective methods of determining functional value of sensibility in the hand. JBJS 40A: 454–466.

Moberg E (1962) Criticism and study of methods for examining sensibility in the hand. Neurology 12: 8–19.

Moberg, E. (1978) Sensibility in reconstructive limb surgery. In: *Symposium on the Neurologic Aspects of Plastic Surgery*, S. Fredericks and G.S. Brody, eds., pp. 30–35, St. Louis: C.V. Mosby.

Nakada M (1993) Localization of a constant-touch and moving-touch stimulus in the hand. J Hand Ther 6: 23–28.

Nicholson OR, Seddon HJ (1957) Nerve repair in civil practice. British Medical Journal 2: 1065–1071.

Nitschke JE, McMeeken JM, Burry HC, Matyas TA (1999) When is a change a genuine change? A clinically meaningful interpretation of grip strength measurements in healthy and disabled women. J Hand Ther 12: 25–30.

Norrsell U, Finger S, Lajonchere C (1999) Cutaneous sensory spots and the "law of specific nerve energies": History and development of ideas. Brain Res Bull 48: 457–465.

Novak CB, Kelly L, Mackinnon SE (1992) Sensory recovery after median nerve grafting. J Hand Surg 17A: 59–68*.

Novak CB, Mackinnon S, Kelly L (1993a) Correlation of two-point discrimination and hand function following median nerve injury. Ann Plas Surg 31: 495–498.

Novak CB, Mackinnon SE, Williams JI, Kelly L (1993b) Establishment of reliability in the evaluation of hand sensibility. Plast Reconstr Surg 92: 311–322.

Novak CB (2001) Evaluation of hand sensibility: a review. J Hand Ther 14: 266–272.

Onne L (1962) Recovery of sensibility and sudomotor activity in the hand after nerve suture. Acta Chir Scand [Suppl] 300: 1–69.

Peolsson A, Hedlund R, Oberg B (2001) Intra- and inter-tester reliability and reference values for hand strength. J Rehab Med 33: 36–41.

Rosén B (1996) Recovery of sensory and motor function after nerve repair. J Hand Ther 9: 315–327.

Rosén B, Lundborg G (1998) A new tactile gnosis instrument in sensibility testing. J Hand Ther 11: 251–257.

Rosén B, Jerosch-Herold C (2000) Comparing the responsiveness over time of two tactile gnosis tests: two point discrimination and STI-test. Brit J Hand Ther 5: 114–119.

Rosén B (2003) Inter-tester reliability of a tactile gnosis test: the STI test. Brit J Hand Ther 8: 98–101.

Rosén B, Dahlin LB, Lundborg G (2000) Assessment of functional outcome after nerve repair in a longitudinal cohort. Scand J Plast Reconstr Surg Hand Surg 34: 71–78.

Rosén B, Lundborg G (2000) A model instrument for the documentation of outcome after nerve repair. J Hand Surg 25A: 535–543.

Rozental TD, Beredjiklian PK, Guyette TM, Weiland AJ (2000) Intra- and interobserver reliability of sensibility testing in asymptomatic individuals. Ann Plas Surg 44: 605–609.

Sackett DL, Rosenberg WM, Gray JA, Haynes RB, Richardson WS (1996) Editorial: Evidence based medicine: What it is and what it isn't. British Medical Journal 312: 71–72.

Sakellarides H (1962) A follow-up study of 172 peripheral nerve injuries in the upper extremity in civilians. JBJS 44-A: 140–148.

Sapega AA (1990) Muscle performance evaluation in orthopaedic practice. JBJS 72-A: 1562–1574.

Scarfone H, McComas AJ, Pape K, Newberry R (1999) Denervation and reinnervation in congenital brachial palsy. Muscle Nerve 22: 600–607.

Schreuders TA, Roebroeck M, Van der Kar TJ, Soeters JN, Hovius SE, Stam HJ (2000) Strength of the intrinsic muscles of the hand measured with a hand-held dynamometer: Reliability in patients with ulnar and median nerve paralysis. J.Hand Surg.[Br.Eur.] 25B: 560–565.

Schreuders TAR, Roebroeck ME, Jaquet JB, Hovius SER, Stam HJ (2004) Measuring the strength of the intrinsic muscles of the hand in patients with ulnar and median nerve injuries: Reliability of the Rotterdam Intrinsic Hand Myometer (RIHM). J Hand Surg 29A: 318–324.

Schwartz S, Cohen ME, Herbison GJ, Shah A (1992) Relationship between two measures of upper extremity strength: Manual muscle test compared to hand-held myometry. Arch Phys Med Rehab 73: 1063–1068.

Shauver MJ, Chung KC (2009) The minimal clinically important difference of the Michigan hand outcomes questionnaire. J Hand Surg Am 34: 509–514.

Siao P, Cros DP (2003) Quantitative sensory testing. Phys Med Rehab Clin N Am 14: 261–286.

Sollerman C, Ejeskar A (1995) Sollerman hand function test. Scand J Plas Reconstr Hand Surg 29: 167–176.

Spindler KP, Kuhn J, Dunn W, Matthews C, Harrell FE, Dittus RS (2005) Reading and reviewing the orthopaedic literature: A systematic, evidence-based medicine approach. J Am Acad Orthop Surg 13: 220–229.

Strickland, J., R. Idler, and J. Del Signore (1991) Ulnar nerve repair. In: *Operative Nerve Repair and Reconstruction*, R. Gelberman, ed., pp. 425–436, Philadelphia: Lippincott.

Tallis R, Staniforth P, Fisher TR (1978) Neurophysiological studies of autogenous sural nerve grafts. J Neurol Neurosurg Psychiatry 41: 677–683.

Tawney G (1895) The perception of two points not the space-threshold. Psychol Rev 2: 585–593.

Van Boven RW, Johnson KO (1994a) The limit of tactile spatial resolution in humans: grating orientation discrimination at the lip, tongue, and finger. Neurology 44: 2361–2366.

Van Boven RW, Johnson KO (1994b) A psychophysical study of the mechanisms of sensory recovery following nerve injury in humans. Brain 117: 149–167.

Van de Kar THJ, Jaquet JB, Meulstee J, Molenaar CBH, Schimsheimer RJ, Hovius SER (2002) Clinical value of electrodiagnostic testing following repair of peripheral nerve lesions: A prospective study. J Hand Surg 27B: 345–349.

Van Vliet D, Novak C, Mackinnon SE (1993) Duration of contact time alters cutaneous pressure threshold measurements. Ann Plas Surg 31: 335–339.

Vega-Bermudez F, Johnson KO (1991) Spatial structure of primary afferent receptive fields in the somatosensory system. Soc Nsci Abst 17: 840. (Abstract)

von Prince K, Butler B (1967) Measuring sensory function of the hand in peripheral nerve injuries. Am J Occup Ther 21: 385–395.

Vordemvenne T, Langer M, Ochman S, Raschke M, Schult M (2007) Long-term results after primary microsurgical repair of ulnar and median nerve injuries: A comparison of common score systems. Clin Neurol Nsurg 109: 263–271.

Weber, E.H. (1978) *The Sense of Touch*. H.E. Ross and D.J. Murray, trans., London: Academic Press.

Weinstein, S. (1968) Intensive and extensive aspects of tactile sensitivity as a function of body part, sex, and laterality. In: *The Skin Senses*, D. Kenshalo, ed., pp. 195–222, New York: Plenum Press.

Weinstein S (1993) Fifty years of somatosensory research: From the Semmes-Weinstein monofilaments to the Weinstein Enhanced Sensory Test. J Hand Ther 6: 11–28.

Werner JL, Omer GE (1970) Evaluating cutaneous pressure sensation of the hand. Am J Occup Ther 24: 347–356.

Woodhall, B. and G. Beebe, eds. (1956) *Peripheral Nerve Regeneration: A Follow-up Study of 3656 WW II Injuries*. Washington, DC: US Government Printing Office.

Wynn Parry CB, Salter M (1976) Sensory re-education after median nerve lesions. Hand 8: 250–257.

Zachary RB, Holmes W (1946) Primary suture of nerves. SG&O 82: 632–651.

5

CLINICAL NERVE REPAIR
AND GRAFTING

THE ANATOMY of the median, ulnar, radial, accessory, facial, and sciatic nerves is described as a basis for the discussion of outcomes. Clinical outcomes are derived from a meta-analysis of the literature, as well as from well-documented clinical series that focus on a specific question. Analysis of median and ulnar nerve repair and grafting established that (1) Age is the primary determinant of outcome after neural repair or grafting, (2) The proximo-distal level of injury influences motor but not sensory recovery, (3) Delay in repair adversely affects outcome, (4) Functional recovery decreases as the severity of injury to the nerve increases, (5) The use of the operating microscope and microsutures improves the results of nerve repair, (6) Functional restoration after nerve grafting deteriorates as graft length increases, and (7) The outcome of nerve grafting is equal to that of nerve repair in distal nerves that serve a single function. Including additional nerves in the analysis revealed that (1) False sensory localization after median nerve repair and synkinesis after facial nerve repair suggest the absence of

topographic specificity in both sensory and motor regeneration; (2) Results of radial nerve repair are consistent with loss of motor axons into proximal muscles, compromising the reinnervation of distal muscles; and (3) The regeneration possible in the sciatic nerve indicates that regeneration from the brachial plexus to the hand should be physiologically possible. Many of these clinical findings can be restated biologically in terms of intraneural organization, the effects of denervation time on regeneration, and age-related changes in gene expression. This restatement facilitates the design of strategies to improve the persistently disappointing results of nerve repair and grafting.

INTRODUCTION

This chapter summarizes published results of peripheral nerve repair and grafting. These results are then analyzed with two goals in mind. First, it is important to realize where our therapies are effective and where they remain lacking, so that we can focus research efforts on the areas of greatest need. Second, as a prerequisite for experimentation, clinical findings are restated in biologic terms. The outcome of each nerve repair is modified by a series of primary clinical variables such as patient age, level of injury, and delay in treatment. Clinical variables must then be expressed in biologic terms, such as severity of injury to the neuron, regeneration speed, or duration of pathway and end organ denervation. Several sections of this chapter include attempts to use clinical data to define at least some of these biological variables. Once identified, they can be subject to experimentation to define both their relative influences and the nature of their underlying mechanisms. Chapter 7, a review of experimental outcomes, will show which biologic variables have been subject to experimental analysis and what we have learned about their role in shaping outcomes.

In 1972, Paul Brown summarized what he believed to be the factors influencing the outcome of nerve repair: (1) type of nerve; (2) age of patient; (3) level of injury; (4) length of defect; (5) associated injuries; (6) surgical technique; and (7) delay till surgery. Evidence, largely in favor of the action of these factors, has been deduced from many subsequent clinical series. However, published reports vary widely in quality. Analysis of any one variable can be valid only when the impact of the others has been controlled for or eliminated. Unfortunately, isolation of one variable is difficult when publications are compromised by such factors as inclusion of partial injuries, inclusion of data from all age groups without stratification by age, or evaluation of results by idiosyncratic grading schemes (reviewed in Brushart, 1998). In this review, two strategies have been used to overcome these shortcomings. Most published data on end-to-end nerve suture have been summarized by grouping strategies, selected by their authors to emphasize the effect of a particular variable such as age. When these groups have been carefully defined, it is possible to extract data to evaluate the impact of a single variable. For instance, this review begins by summarizing the results of primary repair of sharp median nerve lacerations at wrist and distal forearm levels in adults in order to minimize the consequences of delay, length of defect, associated injuries, level of injury, and patient age. The results of nerve grafting, in contrast, have often been published with variables such as age, delay to repair, and gap length listed in tabular form, permitting meta-analysis to reveal the influence of each variable.

The median, ulnar, and digital nerves are addressed first, as they are represented by the bulk of available reports and provide the most information on the variables mentioned above. Other nerves are included to examine additional issues, such as the clues provided by the sciatic nerve on the maximum distance over which peripheral axons may regenerate, and by the facial nerve on the specificity of muscle reinnervation. Data from the brachial plexus are used sparingly, as it is difficult to isolate the effects of a single factor in a system with so many components, each of which may be injured to a different degree. In each instance, data have been chosen to illustrate a specific biologic principle; no attempt has been made to provide an exhaustive clinical review.

In this chapter, results are graded according to the MRC scale (Chapter 4). Although this grading system is moderately subjective, it has been used in the majority of published clinical reports. In one recent study, the results of MRC grading were found to be in excellent agreement with those obtained using the Rosén instrument (Vordemvenne et al., 2007). The following analysis contains several comparisons in which outcomes are characterized by the number of patients achieving levels <S3, S3, S3+, or S4 in the sensory system and levels <M3, M3, M4, or M5 in the motor system. The long linear model homogeneity test and Chi Square test were first applied to ascertain whether there were indeed differences in overall patient distribution between the groups to be compared. If the groups were found to be different, two-sample binomial tests were then applied to compare the groups at each level of outcome, i.e., did the proportion of patients achieving S3 differ between young patients and old patients. Sufficient information was available on individual cases of nerve grafting to allow multivariant analysis of the impact of age, gap length, and delay on outcome.

The terminology applied to peripheral nerve surgery may be confusing. Some authors use the term "repair" to include both end-to-end nerve suture and nerve grafting. In this text, the terms "nerve repair" and "nerve suture" will be used interchangeably to describe the reunion of cut nerve ends with microsuture. Although we are not actually repairing the nerve, this term has gained currency through over a century of use. If the ends are held together with some other material, the name of this material would be added to the description, e.g., fibrin glue repair. The more cumbersome term "end-to-end nerve suture," though clearly descriptive, will be reserved for comparisons involving procedures such as end-to-side repair. The term "nerve grafting" is unambiguous, and refers to the bridging of a nerve gap with a portion of peripheral nerve taken from elsewhere on the patient. If another material is used to bridge the gap, this material will be named, such as allograft or muscle graft.

The majority of p values presented in this chapter result from secondary analyses of published data. However, statistical information is often provided in more recent publications. To differentiate between the two, the abbreviation PA will stand for "published analysis," that already available in the literature, and AA will stand for "author's analysis," that performed specifically for this text. All clinical papers provide Level IV evidence (Chapter 4, Table 4-4) unless specified otherwise.

THE MEDIAN AND ULNAR NERVES AND THEIR DIGITAL TRIBUTARIES

Anatomy

The median nerve is formed by the juncture of the medial and lateral chords of the brachial plexus. As a result of this broad origin, it receives axons from C6, C7, C8, and T1 roots. The nerve descends through the arm anterior to the medial intermuscular plane, giving off no significant branches above the elbow. It traverses the elbow joint capsule between the pronator teres medially and the biceps tendon laterally, then enters the forearm between the heads of the pronator teres (Figure 5-1). Branches in the elbow area supply the pronator teres, flexor carpi radialis, and palmaris longus muscles, and the anterior interosseous nerve. The latter continues distally to innervate the radial profundus muscles, the flexor pollicis longus, and the pronator quadratus. The median nerve continues to the wrist in the plane between the profundus and sublimis muscles, innervating the sublimis as it goes. A palmar cutaneous branch is also given off proximal to the wrist. The median nerve enters the hand through the carpal tunnel (Figure 5-2). Immediately distal to the tunnel, the recurrent motor branch ramifies to innervate the flexor pollicis brevis, abductor policis brevis, and opponens pollicis. After giving off the motor branch, the nerve arborizes to form the common digital nerves and minute branches to the radial lumbrical muscles (summarized from Sunderland, 1978).

The ulnar nerve arises from the medial cord of the brachial plexus, receiving contributions from the C8 and T1 cervical roots. It enters the arm adjacent to the coracobrachialis on the anterior aspect of the medial intermuscular septum. After passing the humeral insertion of the coracobrachialis, it penetrates the septum from anterior to posterior and continues distally on the anteromedial surface of the triceps. At the elbow, the nerve is confined within the cubital tunnel posterior to the medial humeral epicondyle (Figure 5-3). It emerges from the tunnel distally to enter the forearm between the two heads of the flexor carpi ulnaris, then courses to the wrist between the flexor carpi ulnaris anteriorly and the flexor digitorum profundus posteriorly. The flexor carpi ulnaris usually receives 2–4 muscular branches just distal to the epicondyle, and the flexor digitorum profundus to the ring and small fingers receives a single branch immediately thereafter. The dorsal cutaneous nerve, which innervates the ulnar territory on the dorsum of the hand, arises 5–10 cm proximal to the wrist and spirals distally and dorsally around the ulna.

The ulnar nerve enters the hand through Guyon's canal (Figure 5-4). This passageway lies superficial to the transverse carpal and piso-hamate ligaments, deep to the palmaris brevis, and is bounded ulnarly by the pisiform and radially by the hook of the hamate. The nerve splits into superficial (cutaneous) and deep (muscular) divisions within the canal. Branches to the hypothenar muscles also arise in this area. The abductor digiti minimi receives one or two branches from the ulnar trunk or its deep branch, after which the flexor digiti minimi and opponens digiti minimi are supplied from the deep branch.

Upon exiting Guyon's canal, the superficial branch divides into a palmar digital branch to the ulnar side of the small finger and a common digital branch to the fourth webspace. The deep branch spirals deep and radialward around the hook of the hamate, passing between the abductor and flexor digiti minimi. It then penetrates the opponens digiti minimi to lie beneath the profundus tendons and directly on the interosseous muscles, which it innervates sequentially as it passes radialward across the palm. The third and fourth lumbrical muscles are usually innervated from the subjacent interosseous branches, and the adductor pollicis and flexor pollicis brevis (ulnar head) from the terminal fibers of the deep branch (summarized from Sunderland, 1978).

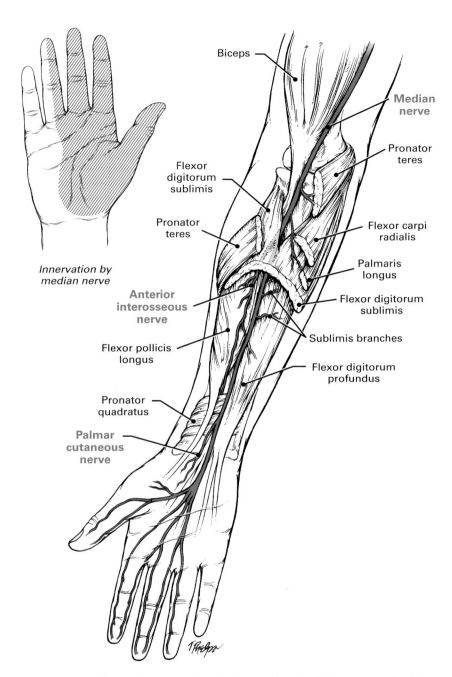

Biceps

Median
nerve

Pronator
teres

Flexor
digitorum
sublimis

Pronator
teres

Flexor carpi
radialis

Palmaris
longus

Flexor digitorum
sublimis

*Innervation by
median nerve*

Anterior
interosseous
nerve

Sublimis branches

Flexor pollicis
longus

Flexor digitorum
profundus

Pronator
quadratus

Palmar
cutaneous
nerve

FIGURE 5-1   The course of the median nerve from distal arm to hand and the structures that it innervates in the forearm. The bellies and distal tendons of the flexor carpi radialis, palmaris longus, and flexor digitorum sublimis have been cut away to expose the median nerve in the mid and distal forearm. The entire flexor digitorum profundus system is shown, even though the ulnar portion is innervated by the ulnar nerve. The anatomy portrayed in this and subsequent plates is described in detail in the text.

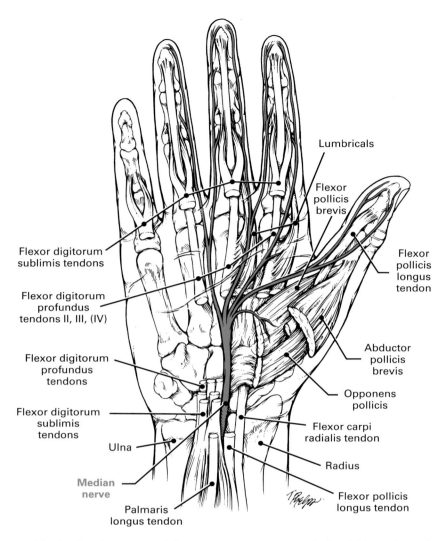

Lumbricals

Flexor pollicis brevis

Flexor pollicis longus tendon

Flexor digitorum sublimis tendons

Flexor digitorum profundus tendons II, III, (IV)

Flexor digitorum profundus tendons

Abductor pollicis brevis

Opponens pollicis

Flexor digitorum sublimis tendons

Flexor carpi radialis tendon

Ulna

Radius

Median nerve

Flexor pollicis longus tendon

Palmaris longus tendon

FIGURE 5-2   The distal median nerve and the structures it innervates in the hand. The tendons of median-innervated long flexors and the origins of median-innervated thenar muscles have been cut away to expose the palmar area. The lumbricals to the index and middle fingers are innervated by branches of the common digital nerves.

The digital nerves are the terminal branches of the median and ulnar nerves in the hand (Figures 5-2, 5-4). At its point of arborization in the palm the median nerve provides a short common digital nerve that rapidly divides into the two digital nerves to the thumb, a single digital nerve to the radial aspect of the index finger, and common digital nerves that bifurcate to serve both sides of the second and third webspaces. The ulnar nerve supplies a common digital nerve to the fourth webspace and a single nerve to the ulnar aspect of the small finger.

The digital nerves supply the entire cutaneous territory they traverse, so they are constantly giving off small branches to overlying skin. A dorsal digital branch is given off distal to the metacarpophalyngeal joint (knuckle joint) in the fingers, and serves the dorso-lateral aspect of the digit and the dorsal surface of a variable portion of the digit tip.

Median and Ulnar Nerve Repair

Review of the current literature identified 10 clinical series from which it was possible to extract cases

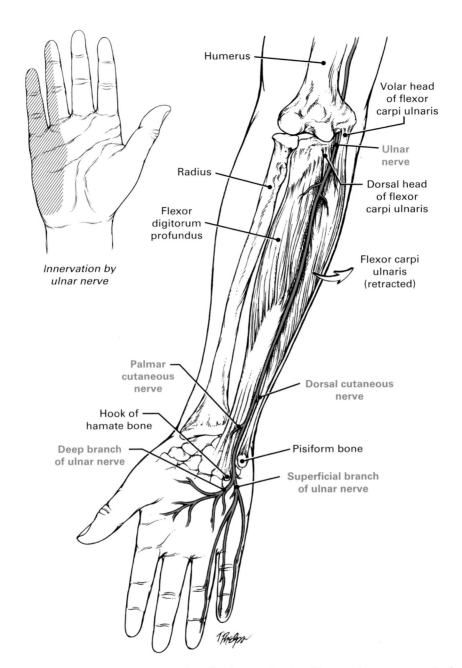

Innervation by
ulnar nerve

FIGURE 5-3 The course of the ulnar nerve from distal arm to hand and the muscles it innervates in the forearm. The belly of the flexor carpi ulnaris has been retracted ulnarly to reveal the nerve beneath it.

that met strict criteria for standardization (Lijftogt et al., 1987; Jongen, Van Twisk, 1988; Rogers et al., 1990; Birch, 1991; Strickland et al., 1991; Chassard et al., 1993; Imai et al., 1996 [evidence level 3]; Rosen, 1996; Kato et al., 1998; Selma et al., 1998). To obtain adequate numbers, series were included, as noted, if one criterion was violated to a minor degree. These criteria were: (1) age at least 17 years (except Birch, 1991, which included patients down to age 15), (2) minimum follow-up of 2 years (except Jongen, Van Twisk, 1988, and Chassard et al., 1993), (3) sharp injury, (4) wrist

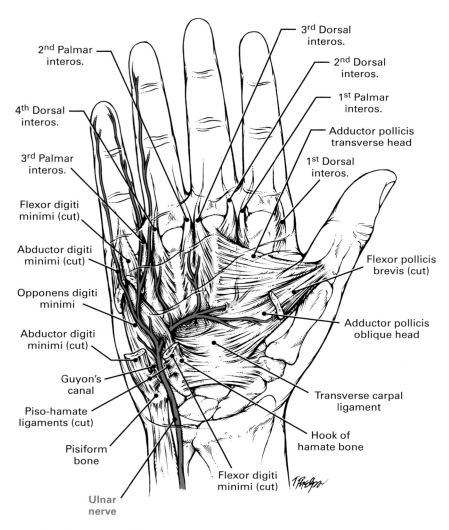

2nd Palmar
interos.

4th Dorsal
interos.

3rd Palmar
interos.

Flexor digiti
minimi (cut)

Abductor digiti
minimi (cut)

Opponens digiti
minimi

Abductor digiti
minimi (cut)

Guyon's
canal

Piso-hamate
ligaments (cut)

Pisiform
bone

Ulnar
nerve

Flexor digiti
minimi (cut)

3rd Dorsal
interos.

2nd Dorsal
interos.

1st Palmar
interos.

Adductor pollicis
transverse head

1st Dorsal
interos.

Flexor pollicis
brevis (cut)

Adductor pollicis
oblique head

Transverse carpal
ligament

Hook of
hamate bone

FIGURE 5-4   The ulnar nerve and the structures innervated by it in the hand. The lumbrical muscles to the ring and small fingers, innervated by the ulnar nerve, are not shown. The bellies of the abductor digiti minimi and flexor digiti minimi have been cut away to expose deeper structures.

and distal forearm levels, (5) primary or delayed primary repair, and (6) use of the operating microscope. These criteria were chosen to isolate properties intrinsic to the median and ulnar nerves and minimize confounding variables. When the results of cases that met these criteria were compared (Figure 5-5), no significant differences were found between median and ulnar nerves at any level of sensory or motor recovery. Overall, roughly 10% of patients achieve near-normal function of S4, M5, and roughly 60% will recover at least to the S3+, M4 level.

The results of treating distal median and ulnar nerve injuries have been compared in a variety of settings. Analysis of 48 median and 84 ulnar nerve grafts performed on young adults during the recent Balkan conflict revealed no difference in either sensory or motor recovery as graded on a modified MRC scale (Roganovic, Pavlicevic, 2006). Evaluating a more diverse group that included patients of all ages treated with repair or graft, Rosén and Lundborg (2000) found no difference in sensory outcomes, but significantly better motor function in the median nerve. A recent, similarly inclusive

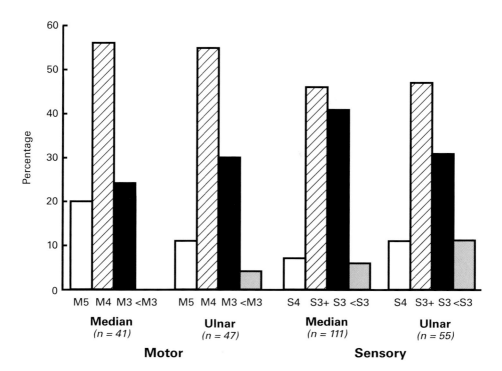

FIGURE 5-5   The results of primary and delayed primary median and ulnar nerve repair after laceration at wrist or distal forearm level in adults followed for a minimum of 2 years. Outcomes are graded on the MRC scale as modified by Mackinnon and Dellon (1988). There are no significant differences between median and ulnar nerve outcomes.

meta-analysis revealed an even greater difference in motor outcomes, but again no difference in sensory recovery (Ruijs et al., 2005). Overall recovery as graded on the LSU scale (Chapter 4) was better for the median nerve, though significance was not determined (Kim et al., 2001b, 2003a). Median and ulnar outcomes were thus similar in adults with either repair (the current analysis) or graft (Roganovic, Pavlicevic, 2006), but series that included children tended to favor the median over the ulnar (Rosén, Lundborg, 2000; Kim et al., 2001b, 2003a; Ruijs et al., 2005). Prospective analysis of median and ulnar repairs with validated instruments such as that described by Rosén and Lundborg should help clarify the possibility that motor outcomes differ more in children than in adults.

Age Is a Primary Determinant of Recovery

The effect of age on the outcome of nerve repair was first noted by Seddon, who observed that "In children recovery was rather better than in adults" (Nicholson, Seddon, 1957, p1070). Thorough examination of sensory recovery by Onne (1962) provided the strongest early confirmation of this trend. By using his carefully tabulated data it is possible to compare patients above and below the age of 21 with repair of sharp distal median or ulnar nerve lacerations performed within 6 months of injury and subjected to long-term follow-up. The operating microscope was not used in these cases. Juveniles achieved a 2-point discrimination of 6 mm or less in 59% of cases, whereas this level of function was achieved by only 5% of adults (p = 0.0, AA). A 2-point discrimination of 7–15 mm was reached by 38% of children and 10% of adults (p = 0.03, AA). Sensory recovery was thus dramatically better in children than in adults. Similar findings were obtained when the results of microscopic median nerve suture were stratified by age (Figure 5-6). The adult median nerve results depicted in Figure 5-5 were compared with those from juveniles extracted from the same clinical series and additional cases

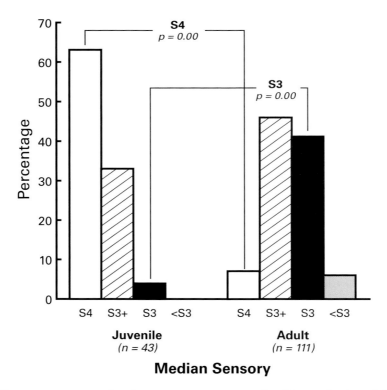

Median Sensory

FIGURE 5-6   The sensory outcome of median nerve repair at wrist or distal forearm levels in children and adults. Recovery of 2-point discrimination of 6 mm or less was achieved by 63% of children and only 7% of adults, while failure to regain 2-point discrimination of at least 15 mm was far more common in adults.

from a series focusing on children (Tajima, Imai, 1989). Recovery of 2-point discrimination of 6 mm or less (S4) was achieved by 63% of children and only 7% of adults (p = 0.00, AA). Conversely, S3 was obtained by 4% of juveniles and 41% of adults (p = 0.00, AA). A similarly large age effect was found in both a recent clinical series (Vordemvenne et al., 2007) and in a meta-analysis of ulnar and median nerve outcomes (Ruijs et al., 2005).

The digital nerve is an ideal model in which to isolate the impact of age on sensory recovery because axons are only required to regenerate over short distances, there are no tributary branches to other areas, and sensory pathways cannot be taken up by misdirected motor axons; none are present at this level of the nerve. Three published series of microscopic digital nerve repairs allow detailed stratification of age and 2-point discrimination and were thus combined for analysis (Altissimi et al., 1991; Efstathopoulos et al., 1995; Weinzweig et al., 2000) (Figure 5-7). Dramatic differences in the

proportion of patients achieving a 2-point discrimination of 6 mm or less were found between juveniles ages 1–10 and both older children and young adults (ages 11–40, p = 0.0, AA) and older adults (ages >40, p = 0.0, AA). Given the robust regeneration still present in members of the middle age group, these differences imply that juvenile axons are better at finding appropriate end organ targets, or, in the absence of such target selectivity, the juvenile CNS is better at adapting to miswired distal connections.

The impact of age on motor function is clearly documented in the large series of ulnar nerve repairs presented by Gaul (1982). The outcome of each repair was expressed as the key pinch (tip of thumb to side of index finger) strength in the operated extremity as a percentage of that in the opposite, normal extremity. Repairs performed in the arm restored a mean of 33% of the contralateral pinch strength in adults (n = 10), while juveniles (n = 5) did twice as well at 65%. Juveniles (n = 10) also

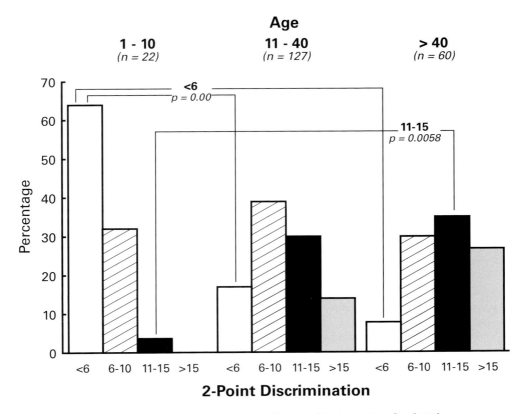

Age

| 1 - 10 | 11 - 40 | > 40 |
| *(n = 22)* | *(n = 127)* | *(n = 60)* |

FIGURE 5-7   The effect of patient age on the recovery of 2-point discrimination after digital nerve repair. Juveniles fared significantly better than either teenagers or adults.

fared better than adults (n = 14) after repairs in the forearm. Regression analysis showed the effect of age to be significant (p = 0.013, AA) and independent of level of injury.

The powerful effect of patient age on the outcome of nerve repair has two important consequences for the study of regeneration. First, patient age must be rigorously controlled before data from a clinical series can be used to examine the importance of other variables. Second, we are given, in juveniles, a model in which the outcome of regeneration is often excellent. If a treatment could routinely produce similar results in adults, it would be considered a significant improvement over current therapy. A potential therapeutic strategy would thus be to identify the components of the regeneration process that deteriorate with age, and to improve their performance in adults.

PROXIMO-DISTAL LESION LEVEL INFLUENCES MOTOR BUT NOT SENSORY RECOVERY

In an early study of civilian median and ulnar nerve injuries, Seddon suggested that injury level might influence outcome (Nicholson, Seddon, 1957). S3 was achieved in 29% of high injuries and 40% of low injuries, and S3+ in 14% of high injuries and 25% of low injuries. However, the small number of proximal injuries precludes statistical analysis. A large modern series of ulnar and median repairs and grafts in patients of all ages showed no impact of proximo-distal level of injury on surgical result (Kline, Hudson, 1995). Patients were evaluated by the LSU scale, in which a Grade III result signifies the following: median motor-pronation, wrist and finger flexion against gravity and some resistance, some distal muscles contract against gravity; ulnar motor-flexor carpi ulnaris and small finger profundus contract against gravity and some resistance, some distal muscles contract against gravity; sensory-response to touch and pin in autonomous zone of nerve (the area served exclusively by that nerve without overlap from its neighbors), with sensation mislocalized and not normal, some overresponse present. Grade III was reached by 15/20 (75%) of patients with proximal lesions, 27/35 (77%) of those with elbow and forearm lesions, and 24/31 (77%) of those injured at the wrist. It is certainly possible, however, that comparison of Grade IV or V outcomes could disclose differences masked by placing the cutoff at Grade III.

Narrowing inclusion criteria to focus on the effects of lesion level improves the power of analysis. There are few reports of simple nerve laceration in the proximal extremity to compare with the ample data on distal laceration, whereas reports of grafting procedures are more evenly distributed. Outcomes from adult median and ulnar grafting procedures

were thus compared to minimize the effects of age and type of lesion on the analysis (Figure 5-8). Since graft length was not taken into account, data could be extracted from several publications (Millesi et al., 1972, 1976; Moneim, 1982; Stellini, 1982; Lijftogt et al., 1987; Frykman, Cally, 1988; Birch, 1991; Trumble et al., 1995). This analysis revealed that lesion level did not influence sensory recovery in this population. Motor recovery, however, was more sensitive to the level of injury. Patients with distal lesions were more likely to recover to M4 (p = 0.04, AA), and patients with proximal lesions more often failed to achieve M3 function (p = 0.0003, AA). A similar effect of proximo-distal location on motor but not sensory recovery was found in a recent meta-analysis of median and ulnar nerve repairs that included patients of all ages (Ruijs et al., 2005).

The relationship between lesion level and motor recovery is further clarified by additional reports that could not be included in this analysis. In his review of ulnar nerve repairs, Gaul (1982) expressed each result as a ratio of pinch strength

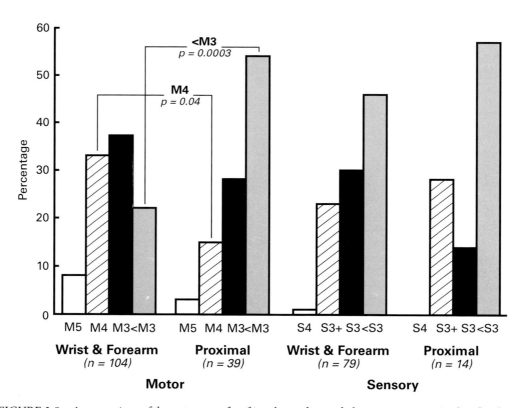

FIGURE 5-8 A comparison of the outcomes of grafting the median and ulnar nerves at proximal or distal levels. Lesion level did not affect sensory recovery, but had a significant impact on motor recovery.

in the operated extremity to that in the opposite, uninjured extremity. Adults recovered to a mean of 60% after distal nerve repair (n = 14), but to a mean of only 33% after proximal repair (n = 10; p = 0.009, AA). Similarly, the outcome of median nerve grafts scored on an MRC scale modified to include patient satisfaction was good or excellent in 10% of proximal injuries, 33% of intermediate-level injuries, and 69% of distal injuries (Roganovic, 2005). Lesion level is widely assumed to be a determinant of outcome in nerve repair. A prominent review of factors influencing outcome cited 13 articles as evidence of this effect (Steinberg, Koman, 1991). Only 2 of these publications took patient age into account, however, and none provided statistical analysis of their data. The current summary of grafting results (Figure 5-8) and the series discussed above (Gaul, 1982; Roganovic, 2005; Ruijs et al., 2005) provide more concrete evidence for this assumption.

A variety of factors could compromise functional restoration after proximal lesions. Proximal injury may have more severe consequences for the neuron by amputating a greater percentage of its volume, and by forcing it to sustain regeneration for a longer period of time to reach the periphery. Proximal tributaries, usually to large muscles, may "siphon off" regenerating axons, decreasing the population of axons available to continue distally. Additionally, increasing the time during which distal pathway and end organs are denervated will diminish the effectiveness of their function once axons arrive (Chapter 9). Any one of these mechanisms could have a more pronounced effect in the motor system, resulting in the clinical observations described above.

DELAY IN TREATMENT COMPROMISES OUTCOME

Although it is relatively easy to demonstrate that delay compromises outcome, it is more difficult to ascertain why. This difficulty is exemplified by three clinical series that specifically examine the effects of delayed treatment. In one series, repair or grafting of median and ulnar nerves failed in 3/32 (9%) of patients when performed within 6 months, but failed in 9/28 (32%) if delayed for more than 6 months (p < 0.01, AA; Birch, 1991). Digital nerve repair and grafting was shown to be similarly sensitive to delay. Digital nerves repaired within 3 months of injury achieved S4 sensibility in 19/34 (56%), but those repaired after 12 months did so in only 5/66 (8%, p = 0.01, PA; Kallio, 1993). In a third

series, secondary ulnar nerve repair or grafting was followed by better motor recovery if performed within 3 months (p <= 0.05, PA; Barrios et al., 1989). Unlike the first two series, however, the third provides sufficient data to ascertain that delay was substantially longer in graft than in repair cases. Thus, although these publications clearly establish that delay is harmful, they cannot help us distinguish between the effects of primary biological variables (progressive deterioration of neuron, pathway, and end organ) and secondary surgical variables (end-to-end repair vs. grafting). When a nerve is transected, its elastic components draw the cut ends apart. If surgery is performed promptly, this elastic retraction can be overcome, and direct suture of the nerve ends is often possible. Prolonged delay, in contrast, allows progressive intraneural scarring that fixes the retraction in place, preventing the ends from being brought back together again (Millesi, 1986). As a result, even sharp lacerations may require grafting after treatment delay of several months.

The biological processes inherent in delay can be evaluated more selectively by reviewing series limited to either direct repair or grafting. In a study of end-to-end median and ulnar nerve suture, Marsh (1990) noted that increasing delay correlated with decreasing ability to perform a battery of functional tests (p <= 0.005, PA). Similarly, Trumble demonstrated that the delay before nerve grafting correlated with the percentage of normal strength regained (p = 0.05, PA; Trumble et al., 1995). Delay is thus important for biological as well as surgical reasons.

FUNCTION DECREASES WITH INCREASING VIOLENCE OF INJURY

Severity of injury is even more difficult to isolate as a biologic factor than is delay of treatment. The primary variable is the extent of damage to the nerve itself. Sharp laceration directly injures only a few millimeters of nerve. When laceration accompanies fracture, skeletal stability is lost and the nerve is stretched before it gives way, extending the zone of injury both proximally and distally. The most extensive damage is caused by high velocity gunshot wounds; a momentary shock wave violently distorts the nerve, injuring it far above and below the site of projectile contact. Secondary variables include both biological and clinical factors. Devascularization and scarring of surrounding tissues may compromise neural blood supply and result in gradual constriction of the nerve, preventing regeneration. The nerve may be subject to external trauma after soft tissue protection is lost. When nerve is immobilized by scar, it can no longer respond to joint motion by gliding through supple tissues to redistribute tension (Millesi, 1986). Focusing this tension on the site of injury can cause further damage to this compromised area. Clinically, more extensive injury is more likely to be treated by nerve grafting than by simple repair and to receive definitive treatment on a delayed basis, introducing new variables.

The influence of injury severity on outcome is demonstrated convincingly by the large series of Vietnam-era nerve injuries treated at the Brooke Army Hand Center and reported by Dr. George Omer (1974). In the patients treated with end-to-end suture, good clinical function was restored to 33/75 (44%) of patients with lacerations, 10/32 (31%) of those with low velocity gunshot wounds, and 7/35 (20%) suffering from high velocity wounds. Even this series has confounding variables, as lacerations received definitive treatment more promptly than gunshot wounds.

The importance of injury severity may be further appreciated by returning to the microcosm of the digital nerve. Outcomes experienced by adults undergoing microscopic repair of digital nerves were extracted from 3 clinical reports (Buncke, 1972; Sullivan, 1985; Weinzweig et al., 2000). Two-point discrimination of 6 mm or less was restored to 37/91 (41%) of fingers after sharp laceration, but to only 5/51 (10%) after transections with a crushing component ($p = 0.0001$, AA). Extension of tissue damage beyond the site of transection thus compromises functional outcomes.

Successful reconstruction of severely traumatized peripheral nerve depends on accurate assessment of the degree of nerve injury. Traditionally, this assessment was made by delaying treatment to allow compromised nerve to declare itself. The process of decision-making can often proceed more quickly and more accurately when intra-operative electrophysiologic testing is used to confirm early regeneration and to separate healthy from diseased portions of a nerve (Kline, Happel, 1993). Even so, this technique requires a delay to allow for early regeneration, and cannot assess the quality of portions of the distal stump that have not yet been challenged by regenerating axons. What is clearly needed is a way to identify nerve that cannot support regeneration, but in a time-frame of days to weeks. Recent advances in peripheral nerve imaging

(Dailey et al., 1997) suggest that an MRI-based technique could be developed to satisfy these requirements. The sooner that decisions are made, the shorter the delay to definitive treatment will be. The more accurate the resection of diseased nerve, the better the chance of returning axons to the periphery. A rapid, accurate diagnostic technique would be of great benefit to many patients.

SURGICAL TECHNIQUE INFLUENCES RECOVERY FROM NERVE REPAIR

The technique used to join nerve ends together has evolved significantly since the first large series of civilian nerve injuries were reported after World War II (Nicholson, Seddon, 1957; Larsen, Posch, 1958; Stromberg et al., 1961; Onne, 1962; Sakellarides, 1962). As the operating microscope and fine microsutures evolved together, it is impossible to define their relative contributions to the overall improvement that accompanied their combined use. This improvement is demonstrated by comparison of the data on modern median and ulnar nerve repair (Figure 5-5) with data obtained from historical controls in which the microscope and microsutures were not used (Figure 5-9). Sensory recovery after median nerve repair (Onne, 1962) and motor recovery after ulnar repair (Nicholson, Seddon, 1957) were most extensively chronicled in the older publications. Recovery to S3+, seen in 2/15 (13%) of median nerves sutured without the microscope or microsutures, was found in 51/111 (46%) of those sutured with modern technique ($p = 0.0163$, AA). Ulnar motor function never reached M5 after 60 repairs performed without the microscope, but did so in 5/47 (11%) when the microscope was used ($p = 0.00$, AA). This analysis confirms that development of microsutures and the operating microscope have clearly benefited patients with distal median and ulnar nerve injuries.

To the naked eye, the cut surface of a transected peripheral nerve presents a fairly uniform appearance. To the microsurgeon, it looks more like an electrical cable, with bundles of wires, or fascicles, contained within an outer covering, the epineurium (Chapter 1; Figure 5-10). Selective reunion of these neuronal subunits was discussed early in the twentieth century, long before the necessary tools were available (Langley, Hashimoto, 1917). Once microsurgical instruments became available, it was only natural that surgeons would rise to the challenge of reuniting cut fascicles, either individually or in

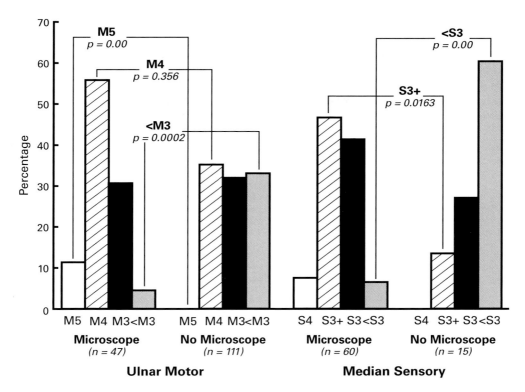

FIGURE 5-9 The results of median and ulnar nerve repairs with and without the aid of the operating microscope. The analysis is limited to median sensory and ulnar motor function, as these were documented most thoroughly in early reports. Use of the operating microscope and microsurgical technique clearly benefited both sensory and motor outcomes.

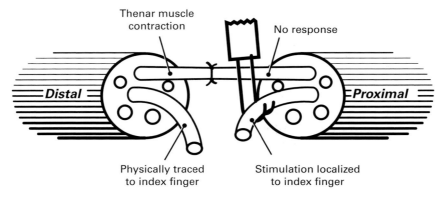

FIGURE 5-10 Selective fascicular reunion. A proximal fascicle that did not produce a sensory response when stimulated, and is thus presumed to be predominately motor, has already been matched with a distal fascicle that could be traced to muscle. Stimulation of the proximal fascicle on the electrode produced sensation referred to the index finger. This fascicle will be matched with a distal fascicle that can be anatomically traced to the index finger.

groups. Working at the fascicular level of digital nerves did not enhance restoration of sensibility (Young et al., 1981 [evidence level 1]; Tupper et al., 1988). In retrospect this is not surprising, as the presumed goal of fascicular repair is to guide regenerating axons to appropriate distal pathways while excluding axons that belong in other pathways. Since all fascicles of a given digital nerve carry purely cutaneous axons to a small topographic area, there is little to distinguish one fascicle from another and little expectation of sensory compromise if fascicles are mismatched. Excellent sensibility can even be obtained when fascicular anatomy is eliminated altogether by substituting a hollow tube for a nerve graft (Weber et al., 2000 [evidence level 2]).

A more challenging test of the concept of selective fascicular reunion is provided by repair of the median and ulnar nerves. In these nerves, fascicles carry both sensory and motor fibers to a variety of destinations, so the likelihood of mismatch and functional compromise is greater. Electrophysiologic and histological techniques have been devised to aid in the process of fascicular matching (Figure 5-10). Electrical stimulation of single fascicles in the awake patient permits characterization of proximal sensory and distal motor fascicles. Stimulation of cutaneous fascicles in the proximal stump, which are still connected to the brain, allows the patient to identify their normal site of termination (e.g., the index finger). Stimulation of motor fascicles in the distal stump results in visible contraction of the muscle served by that fascicle if performed within 24 hours of injury. Using this technique, Gaul restored 60% of normal pinch strength to 6/7 patients with ulnar nerve injuries, and 80% of opposition strength to 7/11 patients with median injuries (Gaul, 1986). Similarly, Jabaley was able to restore M5 function to 8/15 patients with a variety of upper extremity nerve injuries, having identified predominately motor or sensory fascicles with confidence in each case (Jabaley, 1991). When adults with complete median or ulnar injuries are extracted from the series presented by Kato (Kato et al., 1998), M5 recovery is achieved by 5/16 and S4 by 8/16. All grades of M5 were assigned to the median nerve in this series, suggesting that undamaged residual thenar function could have artificially inflated motor recovery.

Intra-operative histologic staining of nerve biopsies to identify motor fascicles through the presence of the enzyme acetylcholinesterase was described many years ago (Gruber et al., 1976). Application of this technique to 11 patients with median and/or ulnar nerve injury improved median but not ulnar sensory recovery, and had no significant effect on motor function (Deutinger et al., 1993 [evidence level 3]). Overall, these series compare favorably with the results expected for median and ulnar repair in adults (Figure 5-5), suggesting that correct fascicular alignment improves outcome. Prospective evaluation of fascicular alignment techniques is thus an appropriate goal for future clinical studies.

FAULTY SENSORY LOCALIZATION: SENSORY REGENERATION LACKS TOPOGRAPHIC SPECIFICITY

When tactile stimulation is perceived not in the area of contact but in a different location, the phenomenon is called "faulty sensory localization." This perceptual abnormality was first described by John Mitchell, a neurologist who examined survivors of the American Civil War previously treated for nerve injuries by his father, Silas Weir Mitchell (Mitchell, 1895). He did not attempt to explain these observations himself, but consulted W. H. Howell of Johns Hopkins, who ventured that "some of the bundles from the central end might take a wrong route and reach a wrong termination ... then the impulses aroused by stimulation of the peripheral endings would call forth sensations which previous experience had localized in a different region; and this mis-reference of sensation might or might not be overcome by future training" (Mitchell, 1895, p239). Further study of faulty localization in the early twentieth century resulted in a consensus that it could only be caused by nerve injury followed by misdirected regeneration (reviewed in Hawkins, 1948). In the modern era, faulty sensory localization was studied in greater detail by Hallin and coworkers (Hallin et al., 1981). Methodical clinical examination revealed the true extent of mislocalization and confirmed its presence to equal degrees in young and old patients (Figure 5-11). On the basis of intraneural electrophysiology, Hallin et al. suggested that "fibers growing out from the fascicles of the sectioned nerve do not only innervate coherent skin areas as they originally did, but tend to spread out to innervate separate skin patches" (Hallin et al., 1981, p104).

Mislocalization of sensory stimuli is a common experience during the early stages of sensory recovery. So common, in fact, that the MRC definition of S3+ includes the observation that "localization of the

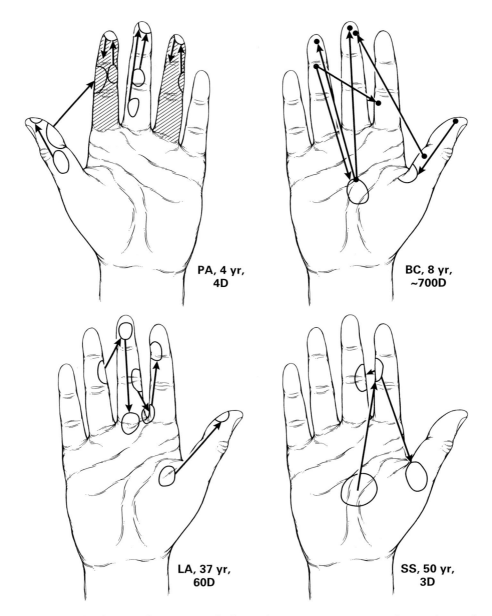

FIGURE 5-11 Mislocalization of sensory stimuli after median nerve repair. Arrows indicate reference from the area stimulated to the area where the stimulus was perceived. Patient PA referred touch of the index and ring finger tips to the entire digit as indicated by the diagonal hatching. Each caption provides patient initials, age at injury, and the delay between injury and nerve repair. Reproduced with permission from Hallin et al., 1981.

stimulus is good" (Table 4-2), in tacit contradistinction to the lower grades, in which localization is poor. A patient's ability to localize stimuli is reported in few publications on nerve repair. Wynn Parry noted that "incorrect localisation is inevitable when re-innervation occurs after nerve suture," but felt that sensory reeducation could restore the ability to localize to

"near perfect" levels (Wynn Parry, Salter, 1976, p252). Marsh (1990) examined 21 patients for ability to localize stimuli after median or ulnar nerve repair and found that, although most did well, several patients demonstrated significant impairment. In response to the ease with which Marsh's patients localized stimuli to relatively large areas, Jerosch-Herold (2000) made the test more difficult by dividing the pulp of the distal phalynx into quadrants and testing each separately. In a study of 41 patients with median nerve injury, a mean of only 56% of stimuli were correctly localized (Jerosch-Herold, 2000). Further evaluation of this testing pattern revealed excellent test-retest reliability and ability to discriminate normal from injured median nerves (Jerosch-Herold et al., 2006).

The prevalence of mislocalization and its importance to sensory function have yet to be established. When faulty localization is sought out, it is found commonly during the early stages of reinnervation. It may become less prominent during later stages, and may be improved by sensory reeducation. These observations suggest that as more and more sensory axons reinnervate a given area, the CNS is able to select inputs to form a meaningful pattern, suppressing discordant information. Close examination of Figure 5-11 also suggests a lack of one-to-one correspondence between sensation (what is detected) and sensibility (what we experience). The physical distance between actual and perceived stimuli in these diagrams is always substantial: tip to base of digit, digit to palm, one digit to another. With the exception of these large shifts, sensibility in other areas remains well localized. One would, however, expect projection errors to come in all magnitudes. The discrepancy between observation and expectation suggests either that axons are able to correct small projection errors and return to appropriate areas (less likely), or that these smaller errors occur but can be suppressed (more likely; Chapter 11).

Faulty sensory localization can be detected after nerve repair in both adults and children (Figure 5-11). Multiple regression analysis of factors contributing to outcome after peripheral nerve repair confirms that faulty localization is not a factor of age (Jerosch-Herold, 2000), and that the ability to localize remains as a valid predictor of function when the effects of age have been eliminated (Marsh, 1990). In terms of human biology, this analysis suggests that regenerating sensory axons cannot selectively reinnervate the areas of skin they once served, and that this inability compromises outcome in both adults and children. In other words, cutaneous reinnervation lacks topographic specificity (Chapter 10). Furthermore, although clinical observation suggests a central mechanism to suppress or redirect input from small projection errors, gross errors persist regardless of age. The ability to correct for these large errors is therefore not one of the beneficial effects of young age on the outcome of nerve repair.

Median and Ulnar Nerve Grafting

Data on adults followed for a minimum of 2 years after ulnar or median nerve grafting at wrist or forearm level were extracted from several publications (Millesi et al., 1972, 1976; Moneim, 1982; Stellini, 1982; Lijftogt et al., 1987; Frykman, Cally, 1988; Birch, 1991; Novak et al., 1992; Trumble et al., 1995) (Figure 5-12). No significant differences between median and ulnar outcomes were noted, except for more frequent restitution of M5 function in the median nerve. As discussed previously, residual thenar function supplied by radial and ulnar nerves may be responsible for this discrepancy.

The results of grafting the ulnar and median nerves were then evaluated in the context of end-to-end nerve repair. The frequency with which patients achieved function of M4, S3+ or better after nerve repair (Figure 5-5) was compared with the frequency of this level of recovery after grafting (Figure 5-12). Sensory and motor recovery were superior after repair in both median and ulnar nerves (p <= 0.02, AA). Millesi's assertion that "interfascicular nerve-grafting gives results which are at least as good as those after epineurial suture" (Millesi et al., 1976, p209) was based on comparison of grafting results with two early series of nerve repairs performed without the microscope (Nicholson, Seddon, 1957; Sakellarides, 1962). Now that adequate data are available for comparison of microscopic grafting with microscopic nerve repair, grafting can be viewed in a more realistic context; the average graft is not as good as the average repair. Equally important from a biological viewpoint, however, is the finding that the best graft can be better than the average repair. This is exemplified by a series of patients in whom median nerve grafting included carpal tunnel release, exclusion of the thenar muscle branch from the distal graft juncture, and extensive postoperative sensory reeducation. Eleven of 14 patients treated in this fashion achieved S3+ or better, demonstrating the potential of nerve grafting under ideal circumstances (Novak et al., 1992).

NERVE GRAFTING: ANALYSIS OF VARIABLES

The variables that contribute to the final outcome of nerve grafting can be broken down into the clinical and the biologic. Clinically, nerve grafting is more likely to be performed after severe injury, or for

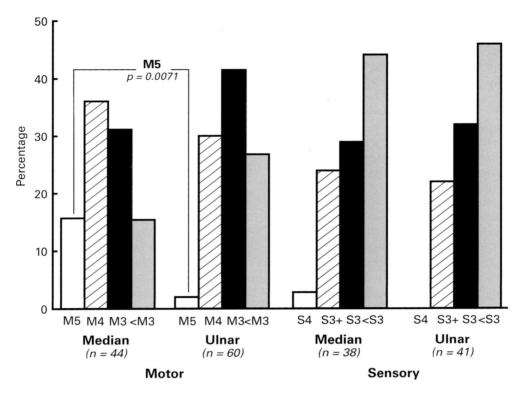

FIGURE 5-12   Results of grafting the median or ulnar nerve at wrist or forearm level after a minimum of 2 years follow-up. Motor function was better in the median nerve, though this difference may reflect the contributions of uninjured neuromuscular units to thumb abduction.

simple transection that has been left untreated for several months. As has been shown previously, both severity of injury and delay of treatment compromise outcome after repair, and would be expected to do so after grafting as well. Biologically, nerve grafting introduces factors not encountered after nerve repair: graft revascularization to maintain viability, passage of axons across two suture lines, and substantial anatomical mismatch between host and graft nerve segments at both ends of the graft.

Review of published results identified 67 cases of median or ulnar nerve grafting in which adequate information was provided on patient age, delay between injury and surgery, length of graft, nerve treated, and outcome (Millesi et al., 1972; Moneim, 1982; Frykman, Cally, 1988; Trumble et al., 1995). Data from these cases were subjected to multiple regression analysis to evaluate the isolated effects of each variable. The effects of age were overwhelming; delay, graft length, and nerve (median vs. ulnar) were not found to influence outcome significantly. When nerve identity was

removed from the analysis, the result was the same. It is likely, given the number of variables in the system that must be accounted for, that inclusion of more cases will eventually demonstrate the significance of factors other than age. Nonetheless, this analysis strongly emphasizes the relative importance of age over all other variables.

More specific information on the impact of gap length is provided by two carefully analyzed groups of patients. Novak et al. (1992, p65) applied Spearman rank analysis to the outcomes of 14 median nerve grafts of length 1–12 cm in adults and observed "assessment of correlational relationships between graft length and object identification revealed r = 0.66 (p < 0.020) with large objects and r = 0.74 (p = 0.006) with small objects." Trumble et al. (1995) used a force transducer to quantify the strength regained after grafting gaps of 2.5–11 cm in radial, median, or ulnar nerves and found a significant correlation between strength of the reinnervated limb, as a percentage of the opposite, normal limb, and graft length. These studies benefit from the limitation of extraneous variables and examination of a wide range of graft lengths. The variables examined, the ability to identify a series of objects with the hand (Novak et al., 1992) and the objective strength of reinnervated muscle (Trumble et al., 1995), are not routinely presented in follow-up studies and were thus not included in the regression analysis described above. Objective determination of muscle strength, normalized by comparison with the opposite limb, also introduces a new level of precision to motor testing, and thus increases the power of correlational analysis.

Graft length might influence regeneration in several ways. Longer grafts may be harder to revascularize (Chapter 8). Graft anatomy may also play a role. Cutaneous nerve, the usual source of graft, often gives off small tributaries. These can be identified and dissected off short grafts, but this process becomes increasingly difficult with long grafts. Obligatory loss of axons from longer grafts may thus compromise distal stump reinnervation. The longer the graft, the longer it will take regenerating axons to reach the second suture line. If this suture line becomes progressively scarred in the absence of crossing axons, it may be a time-sensitive impediment to regeneration. Finally, a secondary anatomical factor may also contribute. As fascicles travel down a nerve they intermix, exchanging axons through intraneural plexi (Chapter 1). The cross-sectional anatomy of the nerve is thus changing constantly. The longer the piece of nerve resected, the more difficult it becomes to identify and reconnect equivalent areas of proximal and distal stumps.

Further insight into the biology of nerve grafting may be obtained from analysis of the large number of digital nerve repairs and grafts reported (Buncke, 1972; McFarlane, Mayer, 1976; Tenny, Lewis, 1984; Sullivan, 1985; Nunley et al., 1989; Weinzweig et al., 2000) (Figure 5-13). Sensory axon regeneration through grafts up to 15 mm in length restored sensibility indistinguishable from that found after end-to-end repair of simple lacerations. Only when grafts were longer than 15 mm did they become less likely than repairs to restore 2-point discrimination

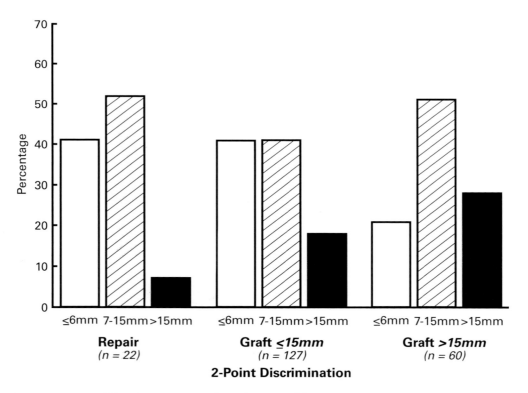

FIGURE 5-13   Sensibility after repair or grafting of transected digital nerves. Regeneration through grafts up to 15 mm in length restored sensibility indistinguishable from that found after end-to-end suture of sharp lacerations, whereas longer grafts fared less well.

of 6 mm or better (p = 0.0269 AA). The anatomical match between digital nerve and graft sources such as the sural nerve is excellent, minimizing a prominent variable that may compromise the grafting of larger nerves. The digital nerve carries only cutaneous axons destined for a small area, eliminating the risk from mismatch of axons and their distal pathways. No matter where a regenerating axon enters the distal stump, it is likely to provide useful function. In larger nerves that contain both cutaneous and motor axons destined for a variety of locations, such as the median and ulnar, the risk of mismatch is far greater. For instance, motor axons that are misdirected to skin will provide no function, and will block appropriate axons from the pathways they occupy. In the digital nerve, when these organizational factors are minimized, it is clear that interposition of a second suture line is not in itself harmful. Function after grafting of more complex nerves, where intraneural organization is crucial, is thus likely to be degraded by increased misdirection at a second suture line.

THE ACCESSORY AND FACIAL NERVES

Topographic Specificity during Muscle Reinnervation

The term "topographic specificity" refers to the ability of axons normally serving a particular area of the body to regenerate with precision to that area after they are injured (Chapter 9). Examination of the outcome of accessory nerve injury will establish the best case scenario for proximal motor nerve regeneration, as all injured axons project to a single muscle, the trapezius. They will thus reach the topographically correct target no matter how much axonal misdirection occurs at the suture line. The extra-temporal facial nerve is also a proximal motor nerve. In stark contrast to the simplicity of the accessory nerve, the facial nerve innervates a complex system of facial muscles. In this case, a failure of topographic specificity will manifest itself as synkinesis, or co-contraction of separate muscles. Axons centrally wired to control one muscle will now control several, often antagonistic muscles; a demand for function of one muscle will lead to co-contraction of several, leading to obvious facial distortion and deformity.

The XI cranial or spinal accessory nerve exits the skull with the vagus nerve through the jugular foramen. It innervates the sternocleidomastoid muscle below the transverse process of the first cervical vertebra, either passing beneath or penetrating the sternocleidomastoid at the junction of its upper and middle thirds (Figure 5-14). The nerve is quite superficial as it descends across the posterior triangle of the neck to innervate the trapezius. It is in this area that it is often subject to iatrogenic injury during tumor excision or lymph node biopsy.

Injury of the accessory nerve in the posterior triangle of the neck results in inability to elevate, or "shrug," the shoulder. Additionally, loss of scapular stabilization and rotation, both functions of the trapezius muscle, result in inability to abduct the shoulder beyond 90°. Transection of the accessory nerve provides an ideal test of the outcome of motor nerve repair. The nerve is short, ensuring that axons will reinnervate muscle soon after entering the distal nerve stump. The injury, usually the result of surgery, is fairly standardized in both its extent and location within the posterior triangle of the neck. At this level the nerve carries fibers to only one target, the trapezius muscle, so most axons that cross the repair site should contact muscle and have a positive impact on function.

The outcome of repair or grafting of the accessory nerve after iatrogenic injury is often excellent. In spite of delays in treatment of up to 1 year, 21/27 (78%) of adult patients in four comparable series regained a full 180° of shoulder abduction (Ogino et al., 1991; Nakamichi, Tachibana, 1998; Novak, Mackinnin, 2002; Chandawarkar et al., 2003). In the largest single series reported, spanning a 23-year period, 77% of 84 patients were able to abduct at least 90° (Kim et al., 2003b). When topographic specificity is minimized as a factor, as it is with repair of the accessory nerve, the results of proximal motor nerve regeneration can thus be excellent, even when a graft is required.

The anatomy of the facial nerve is far more complex than that of the accessory nerve (Figure 5-15). The motor portion of the facial nerve leaves the temporal bone through the stylomastoid foramen. It rapidly penetrates the parotid gland, where it ramifies into six to eight tributaries. These branches exit the parotid in a variety of patterns, complicated further by plexiform interconnections among them (Shapiro, 1954). Examination of the nerve in cross section reveals some consistent fiber localization (Meissl, 1977), but fascicular variability predominates. The overall picture is thus one of marked intermingling of fibers destined for the 17 separate muscles innervated by the facial nerve.

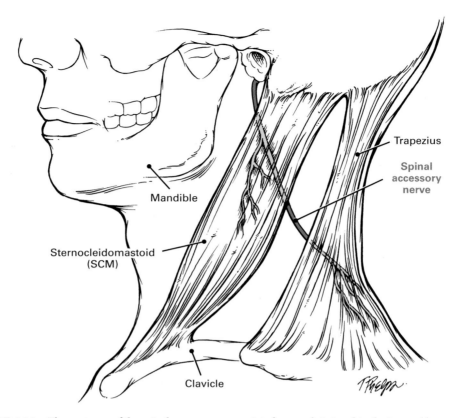

FIGURE 5-14 The anatomy of the spinal accessory nerve. It is frequently injured in the interval between the sternocleidomastoid and trapezius muscles during lymph node biopsy.

The grading of facial muscle function is by necessity more subjective than grading of extremity muscles, as it is performed entirely on the basis of inspection. The scale devised by House and Brackmann (House, Brackmann, 1985) is used frequently for this purpose. Grade I describes normal facial function. A Grade II result is characterized by normal symmetry and tone at rest, complete eye closure with minimal effort, slight asymmetry of the mouth, moderate to good forehead function, and only slight synkinesis. Patients with a Grade III result have significant dysfunction, with an obvious difference between injured and uninjured sides of the face, synkinesis (Figure 5-16), and contracture and/or hemifacial spasm. The eye can be closed only with effort, there is only slight to moderate movement of the forehead, and the mouth is weak even with maximal effort. Grades IV and V describe progressively less function; Grade VI is no function at all.

Four comparable publications graded the results of individual facial nerve repair and grafting procedures with the House-Brackmann scale, permitting analysis of their combined results (Stephanian et al., 1992; Green et al., 1994; Saeed, Ramsden, 1996; Falcioni et al., 2003). No cases regained function to the Grade I or Grade II level. Grade III function, which includes significant dysfunction and synkinesis, was restored in 10/12 (83%) of patients after end-to-end nerve repair, but in only 48/101 (48%) of patients who underwent nerve grafting procedures. These results differ from those of accessory nerve repair in two ways. First, overall muscle strength appears to be significantly diminished after facial nerve regeneration, unlike the robust trapezius strength recovered through the accessory nerve. This difference could reflect the death of significant numbers of facial motoneurons in response to a more proximal transection injury, decreased regenerative potential of motoneurons that normally serve small, delicate facial muscles as opposed to those serving the massive motor units of the trapezius, or changes within the muscles themselves. Second,

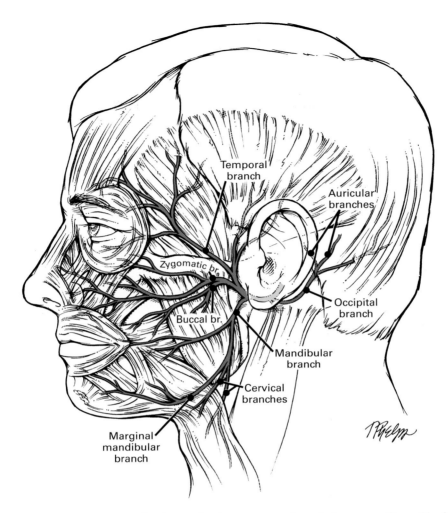

FIGURE 5-15   The anatomy of the facial nerve distal to its passage through the temporal bone. The facial nerve ramifies in a variable pattern to innervate 17 separate muscles. Fine coordination of these muscles is needed to produce facial expression.

the observation of synkinesis after facial nerve repair clearly indicates that motoneurons centrally wired to produce one function have reinnervated muscles that produce other, often opposing functions.

Spector et al. (1991) focused on the issue of synkinesis in their review of a large series of facial nerve reconstructions. End-to-end nerve repair of the facial nerve trunk restored facial symmetry and tone in 10/10 cases, but synkinesis was present in 7 of these. When the major components of the nerve were separated and repaired individually, symmetry and tone were again restored, but only 2/8 results were compromised by synkinesis. In marked contrast,

nerve grafting resulted in synkinesis in 22/23 patients. These results suggest a correlation between axonal alignment in proximal and distal stumps and the resulting specificity of facial muscle reinnervation. The more precise alignment obtained by selective reunion of fascicular groups minimized synkinesis, while the enhanced randomness imposed by axons crossing repair sites at each end of a graft increased it. The topographic specificity of muscle reinnervation thus appears to be under some degree of mechanical control. Conversely, the facial nerve experience provides no evidence that motor axons can "find their way" to the correct muscle. Of further

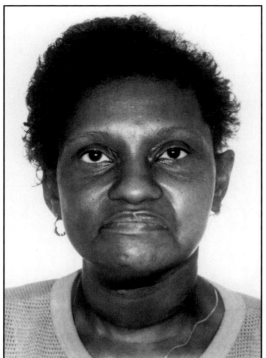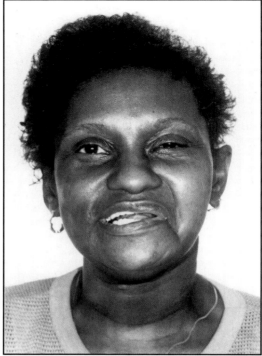

FIGURE 5-16   Synkinesis of the facial muscles after facial nerve transection and repair. Left—the face at rest. Right—the patient is attempting to smile. The reinnervated left side of the face is distorted by uncoordinated activity of the facial muscles that have been reinnervated by topographically inappropriate motoneurons. Reprinted with permission from Spector et al., 1991.

interest is the observation by Spector et al. (1991) that an excellent result at 9–18 months postoperatively could then deteriorate as reinnervation continued and synkinesis became more prominent. In four cases this process was so severe that hemifacial spasm resulted. This implies that even late-arriving motor axons are not capable of reinnervating correct muscle targets under clinical conditions. Overall, motor axons regenerating in the adult appear to have little if any intrinsic ability to return to their topographically correct muscle target. This lack of topographically specific muscle reinnervation is also a frequent consequence of obstetrical brachial plexus palsy, indicating that it is not a property of regeneration in the young that is lost with aging (Chuang et al., 1998). Restoration of topographic specificity is thus an appropriate surgical goal in situations where axons serving specific motor functions can be identified and matched in proximal and distal nerve stumps, in both adults and children.

THE RADIAL NERVE

Loss of Axons into Proximal Nerve Branches May Compromise Distal Reinnervation

After proximal nerve repair, reinnervation of muscles near the repair site will diminish the axon population available to more distal structures. However, the precise impact of this phenomenon is difficult to measure. This is because the consequences of axon loss into a proximal tributary can only be appreciated once the remaining axons have reinnervated their distal targets, permitting assessment of functional deficits. In the median and ulnar nerves, the effects of diverting axons to proximal forearm branches cannot be tested until the remaining axons have grown an additional 20 cm to reinnervate the hand. Those axons that remain in the nerve trunk and regenerate toward the hand will be subject to additional variables, such as the progressive inability of denervated Schwann cells to support regeneration (Hoke et al., 2002). Compromised distal reinnervation in this setting could thus reflect either axon loss into proximal branches, or failure of the remaining axons to complete their journey.

The radial nerve trunk gives off branches near the elbow in a manner similar to the median and ulnar nerves, but it distributes its terminal muscular branches in the proximal forearm rather than in the hand. Axons are not required to regenerate over long distances between proximal and distal branch points. Any difference in outcome between lesions above and below the proximal branches is thus more likely to result from diverting axons into proximal tributaries, and less likely to be the consequence of attrition in long forearm pathways. Consequently, the radial nerve is an appropriate model in which to investigate the impact of proximal branch reinnervation on distal function.

The radial nerve arises from the brachial plexus as the distal extension of the posterior cord. It receives fibers from the fifth, sixth, seventh, and eighth cervical levels. The nerve enters the arm between the long and medial heads of the triceps, then courses distally between the medial and lateral heads of the triceps within the spiral groove of the humerus. Beginning medial to the humeral head, it spirals around the posterior aspect of the humeral shaft, eventually penetrating the lateral intermuscular septum at the junction of the middle and lower thirds of the humerus. During this passage it gives off branches to the triceps and the posterior cutaneous nerves of the arm and forearm. The radial nerve approaches the elbow in a plane anterior to the brachialis and lateral to the muscles arising from the supracondylar ridge of the humerus: the brachioradialis, extensor carpi radialis longus, and extensor carpi radialis brevis (Figure 5-17). These muscles are innervated sequentially in the area of the lateral epicondyle. At the anterior elbow capsule the nerve bifurcates into its terminal branches, the superficial radial nerve and the posterior interosseous nerve (PIN). The former travels distally beneath the brachioradialis muscle as far as the wrist, where it ramifies to innervate the dorso-radial hand and the dorsal aspects of the thumb, index, and middle fingers. The PIN enters the dorsal forearm by spiraling around the proximal radius between the heads of the supinator muscle. The sequential order of muscle innervation from the PIN is often: supinator, extensor digitorum

communis and extensor carpi ulnaris in equal frequency, abductor pollicis longus, extensor digiti minimi, extensor pollicis longus, extensor pollicis brevis, and extensor indicis proprius. This pattern is subject to great variability, and deviations in the order of muscle reinnervation by regenerating axons should be expected (summarized from Sunderland, 1978).

The outcome of radial nerve lesions was documented by proximo-distal level in a recent series of 260 radial nerve repairs and grafts (Shergill et al., 2001). Results were graded by the MRC scale, assigning a rating of "good" to those with return of proximal muscle strength to M5 or M4 and distal strength to M3. In the context of this analysis, patients rated "good" regained strong wrist extension and the ability to extend the thumb and digits against some resistance. Repair or grafting of radial nerve injuries distal to the triceps innervation and proximal to the PIN restored good function to 69/221 patients (31%), while 16/18 injuries to the PIN itself (89%) recovered to this degree. In patients with more proximal lesions, reinnervation of cutaneous and muscle branches in the elbow area is thus likely to have compromised the function of distal musculature, reducing the percentage of patients achieving M3 by 58%. A similar analysis by level using the LSU series of radial and posterior interosseous nerve repairs showed little difference between intermediate and distal levels (Kim et al., 2001a; 2006). These patients were reported as the percentage reaching Grade III on the LSU scale, which does not require any EPL function, so a difference between intermediate and low levels could have been masked by the technique of analysis and recording. Excellent PIN recovery is confirmed by the experience of other authors (Young et al., 1990; Roganovic, Petkovic, 2004). Referring back to the combined series of median and ulnar nerve grafts presented earlier (Figure 5-12), M3 strength was restored in 18/39 high lesions (47%) and 81/104 low lesions (78%), a difference of 31%. There was no statistically significant difference between the disto-proximal decline in outcome after radial nerve repair (58%) and that after median or ulnar grafting (31%). The effect of reinnervating proximal branches with little additional nerve length in the radial nerve was thus at least as great as the combined impact of reinnervating proximal branches and traversing long pathways in the median and ulnar nerves.

The hypothesis that proximal branches may "steal" axons from distal tributaries (Figure 5-18)

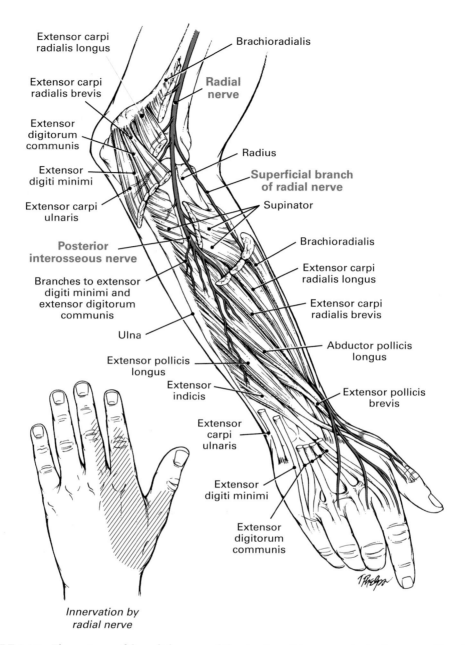

Extensor carpi
radialis longus

Extensor carpi
radialis brevis

Extensor
digitorum
communis

Extensor
digiti minimi

Extensor carpi
ulnaris

**Posterior
interosseous nerve**

Branches to extensor
digiti minimi and
extensor digitorum
communis

Ulna

Extensor pollicis
longus

Extensor
indicis

Extensor
carpi
ulnaris

Extensor
digiti minimi

Extensor
digitorum
communis

Brachioradialis

**Radial
nerve**

Radius

**Superficial branch
of radial nerve**

Supinator

Brachioradialis

Extensor carpi
radialis longus

Extensor carpi
radialis brevis

Abductor pollicis
longus

Extensor pollicis
brevis

*Innervation by
radial nerve*

FIGURE 5-17   The anatomy of the radial nerve and the structures it innervates in the forearm and hand. The bellies of radial-innervated muscles of the mobile wad—the brachioradialis, extensor carpi radialis longus, and extensor carpi radialis brevis—as well as those of the extensor carpi ulnaris and digital extensors, have been removed to expose the deep muscles of the dorsal forearm. The superficial, cutaneous branch of the radial nerve traverses the forearm beneath the brachioradialis, then emerges at the wrist level to innervate the dorso-radial hand.

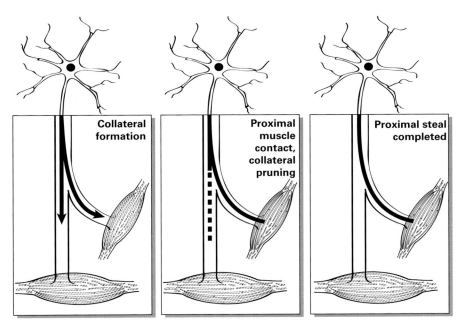

FIGURE 5-18   The Proximal Steal Hypothesis. If motoneurons regenerating to distal targets have a collateral in a branch to more proximal muscle, this collateral may become established, resulting in the pruning of the longer projection. Proximal muscles will tend to be reinnervated at the expense of their distal partners.

is further substantiated by observation of the recovery of individual muscles served by the PIN. Two smaller series in which cases are individually described clearly document that the distal-most muscles reinnervated through the PIN, the extensors of the thumb and index finger, may not regain function even after prolonged intervals (Fisher, McGeoch, 1985; Zook et al., 1989). Why do we not observe the converse, poor reinnervation of proximal PIN muscles in the presence of strong thumb extension? It is well documented that regenerating motor axons generate multiple collateral sprouts that branch extensively at the repair site to enter pathways leading to several muscles (Chapter 9). This observation raises the possibility that successful contact with a proximal muscle by one collateral leads to pruning of its sibling collaterals still on route to more distal muscles. Given that insufficient axons cross the suture line to restore the distal stump to normal, the remaining axons will tend to reinnervate the muscles they contact first at the expense of those farthest downstream. This hypothesis invites both more detailed clinical observation and experimental verification. If it predicts the behavior of motor axons correctly, then strategies to exclude or

reroute proximal motor tributaries may be a valid strategy for improving distal reinnervation.

THE SCIATIC NERVE

The Limits to Regeneration

The sciatic nerve is by far the longest in the body. Although it has a reputation for poor recovery after injury, the results of repair under optimal circumstances establish that axons can regenerate over great distances.

The sciatic nerve receives contributions from L4, L5, S1, S2, and S3 before exiting the pelvis through the sciatic notch. In the gluteal region it lies beneath the gluteus maximus, curving laterally around the ischial tuberosity to enter the thigh. It descends vertically down the posterior thigh on the surface of the adductor magnus and under cover of the hamstring muscles, extensors of the hip and flexors of the knee that it innervates. The sciatic nerve splits into tibial and peroneal divisions as it approaches the knee, having already traveled 35–40 cm since leaving the pelvis. The tibial division continues distally beneath the gastroc/soleus, innervating the sural cutaneous nerve and muscles that plantarflex (straighten) the ankle, invert the ankle (toe in), and flex the toes. It curves posterior to the medial malleolus of the ankle to supply skin on the sole of the foot and small muscles of the foot through the medial and lateral plantar nerves. After leaving the knee, the nerve travels an additional 45–50 cm before reaching the ankle. The peroneal division enters the lower leg by curving anteriorly around the neck of the fibula, where it divides into superficial and deep branches. The superficial branch courses distally beneath the peroneii, muscles that dorsiflex (bend) and evert (toe out) the ankle, which it innervates before reaching the foot to supply sensation to the dorsal and lateral aspect of the foot and toes. The deep branch supplies the remaining dorsiflexors of the ankle and toes and the skin of the first webspace.

Sciatic nerve injuries are relatively uncommon, and only one large series of cases has been published (Kim et al., 2004). Results were expressed as the number of patients reaching LSU grade III or better. The tibial and peroneal divisions are graded separately. Tibial grade III requires ankle plantarflexion against gravity and some resistance (gastroc/soleus), trace or better ankle inversion (tibialis posterior), and response to touch and pain on the sole of the foot with sensory mislocalization, sensation not normal with some overresponse present. Peroneal grade III mandates ankle eversion and dorsiflexion against some resistance (peroneii and tibialis anterior), though function of the toes is usually absent. These criteria were met after repair or graft of thigh level lacerations in 22/26 (85%) of tibial divisions and 18/26 (69%) of peroneal divisions. In the majority of cases, motor axons thus regenerated 40–50 cm and cutaneous axons regenerated 50–70 cm.

As even a single case can help define the limits of possibility, exceptional case reports may be worthy of note. One such case was presented by Sunderland (Sunderland et al., 1993) not long before his death. The sciatic nerve of a 23-year-old man was lacerated by a propeller at buttock level. The nerve was repaired anatomically under no tension, as the femur was shortened during fracture fixation. Seven years later, function of the knee and plantar flexion and inversion of the foot were normal. The peroneii and tibialis anterior could contract against strong resistance, and the digital flexors against moderate resistance. The patient could stand on tiptoe unaided. The dorsum of the foot was sensitive to pinprick and light touch, but application of these stimuli to the sole of the foot resulted in a blunt, mildly unpleasant sensation. By following Tinel's sign (a tingling produced by tapping directly over the tips of regenerating axons), Sunderland estimated that axons regenerated at 2.6 mm/day in the thigh, 1.2 mm/day in the proximal 3/4 of the lower leg, and 0.9 mm/day in the distal 1/4 of the lower leg. He calculated that in this case motor axons grew at least 70 cm, and sensory axons grew at least 90 cm.

The sciatic nerve experience thus indicates that both motor and sensory axons are capable of regenerating over great distances. These results are even more remarkable when one considers that the distance traversed by regenerating adult sciatic axons is at least an order of magnitude greater than that encountered during their development. A neuron's ability to elongate after injury is thus not restricted by the distance it traversed on its developmental journey.

CONCLUSIONS

Adequacy of Current Therapy

How well does suture of transected peripheral nerve restore lost function? Only 10% of adults will regain near-normal function after median or ulnar nerve repair, though a full 60% will regain useful function. Unfortunately, that leaves 9 of 10 without fine sensory discrimination and coordination, and 4 of 10 without the rudimentary function needed for gross manual activity. These failures are especially significant, as they often occur in otherwise healthy individuals whose capacity for work and recreation is substantially reduced by this single factor.

How well does nerve grafting restore function? In aggregate, the results of median and ulnar nerve grafting do not equal those of end-to-end repair. However, grafting of terminal nerves that serve a single or closely related functions can be as effective as direct nerve repair. This observation suggests that grafts may compromise outcome through their effects on axonal organization in addition to any potential effects on regeneration per se.

Adequacy of Reporting

Hundreds of reported cases could not contribute to the analysis in this chapter because they were presented with insufficient detail to isolate important variables. Many more were presented with enough information to shed light on one or more specific issues, but not enough to be included in a meta-analysis. Valuable clinical data could be used far more effectively if reports of the outcome of nerve repair and reconstruction included a full set of data on each patient as a supplement. This would facilitate a more powerful analysis than is currently possible, and support decision-making with far greater confidence when multiple treatment options are available.

Restatement of Clinical Variables in Biologic Terms

Patient age is clearly the most important clinical variable that influences the outcome of peripheral nerve surgery. In the premicrosurgery era, age was found to correlate with recovery of 2-point discrimination. Review of surgery performed with modern techniques confirms this finding in both the median nerve and the digital nerve. Restoration of ulnar motor function is also strongly age-dependent. The outcome of nerve grafting is similarly affected; when a large series of grafting procedures was analyzed for this chapter, age emerged as the only significant variable. Youth cannot, however, prevent or compensate for large pathfinding errors that result in synkinesis or faulty sensory localization.

A variety of biological factors could possibly contribute to the age effect. Limbs are shorter in the young and regeneration occurs more rapidly, both decreasing the time needed for end organ reinnervation. The young might retain developmental cues that enhance the specificity of distal stump reinnervation. End organs themselves might retain qualities that influence their pattern and specificity of reinnervation. Although the consequences of gross pathfinding errors cannot be eliminated, central correction for smaller errors may occur more readily in the young. The potential therefore exists to improve adult outcomes by determining which regeneration components are most age-sensitive and enhancing their performance in adults.

Three prominent clinical variables—location of injury, surgical technique, and length of nerve defect—exert their effects to varying degrees through the biological variable of intraneural organization. The location of the injury defines the degree of functional localization within a nerve, progressing from diffuse at proximal levels to more precise distally. The extent to which the surgeon can influence outcome by precise matching of nerve fascicles varies according to the proximo-distal localization of

discrete functions within these fascicles. As the size of a nerve gap increases, the physical correspondence of functionally related axons on the cut surfaces of the proximal and distal stumps will diminish, making it progressively more difficult to direct axons to appropriate targets.

Excellent results are often obtained by repairing nerves that serve a single or a few functionally related targets, such as the digital nerve (sensory) and the accessory and posterior interosseous nerves (motor). The results of repair deteriorate as the internal complexity of the nerve increases, as demonstrated by persistence of false sensory localization after median nerve repair, lack of individual digital control after distal ulnar nerve repair, and disabling synkinesis after facial nerve repair. The contributions to these phenomena of distance from neuron to injury and distance from injury to target can be canceled out by comparing nerves of similar length but differing internal organization. In the facial and accessory nerves, an ideal pairing from this perspective, functional restoration is inversely proportional to organizational complexity. Similarly, one may compare the results of repairing a single nerve above or below prominent branching points. Repair of radial nerve tributaries such as the PIN is clearly more effective than repair of the radial nerve trunk a short distance proximally.

The relationship between intraneural complexity and the outcome of surgery is confirmed by analysis of grafting procedures. Grafting the digital and accessory nerves often produces results equal to those of nerve repair, while grafting the more complex median, ulnar, and facial nerves does not routinely match this standard. The inverse relationship between intraneural complexity and the outcome of repair suggests that regenerating axons, both sensory and motor, lack an intrinsic mechanism to guide them back to the patch of skin or particular muscle that they innervated previously. In other words, both sensory and motor axon regeneration appear to lack topographic specificity.

A final clinical variable, time, plays a critical role in regeneration. The importance of time as a variable is demonstrated most clearly by analysis of the deleterious effects of delay in treatment, a time span that can be quantified precisely. Time also functions routinely as a consequence of distance, such as the length of nerve that separates the site of nerve injury from denervated end organs. The equation governing this effect is Denervation Time = Repair Delay + (Regeneration Speed x Distance to End Organ).

All components of the peripheral nervous system deteriorate to varying degrees and at varying speeds once they are denervated. Atrophy of skin and subcutaneous tissue, stiffness of joints, and degeneration of cutaneous and muscle end organs were readily appreciated by clinicians (Sunderland, 1978). More recent experimental work has emphasized the limitations that are also imposed on regeneration by prolonged neuronal axotomy and pathway denervation (Fu, Gordon, 1995a,b; Chapter 9).

Two distinct therapeutic strategies will be necessary to offset the effects of time on regeneration. First, accelerating the speed of regeneration will decrease the time needed to reinnervate distal pathway and end organ. Theoretically, of course, reinnervation time could be eliminated by fusing axons of the proximal and distal stump, obviating the need for regeneration to occur at all. In the absence of this ultimate "cure" for nerve injury, techniques of preventing pathway and end organ atrophy by maintaining expression of appropriate genes will soften the impact of time on functional outcomes.

REFERENCES

Altissimi M, Mancini GB, Azzara A (1991) Results of primary repair of digital nerves. J Hand Surg 16B: 546–547.

Barrios C, Amillo S, de Pablos J, Canadell J (1989) Secondary repair of ulnar nerve injury. Acta Orthop Scand 61: 46–49.

Birch R (1991) Repair of median and ulnar nerves. JBJS 73B: 154–157.

Brushart, T. (1998) Nerve repair and grafting. In: *Green's Operative Hand Surgery*, Vol. 4, D. Green, R. Hotchkiss and W. Pederson, eds., pp. 1381–1403, New York: Churchill Livingston.

Buncke HJ (1972) Digital nerve repairs. Surg Clin NA 52: 1267–1285.

Chandawarkar R, Cervino L, Pennington G (2003) Management of iatrogenic injury to the spinal accessory nerve. Plast Reconstr Surg 111: 611–617.

Chassard M, Pham E, Comtet JJ (1993) Two-point discrimination tests versus functional sensory recovery in both median and ulnar nerve complete transections. J Hand Surg 18B: 790–796.

Chuang DCC, Ma HS, Wei FC (1998) A new evaluation system to predict the sequelae of late obstetric brachial plexus palsy. Plast Reconstr Surg 101: 673–685.

Dailey AT, Tsuruda JS, Filler AG, Maravilla KR, Goodkin R, Kliot M (1997) Magnetic resonance neurography of peripheral nerve degeneration and regeneration. Lancet 350: 1221–1222.

Deutinger M, Girsch W, Burggasser G, Windisch A, Joshi D, Mayr N, Freilinger G (1993) Peripheral nerve repair in the hand with and without motor sensory differentiation. J Hand Surg 18A: 426–432.

Efstathopoulos D, Gerostathopoulos N, Misitzis D, Bouchlis G, Anagnostou S, Daoutis N (1995) Clinical assessment of primary digital nerve repair. Acta Orthop Scand Suppl 264: 45–47.

Falcioni M, Taibah A, Russo A, Piccirillo E, Sanna M (2003) Facial nerve grafting. Otol Neurotol 24: 486–489.

Fisher TR, McGeoch CM (1985) Severe injuries of the radial nerve treated by sural nerve grafting. Injury 16: 411–412.

Frykman GK, Cally D (1988) Interfascicular nerve grafting. OCNA 19: 71–80.

Fu SY, Gordon T (1995a) Contributing factors to poor functional recovery after delayed nerve repair: prolonged denervation. J Neurosci 15: 3886–3895.

Fu SY, Gordon T (1995b) Contributing factors to poor functional recovery after delayed nerve repair: Prolonged axotomy. J Neurosci 15: 3876–3885.

Gaul JS (1982) Intrinsic motor recovery: a long-term study of ulnar nerve repair. J Hand Surg 7: 502–508.

Gaul JS (1986) Electrical fascicle identification as an adjunct to nerve repair. Hand Clinics 2: 709–722.

Green JD, Shelton C, Brackmann DE (1994) Surgical management of iatrogenic facial nerve injuries. Otolaryngol Head Neck Surg 111: 606–610.

Gruber H, Freilinger G, Holle J, Mandl H (1976) Identification of motor and sensory funiculi in cut nerves and their selective reunion. Brit J Plas Surg 29: 70–73.

Hallin RG, Wiesenfeld Z, Lindblom U (1981) Neurophysiological studies on patients with sutured median nerves: faulty sensory localization after nerve regeneration and its physiological correlates. Exp Neurol 73: 90–106.

Hawkins GL (1948) Faulty sensory localization in nerve regeneration. J Neurosurg 5: 11–18.

Hoke A, Gordon T, Zochodne DW, Sulaiman OAR (2002) A decline in glial cell-line-derived neurotrophic factor expression is associated with impaired regeneration after long-term Schwann cell denervation. Exp Neurol 173: 77–85.

House JW, Brackmann DE (1985) Facial nerve grading system. Otolaryngol Head Neck Surg 93: 146–147.

Imai H, Tajima T, Natsumi Y (1996) Successful reeducation of functional sensibility after median nerve repair at the wrist. J Hand Surg 16A: 60–65.

Jabaley, M.E. (1991) Electrical nerve stimulation in the awake patient. In: *Operative Nerve Repair and Reconstruction*, R.H. Gelberman, ed., pp. 241–257, Philadelphia: Lippincott.

Jerosch-Herold C (2000) Should sensory function after median nerve injury and repair be quantified using two-point discrimination as the critical measure? Scand J Plast Reconstr Surg Hand Surg 34: 339–343.

Jerosch-Herold C, Rosen B, Shepstone L (2006) The reliability and validity of the locognosia test after injuries to peripheral nerves in the hand. JBJS 88B: 1048–1052.

Jongen S, Van Twisk R (1988) Results of primary repair of ulnar and median nerve injuries at the wrist: an evaluation of sensibility and motor recovery. Neth J Surg 40: 86–89.

Kallio PK (1993) The results of secondary repair of 254 digital nerves. J Hand Surg 18B: 327–330.

Kato H, Minami A, Kobayashi M, Takahara M, Ogino T (1998) Functional results of low median and ulnar nerve repair with intraneural fascicular dissection and electrical fascicular orientation. J Hand Surg 23A: 471–482.

Kim DH, Kam AC, Chandika P, Tiel RL, Kline DG (2001a) Surgical management and outcome in patients with radial nerve lesions. J Neurosurg 95: 573–583.

Kim DH, Kam AC, Chandika P, Tiel RL, Kline DG (2001b) Surgical management and outcomes in patients with median nerve lesions. J Neurosurg 95: 584–594.

Kim DH, Han K, Tiel RL, Murovic JA, Kline DG (2003a) Surgical outcomes of 654 ulnar nerve lesions. J Neurosurg 98: 993–1004.

Kim DH, Cho YJ, Tiel RL, Kline DG (2003b) Surgical outcomes of 111 spinal accessory nerve injuries. Neurosurgery 53: 1106–1112.

Kim DH, Murovic JA, Tiel R, Kline DG (2004) Management and outcomes in 353 surgically treated sciatic nerve lesions. J Neurosurg 101: 8–17.

Kline DG, Happel LT (1993) A quarter century's experience with intraoperative nerve action potential recording. Can J Neurol Sci 20: 3–10.

Kline, D.G. and A.R. Hudson. (1995) *Nerve Injuries*, Philadelphia: Saunders.

Langley JN, Hashimoto M (1917) On the suture of separate nerve bundles in a nerve trunk and on internal nerve plexuses. J Physiol 51: 318–345.

Larsen RD, Posch JL (1958) Nerve injuries in the upper extremity. Arch Surg 77: 469–482.

Lijftogt H, Dijkstra R, Storm van Leeuwen J (1987) Results of microsurgical treatment of nerve injuries of the wrist. Neth J Surg 39: 170–174.

Mackinnon, S.E. and A.L. Dellon. (1988) *Surgery of the Peripheral Nerve*, New York: Thieme.

Marsh D (1990) The validation of measures of outcome following suture of divided peripheral nerves supplying the hand. J Hand Surg 15-B: 25–34.

McFarlane RM, Mayer JR (1976) Digital nerve grafts with the lateral antebrachial cutaneous nerve. J Hand Surg 1: 169–173.

Meissl, G. (1977) Facial nerve suture. In: *Facial Nerve Surgery*, U. Fisch, ed., pp. 209–215, Birmingham, AL: Aesculapius.

Millesi H, Meissl G, Berger A (1972) The interfascicular nerve-grafting of the median and ulnar nerves. JBJS 54-A: 727–750.

Millesi H, Meissl G, Berger A (1976) Further experience with interfascicular grafting of the median, ulnar, and radial nerves. JBJS 58-A: 209–218.

Millesi H (1986) The nerve gap: theory and clinical practice. Hand Clinics 2: 651–663.

Mitchell, J.K. (1895) *Remote Consequences of Injuries of Nerves, and Their Treatment: An Examination of the Present Condition of Wounds Received 1863–5, with Additional Illustrative Cases*, Philadelphia: Lea Brothers.

Moneim MS (1982) Interfascicular nerve grafting. Clin Orthop 163: 65–74.

Nakamichi K, Tachibana S (1998) Iatrogenic injury to the spinal accessory nerve. JBJS 80-A: 1616–1620.

Nicholson OR, Seddon HJ (1957) Nerve repair in civil practice. British Medical Journal 2: 1065–1071.

Novak CB, Kelly L, Mackinnon SE (1992) Sensory recovery after median nerve grafting. J Hand Surg 17A: 59–68*.

Novak CB, Mackinnon SE (2002) Patient outcome after surgical management of an accessory nerve injury. Otolaryngol Head Neck Surg 127: 221–224.

Nunley JA, Ugino MR, Goldner R, Regan N, Urbaniak JR (1989) Use of the anterior branch of the medial antebrachial cutaneous nerve as a graft for the repair of defects of the digital nerve. JBJS 71-A: 563–567.

Ogino T, Sugawara M, Minami A, Kato H, Ohnishi N (1991) Accessory nerve injury: conservative or surgical treatment? J Hand Surg 16B: 531–536.

Omer GE (1974) Injuries to nerves of the upper extremity. JBJS 56-A: 1615–1624.

Onne L (1962) Recovery of sensibility and sudomotor activity in the hand after nerve suture. Acta Chir Scand [Suppl] 300: 1–69.

Roganovic Z, Petkovic S (2004) Missile severances of the radial nerve. Results of 131 repairs. Acta Neurochir 146: 1185–1192.

Roganovic Z (2005) Missile-caused median nerve injuries: results of 81 repairs. Surg Neurol 63: 410–419.

Roganovic Z, Pavlicevic G (2006) Difference in recovery potential of peripheral nerves after graft repairs. Neurosurgery 59: 621–633.

Rogers G, Henshall A, Sach R, Wallis K (1990) Simultaneous laceration of the median and ulnar nerves with flexor tendons at the wrist. J Hand Surg 15-A: 990–995.

Rosén B (1996) Recovery of sensory and motor function after nerve repair. J Hand Ther 9: 315–327.

Rosén B, Lundborg G (2000) A model instrument for the documentation of outcome after nerve repair. J Hand Surg 25A: 535–543.

Ruijs AC, Jaquet J-B, Kalmijn S, Giele H, Hovius SER (2005) Median and ulnar nerve injuries: A meta-analysis of predictors of motor and sensory recovery after modern microsurgical nerve repair. Plas Recon Surg 116: 484–494.

Saeed SR, Ramsden RT (1996) Rehabilitation of the paralysed face: results of facial nerve surgery. J Laryng Oto 110: 922–925.

Sakellarides H (1962) A follow-up study of 172 peripheral nerve injuries in the upper extremity in civilians. JBJS 44-A: 140–148.

Selma P, Emre O, Oguz P, Ersin N, Oya N (1998) Evaluation of the improvement of sensibility after primary median nerve repair at the wrist. Microsurgery 18: 192–196.

Shapiro, H.H. (1954) *Maxillofacial Anatomy*, Philadelphia: Lippincott.

Shergill G, Bonney G, Munshi P, Birch R (2001) The radial and posterior interosseous nerves. JBJS 83-B: 646–649.

Spector JG, Lee P, Peterein J, Roufa D (1991) Facial nerve regeneration through autologous nerve grafts: a clinical and experimental study. Laryngoscope 101: 537–554.

Steinberg, D.R. and L.A. Koman (1991) Factors affecting the results of peripheral nerve repair. In: *Operative Nerve Repair and Reconstruction*, R. Gelberman, ed., pp. 349–364, Philadelphia: Lippincott.

Stellini L (1982) Interfascicular autologous grafts in the repair of peripheral nerves: eight years experience. Brit J Plas Surg 35: 478–482.

Stephanian E, Sekhar LN, Janecka IP, Hirsch B (1992) Facial nerve repair by interposition nerve graft: results in 22 patients. Neurosurgery 31: 73–77.

Strickland, J., R. Idler, and J. DelSignore. (1991) Ulnar nerve repair. In: *Operative Nerve Repair and Reconstruction*, R. Gelberman, ed., pp. 425–436, Philadelphia: Lippincott.

Stromberg WB Jr, McFarlane RM, Bell J, Koch S, Mason M (1961) Injury of the median and ulnar nerves. JBJS 43-A: 717–730.

Sullivan DJ (1985) Results of digital neurorrhaphy in adults. J Hand Surg [Br Eur] 10B: 41–44.

Sunderland, S. (1978) *Nerves and Nerve Injuries*, New York: Churchill Livingston.

Sunderland S, McArthur RA, Nam DA (1993) Repair of a transected sciatic nerve. A study of nerve regeneration and functional recovery: Report of a case. J Bone Joint Surg [Am] 75A: 911–914.

Tajima T, Imai H (1989) Results of median nerve repair in children. Microsurgery 10: 145–146.

Tenny JR, Lewis RC (1984) Digital nerve grafting for traumatic defects. JBJS 66-A: 1375–1379.

Trumble TE, Kahn U, Vanderhooft E, Bach A (1995) A technique to quantitate motor recovery following nerve grafting. J Hand Surg 20A: 367–372.

Tupper JW, Crick JC, Matteck LR (1988) Fascicular nerve repairs: A comparative study of epineurial and fascicular (perineurial) techniques. OCNA 19: 57–69.

Vordemvenne T, Langer M, Ochman S, Raschke M, Schult M (2007) Long-term results after primary microsurgical repair of ulnar and median nerve injuries: a comparison of common score systems. Clin Neurol Neurosurg 109: 263–271.

Weber RA, Breidenbach WC, Brown RE, Jabaley ME, Mass DP (2000) A randomized prospective study of polyglycolic acid conduits for digital nerve reconstruction in humans. Plast Reconstr Surg 106: 1036–1045.

Weinzweig N, Chin G, Mead M, Stone A, Nagle D, Gonzalez M, Koerber A (2000) Recovery of sensibility after digital neurorrhaphy: a clinical investigation of prognostic factors. Ann Plas Surg 44: 610–617.

Wynn Parry CB, Salter M (1976) Sensory re-education after median nerve lesions. Hand 8: 250–257.

Young C, Hudson A, Richards R (1990) Operative treatment of palsy of the posterior interosseous nerve of the forearm. JBJS 72-A: 1215–1219.

Young L, Wray C, Weeks PM (1981) A randomized prospective comparison of fascicular and epineurial digital nerve repairs. Plast Reconstr Surg 68: 89–92.

Zook E, Hurt AV, Russell RC (1989) Sural nerve grafts for delayed repair of divided posterior interosseous nerves. J Hand Surg 14A: 114–120.

6

DETERMINING
EXPERIMENTAL OUTCOME

THIS CHAPTER describes a variety of measurements that have been used to characterize the outcome of nerve repair in experimental studies. Tests that characterize the process of regeneration, or that cannot be used to compare experimental animals, are described elsewhere. Axon counts and morphometrics, once imprecise, can now be determined from plastic sections at high magnification with the aid of powerful software programs. Electrophysiologic measurements are used frequently to characterize aspects of both sensory and motor axon regeneration, including the specificity of target reinnervation; newer techniques, such as magnetoneurography and motor unit number estimation (MUNE) are providing categories of information not previously available. Precise measurement of force generated by isolated muscles in response to neural stimulation has long been a mainstay of regeneration studies; examination of skin and muscle histology, in contrast, is performed infrequently. Retrograde labeling studies are assuming a central role in determining both the number and identity of neurons

that reinnervate a defined nerve or tissue. Voluntary function has been evaluated most frequently by measuring the walking tracks of rats that have undergone nerve repair. Strong interest in this testing modality has resulted in many refinements in technique and has stimulated the development of video gait analysis. The recent popularity of rat upper extremity models has fostered the development of new tests such as the rat grasping test and the Montoya staircase test. Rat sensory evaluation, developed in the context of pain studies, is less useful for the testing of tactile acuity.

AXON MORPHOLOGY
AND NUMBER

The classic studies of peripheral nerve regeneration performed in the first half of the twentieth century were based on light microscopic examination of 5–10 μm paraffin sections. Counts of myelinated axons varied by as much as 20% depending on staining technique; as a result, reliable quantification of unmyelinated axons was not possible (Aitken et al., 1947; Shawe, 1955). The subsequent development of plastic embedding for electronmicroscopy enhanced the accuracy of counting myelinated axons with the light microscope; electronmicroscopy itself extended this ability to unmyelinated axons. The uniform standard now involves plastic embedding of nerve that has either been fixed in situ, or immobilized in a stretched position before fixation to straighten axons within the perineurium.

In some early studies of plastic-embedded material, counts of both myelinated and unmyelinated axons were made directly from photomontages of electronmicroscopic images (Kline et al., 1981; Jenq, Coggeshall, 1985). More commonly today, myelinated axon number and morphology are determined from light microscopic examination of 0.5–2.0 μm plastic sections of tissue that has been osmicated and counterstained with dyes such as toluidine blue. Low power images are obtained digitally and analyzed with appropriate software to determine the total intrafascicular area of a nerve specimen. Digital images taken at 1,000–2,000x are then modified by specialized software that highlights the darkly labeled myelin. From these images the software counts a sample of myelinated axons and determines, for each axon, the total fiber diameter (diameter outside the myelin sheath) and axon diameter (diameter inside the myelin sheath). Secondary calculations of myelin thickness, g ratio, (axon diameter/total fiber diameter—see Chapter 1), and fiber density are then performed. The percentage of the nerve that is evaluated at high power and the criteria for choosing areas of the nerve to examine vary widely among investigators (Mackinnon, Dellon, 1988; Archibald et al., 1995; Gómez et al., 1996).

The quality of information gained from axon counts may be enhanced by manipulating the axon population under study. For instance, excision of dorsal root ganglia serving a given nerve at the time of nerve repair (Redett et al., 2005) or after a period of regeneration (Luo, Lu, 1996) will ensure that all myelinated axons distal to the repair are motor and not sensory.

ELECTROPHYSIOLOGY

The electrophysiologic parameters that characterize axon performance are elicited by delivering an electrical stimulus to one portion of a nerve and recording the resulting electrical activity from distant nerve or muscle. The compound muscle action potential (CMAP) (Figure 6-1) represents the summation of individual motor unit action potentials, and is expressed in millivolts. The sensory nerve action potential (SNAP) and compound nerve action potential (CNAP), in contrast, result from electrical activity within nerve alone, are recorded in microvolts, and can only be appreciated by averaging the responses to a large number of stimuli.

The CMAP has several salient characteristics (Figure 6-1). Latency is the time elapsed between the stimulus and the first deflection from baseline, thus reflecting the behavior of the most rapidly conducting axons. It includes the time required for the stimulus to travel down the nerve, the delay inherent in neuromuscular transmission, and the time required for the action potential to propagate along the muscle membrane to the recording electrodes. The amplitude of the CMAP in response to maximal stimulation, measured from either baseline-to-peak or peak-to-peak, is often used as an approximate gauge of the number of axons regenerating after nerve repair. CMAP amplitude may be influenced by the number and size of motor units responding to the stimulus, the varying conduction velocities of their axons, and, most importantly, by the substantial increase in motor unit size that often accompanies reinnervation (Gordon et al., 1993; Fugleholm et al., 2000). As regeneration and myelination advance, additional reinnervated muscle fibers are recruited and their response is progressively synchronized, increasing the amplitude of the CMAP toward normal (Madison et al., 1999). A more precise estimation of axon number may be obtained by determining the area under the CMAP curve (Rosen, Jewett, 1980; Archibald et al., 1991).

The CMAP is the direct, peripheral response to electrical stimulation of motor axons. Muscle contraction may also be induced, however, by indirect excitation of motoneurons through reflex pathways. The H Reflex is the electrical equivalent of the monosynaptic stretch reflex. It has a longer latency than the CMAP, as it requires stimulation of IA afferent fibers, proximal conduction of this signal through the dorsal root ganglion (DRG) to the anterior horn of the spinal cord, synaptic transmission from the afferents to motoneurons, and distal conduction through motor axons to muscle. Although more difficult to elicit than the CMAP, it has been evaluated after experimental nerve repair and regeneration (Valero-Cabré, Navarro, 2001; English et al., 2007).

The SNAP is the summation of action potentials traveling within individual sensory axons that were

Compound Motor Action Potential (CMAP)

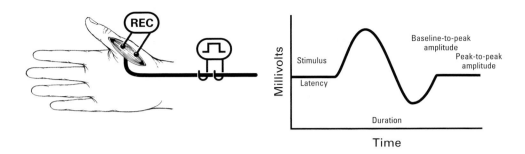

Sensory Nerve Action Potential (SNAP)

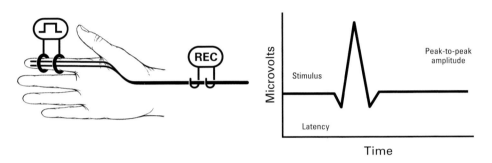

FIGURE 6-1 The compound motor action potential (CMAP) and sensory nerve action potential (SNAP). The CMAP is the summation of motor action potentials that result from proximal stimulation of motor axons. It is a robust signal produced by electrical activity within muscle, and is recorded in millivolts. The SNAP, in contrast, is the summation of action potentials traveling in sensory axons. Averaging techniques are required to separate the SNAP from baseline activity, and it is recorded in microvolts.

stimulated simultaneously by an electrical pulse delivered to the sensory nerve. Its configuration (Figure 6-1) is influenced by the amplitude and duration of these action potentials, the number of axons conducting, the distance covered, and the conduction velocities of the constituent axons. As discussed in Chapter 1, the conduction velocity of both normal and regenerated nerve is determined by nerve fiber diameter and myelin thickness (Cragg, Thomas, 1957, 1964). The latency of the SNAP reflects only the maturation of the most rapidly conducting axons, so its derivative, conduction velocity, will reveal little about the performance of the majority of axons in the nerve. Additionally, the heterogeneity of conduction velocities in sensory nerve, accentuated during regeneration, results in temporal dispersion and decreased amplitude of the SNAP

as the distance between stimulus and recording electrodes is increased (Rosen, Jewett, 1980).

Specialized electrophysiologic techniques have been devised to characterize the progression and outcome of experimental nerve regeneration. The proportion of axons that cross the site of nerve repair was first determined by electrically stimulating the distal stump while recording from small strands of axons dissected from the proximal stump. The percentage of proximal strands that received signals from the distal stump was then used as a measure of regeneration success (Pover, Lisney, 1989). A similar technique of recording from dorsal rootlets while stimulating specific receptors in the skin has been used to quantify the regeneration of specific fiber populations (Burgess et al., 1968). Alternatively, the nerve can be stimulated above and below the repair site while recording far proximally. The areas of the resulting compound action potentials will reflect the number of axons conducting in the proximal, uninjured nerve, and in the reinnervated distal stump. The degree to which proximal axons enter the distal stump is expressed as the "conduction fraction" (Hentz et al., 1991). This information can then be subjected to a "wave decomposition" technique to define the subpopulations of axons that make up the compound action potential, and to determine the contribution of each to the delay of conduction across the nerve repair. The percentage of axons that traverse a nerve repair can also be addressed by magnetoneurography, a technique that measures fluctuations in the magnetic field around a nerve as it conducts an impulse. A wire sensor coil is placed around the nerve proximal to the repair site, the nerve is stimulated distally, and over 1000 stimuli are averaged to improve the signal/noise ratio. The value obtained from regenerated nerve is expressed as a percentage of the value obtained from the contralateral, normal nerve (Kuypers et al., 1998).

Electrophysiologic techniques can also be used to assess the specificity with which axons within a proximal fascicle reinnervate that fascicle on the distal side of the nerve repair (fascicular specificity, Chapter 10) (Valero-Cabré, Navarro, 2002). After sciatic nerve repair and regeneration in the rat, the sciatic nerve is transected proximal to the healed repair and recording electrodes are placed distally in the gastrocnemius and plantar muscles (tibial nerve innervated) and the tibialis anterior muscle (peroneal nerve innervated). The proximal sciatic stump is first stimulated in its entirety, and is then dissected into its peroneal and tibial components, each of which is stimulated individually. To determine the degree of specific reinnervation of each muscle, the CMAP amplitude resulting from stimulation of the correct proximal fascicle is divided by the CMAP amplitude resulting from stimulation of the entire sciatic nerve. A similar technique has been described in which muscle force generation, rather than CMAP amplitude, is the measure of regeneration (Zhao et al., 1992).

Motor unit number estimation (MUNE—Chapter 4) is a potentially valuable electrophysiologic tool for both experimental and clinical regeneration research (Madison et al.1999; Gordon et al., 2007). The stimulus current applied to a reinnervated muscle nerve is increased gradually from threshold, causing distinct incremental increases in CMAP amplitude, each of which corresponds to the recruitment of an additional motor unit. To determine the number of motor units that have been reinnervated, the amplitude of the maximum CMAP is divided by the average amplitude of the first 5–10 motor unit potentials. In the primate median nerve model, Madison et al. (1999) were able to discern nearly all reinnervated thenar motor units individually, so little extrapolation was necessary.

Electromyography, the recording of electrical activity within muscle, has also been used to evaluate experimental nerve repair. Individual muscles fire in a specific pattern during the normal gait cycle; deviations from this pattern can be quantified to characterize the specificity of regeneration after nerve repair (Gramsbergen et al., 2000).

MUSCLE STRENGTH TESTING

Muscle strength testing is usually performed at the end of nerve regeneration experiments, as it most often involves injury to the neuromuscular unit. A fairly standard approach was developed by Bodine et al. (1987) and Totosy de Zepetnek et al. (1992), and has been used by many investigators (e.g., Bolesta et al., 1988; Frey et al., 1990; Evans et al., 1994; Fu, Gordon, 1995; Bodine-Fowler et al., 1997). Bones from which the muscle to be tested originates, as well as joints that it crosses, must be immobilized rigidly. The tendon of insertion, or the patella in the case of the quadriceps muscle (Frey et al., 1990), is connected to a strain gauge, and muscle and nervous tissue are bathed in a warm medium to maintain physiologic temperatures. A brief (0.1–0.2 millisecond) square-wave pulse is then delivered to the innervating nerve to elicit a muscle twitch, the effect of which is measured isometrically as "twitch tension." The amplitude of the twitch tension will depend on several factors discussed in Chapter 3 and recently summarized by Kernell (2006): the degree to which individual muscle fibers are activated by a single action potential, the extent of myosin light-chain phosphorylation, the dynamics of calcium binding to troponin C, and the elasticity of the muscle. The apparatus is adjusted to the muscle length that maximizes isometric twitch tension, and then a supraphysiological rate of stimulation (often 100 Hz) is applied to combine the forces of all activated fibers into a tetanic contraction. In this experimental setting, the tetanic force will be determined by the innervation ratio (number of muscle fibers/motor unit), the mean cross-sectional area of the muscle fibers, and the specific tension, the force per cm^2 of cross-sectional area (Kernell, 2006).

The above technique can be modified to minimize or eliminate its invasiveness, opening the possibility of repeated measurements. Exposure of reinnervated muscle is unnecessary if indirect force measurements are made through a hinged footplate (monkey tibial nerve [Kline et al., 1975]) or loop of thread around a toe (rat tibial nerve [Kerns et al., 1987]). Similarly, stimulation can be delivered through the skin rather than directly to the nerve (Kerns et al., 1987).

MORPHOLOGIC STUDIES OF SKIN AND MUSCLE

The morphologic properties of skin and muscle have been used only occasionally to quantify reinnervation. Functioning sweat glands are mapped in the mouse by injection of pilocarpine to stimulate sweating, followed by localization of the sweat drops on a silicon mold of the foot (Navarro, Kennedy, 1989). The anatomy of axons in the dermis and epidermis is well delineated by immunohistochemical demonstration of protein gene product 9.5 (PGP 9.5). The density of PGP 9.5 immunoreactivity in the skin is highly predictive of sweat gland reinnervation ($r=0.91$, $p<0.001$) (Verdú, Navarro, 1997), but is less closely related to the response to pinprick ($r=0.63$, $p<0.01$). Polymodal C fibers have been mapped by intra-arterial injection of Evans blue, followed by stimulation of the nerve of interest to induce extravasation into the skin (Povlsen et al., 1993).

Muscle reinnervation has been characterized using the technique of glycogen depletion (Totosy de Zepetnek et al., 1992). The physiologic properties of a single motor unit are first defined by isolating and stimulating its motor axon. The motor unit is then fired repeatedly for up to 4 hours to deplete glycogen from its fibers before the muscle is excised, rapidly frozen, and processed with a glycogen stain. The physiologic properties of the motor unit are then correlated with the anatomy and histochemical properties of the fibers that do not stain for glycogen. This elegant technique is a powerful tool for the evaluation of reinnervated muscle, but has limited application to studies of nerve repair as it can only investigate a single motor unit in each muscle.

Muscle weight is a convenient measure of reinnervation (e.g., Rodkey et al., 1980; Shibata et al., 1991; Bodine-Fowler et al., 1997). Denervated muscle atrophies rapidly by proteolytic destruction of muscle fibers, eventually losing up to 85% of its bulk (Gutmann, Zelena, 1962). After 6–10 months, the remaining muscle fibers may occupy less than 5% of their original cross-sectional area; Schmalbruch et al., 1991). Most studies of nerve repair involve wet muscle weight, obtained by excising and weighing the given muscle as rapidly as possible to prevent dehydration. Alternatively, the muscle may be dehydrated thoroughly so that only the weight of the structural components is determined.

RETROGRADE LABELING STUDIES

Retrograde tracing with the enzyme horseradish peroxidase (HRP) was introduced as a neuroanatomical technique in 1971 (Kristensson, Olsson, 1971). HRP that is applied to axons in the periphery is carried by axoplasmic transport to their parent neurons, where it can be demonstrated histochemically. Tissue sections containing these neurons are bathed in a solution of H_2O_2 and a chromogenic aromatic amine that turns color only where HRP is present to catalyze its oxidation. Early HRP techniques produced faint, incomplete labeling of neuron populations. The introduction of 3',5'-tetramethylbenzidine (TMB) as a chromogen, allowing quantitative, dark labeling of exposed neurons (Mesulam, 1978) (Figure 6-2), initiated the modern era of neuroanatomical tracing.

HRP tracing with TMB as chromogen was applied to the study of nerve repair and regeneration not long after its introduction (Brushart, Mesulam, 1980a). Retrograde (from peripheral axon to central neuron) tracing asks the question "Where are the neurons whose axons have been exposed to HRP?" Labeled neurons can be counted and their location defined with reference to known landmarks in the CNS, or within DRGs at given root levels. After repair of a nerve trunk (e.g., rat sciatic) that gives off distal tributaries (tibial, peroneal, sural), the question can be modified to ask, for instance, "To what extent do peroneal nerve axons return to the peroneal nerve after repair of the proximal sciatic trunk?" (Brushart, Mesulam, 1980a). The answer to this question can reveal the specificity with which axons restore appropriate distal connections after a variety of surgical manipulations (Brushart et al., 1983).

The value of data obtained by retrograde tracing is wholly dependent on the successful performance of appropriate experimental controls. In all tracing experiments it is mandatory to demonstrate that proximal transport of the tracer can be limited to the intended pathway. This can be done by applying

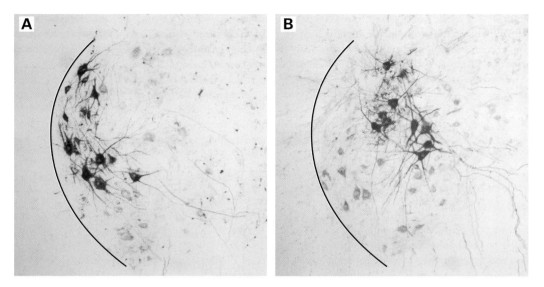

FIGURE 6-2   Retrograde labeling of rat motoneurons with horseradish peroxidase. Labeled motoneurons are dark black, while unlabeled motoneurons are lightly stained with neutral red. The peroneal motoneuron pool, on the left, lies at the lateral margin of the anterior horn of the spinal cord. The tibial pool is more centrally located, adjoining but not overlapping the peroneal pool (see Chapter 3, Figure 3-5 for a map of motoneuron pools in the cat).

the tracer to the tissue to be studied, then interrupting the innervating nerve at a more proximal level. If there is still neuronal labeling, then the tracer has been spread hematogenously or has been picked up by adjacent tissue. This type of unwanted labeling can often be eliminated by physically isolating the area of nerve exposed to the tracer. When tracer is applied by intramuscular or intradermal injection, increasing the risk of diffusion, it may be necessary to denervate adjacent structures through separate, proximal incisions to prevent the transport of label taken up by contaminated tissues (Burke et al., 1977; Brushart, Mesulam, 1980a). It is also important to realize that this type of experiment proves that the tracer *can* be controlled, not that it actually *is* controlled in each experimental animal, so precise standardization of technique is critical to reproducibility.

When a single tracer is used, evaluation of the "correctness" of reinnervation must rely on comparison of the postoperative location of labeled neurons with a separate, normal standard. In the spinal cord this is facilitated by comparing operated and nonoperated, normal sides of the cord; the symmetry of the motoneuron pools serving a given muscle or tributary nerve on right and left sides of the rat is very precise (Brushart, Mesulam, 1980a; Wasserschaff, 1990; English, 2005). In the

first comparison of regeneration specificity after various types of nerve repair (Brushart et al., 1983), neurons were scored as to their medial/lateral position within the spinal cord and on the degree of longitudinal offset of their motoneuron pools (Figure 3-5; Figure 6-2). Of these two criteria, the medial-lateral is probably the most functionally significant, as pools of the antagonistic peroneal and tibial nerves are side-by-side, while pools that overlap on the longitudinal axis serve related functions. Reinnervation of muscle by motoneurons that are wired to fire its antagonists is likely to disrupt function far more than reinnervation by motoneurons programmed for synergistic function. In more recent work longitudinal location of a motoneuron pool within the spinal cord has been represented by a weighted mean position that was defined as "the point from which the sum of distances to all cells located rostrally from it was equal to the sum of the distances to all cells located caudally" (Wasserschaff, 1990, p243). This formulation can be a fairly sensitive measure of specificity when one is evaluating the motoneuron pool of a single muscle in the context of other synergistic muscles served by the same nerve trunk, such that all the motoneurons will lie within a single longitudinal column. Motoneuron location has also been scored by the mean distance to the nearest labeled neuron, a scale that places equal weight on longitudinal and lateral displacement (Galtrey et al., 2007).

Horseradish peroxidase normally enters cells through diffusion. Coupling HRP to a substance that is internalized by active endocytosis, however, such as wheat germ agglutinin (WGA), can increase its uptake by 40-fold (Gonatas et al., 1979). Application of HRP-WGA to cut axons labels not only their parent neurons, but the projections of these neurons within the spinal cord and brainstem (Brushart, Mesulam, 1980b; Brown et al., 1989; Culberson, Brushart, 1989). HRP-WGA is also taken up from the skin after intradermal injection, providing a technique for mapping the dorsal horn projections of a peripheral structure before and after nerve repair (Brushart et al., 1981). Additionally, it provides continuous axonal labeling, and can thus be used to trace the location of a defined group of axons throughout an extremity, or to compare the position of a defined axon population above and below a nerve repair (Brushart, 1991).

Simultaneous Double-Labeling

Once HRP tracing was established as a valuable neuroanatomical technique, the next challenge was to demonstrate collateral projections of a single neuron. This required two separate tracers that both labeled all of the neurons to which they were exposed, that could be applied to different tributary nerves and transported through different pathways to the same parent neuron, and that could then be co-localized in that neuron (Figure 6-3). The process of simultaneous double-labeling from distal tributaries A and B of a repaired nerve asks three questions: (1) Which neurons project their axons only down branch A? (2) What other neurons project their axons only down branch B? and (3) What neurons send axon collaterals to both branch A and B?

The discovery of fluorescent dyes that are carried by axoplasmic transport satisfied the need for multiple tracers (Kuypers et al., 1979), though it was soon recognized that "one can rarely, if ever, label the entire population of neurons projecting down a certain nerve" with fluorescent dyes (Taylor et al., 1983). Additionally, there were problems of rapid fading, limited cellular definition, and diffusion of the dye from labeled neurons (Schmued, Fallon, 1986). Fluoro-Gold, a robust tracer that labeled all neurons to which it was exposed, and with stunning

anatomical detail, surmounted these problems. We initially paired Fluoro-Gold with HRP after determining that it labeled the same number of motoneurons when exposed to the rat femoral nerve, and could be confined to an intended pathway without unwanted uptake by surrounding tissue (Brushart, 1990). Similar quantitative labeling of DRG neurons with Fluoro-Gold was obtained by Baranowski et al. (1992). Combining these two tracers required complicating the histochemical protocol by using a pH change perfusion (Berod et al., 1981), as use of the normal HRP protocol resulted in leakage of Fluoro-Gold from labeled neurons.

The HRP–Fluoro-Gold protocol was time-consuming, as it required a lengthy perfusion, followed by the performance of a histochemical reaction on ordered serial sections. The procedure was later simplified by substituting Fluoro-Ruby for HRP, eliminating the need for any tissue processing after perfusion and sectioning; tissue sections could be taken from the microtome and mounted directly (Al-Majed et al., 2000). Fluoro-Ruby is a conjugate of dextran with the fluorochrome tetramethylrhodamine that can be differentiated from Fluoro-Gold with ease. Under ideal circumstances, when Fluoro-Ruby is applied directly to cut nerve for at least 1 hour, it can label as many neurons as Fluoro-Gold (Novikova et al., 1997; Boyd, Gordon, 2001; internal controls, Brushart lab). This is not always the case, however (Choi et al., 2002), especially after a prolonged regeneration experiment. Fluorescent debris accumulates in motoneurons as rats age, and can mimic the appearance of retrograde label. To compensate for this potential loss of quantitative labeling, the polarity of tracer application is alternated from one experimental preparation to the next, ensuring that a potential difference between the effectiveness of the two tracers will not bias experimental outcome (Brushart et al., 2002).

The simultaneous use of two tracers requires the performance of additional control experiments. An important part of ensuring that tracer is confined to the intended pathway is proving that it is not taken up unintentionally through the other pathway of interest. Proximal transection of each nerve after it has been exposed to tracer should limit labeling to the tracer that is applied to the other, intact nerve. In normal animals, there should be minimal or no double-labeling of neurons, as normal neurons rarely send collaterals down two separate tributary nerves. Additionally, it is important to demonstrate that both tracers label the same neurons and can be

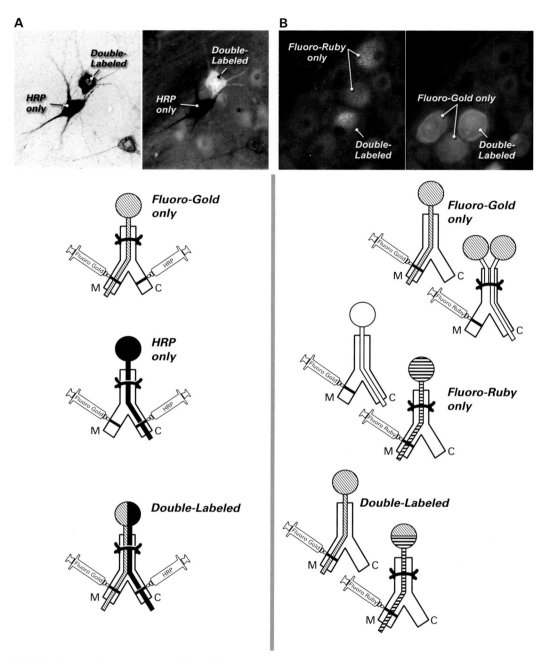

FIGURE 6-3 A. Simultaneous double-labeling with HRP and Fluoro-Gold in the rat femoral nerve model. The photograph in the upper left is taken with transmitted light and shows two HRP-labeled motoneurons. The same neurons are illuminated with fluorescent light on the right, revealing that one of the HRP-containing neurons also contains Fluoro-Gold, and is thus double-labeled. The cartoons below illustrate the three possible outcomes of simultaneous double-labeling; a neuron that projects to either pathway alone will take up only the tracer that is applied to that pathway, while a neuron that projects collaterals to both pathways will take up both tracers and be double-labeled. B. Sequential double-labeling. The photograph on the right shows rat dorsal root ganglion neurons prelabeled with Fluoro-Gold (FG), and that on the left, of the same tissue, shows neurons

(Continues)

visualized in the same cell without difficulty. This is often accomplished by labeling a single, previously uninjured nerve with both tracers and determining the percentage of cells that are double-labeled. In addition to increasing technical complexity, simultaneous double-labeling provides new opportunities for scoring cell location. For instance, English (2005) has described a "laterality index" that represents the number of times that motoneurons labeled from the peroneal nerve are lateral to those labeled from the tibial nerve after mouse sciatic nerve repair.

A crucial aspect of labeling studies is the technique used for cell counting. The established baseline for comparison is the use of ordered serial sections of HRP-labeled tissue, allowing the counter to examine each section in the context of the two adjacent sections, so that each neuron is counted only once (Swett et al., 1986). A more practical alternative is the counting of all labeled cells that contain the nucleus, then using a correction factor to account for the possibility that a split nucleus may appear in two tissue sections (Abercrombie, 1946). Error introduced by this technique will depend on the variability of nuclear size in a neuronal population and the degree to which nuclei change size after neuronal injury. When dealing with α and β motoneurons, this variability is small (Brushart, Mesulam, 1980a). It is therefore perfectly reasonable to apply this approach when comparing control and experimental motoneuron counts within a single experiment or model.

In some models counting every labeled neuron is not practical, and it becomes necessary to examine a representative sample. This process was revolutionized by introduction of stereological counting techniques (Gundersen, 1986). The ensuing debate as to the appropriate role for the stereologic approach was as vituperous as any in science, spawning titles such as "Quantification without Pontification" (Guillery, Herrup, 1997) on the one hand, and

"If You Assume, You Can Make an Ass out of U and Me" (Mayhew, Gundersen, 1996) on the other. The successful application of stereology to nerve regeneration experiments is exemplified by several recent studies (e.g., Dohm et al., 2000; Valero-Cabré et al., 2001).

Sequential Double-Labeling

Sequential double-labeling can provide the most powerful data on regeneration specificity, but is the most technically challenging of the labeling techniques. One tracer is applied to a specific nerve or soft tissue before the test lesion to label neurons that normally innervate that structure (prelabel). A second tracer is then applied to the same area after the lesion has been made proximally and axons have been allowed to regenerate (postlabel). Sequential double-labeling asks the question "What neurons that innervated this tissue originally have regenerated back to it after a nerve lesion?" (Figure 6-3).

The controls for sequential double-labeling are particularly stringent. As was discussed for simultaneous double-labeling, it is important to pick two tracers that label equal numbers of neurons and that can be co-localized readily within a cell. There are, however, several additional criteria for tracer choice. The first tracer should remain within labeled neurons in detectible quantities throughout the experiment, without significant leakage or toxicity. It is crucial to establish that tracer distribution is not altered by the test lesion, as some tracers may leak from injured neurons. Additionally, the prelabel should be cleared from the site of application so that it cannot be taken up by axons that regenerate into the labeled pathway from other sources (Puigdellívol-Sánchez et al., 2003). These neurons could pick up residual prelabel from the pathway, be identified incorrectly as normally innervating the prelabeled structure, and artificially inflate estimates of regeneration specificity. Figure 6-4 illustrates our approach to providing

FIGURE 6-3 (Continued)
postlabeled with Fluoro-Ruby (FR). A single cell has been labeled with both tracers, and is thus double-labeled. The cartoons below illustrate the interpretation of possible outcomes of sequential double-labeling. The rat femoral motor branch was labeled before and after repair of the proximal femoral nerve trunk. Neurons labeled with only FG originally projected to the muscle branch but either failed to regenerate or regenerated elsewhere. Neurons labeled with only FR did not originally innervate the muscle branch, but regenerated into it after repair. Neurons double-labeled with FR and FG both originated in and returned to the muscle branch. Reprinted from Brushart et al., 2005.

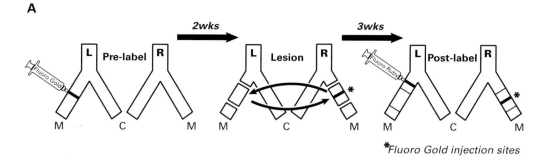

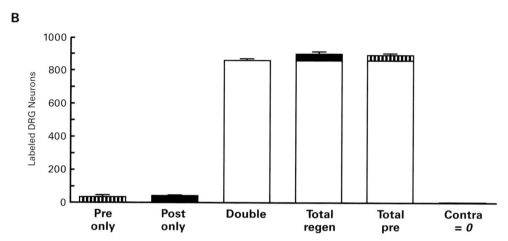

FIGURE 6-4   Controls for sequential double-labeling in the rat femoral nerve model. These evaluate the persistence of the first label (FG) in the pathway over time, the consistency with which both labels (FG and FR) can be demonstrated within the same neurons, and the possibility that regenerating axons might pick up residual of the first label (FG) from the site of prelabeling. The femoral muscle branch was prelabeled with FG to identify those neurons that normally innervate muscle (A). Two weeks later, exchange grafting of right and left muscle branches was performed to inflict a neuronal injury equivalent to that of nerve repair while minimally altering the population of axons in the proximal muscle nerve. This maneuver also allowed previously unlabeled axons on the right side of the animal to grow through the original site of FG injection and pick up any residual tracer. After a regeneration interval of 3 weeks, the muscle branch was labeled a second time to identify neurons that had extended their axons down this branch after repair. The results of this control experiment (B) demonstrate the viability of the sequential labeling technique. The number of double-labeled cells can be viewed either in the context of the total number of cells prelabeled (Total Pre = 96%) or the total number of cells postlabeled (Total regen = 95%). FG thus persists in a high percentage of neurons for 5 weeks, FG and FR can be consistently co-localized in DRG neurons, and FG is completely cleared from the pathway by 2 weeks. Reprinted from Brushart et al., 2005.

appropriate controls for sequential double-labeling with Fluoro-Gold and Fluoro-Ruby. This sequence asks two questions that are often ignored: (1) Does the nerve repair, usually performed 2–3 weeks after administration of the prelabel, result in leakage of prelabel from the cells that contain it? In most cases, controls presented to show that a prelabel remains stable in neurons for the duration of an experiment do not include a test lesion. (2) Does prelabel remain at the site of application long enough to label regenerating axons? In the case of Fluoro-Gold, we found that previously unlabeled axons passing through the prelabeling site were never labeled by residual tracer in the pathway (Brushart et al., 2005). Unfortunately, prolonged exposure to Fluoro-Gold is toxic to neurons (Garrett et al., 1991;

Novikova et al., 1997), so it cannot be recommended for sequential labeling experiments of longer than 6 weeks duration.

The percentage of neurons that are double labeled can be calculated in a variety of ways (Skouras et al., 2002; Brushart et al., 2005; Puigdellivol-Sanchez et al., 2006); Figure 6-4 demonstrates calculation of the percentage obtained with the Fluoro-Gold, Fluoro-Ruby combination, both on the basis of the number of neurons prelabeled (96%) and on the basis of the total number labeled at the end of the experiment (95%).

VOLUNTARY MOTOR FUNCTION

Rat Walking Track Analysis

Evaluation of voluntary function after experimental nerve repair was first attempted by Gutmann, who observed the loss of toe spreading after injury of the rabbit peroneal nerve, but found it difficult to quantify (Gutmann, 1942). In the rat, however, Hasegawa (1978) was able to measure the loss and recovery of toe spread after nerve crush. Stimulated by these observations and by the more general study of rat footprints in neurologic disease (Hruska et al., 1979; Jolicoeur et al., 1979), de Medinaceli formulated the well-known sciatic functional index (SFI) (de Medinaceli et al., 1982). He obtained walking tracks by dipping a rat's foot in photographic developer, then letting the rat walk across x-ray film. After a variety of unilateral sciatic nerve lesions he measured the distance between feet (to other foot—TOF), the print length (PL), the distance between second and fourth toes (intermediate toe spread—IT), and the distance between the first and fifth toes (toe spread—TS). From these he calculated an index of recovery, the SFI, by comparing the measurements of the normal and experimental foot. This formula was derived empirically, and was based on the assumption that all variables were of equal importance (Figure 6-5).

The de Medinaceli formula for calculating the SFI was later altered by eliminating consideration of the distance between feet (TOF) and by modifying the weighting of contributing measurements.

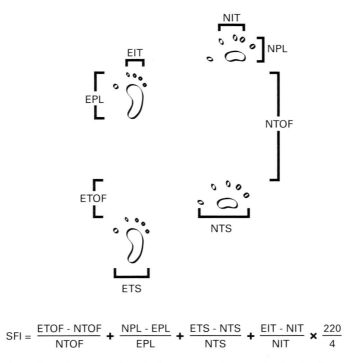

$$SFI = \frac{ETOF - NTOF}{NTOF} + \frac{NPL - EPL}{EPL} + \frac{ETS - NTS}{NTS} + \frac{EIT - NIT}{NIT} \times \frac{220}{4}$$

FIGURE 6-5   The de Medinaceli protocol for calculating sciatic functional index (SFI). NPL—normal print length, EPL—experimental print length, NTS—normal toe spread, ETS—experimental toe spread, NIT—normal intermediate toe spread, EIT—experimental intermediate toe spread, NTOF—normal distance to opposite foot, ETOF—experimental distance to opposite foot.

Initial efforts by Carlton and Goldberg (1986) were reported in abstract form only. Subsequently, Bain et al. (1989) measured the tracks of rats with peroneal, tibial, and sciatic nerve lesions and subjected their results to multiple linear regression analysis. They determined that the distance between feet (TOF) did not predict function, and were able to weight the contribution of each remaining factor to the whole more accurately, adding the letter "E" to identify experimental measurements, and the letter "N" to identify normal ones (SFI = −38.3 (EPL − NPL/NPL) + 109.5 (ETS − NTS/NTS) + 13.3 (EIT − NIT/NIT) − 8.8). When compared with the de Medinaceli and Carlton equations, this formulation gave lower mean values and standard deviations in sham-operated animals, and was able to differentiate peroneal-injured animals from sham controls, which the others could not.

Walking track analysis, though a seminal contribution to the study of nerve repair and regeneration, must be approached with caution. In their initial presentation, de Medinaceli et al. (1982) described a high interobserver correlation when individuals were asked to measure specified tracks (r = 0.98, p < 0.0001). In a later study by Brown et al. (1991) in which observers were shown an entire sequence of prints and given the freedom to pick those to measure, the interobserver reliability decreased somewhat (r = 0.92); paradoxically, the intra-observer reliability was poor (r = 0.53 − 0.76). Numerous technical problems may also compromise the recording and interpretation of rat walking tracks (discussed in Varejao et al., 2001, 2004). Chief among these are the alteration of the footprint by autotomy or contracture. Autotomy, or self-mutilation, varies widely among rat strains (Inbal et al., 1980; Carr et al., 1992) and may be mitigated by both topical and oral medications (discussed in Varejao et al., 2004). Contractures form when the flexion and extension forces across a joint are chronically imbalanced. In the face of significant contracture it is difficult or impossible to measure walking tracks (Dellon, 1989; Hare et al., 1992): in one recent study, it was necessary to operate on 86 rats to obtain meaningful results in 30 (Martins et al., 2006). Exclusion of so many animals can significantly bias the outcome of an experiment, especially when those eliminated for severe contractures are likely to be those with the worst experimental results. Providing a wire mesh for rats to walk across in their cage helps minimize contracture formation (Strasberg et al., 1996).

The risk of autotomy and contracture formation is reduced substantially when only the tibial or peroneal nerve is injured and repaired (Hare et al., 1992). In a manner similar to that used to recalculate the equation for the SFI, Bain et al. (1989) derived equations for a tibial function index (TFI = −37.2 (EPL − NPL)/NPL + 104.4 (ETS − NTS)/NTS + 45.6 (EIT − NIT)/NIT − 8.8) and a peroneal function index (PFI = 174.9 (EPL − NPL)/NPL + 80.3 (ETS − NTS)/NTS − 13.4). Limiting experimental injury to either peroneal or tibial nerve also solves a major shortcoming of the SFI. Whereas the TFI and PFI detect recovery after isolated tibial or peroneal nerve transection and repair, the SFI rarely improves after sciatic nerve transection, regardless of the means of repair (Chapter 7). This discrepancy may be explained by a critical difference between sciatic nerve injury on the one hand, and tibial or peroneal injury on the other; the former introduces the possibility of crossed reinnervation of antagonistic muscles, while the latter does not. The impact of confused reinnervation among synergistic muscles is far less than that of crossed reinnervation of flexors and extensors (Wikholm et al., 1988).

The interpretation of rat walking tracks continues to advance. Recently, Bervar (2000) found that static TS (the distance between the first and fifth toes with the animal stationary) correlates strongly with the SFI after nerve injury (r = 0.9343; p < 0.0001). Substitution of this single measurement for the complex SFI could greatly simplify the evaluation of groups of experimental animals. An even stronger correlation between SFI and static TS was found when the technique was evaluated independently by a second laboratory (r = 0.958, p < 0.001; (Smit et al., 2004). Semiautomated techniques of walking track analysis have also been developed that allow simultaneous calculation of both footprint and gait parameters, as well as estimation of the force applied by each paw (Deumens et al., 2007; Bozkurt et al., 2008).

The principles behind the rat SFI have been extended to the mouse sciatic nerve and the rat upper extremity. Our recently acquired ability to turn off or enhance the activity of specific mouse genes has initiated a quest for gene-function correlations. Both dynamic (Inserra et al., 1998; Yao et al., 1998) and static (Baptista et al., 2006) indices for the mouse have been generated and tested in response to this need. Similarly, attempts to model brachial plexus injuries have stimulated the development of rat upper extremity pawprint analysis (Bontioti et al., 2003). Galtrey and Fawcett (2007) evaluated upper extremity footprints after various degrees of intentional axon misdirection, and found that toe spread accurately reflected lesion severity, but print length did not. Perhaps most important, there is a growing awareness that seemingly identical rats of an inbred strain may differ in their desire to explore and in their response to stress, both of which may introduce unanticipated experimental variables (Van Meeteren et al., 1997a, 1997b; Galtrey, Fawcett, 2007).

In spite of the growing sophistication of walking track analysis, significant limitations remain. As axons regenerate down the sciatic, tibial, or peroneal nerve distal to a transection and repair at thigh level, they will first reinnervate the long flexors and/or extensors of the ankle. The SFI, TFI, or PFI may thus improve in the first 1–2 months as a result of this. As regeneration progresses, however, muscles intrinsic to the foot will be reinnervated, and the balance of forces acting on the toes will be altered. SFI usually plateaus about 3 months after nerve repair (Chapter 7), and only then does it reflect the reinnervation of all muscles involved. Although the progression of SFI is usually followed throughout an experiment, there is thus no basis for comparing values obtained before reinnervation has stabilized. A second shortcoming of the walking track techniques is that the paw is treated as a "black box." Axons go in and function comes out, but there is no data regarding which muscles need to be innervated to what degree to produce a given level of function, or how much axonal misdirection among the various muscles is required to degrade function. As a result, walking track results cannot be used to predict the effects of a given repair technique or treatment on a different neuromuscular system.

VIDEO GAIT ANALYSIS

An alternative to measuring and interpreting rat walking tracks is provided by video analysis of rat walking gait. This can be recorded from beneath, from the side, or simultaneously from the side and beneath by placing an angled mirror below a transparent runway (Westerga, Gramsbergen, 1990). In early studies, the duration of the stance phase, the period during which the foot touches the floor, was found to correlate with both SFI ($r=0.797$) and TS obtained by video analysis ($r=0.822$; both $p < 0.001$) (Walker et al., 1994). A second gait parameter, the ankle angle, was initially defined in the sagittal plane by the intersection of lines passing from knee to ankle and from metatarsal head to ankle (intersection model). The ankle angle at the end of the swing phase, as the foot is about to touch the ground, was found to be a sensitive indicator of peroneal nerve crush that returned to normal by 3 weeks postinjury (Santos et al., 1995). When defined as the difference between the angle formed by the tibial shaft and the ground and the angle formed by the foot and the ground (2-segment model), the ankle angle at midstance differentiated grafted from unrepaired sciatic nerves, whereas the SFI did not (Lin et al., 1996).

The first global analysis of rat gait after nerve injury was performed by Yu and colleagues (2001). Discriminate analysis of 7 primary gait parameters identified those that varied with walking speed, and resulted in the choice of the following primary and derived factors as sensitive indicators of nerve injury: (1) the R:L stance/swing ratio (SS); (2) the ratio of R:L step length (SLR), defined with reference to the middle metacarpal head to eliminate the effects of toe contracture; (3) the ankle angle (intersection model) at the end of stance (ATS); (4) the ankle angle at midstance (AMS); and (5) midline deviation of the trunk (MID). These factors were used to generate functional scores for the sciatic nerve (sciatic score = $12.42 \times$ SS + 10.$29 \times$ATS + $10.58 \times$SLR – 30.86), the tibial nerve (tibial score = $18.53 \times$ SS + $11.5 \times$ATS – 28.75), and the peroneal nerve (peroneal score = $-13.73 \times$ AMS – $8.72 \times$MID + 16). Interobserver variability was described as "negligible"; attempts to correlate the new functional scores with the traditional SFI were defeated by the authors' reported inability to interpret any of the standard footprint recordings after tibial or peroneal nerve injury. In further refinements, Varejao and colleagues defined separate components of the stance phase (Varejao et al., 2002), and showed that these remained abnormal 8 weeks after sciatic crush, even when SFI had returned to normal (Figure 6-6) (Varejao et al., 2003b). They also defined the "toe out angle," the angle between the direction of movement and the axis of the foot, and found that it correlated well with the SFI ($r=0.99$) (Varejao et al., 2003a).

Gait analysis has also been applied to femoral nerve lesions in the mouse. Irintchev and colleagues (2005) filmed mice from the rear during beam walking and defined three parameters that changed significantly after femoral nerve lesion: (1) the heels-tail angle (HTA), the angle between lines

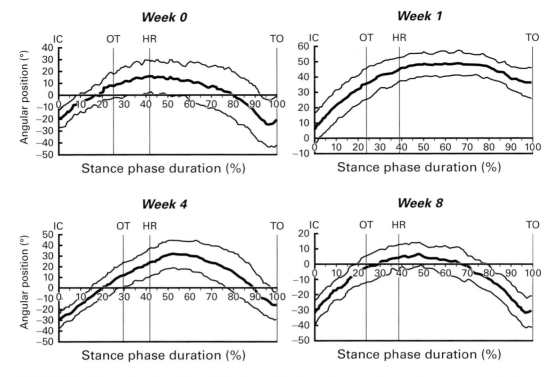

FIGURE 6-6 Kinematic plots of the ankle in the sagittal plane as it moves through the stance phase of gait. The sciatic nerve has been crushed at week 0 and recovers progressively thereafter. Standard deviation is plotted on either side of the mean. IC—initial contact, OT—opposite toe-off, HR—heel rise, TO—toe off. Reprinted with permission from Varejao et al., 2003b.

connecting the heels and the external urethral orifice (females) or anus (males); (2) the foot-base angle (FBA), the angle between the axis of the foot and the floor at the end of stance; and (3) the limb protraction length ratio (PLR), the ratio of the relative lengths of the intact and lesioned limb as the mouse, suspended by its tail, grasps for a pencil (Figure 6-7). Because the absolute values of these parameters varied with mouse sex and age, a recovery index was calculated to facilitate experimental comparisons $(RI = (X_{preop} - X_{denervated}) / (X_{denervated} - X_{reinnervated}) \times 100)$. The recovery index for each of the three parameters differentiated the gait 1 month after femoral crush from that 1 month after femoral transection.

Video gait analysis overcomes the primary limitations of walking track analysis—distortion of the footprint through autotomy or contracture—and is more sensitive to neuromuscular deficits. The accuracy of results may be compromised, however, by motion of the skin, and thus motion of the reference marks, in relation to underlying bone (Westerga, Gramsbergen, 1990; Alexander, Andriacchi, 2001).

In our laboratory this problem is eliminated by surgically anchoring skin directly to bone at the reference points 1 week before rats are acclimatized to the testing apparatus. Little work has been done on intra- and interobserver reliability, especially on the placing of video markers, and the above studies on nerve transection or crush need to be extended to analysis of nerve repair.

UPPER EXTREMITY GRASPING TEST

The grasping test, as initially described, is performed by lowering a rat by the tail until it grasps a wire grid mounted on an electronic balance, and withdrawing the rat until it lets go (Bertelli, Mira, 1995). The maximum force registered on the balance is interpreted as the grip strength. In the rat, the median nerve innervates the digital flexors and the ulnar nerve provides wrist flexion (Bertelli, Mira, 1995; Papalia et al., 2003). The original device was modified by Papalia et al. (2003) to eliminate the tendency

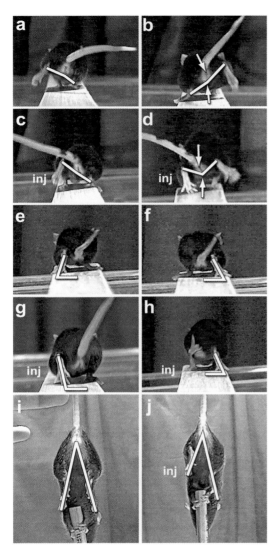

FIGURE 6-7 Mouse femoral nerve gait analysis. Single video frames from recordings of beam walking (a–h) and limb protractions (I and j) in intact animals (a, b, e, f, and I) and animals 7 days after left femoral nerve crush (c, d, g, h, and j). The lines illustrate the heel-tail angle (HTA, a–d), the foot-base angle (FBA, e–h), and the limb lengths used for calculation of the limb protraction length ratio (PLR, I and j). Reproduced with permission from Irintchev et al., 2005.

for rats to walk along the grid and to exert force by flexing their wrist. Although these tests both indicate the progressive return of grip strength, neither has been evaluated for inter- or intra-observer reliability. An apparatus that permits simultaneous evaluation of grip strength in both upper extremities, initially designed to measure the consequences of CNS lesions (Dunnett et al., 1998), has also been adapted for testing after peripheral nerve repair; statistical analysis revealed significant effects of both injury severity and time (Galtrey, Fawcett, 2007). The accuracy of grip strength testing is affected by sampling rate, the nature of the object grasped, the angle of approach, sensory deficits, and body weight (Maurissen et al., 2003). As a result of this variability, these authors recommend that testing results be referred to as "grip performance." Rat motivation also plays a prominent role (Bertelli, Mira, 1995; Papalia et al., 2003); in our laboratory large intra-animal variation from day to day precluded use of the test in Sprague-Dawley rats.

THE MONTOYA STAIRCASE TEST

The staircase test was devised to quantify skilled use of individual rat upper extremities during evaluation of motor systems performance (Montoya et al., 1991). The rat is given narrow access to a descending staircase, each stair containing food pellets in a sunken well (Figure 6-8). In food-deprived rats, grasping ability is determined by the number of pellets removed, and reaching ability by the number of excess pellets knocked down to levels beyond reach. Analysis of performance after a variety of CNS lesions revealed a significant difference among the scores represented by each level (ANOVA; $p < 0.001$). Additional information on the contributions of impairment, recovery, and compensation to the final result can be obtained through more time-consuming video analysis (Whishaw et al., 1997) or by using pellets that are color-coded by level (Kloth et al., 2006).

Neural control of rat upper extremity function cannot be used as a direct model of human motor control. Structurally, the higher primate and human hand muscles are controlled through direct corticomotoneuronal projections, whereas rat muscles are not (Chapter 3). There are, however, indirect projections through the corticospinal tract that control reaching behavior (Li et al., 1997). In the rat, reaching is directed initially by olfaction rather than vision (Whishaw, Tomie, 2007); once the target has been contacted, haptic input is used to adjust the trajectory of subsequent reaching and to adjust grip (Ballermann et al., 2000). It is also important to recognize that rat strains differ significantly in their

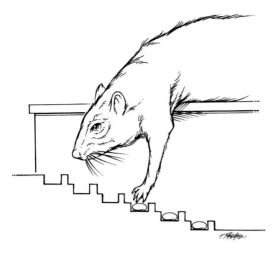

FIGURE 6-8   The Montoya staircase test for rat upper extremity function. The rat is presented with food pellets on a staircase that represents 7 graded stages of reaching difficulty (Montoya, 1991). Access is limited by confining the staircase within a narrow well (not shown). Grasping ability is determined by the number of pellets removed, and reaching ability by the number of excess pellets knocked down to levels beyond reach.

reaching performance. Sprague-Dawley and Lewis rats do poorly in comparison with Long-Evans and Lister hooded rats (Whishaw et al., 2003; Galtrey, Fawcett 2007); Lewis rats performed well in isolated trials (Pagnussat et al., 2009).

REFLEX AND STEREOTYPICAL RESPONSES

Rabbit Toe Spread Test

Gutmann (1942) observed that rabbits could no longer spread their toes after peroneal nerve transection, and found that a toe-spreading reflex could be elicited by partially dropping the animal toward a flat surface. Impaired toe spreading resulted from inaction of the peroneal II, III, and IV muscles that spread the second, third, and fourth toes respectively. Gutmann formulated a scale to describe the progressive recovery of this function: Degree 1, minimal spreading of fourth toe alone; Degree 2, slight spreading of all three toes; Degree 3, spreading of all three toes less forcefully than normal; and Degree 4, full, normal spreading of all three toes. This test was recently found to discriminate the time

required for muscle reinnervation after peroneal nerve lesions made only 1 cm from one another, and is thus a sensitive indicator of the onset of motor recovery (Schmitz, Beer, 2001).

Extensor Postural Thrust

The extensor postural thrust (EPT) was first measured in a study of the effects of local anesthesia on rat sensory and motor performance (Thalhammer et al., 1995). The rat is grasped by the examiner and lowered onto a balance, which it will contact with the ankle extended. The force required to then flatten the foot on the balance is the EPT. In a comparative test of EPT and SFI, the recovery curves were quite similar, though no r values were calculated (Hadlock et al., 1999).

Rat Grooming Test

The rat responds to dropping water onto its snout with a sweeping movement of the paw that requires elbow and shoulder flexion. Bertelli has devised a grading system that scores the completeness of this motion as an index of recovery after experimental brachial plexus reconstruction (Bertelli, Mira, 1993). This test has not been validated, and has been replaced by the grasping test in Bertelli's more recent investigations (Bertelli et al., 2004, 2005).

Facial Nerve Function

The rat facial nerve, with its many muscle branches, is an ideal model for the study of motor reinnervation (Angelov et al., 1996). The rat explores its often dark environment by rhythmically "whisking" its vibrissae (whiskers), an activity controlled by fibers within the buccal branch of the facial nerve. Normal whisking consists of a cycle of vibrissal protraction and retraction repeated 5–11 times per second. After facial nerve injury, the vibrissae assume a caudal, retracted position and no longer move. With progressive reinnervation, the position and motion of the vibrissae are restored (Figure 6-9). Whisking performance is analyzed from video clips selected on the basis of animal head position, whisking frequency, and degree of protraction (Guntinas-Lichius et al., 2001) and is thus somewhat subjective. The parameters measured are protraction angle, whisking frequency, whisking amplitude, and angular velocity and acceleration during protraction. Rat facial nerve function may also be evaluated by

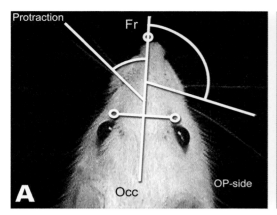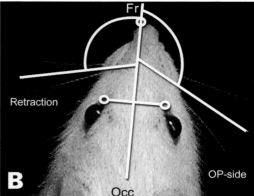

FIGURE 6-9   Analysis of rat whisking behavior. Protraction (above) and retraction (below) of selected whiskers is viewed from above with reference to the fronto- (Fr) occipital (Occ) line. There is a full range of motion on the left, normal, side; little motion occurs on the right, operated side. Reprinted with permission from Guntinas-Lichius et al., 2002.

measuring the degree of eye closure in response to an air puff on the cornea (Choi, Raisman, 2005). Facial nerve recovery in the monkey has been evaluated by measuring the oral commissural angle on video recordings of facial movement (Hontanilla et al., 2006).

EVALUATION OF SENSORY FUNCTION

The extensive use of the rat sciatic nerve to model neuropathic pain has resulted in the development of tests for normal physiologic pain, for allodynia, a painful response to a normally nonpainful stimulus, and for hyperpathia, an increased response to an already painful stimulus. Physiologic pain has been tested by delivering electric shocks to the rat foot. The output of a 540 Volt AC source is adjusted by controlling impedance to produce a current of between 0.1 and 0.6 mA when the skin completes the circuit between two stimulating electrodes (De Koning et al., 1986). A rat with intact sensation will withdraw immediately from even the smallest stimulus. No withdrawal in response to a stimulus of 0.6 mA indicates total loss of sensation, and response to stimuli of 0.3 mA and above a 50% loss of sensation (Hoogeveen et al., 1992). Alternatively, a "pinprick score" can be derived by testing five areas on the plantar surface of the paw with a blunt needle and scoring the response as none, reduced, or normal (Lago, Navarro, 2006). Neither of these tests has been validated.

Allodynia is often evaluated with Semmes-Weinstein filaments (Chapter 4) or a modification thereof. Animals are tested in an enclosure with a wire mesh floor so that the sole of the foot can be contacted by filaments introduced from below. Withdrawal of the foot is scored as a positive response. Two paradigms have been described for routine sensory testing: the up-down method (Dixon, 1980; Chaplan et al., 1994) and the response incidence method (Kim, Chung, 1992; Kinnman, Levine, 1995). With the up-down method, a series of six monofilaments is used, beginning with one near the middle of the range. If a positive response is observed, the next smaller filament is applied; If the rat fails to respond, the next higher force is applied. The pattern of positive and negative responses is converted to a 50% threshold value by using a formula derived by Dixon (1980). Comparison of results obtained by experienced investigators with this method revealed high interobserver reliability ($p = 0.006$) (Chaplan et al., 1994). The response incidence method employs the same six monofilaments, always beginning with the weakest and progressing to the strongest. Each filament is applied 5 times for 1 second, and the number of trials eliciting withdrawal is used to estimate the incidence of response.

Heat is the stimulus most commonly used to elicit hyperpathic pain. The response to heat is frequently evaluated by focusing a light source through a glass-bottomed chamber onto the sole of the foot (Hargreaves et al., 1988). The latency between the onset of stimulation and withdrawal of the foot is measured five times at 5-minute intervals, and expressed as a mean. Alternatively, heat may be applied directly to the foot with a hot probe (Thalhammer et al., 1995), or the rat may be placed on a hot plate (Dowdall et al., 2005). Sensitivity to cold has also been evaluated, though less frequently (Lindsey et al., 2000; Galtrey, Fawcett, 2007).

CONCLUSIONS

This chapter has described many of the techniques used to quantify the outcome of experimental nerve repair. When evaluating a particular technique, it is important to ask: (1) How accurately and reproducibly does this test measure the target variable? (2) What does this variable mean in the context of nerve regeneration? Clearly, some of the techniques described have been scrutinized and validated to various degrees, while others have been used by one or two labs without determination of their sensitivity, specificity, or reproducibility. A second factor that often receives insufficient emphasis when evaluating the efficacy of a technique is the adequacy of control experiments. This is especially true for retrograde labeling, where outcomes are highly dependent on both the choice of retrograde tracers and the technique used to apply them. For instance, when the popular tracer Fast Blue was used to prelabel motoneurons before nerve repair, experimental counts of Fast Blue–labeled neurons were elevated by 20–40% over counts obtained by labeling contralateral, normal control nerves at the end of the experiment (Brushart, unpublished results). This phenomenon has been attributed to retention of tracer in the prelabeled pathway (Puigdellivol-Sanchez et al., 2003).

The relative importance of individual tests in characterizing the outcome of nerve repair is still being discussed. Axon counts, for instance, are limited in their significance by the failure of some axons to cross a repair, and by the variable propensity of others to sprout collaterals in a pathway-dependent manner; they are not an accurate indication of the number of neurons that have regenerated. Similarly, the strength of muscle contraction in response to electrical stimulation of its proper nerve is only a measure of possibility; the ultimate usefulness of this muscle will depend on the organization and connections of the motoneurons that drive it. One may encounter both extremes of this limitation in the treatment of neonatal brachial plexus injuries.

Ample innervation of elbow flexors and extensors, but with crossed reinnervation, results in frequent co-contractions that hypertrophy muscle but severely limit motor control. At the other extreme, muscles that respond to nerve stimulation during surgery may never contract spontaneously because the necessary inputs cannot be fired together on a voluntary basis.

Two important questions arise from the catalog of techniques described in this chapter: (1) Which of the individual physiologic and morphometric parameters can be used to predict function? and (2) What tests can be combined to provide the fullest characterization of experimental outcome? These questions will be addressed in Chapter 7, a review of experimental outcomes with the goal of correlating outcome measures to establish a grading scale for results.

REFERENCES

Abercrombie M (1946) Estimation of nuclear population from microtome sections. Anat Rec 94: 239–247.

Aitken JT, Sharman M, Young JZ (1947) Maturation of regenerating nerve fibers with various peripheral connexions. J Anat 81: 1–22.

Al-Majed AA, Neumann CM, Brushart TM, Gordon T (2000) Brief electrical stimulation promotes the speed and accuracy of motor axonal regeneration. J Neurosci 20: 2602–2608.

Alexander EJ, Andriacchi TP (2001) Correcting for deformation in skin-based marker systems. J Biomech 34: 355–361.

Angelov DN, Neiss WF, Streppel M, Andermahr J, Mader K, Stennert E (1996) Nimodipine accelerates axonal sprouting after surgical repair of rat facial nerve. J Neurosci 16: 1041–1048.

Archibald SJ, Krarup C, Shefner J, Li S-T, Madison R (1991) A collagen-based nerve guide conduit for peripheral nerve repair: an electrophysiological study of nerve regeneration in rodents and nonhuman primates. J Comp Neurol 306: 685–696.

Archibald SJ, Shefner J, Krarup C, Madison RD (1995) Monkey median nerve repaired by nerve graft or collagen nerve guide tube. J Neurosci 15: 4109–4123.

Bain J, Mackinnon S, Hunter D (1989) Functional evaluation of complete sciatic, peroneal, and posterior tibial nerve lesions in the rat. PRS 83: 129–138.

Ballermann M, Tompkins G, Whishaw IQ (2000) Skilled forelimb reaching for pasta guided by tactile input in the rat as measured by accuracy, spatial adjustments, and force. Behav Brain Res 109: 49–57.

Baptista AF, Gomes JR, Oliveira JT, Santos SM, Vannier-Santos MA, Martinez AM (2006) A new approach to assess function after sciatic nerve lesion in the mouse-adaptation of the sciatic static index. J Neurosci Methods 161: 259–264.

Baranowski AP, Anand U, McMahon SB (1992) Retrograde labelling of dorsal root ganglion cells in the rat: a quantitative and morphological comparison of Fluoro-Gold with horseradish peroxidase labelling. Neurosci Lett 141: 53–56.

Berod A, Hartman BK, Pujol JF (1981) Importance of fixation in immunohistochemistry: use of formaldehyde solutions at variable pH for the localization of tyrosine hydroxylase. J Histochem Cytochem 29: 844–850.

Bertelli JA, Mira JC (1993) Behavioral evaluating methods in the objective clinical assessment of motor function after experimental brachial plexus reconstruction in the rat. J Neurosci Methods 46: 203–208.

Bertelli JA, Mira JC (1995) The grasping test: a simple behavioral method for objective quantitative assessment of peripheral nerve regeneration in the rat. J Neurosci Methods 58: 151–155.

Bertelli JA, Dos Santos ARS, Taleb M, Calixto JB, Mira JC, Ghizoni MF (2004) Long interpositional nerve graft consistently induces incomplete motor and sensory recovery in the rat: an experimental model to test nerve repair. J Neurosci Methods 134: 75–80.

Bertelli JA, Taleb M, Mira JC, Ghizoni MF (2005) Variation in nerve autograft length increases fibre misdirection and decreases pruning effectiveness: an experimental study in the rat median nerve. Neurol Res 27: 657–665.

Bervar M (2000) Video analysis of standing: an alternative footprint analysis to assess functional loss following injury to the rat sciatic nerve. J Neurosci Methods 102: 109–116.

Bodine SC, Roy RR, Eldred E, Edgerton VR (1987) Maximal force as a function of anatomical features of motor units in the cat tibialis anterior. J Neurophysiol 57: 1730–1745.

Bodine-Fowler S, Meyer S, Moskovitz A, Abrams R, Botte MJ (1997) Inaccurate projection of rat soleus motoneurons: a comparison of nerve repair techniques. Muscle & Nerve 20: 29–37.

Bolesta MJ, Garrett WE Jr., Ribbeck BM, Glisson RR, Seaber AV, Goldner JL (1988) Immediate and delayed neurorrhaphy in a rabbit model: a functional, histologic, and biochemical comparison. J Hand Surg 13A: 364–369.

Bontioti EN, Kanje M, Dahlin LB (2003) Regeneration and functional recovery in the upper extremity of rats after various types of nerve injuries. JPNS 8: 159–168.

Boyd JG, Gordon T (2001) The neurotrophin receptors, trkB and p75, differentially regulate motor axonal regeneration. J Neurobiol 49: 314–325.

Bozkurt A, Deumens R, Scheffel J, O'Dey DM, Weis J, Joosten EA, Fuhrmann T, Brook GA, Pallua N (2008) CatWalk gait analysis in assessment of functional recovery after sciatic nerve injury. J Neurosci Methods 173:91–98.

Brown CJ, Evans PJ, Mackinnon SE, Bain JR, Makino AP, Hunter RT, Hare G (1991) Inter- and intraobserver reliability of walking-track analysis used to assess sciatic nerve function in rats. Microsurgery 12: 76–79.

Brown PB, Brushart TM, Ritz LA (1989) Somatotopy of digital nerve projections to the dorsal horn in the monkey. Somatosens Motor Res 6(3): 309–317.

Brushart TM, Mesulam MM (1980a) Alteration in connections between muscle and anterior horn motoneurons after peripheral nerve repair. Science 208: 603–605.

Brushart TM, Mesulam MM (1980b) Transganglionic demonstration of central sensory projections from skin and muscle with HRP-lectin conjugates. Neurosci Lett 17: 1–6.

Brushart TM, Henry EW, Mesulam MM (1981) Reorganization of muscle afferent projections accompanies peripheral nerve regeneration. Neuroscience 6: 2053–2061.

Brushart TM, Tarlov EC, Mesulam MM (1983) Specificity of muscle reinnervation after epineurial and individual fascicular suture of the rat sciatic nerve. J Hand Surg 8: 248–253.

Brushart TM (1990) Preferential motor reinnervation: a sequential double-labeling study. Restor Neurol Neurosci 1: 281–287.

Brushart TM (1991) The central course of digital axons within the median nerve of macaca mulatta. J Comp Neurol 311:197–209.

Brushart TM, Hoffman PN, Royall RM, Murinson BB, Witzel C, Gordon T (2002) Electrical stimulation promotes motoneuron regeneration without increasing its speed or conditioning the neuron. J Neurosci 22: 6631–6638.

Brushart TM, Jari R, Verge V, Rohde C, Gordon T (2005) Electrical stimulation restores the specificity of sensory axon regeneration. Exp Neurol 194: 221–229.

Burgess PR, Petit D, Warren RW (1968) Receptor types in cat hairy skin supplied by myelinated fibers. J Neurophysiol 31: 833–848.

Burke RE, Strick PL, Kanda K, Kim CC, Walmsley B (1977) Anatomy of medial gastrocnemius and soleus motor nuclei in cat spinal cord. J Neurophysiol 40: 667–680.

Carlton JM, Goldberg NH (1986) Quantitating integrated muscle function following reinnervation. Surgical Forum 37: 611–612.

Carr MM, Best TJ, Mackinnon SE, Evans PJ (1992) Strain differences in autotomy in rats undergoing sciatic nerve transection or repair. Ann Plas Surg 28: 538–544.

Chaplan SR, Bach FW, Pogrel JW, Chung JM, Yaksh TL (1994) Quantitative assessment of tactile allodynia in the rat paw. J Neurosci Methods 53: 55–63.

Choi D, Li D, Raisman G (2002) Fluorescent retrograde neuronal tracers that label the rat facial nucleus: a comparison of Fast Blue, Fluoro-ruby, Fluoro-emerald, Fluoro-Gold and DiI. J Neurosci Methods 117: 167–172.

Choi D, Raisman G (2005) Disorganization of the facial nucleus after nerve lesioning and regeneration in the rat: Effects of transplanting candidate reparative cells to the site of injury. Neurosurgery 56: 1093–1099.

Cragg BG, Thomas PK (1957) The relationship between conduction velocity and the diameter and internodal length of peripheral nerve fibers. J Physiol 136: 606.

Cragg BG, Thomas PK (1964) The conduction velocity of regenerated peripheral nerve fibers. J Physiol 171: 164.

Culberson JL, Brushart TM (1989) Somatotopy of digital nerve projections to the cuneate nucleus in the monkey. Somatosens Motor Res 6(3): 319–330.

De Koning P, Brakkee JH, Gispen WH (1986) Methods for producing a reproducible crush in the sciatic and tibial nerve of the rat and rapid and precise testing of return of sensory function. J Neurol Sci 74: 237–246.

Dellon AL (1989) Sciatic nerve regeneration in the rat: validity of walking track assessment in the presence of chronic contractures. Microsurgery 10: 220–225.

de Medinaceli L, Freed WJ, Wyatt RJ (1982) An index of the functional condition of the rat sciatic nerve based on measurements made from walking tracks. Exp Neurol 77: 634–643.

Deumens R, Jaken RJ, Marcus MA, Joosten EA (2007) The CatWalk gait analysis in assessment of both dynamic and static gait changes after adult rat sciatic nerve resection. J Neurosci Methods 164:120–130.

Dixon WJ (1980) Efficient analysis of experimental observations. Annu Rev Pharmacol Toxicol 20: 441–462.

Dohm S, Streppel M, Guntinas-Lichius O, Pesheva P, Probstmeier R, Walther M, Neiss W, Stennert E, Angelov DN (2000) Local application of extracellular matrix proteins fails to reduce the number of axonal branches after varying reconstructive surgery on rat facial nerve. Restor Neurol Neurosci 16: 117–126.

Dowdall T, Robinson I, Meert TF (2005) Comparison of five different rat models of peripheral nerve injury. Pharmacol Biochem Behav 80: 93–108.

Dunnett SB, Torres EM, Annett LE (1998) A lateralised grip strength test to evaluate unilateral nigrostriatal lesions in rats. Neurosci. Lett. 246: 1–4.

English AW (2005) Enhancing axon regeneration in peripheral nerves also increases functionally inappropriate reinnervation of targets. J Comp Neurol 490: 427–441.

English AW, Chen Y, Carp J, Wolpaw JR, Chen XY (2007) Recovery of electromyographic activity after transection and surgical repair of the rat sciatic nerve. J.Neurophysiol. 97: 1127–1134.

Evans PJ, Awerbuck DC, Mackinnon SE, Wade JA, McKee NH (1994) Isometric contractile function following nerve grafting: a study of graft storage. Muscle & Nerve 17: 1190–1200.

Frey M, Gruber H, Happak W, Girsch W, Gruber I, Koller R (1990) Ipsilateral and cross-over elongation of the motor nerve by nerve grafting: an experimental study in sheep. Plast Reconstr Surg 85: 77–89.

Fu SY, Gordon T (1995) Contributing factors to poor functional recovery after delayed nerve repair: prolonged axotomy. J Neurosci 15: 3876–3885.

Fugleholm K, Schmalbruch H, Krarup C (2000) Post reinnervation maturation of myelinated nerve fibers in the cat tibial nerve: chronic electrophysical and morphometric studies. JPNS 5: 82–95.

Galtrey CM, Fawcett J (2007) Characterization of tests of functional recovery after median and ulnar nerve injury and repair in the rat forelimb. JPNS 12: 11–27.

Galtrey CM, Asher RA, Nothais F, Fawcett JW (2007) Promoting plasticity in the spinal cord with chondroitinase improves functional recovery after peripheral nerve repair. Brain 130: 926–939.

Garrett WT, McBride R, Williams JK, Feringa ER (1991) Fluoro-Gold's toxicity makes it inferior to True Blue for long-term studies of dorsal root ganglion neurons and motoneurons. Neurosci Lett 128:137–139.

Gómez N, Cuadras J, Butí M, Navarro X (1996) Histologic assessment of sciatic nerve regeneration following resection and graft or tube repair in the mouse. Restor Neurol Neurosci 10: 187–196.

Gonatas NK, Harper C, Mizutani T, Gonatas JO (1979) Superior sensitivity of conjugates of horseradish peroxidase with wheat germ agglutinin for studies of retrograde axonal transport. J Histochem Cytochem 27: 728–734.

Gordon T, Yang JF, Ayer K, Stein RB, Tyreman N (1993) Recovery potential of muscle after partial denervation: a comparison between rats and humans. Brain Res Bull 30: 477–482.

Gordon T, Brushart TM, Amirjani N, Chan KM (2007) The potential of electrical stimulation to promote functional recovery after peripheral nerve injury: comparisons between rats and humans. Acta Neurochir Suppl 100: 3–11.

Gramsbergen A, Ijkema-Passen J, Meek M. F. (2000) Sciatic nerve transection in the adult rat: Abnormal EMG patterns during locomotion by aberrant innervation of hindlimb muscles. Exp Neurol 161: 183–193.

Guillery R, Herrup K (1997) Quantification without pontification: choosing a method for counting objects in sectioned tissues. J Comp Neurol 386: 2–7.

Gundersen HJ (1986) Stereology of arbitrary particles. J Microsc 143: 3–45.

Guntinas-Lichius O, Angelov DN, Tomov TL, Dramiga J, Neiss WF, Wewetzer K (2001) Transplantation of olfactory ensheathing cells stimulates the collateral sprouting from axotomized adult rat facial motoneurons. Exp Neurol 172: 70–80.

Guntinas-Lichius O, Wewetzer K, Tomov TL, Azzolin N, Kazemi S, Streppel M, Neiss WF, Angelov DN (2002) Transplantation of olfactory mucosa minimizes axonal branching and promotes the recovery of vibrissae motor performance after facial nerve repair in rats. J Neurosci 22: 7121–7131.

Gutmann E (1942) Factors affecting recovery of motor function after nerve lesions. J Neurol Psych 5: 117–129.

Gutmann E, Zelena J (1962) Morphological changes in denervated muscle. The Denervated Muscle. Prague, Czechoslovak Academy of Science Publishing House: 57–98.

Hadlock T, Koka R, Vacanti JP, Cheney ML (1999) A comparison of assessments of functional recovery in the rat. JPNS 4: 258–264.

Hare GM, Evans PJ, Mackinnon SE, Best TJ, Bain JR, Szalai JP, Hunter DA (1992) Walking track analysis: a long-term assessment of peripheral nerve recovery. Plast Reconstr Surg 89: 251–258.

Hargreaves K, Dubner R, Brown F, Flores C, Joris J (1988) A new and sensitive method for measuring thermal nociception in cutaneous hyperalgesia. Pain 32: 77–88.

Hasegawa K (1978) A new method of measuring functional recovery after crushing the peripheral nerves in unanesthetized and unrestrained rats. Experientia 34: 272–273.

Hentz VR, Rosen J, Xiao S-J, McGill KC, Abraham G (1991) A comparison of suture and tubulization nerve repair techniques in a primate. J Hand Surg 16A: 251–261.

Hontanilla B, Auba C, Arcocha J, Gorria O (2006) Nerve regeneration through nerve autografts and cold preserved allografts using tacrolimus (FK506) in a facial paralysis model: a topographical and neurophysiological study in monkeys. Neurosurgery 58: 768–779.

Hoogeveen JH, Troost D, Wondergem J, van der Kracht AH, Haveman J (1992) Hyperthermic injury versus crush injury in the rat sciatic nerve: a comparative functional, histopathological and morphometrical study. J Neurol Sci 108: 55–64.

Hruska RE, Kennedy S, Silbergeld EK (1979) Quantitative aspects of normal locomotion in rats. Life Sci 25: 171–180.

Inbal R, Devor M, Tuchendler O, Lieblich I (1980) Autotomy following nerve injury: genetic factors in the development of chronic pain. Pain 9: 327–337.

Inserra MM, Bloch DA, Terris DJ (1998) Functional indices for sciatic, peroneal, and posterior tibial nerve lesions in the mouse. Microsurgery 18: 119–124.

Irintchev A, Simova O, Eberhardt KA, Morellini F, Schachner M (2005) Impacts of lesion severity and tyrosine kinase receptor B deficiency on functional outcome of femoral nerve injury assessed by a novel single-frame motion analysis in mice. Eur J Neurosci 22: 802–808.

Jenq C-B, Coggeshall RE (1985) Long-term patterns of axon regeneration in the sciatic nerve and its tributaries. Brain Res 345: 34–44.

Jolicoeur FB, Rondeau DB, Hamel E, Butterworth RF, Barbeau A (1979) Measurement of ataxia and related neurological signs in the laboratory rat. Can J Neurol Sci 6: 209–215.

Kernell, D. (2006) Muscle unit properties and specializations. In: *The Motoneurone and Its Muscle Fibers*, pp. 29–65, Oxford: Oxford University Press.

Kerns JM, Fakhouri AJ, Pavkovic IM (1987) A twitch tension method to assess motor nerve function. J Neurosci Methods 19: 217–223.

Kim SH, Chung JM (1992) An experimental model for peripheral neuropathy produced by segmental spinal nerve ligation in the rat. Pain 50: 355–363.

Kinnman E, Levine JD (1995) Sensory and sympathetic contributions to nerve injury-induced sensory abnormalities in the rat. Neuroscience 64: 751–767.

Kline DG, Hudson AR, Hackett ER, Bratton BR (1975) Progression of partial experimental injury to peripheral nerve. J Neurosurg 42: 1–14.

Kline DG, Hudson AR, Lassmann H (1981) Experimental study of fascicular nerve repair with and without epineurial closure. J Neurosurg 54: 513–520.

Kloth V, Klein A, Loettrich D, Nikkhah G (2006) Colour-coded pellets increase the sensitivity of the staircase test to differentiate skilled forelimb performances of control and 6-hydroxydopamine lesioned rats. Brain Res Bull 70: 68–80.

Kristensson K, Olsson Y (1971) Uptake and retrograde axonal transport of peroxidase in hypoglossal neurones. Acta Neuropath 19: 1–9.

Kuypers HG, Bentivoglio M, van der Kooy D, Catsman-Berrevoets CE (1979) Retrograde transport of bisbenzimide and propidium iodide through axons to their parent cell bodies. Neurosci Lett 12: 1–7.

Kuypers PDL, Van Egeraat JM, Van Briemen LJ, Godschalk M, Hovius SER (1998) A magnetic evaluation of peripheral nerve regeneration: II. The signal amplitude in the distal segment in relation to functional recovery. Muscle & Nerve 21: 750–755.

Lago N, Navarro X (2006) Correlation between target reinnervation and distribution of motor axons in the injured rat sciatic nerve. J Neurotrauma 23: 227–240.

Li Y, Field P, Raisman G (1997) Repair of adult rat corticospinal tract by transplants of olfactory ensheathing cells. Science 277: 2000–2002.

Lin F-M, Pan Y-C, Hom C, Sabbahi M, Shenaq S (1996) Ankle stance angle: a functional index for the evaluation of sciatic nerve recovery after complete transection. J Recon Micro 12: 173–177.

Lindsey AE, LoVerso RL, Tovar CA, Beattie MS, Bresnahan JC (2000) An analysis of changes in sensory thresholds to mild tactile and cold stimuli after experimental spinal cord injury in the rat. Neurorehab Neural Repair 14: 287–300.

Luo ZJ, Lu SB (1996) Selective reinnervation of regenerating mixed nerve fibres across a silicone tube gap: further experimental evidence of neurotropism. J Hand Surg [Br Eur] 21B: 660–663.

Mackinnon S, Dellon AL (1988) A comparison of nerve regeneration across a sural nerve graft and a vascularized pseudosheath. J Hand Surg 13A: 935–942.

Madison RD, Archibald SJ, Lacin R, Krarup C (1999) Factors contributing to preferential motor reinnervation in the primate peripheral nervous system. J Neurosci 19: 11007–11016.

Martins RS, Siqueira MG, da Silva CF, Plese JP (2006) Correlation between parameters of electrophysiological, histomorphometric and sciatic functional index evaluations after sciatic nerve repair. Arq Neuropsiquiatr 64: 750–756.

Maurissen JP, Marable BR, Andrus A, Stebbins KE (2003) Factors affecting grip strength testing. Neurotox Terat 25: 543–553.

Mayhew TM, Gundersen HJ (1996) If you assume, you can make an ass out of u and me: a decade of the disector for stereological counting of particles in 3D space. J Anat 188: 1–15.

Mesulam MM (1978) Tetramethyl benzidine for horseradish peroxidase neurohistochemistry: a non-carcinogenic blue reaction product with superior sensitivity for visualizing neural afferents and efferents. J Histochem Cytochem 26: 106–117.

Montoya CP, Campbell-Hope LJ, Pemberton KD, Dunnett SB (1991) The "staircase test": a measure of independent forelimb reaching and grasping abilities in rats. J Neurosci Methods 36: 219–228.

Navarro X, Kennedy WR (1989) Sweat gland reinnervation by sudomotor regeneration after different types of lesions and graft repairs. Exp Neurol 104: 229–234.

Novikova L, Novikov L, Kellerth JO (1997) Persistent neuronal labeling by retrograde fluorescent tracers: A comparison between Fast Blue, Fluoro-Gold and various dextran conjugates. J Neurosci Methods 74: 9–15.

Pagnussat A, Michaelsen SM, Achaval M, Netto CA (2009) Skilled forelimb reaching in Wistar rats: evaluation by means of Montoya staircase test. J Neurosci Methods 177: 115–121.

Papalia I, Tos P, D'Alcontres FS, Battiston B, Geuna S (2003) On the use of the grasping test in the rat median nerve model: a re-appraisal of its efficacy for quantitative assessment of motor function recovery. J Neurosci Methods 127: 43–47.

Pover C, Lisney SJ (1989) Influence of autograft size on peripheral nerve regeneration in cats. J Neurol Sci 90: 179–185.

Povlsen B, Hildebrand C, Wiesenfeld-Hallin Z, Stankovic N (1993) Functional projection of regenerated rat sural nerve axons to the hindpaw skin after sciatic nerve lesions. Exp Neurol 119: 99–106.

Puigdellívol-Sanchez A, Prats-Galino A, Molander C (2006) Estimations of topographically correct regeneration to nerve branches and skin after peripheral nerve injury and repair. Brain Res 1048: 49.

Puigdellívol-Sánchez A, Prats-Galino A, Ruano-Gil D, Molander C (2003) Persistence of tracer in the application site: a potential confounding factor in nerve regeneration studies. J Neurosci Methods 127: 105–110.

Redett R, Jari R, Crawford T, Chen Y-G, Rohde C, Brushart T (2005) Peripheral pathways regulate motoneuron collateral dynamics. J Neurosci 25: 9406–9412.

Rodkey WG, Cabaud E, McCarroll HR (1980) Neurorrhaphy after loss of a nerve segment: comparison of epineurial suture under tension versus multiple nerve grafts. J Hand Surg 5: 366–371.

Rosen, J.M. and D.L. Jewett (1980) Physiological methods of evaluating experimental nerve repairs. In: *Nerve Repair and Regeneration*, D.L. Jewett and H.R. McCarroll, eds., pp. 150–161, St. Louis: Mosby.

Santos PM, Williams SL, Thomas SS (1995) Neuromuscular evaluation using rat gait analysis. J Neurosci Methods 61: 79–84.

Schmalbruch H, Al-Amood WS, Lewis DM (1991) Morphology of long-term denervated rat soleus muscle and the effect of chronic electrical stimulation. J Physiol.(Lond.) 441: 233–241.

Schmitz HC, Beer GM (2001) The toe-spreading reflex of the rabbit revisited-functional evaluation of complete peroneal nerve lesions. Lab Anim 35: 340–345.

Schmued LC, Fallon J (1986) Fluoro-gold, a new fluorescent retrograde axonal tracer with numerous unique properties. Brain Res 377: 147–154.

Shawe GDH (1955) On the number of branches formed by regenerating nerve-fibers. Brit J Surg 42: 474–488.

Shibata M, Breidenbach W, Ogden L, Firrell J (1991) Comparison of one- and two-stage nerve grafting of the rabbit median nerve. J Hand Surg 16A: 262–268.

Skouras E, Popratiloff A, Guntinas-Lichius O, Streppel M, Rehm KE, Neiss W, Angelov DN (2002) Altered sensory input improves the accuracy of muscle reinnervation. Restor Neurol Neurosci 20: 1–14.

Smit X, Van Neck JW, Ebeli MJ, Hovius SE (2004) Static footprint analysis: a time-saving functional evaluation of nerve repair in rats. Scand J Plas Reconstr Hand Surg 38: 321–325.

Strasberg SR, Watanabe O, Mackinnon SE, Tarasidis G, Hertl MC, Wells MR (1996) Wire mesh as a post-operative physiotherapy assistive device following peripheral nerve graft repair in the rat. JPNS 1: 73–76.

Swett J, Wikholm RP, Blanks RH, Swett A, Conley LC (1986) Motoneurons of the rat sciatic nerve. Exp Neurol 93: 227–252.

Taylor DC, Pierau Fr-K, Schmid H (1983) The use of fluorescent tracers in the peripheral sensory nervous system. J Neurosci Methods 8: 211–224.

Thalhammer JG, Vladimirova M, Bershadsky B, Strichartz GR (1995) Neurologic evaluation of the rat during sciatic nerve block with lidocaine. Anesthesiology 82: 1013–1025.

Totosy de Zepetnek JE, Zung HV, Erdebil S, Gordon T (1992) Innervation ratio is an important determinant of force in normal and reinnervated rat tibialis anterior muscles. J Neurophysiol 67: 1385–1403.

Valero-Cabre A, Navarro X (2001) H reflex restitution and facilitation after different types of peripheral nerve injury and repair. Brain Res 919(2): 302–312.

Valero-Cabre A, Tsironis K, Skouras E, Perego G, Navarro X, Neiss WF (2001) Superior muscle reinnervation after autologous nerve graft or poly-L-lactide-_-caprolactone (PLC) tube implantation in comparison to silicone tube repair. J.Neurosci.Res. 63: 214–223.

Valero-Cabré A, Navarro X (2002) Functional impact of axonal misdirection after peripheral nerve injuries followed by graft or tube repair. J Neurotrauma 19: 1475–1485.

Van Meeteren NLU, Brakkee JH, Helders PJM, Croiset G, Gispen WH, Wiegant VM (1997a) Recovery of function after sciatic nerve crush lesion in rats selected for diverging locomotor activity in the open field. Neurosci Lett 238: 131–134.

Van Meeteren NLU, Brakkee JH, Helders PJM, Wiegant VM, Gispen WH (1997b) Functional recovery from sciatic nerve crush lesion in the rat correlates with individual differences in responses to chronic intermittent stress. J Neurosci Res 48: 524–532.

Varejão AS, Cabrita AM, Geuna S, Melo-Pinto P, Filipe VM, Gramsbergen A, Meek MF (2003a) Toe out angle: a functional index for the evaluation of sciatic nerve recovery in the rat model. Exp Neurol 183: 695–699.

Varejão AS, Cabrita AM, Meek MF, Bulas-Cruz J, Filipe VM, Gabriel RC, Ferreira AJ, Geuna S, Winter DA (2003b) Ankle kinematics to evaluate functional recovery in crushed rat sciatic nerve. Muscle & Nerve 27: 706–714.

Varejão ASP, Meek MF, Ferreira AJA, Patrício JAB, Cabrita AMS (2001) Functional evaluation of peripheral nerve regeneration in the rat: walking track analysis. J Neurosci Methods 108: 1–9.

Varejão ASP, Cabrita AM, Meek MF, Bulas-Cruz J, Gabriel RC, Filipe VM, Melo-Pinto P, Winter DA (2002) Motion of the foot and ankle during the stance phase in rats. Muscle & Nerve 26: 630–635.

Varejão ASP, Melo-Pinto P, Meek MF, Filipe VA, Bulas-Cruz J (2004) Methods for the experimental functional assessment of rat sciatic nerve regeneration. Neurol Res 26: 186–194.

Verdú E, Navarro X (1997) Comparison of immunohistochemical and functional reinnervation of skin and muscle after peripheral nerve injury. Exp Neurol 146: 187–198.

Walker JL, Evans J, Meade P, Resig P, Sisken B (1994) Gait-stance duration as a measure of injury and recovery in the rat sciatic nerve model. J Neurosci Methods 52: 47–52.

Wasserschaff M (1990) Coordination of reinnervated muscle and reorganization of spinal cord motoneurons after nerve transection in mice. Brain Res 515: 241–246.

Westerga J, Gramsbergen A (1990) Development of locomotion in the rat. Dev Brain Res 57: 163–174.

Whishaw I, Woodward NC, Miklyaeva E, Pellis SM (1997) Analysis of limb use by control rats and unilateral DA-depleted rats in the Montoya staircase test: movements, impairments and compensatory strategies. Behav Brain Res 89: 167–177.

Whishaw IQ, Gorny B, Foroud A, Kleim JA (2003) Long-Evans and Sprague-Dawley rats have similar skilled reaching success and limb representations in motor cortex but different movements: some cautionary insights into the selection of rat strains for neurobiological motor research. Behav Brain Res 145: 221–232.

Whishaw IQ, Tomie JA (2007) Olfaction directs skilled forearm reaching in the rat. Behav Brain Res 177: 322–328.

Wikholm R, Swett J, Torigoe Y, Blanks R (1988) Repair of severed peripheral nerve: a superior anatomic and functional recovery with a new "reconnection" technique. J Otol Head & Neck Surg 99: 353–361.

Yao M, Inserra MM, Duh MJ, Terris D (1998) A longitudinal, functional study of peripheral nerve recovery in the mouse. The Laryngoscope 108: 1141–1145.

Yu P, Matloub HS, Sanger JR, Narini P (2001) Gait analysis in rats with peripheral nerve injury. Muscle & Nerve 24: 231–239.

Zhao Q, Dahlin L, Kanje M, Lundborg G (1992) Specificity of muscle reinnervation following repair of the transected sciatic nerve. J Hand Surg 17B: 257–261.

7

OUTCOMES OF EXPERIMENTAL NERVE REPAIR AND GRAFTING

THIS CHAPTER presents experimental results obtained with the evaluation techniques described in Chapter 6, and will be most informative after review of that material. Morphometric studies characterize nerve proximal to a repair as containing increased numbers of axons with reduced mean diameters. Distally, axon numbers may double in the months after repair, returning to normal in the rat only after 18 months, though diameters are still reduced. Short nerve grafts resemble nerve repairs; longer grafts are characterized by a significant drop-off in fiber number across the distal graft juncture. Electrophysiologic determinations reveal that compound motor action potential (CMAP) of reinnervated nerve may return to normal after nerve repair, nerve conduction velocity (NCV) is reduced by 25–50%, and the compound nerve action potential (CNAP) often remains below 50% of normal. Walking electromyogram (EMG) patterns after rodent sciatic nerve repair become disordered and asynchronous. Nerve grafting reduces CMAP in a length-dependent fashion, with reduction in other parameters similar to

those seen after nerve repair. Tetanic force generated by reinnervated muscle may reach 70–80% of normal, though values as low as 20–30% have been reported in the primate. The correlation between muscle weight and muscle force is highly model-dependent. Histologic reinnervation of skin varies by sensory modality, with type I fibers less successful than C fibers. Identification of reinnervating neurons with a single retrograde tracer documents both a reduction in their number and reinnervation of muscle by motoneurons that previously served other muscles. When two tracers are used simultaneously, it is possible to identify neurons that project collaterals to anatomically distinct locations. The sequential use of two tracers to identify neurons that regenerate back to their previous target unmasks a substantial failure of topographic specificity during regeneration. The sciatic functional index (SFI) and its variants return to normal after lesions that spare the Schwann cell basal lamina, but not after transection injuries. Analysis of gait provides a more complex view of function, revealing abnormalities that are not reflected in the SFI. As the rat upper extremity becomes a more popular model, tests such as the Montoya staircase test are being used to evaluate complex grasping function. The quantification of pain sensation has been studied extensively in the rat, but sensitivity to touch can only be approximated. A new experimental outcomes scale is based on the correlations among outcome measures: Category 4, regeneration has occurred; Category 3, end organs are reinnervated; Category 2, regeneration is specific; Category 1, voluntary function is restored. Measures at Grade II predict function, whereas those at Grades III and IV can predict function only under special circumstances. Experiments designed to solve clinical problems have rarely done so, but do provide information crucial to our understanding of the pathophysiology of nerve repair.

AXON COUNTS AND MORPHOLOGY

Nerve Repair—Proximal Stump

Axotomy and nerve repair modify the properties of axons both proximal and distal to the transection. In the 1940s, examining paraffin sections, Gutmann and Sanders (1943) noted a prolonged reduction in fiber (axon + myelin) diameter in the proximal segment of repaired rabbit peroneal nerve. This atrophy was later confirmed by an electronmicroscopic study of ligated cat nerve (Gillespie, Stein, 1983). A linear relationship was found between reductions in axon and fiber diameter, with axonal area decreasing relatively more than total fiber area. The mean diameter of fibers proximal to rat sciatic nerve repair remains at only 75% of normal for up to 24 months (Mackinnon et al., 1991) (Figure 7-1). These changes were examined further in the proximal segments of rabbit peroneal nerves that had been transected and sutured 12 weeks previously (Walbeehm et al., 2003). The population of large fibers (10–15 μm diameter) decreased by 70%, while the population of small fibers (2–5 μm diameter) increased by 35%; myelin thickness and g-ratio (axon diameter/total fiber diameter) did not change significantly in this model.

Nerve injury affects not only the caliber of proximal stump axons, but also their number (Gutmann, Sanders, 1943). After suture of the transected rat sciatic nerve, there is a prolonged rise in proximal axon counts (Mackinnon et al., 1991) (Figure 7-1). Numbers are increased by 40% over controls at 6 months, not decreasing to normal until 24 months.

The potential contributions of proximal sprouting and retrograde axon growth to this phenomenon will be discussed in Chapter 9.

Nerve Repair—Distal Stump

The distal nerve stump has been the primary focus of morphologic studies. Early evaluations of paraffin-embedded material showed reinnervated nerve to be populated by more, smaller axons than the normal proximal stump (Gutman, Sanders, 1943; Sanders, Young, 1944; Shawe, 1955). These observations have been refined by examination of plastic sections. In a longitudinal study of regeneration after rat sciatic nerve repair, Mackinnon and her coworkers found mean axon diameter to be 45% of normal after 1 month, increasing to 70% after 2 years (Mackinnon et al., 1991) (Figure 7-1). In the rat femoral nerve, motor axons that have reinnervated muscle attain significantly greater diameters than do those that project incorrectly to skin (Redett et al., 2005) (Figure 7-2). In the cat, maximum fiber diameter reaches 80–85% of normal after 6–10 months of regeneration (Fugleholm et al., 2000). The distribution of fiber sizes is still markedly distorted 2 cm distal to sciatic nerve repair performed 100–150 days previously (Wolthers et al., 2005) (Figure 7-3); the bimodal distribution of fiber diameters is lost, with substantial increases in the number of 2- and 3-μm fibers and decreases in those 6–12 μm. In the cat model, the reduction in diameter is fairly consistent throughout the entire distal stump (Fugleholm et al., 2000) (Figure 7-4).

The number of myelinated fibers 1 cm distal to rat sciatic repair rises to a maximum of 175% of normal at 3 months, returning to normal only after 24 months have elapsed (Mackinnon et al., 1991) (Figure 7-1). Approximately 1/4 of these are motor fibers, a distribution similar to that in normal sciatic nerve (Lago, Navarro, 2006). Examination of long-term reinnervated cat nerve at several levels reveals that axon numbers remain higher near the repair but then decrease and are consistent from 2 to 10 cm distally (Fugleholm et al., 2000) (Figure 7-4). Eight weeks after rat femoral nerve repair, motoneurons support twice as many myelinated collaterals in muscle nerve as they do in cutaneous nerve, a differential that persists even when end organ contact is denied (Redett et al., 2005) (Figure 7-2). Clearly, axon counts cannot be used to quantify regeneration for at least one year after nerve repair in the rat.

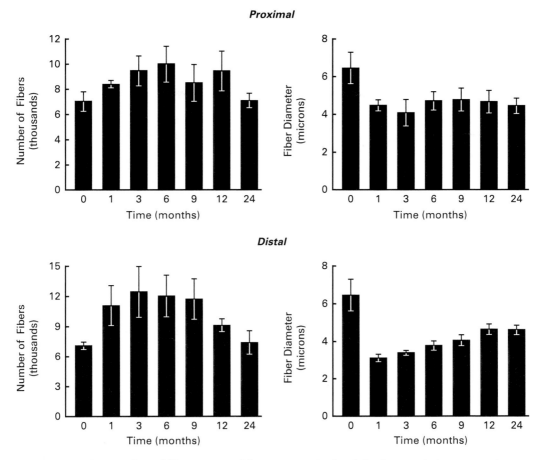

FIGURE 7-1   Mean myelinated fiber counts and diameters proximal and distal to rat sciatic nerve repair. The mean number of fibers proximal to the repair was significantly elevated from 1 to 12 months after surgery ($p < 0.01$). The mean diameter of these fibers was always significantly less than normal ($p < 0.01$). In the distal stump, the mean number of fibers was significantly elevated from 1 to 12 months ($p < 0.01$), returning to near normal by 24 months. The mean diameter of these distal fibers was significantly reduced throughout the study ($p < 0.001$). Reproduced with permission from Mackinnon et al., 1991.

Nerve Grafting

Axon morphometrics have been studied less frequently after nerve grafting. In the mouse, Gomez et al. (1996) found a linear decrease in myelinated axon number across short, 4-mm sciatic nerve grafts, with 4,835 axons in the proximal stump, 4,044 axons at midgraft, and 3,337 in the distal stump. Axon diameters in proximal stump and graft were the same at 2.9 μm, but decreased in the distal stump to 2.3 μm, and g ratios were consistently 0.6. Morphologic evaluation of 3-cm rabbit median nerve grafts after 24 weeks of regeneration revealed a steeper linear decline in axon number across the

graft, with a slight additional decline in the distal pathway (Shibata et al., 1988) (Figure 7-5). In this instance, axon diameter was maintained across the graft, not decreasing until further distally.

The most thorough analysis of axon morphology after nerve grafting was performed on a group of monkeys that had undergone 3-cm median nerve grafts 2 years previously (Archibald et al., 1995). The number of myelinated axons was significantly elevated in the distal stump, suggesting that these short grafts were functionally similar to nerve repairs. Three-dimensional plots of fiber diameter and g ratio in normal monkey nerve (Figure 7-6) revealed a distinctly bimodal distribution. Reinnervated

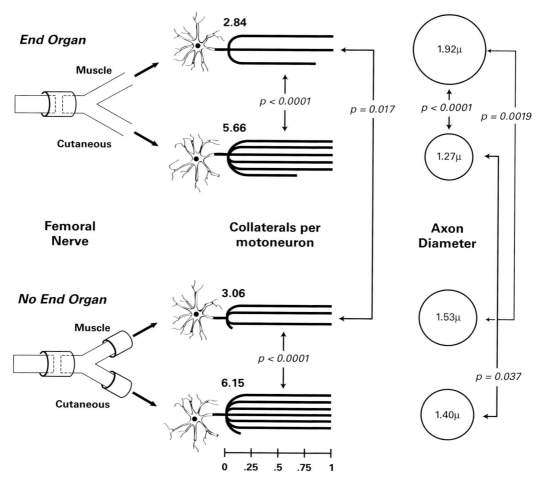

FIGURE 7-2 The number of collaterals per motoneuron and their diameters 8 weeks after rat femoral nerve repair. The upper half of the diagram displays the consequences when end organ contact is permitted, and the lower half displays the corresponding data when end organ contact is denied. Significantly more collaterals per neuron are maintained in cutaneous nerve than in motor nerve, and their number in this "incorrect" pathway is not influenced by the presence or absence of contact with skin. In contrast, motoneurons that project to muscle nerve maintain significantly more collaterals if muscle contact is denied. Increased collateralization thus appears to reflect negatively on the appropriateness of the distal pathway. Motor axon diameter is a less sensitive measure of environment, differing significantly between cutaneous and muscle nerve only when muscle reinnervation is permitted. Reprinted from Redett et al., 2005.

distal stump was characterized by lower fiber diameters and higher g ratios, with evidence of a return to bimodal distribution previously undetected by less rigorous analyses. The longest grafts studied, up to 30 cm in length, have been performed in the sheep (Frey et al., 1990; Rab et al., 1998). Depending on the experimental circumstances, the drop-off in myelinated axon number across the distal juncture was anywhere from 20 to 50%, with fibers maintaining increased diameters in the reinnervated distal stump, which in this model is a muscle nerve. If the axon is still capable of increasing in diameter, in spite of its narrowing within the graft, then the graft Schwann cell must be implicated as a limiting factor. A similar decrease in axon caliber within short nerve grafts containing defective Schwann cells, followed by increase in axon caliber when axons reentered normal nerve, was demonstrated by Aguayo et al. (1977) in the mouse.

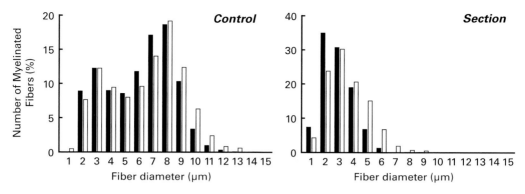

FIGURE 7-3   Distribution of myelinated fiber diameters in the normal rat sciatic nerve (left) and 20mm distal to transection and repair (right). Values obtained 100 days after surgery are represented by solid bars, and those obtained after 150 days by open bars. Axons are in the process of maturing and the normal bimodal size distribution is not seen. Reprinted with permission from Wolthers et al., 2005.

Correlations

Attempts to correlate the total number of myelinated axons in the distal stump after nerve repair or grafting with other outcome measures have been largely unsuccessful. A long-term study of 96 rats with various degrees of regeneration after tibial

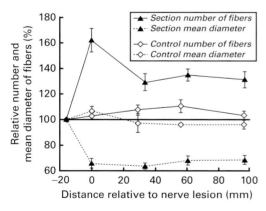

FIGURE 7-4   Relative numbers (solid lines) and relative mean diameters (dashed lines) of myelinated nerve fibers along the cat tibial nerve in reference to the site of surgical transection and repair. Measurements were obtained from specimens harvested between 178 and 297 days after surgery; the opposite, unoperated tibial nerves were used as controls. Reduction in fiber number occurs between 2 and 3 cm distal to the repair, while diameter remains reduced throughout the distal pathway. Reprinted with permission from Fugleholm et al., 2000.

nerve grafting found no relationship between myelinated axon counts and either electrophysiological or walking track parameters (Munro et al., 1998). A smaller evaluation of rat sciatic repairs after 12 weeks of regeneration resulted in similar conclusions (Martins et al., 2006), while a 12-week follow-up of both repair and grafting elicited a weakly negative correlation between axon number and muscle weight (Kanaya et al., 1996; r = –0.50). Similarly, the number of myelinated fibers in the

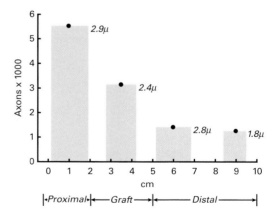

FIGURE 7-5   Mean myelinated fiber number and diameter along the rabbit median nerve 24 weeks after placement of a 3-cm nerve graft. The mean fiber diameter is represented on an arbitrary scale by the relative width of the vertical bar beneath each data point. Figure based on data provided in Shibata et al., 1988.

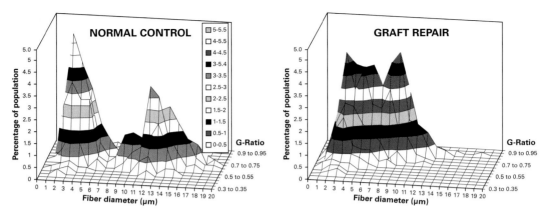

FIGURE 7-6 Three-dimensional plots representing the combined relationship of the frequency distributions of fiber diameter and g-ratio in monkey median nerve 2 cm distal to a 5-mm graft. Each vertical contour represents 0.5% of the total fiber population. Normal nerve has two completely separate peaks and thus a bimodal distribution. Reinnervated nerve has a more monolithic profile, yet two distinct peaks are seen, demonstrating the partial return of a bimodal fiber distribution that was not detected with two-dimensional analysis. Reprinted with permission from Archibald et al., 1995.

distal stump 60 days after a variety of rat sciatic lesions correlated negatively with gastrocnemius CMAP ($r = -0.781$) and SFI ($r = -0.822$) (Lago, Navarro, 2006). These relationships are consistent with the observation that motoneurons support twice as many myelinated axon collaterals in cutaneous nerve as they do in muscle nerve; relatively high axon counts may thus be a paradoxical sign of regeneration failure (Redett et al., 2005).

Meaningful correlations have related various outcome measures to defined subpopulations of axons. The CNAP correlated with the number of distal stump axons over 7 μm in diameter in a longitudinal examination of cat tibial nerve repair (Fugleholm et al., 2000; $r = 0.8438$; $p < 0.001$), while proximal stump nerve compound action current (NCAC) correlated with the number of axons 10–15 μm in diameter (Walbeehm et al., 2003; $r = 0.85$; $p < 0.01$). The number of axons in the nerve to rectus femoris after regeneration through a 30-cm graft in the sheep was highly correlated with the resulting tetanic contraction force (Frey et al., 1990; $r = 1.0$; $p < 0.001$).

The relationship between axon morphometry and other measures of outcome follows a similar pattern to that of axon number, with little positive evidence when an entire population is considered, but significant correlations when specific subsets of axons are examined. Munro et al. (1998), cited

above, found no correlation between mean axon diameter and other parameters. Martins et al. (2006) did find a weak correlation between mean axon diameter and SFI ($r = 0.50$), but the exclusion of 65% of the animals that were entered into the study indicates that SFI readings may be biased by exclusion of all the worst results, those animals with contracture or pain leading to self-mutilation. A similarly weak correlation was found between the ratio of myelin thickness to axon diameter and SFI as determined by de Medinaceli ($r = 0.53$), but not as determined by Bain et al. ($r = 0.24$) (Kanaya et al., 1996) (see Chapter 6 for formulae). The one more substantial positive correlation ($r = 0.7879$) relates the NCV of reinnervated cat tibial nerve to maximum fiber diameter (Fugleholm et al., 2000).

Overall, it appears that the morphometry of strictly defined axon populations can be correlated with their electrophysiologic properties, as one might expect on the basis of the interrelationship of axonal form and function described in Chapter 1. Axon numbers demonstrate that regeneration has occurred, but little more can be surmised unless the population has been selected by specific morphologic criteria or by passage through a filter such as a 30-cm nerve graft. To date there is little justification for attempting to predict voluntary function on the basis of axon number or morphology.

ELECTROPHYSIOLOGY

Nerve Repair

The electrophysiologic consequences of nerve repair and regeneration have been studied extensively in the rat and cat. The CMAP has been recorded as 60 mV from the normal rat gastrocnemius muscle and 8 mV from the smaller plantar muscles of the foot. Ninety days after sciatic nerve repair, the gastrocnemius CMAP returned to 50–70% of normal and the plantar CMAP to 30–35% of normal, with latencies increased 140% and 175% respectively (Valero-Cabré, Navarro, 2001; Valero-Cabré et al., 2004). In both sets of experiments the gastrocnemius CMAP was not altered by purposefully misaligning the repair, demonstrating that CMAP is independent of the topographic specificity of regeneration. In the cat, the normal plantar muscle CMAP is 5–15 mV, and it returns to this value by 300 days after nerve repair (Fugleholm et al., 2000) (Figure 7-7). The CNAP, recorded from nerve rather than from muscle, was found to be 175 uV in the rat tibial nerve, decreasing to 15 mV in the digital nerve of the foot (Lago, Navarro, 2006). These values were still reduced by two-thirds 60 days after sciatic nerve repair. In the cat, the normal tibial CNAP is 100–500 uV, and only returns to 1/3 of this value even 300 days after nerve repair (Fugleholm et al., 2000) (Figure 7-7). CMAP thus recovers more thoroughly than CNAP. The basis for this discrepancy, including temporal dispersion of impulses within regenerating nerve, is discussed in Chapter 6.

NCV is not static throughout the life of a rat, but increases at 0.5 m/s/week as the rat matures and its nodes of Ranvier become more widely spaced (Wolthers et al., 2005). To account for these changes during the course of an experiment, and to permit comparison with other indices of recovery such as the SFI, Wolthers and colleagues (2005) convert CV to a "CV Index," calculated as : Experimental CV – Normal CV/Normal CV x 100. Recorded absolute values of rat sciatic CV vary from 40 to 80 m/s (Meyer et al., 1997; Wolthers et al., 2005), and of cat tibial nerve CV from 70 to 100 m/s (Fugleholm et al., 2000). After sciatic nerve repair these values return to 50% of normal by 16 weeks in the rat (Meyer et al., 1997) and to 60–70% of normal after 300 days in the cat (Fugleholm et al., 2000). Although normal sensory conduction is 20% faster than motor conduction in the cat, as a result of rapid conduction in Ia and Ib afferents, the two are comparable after regeneration, suggesting that sensory fibers do not recover as fully as motor (Fugleholm et al., 2000).

Electrophysiologic measures of nerve regeneration that are used less frequently to assess the outcome of nerve repair include EMG, measurement of the H reflex, magneto-neurographic evaluation of NCAC, and determination of conduction fraction (CF) and mean added delay (MAD). Implantation of EMG needles in the antagonistic rat gastrocnemius and tibialis anterior muscles reveals a burst of activity in the gastrocnemius at the onset of and during the stance phase of gait, and a burst in tibialis anterior at the onset of swing (Figure 7-8). After sciatic nerve repair, EMG patterns are markedly abnormal, with more irregular and often overlapping activity, suggesting that these animals cannot compensate centrally for peripheral miswiring (Gramsbergen et al., 2000). The H reflex in the rat returns approximately 1 week after muscle reinnervation can be detected, but in awake animals the amplitude of the presumed H reflex remains small and never approaches preinjury levels (English et al., 2007). In anesthestized rats, in contrast, H reflex excitability is initially 3–4 times greater than normal, decreasing toward baseline with progressive reinnervation (Valero-Cabré, Navarro, 2001). In this study H reflex determinations did not differentiate between sciatic nerve repairs with correct or reversed alignment, and thus appear to be independent of the topographic specificity of regeneration. NCAC in the rabbit peroneal nerve decreases to 60% of normal in the proximal stump, consistent with a reduction in axon diameters (Walbeehm et al., 2003), and returns only to 25% of normal in the distal stump after 36 weeks (Kuypers et al., 1998). In the monkey median and ulnar nerves, 75–80% of proximal axons were found to conduct across the repair site by 32 weeks after repair, adding a delay of 0.86 m/s after epineurial suture and 0.42 m/s after fascicular suture (Hentz et al., 1991; p < 0.05). The authors conclude that "fascicular suture was associated with an improved repair site milieu compared with epineurial suture"(p258).

Nerve Grafting

The electrophysiology of nerve grafting has been studied only sporadically. In the rat, CMAP amplitude 90 days after placement of an 8-mm sciatic grafts returns to 39% of normal in the gastrocnemius, to 42% in the tibialis anterior, and to 22% in

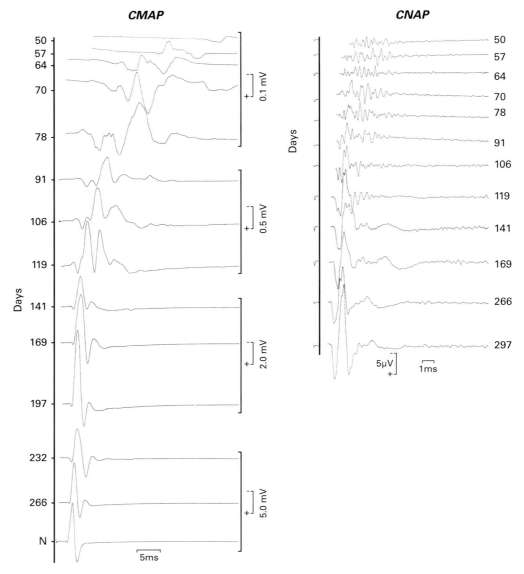

FIGURE 7-7 *Left.* Recovery of CMAP recorded from plantar muscle at progressive intervals after transection and repair of the cat tibial nerve. Note the changing scale at the right margin. The earliest CMAPs are dispersed and represent the asynchronous firing of only a few motor units. As reinnervation progresses and neuromuscular connections mature, an increasing number of motor units are firing with progressively greater synchronization. *Right.* Sequential changes in the CNAP of the same nerves, with progressive decrease in latency, increase in amplitude, and synchronization of impulses as fibers mature. Reprinted with permission from Fugleholm et al., 2000.

the plantar muscles (Valero-Cabré et al., 2001). Breakdown of the regenerate into constituent fiber populations reveals that the number of fibers conducting in the A-alpha distribution increases substantially after grafting, while the number in the A-beta category remains relatively constant (Vleggeert-Lankamp et al., 2004). In the cat, the conduction velocity of A-beta fibers in the sural nerve proximal to a 30-mm graft is reduced by 10% even after 1 year (Pover, Lisney, 1989). Conduction velocities distal to the graft are further reduced by 51% for both A-beta and A-gamma fibers.

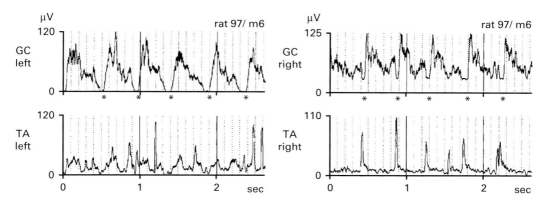

FIGURE 7-8 EMG records from an individual rat after grafting the left sciatic nerve. Asterisks indicate the onset of stance phase. In the right leg, the normal gastrocnemius muscle (GC) fires throughout the stance phase, while the tibialis anterior (TA) fires a short burst at the beginning of swing phase. In the left, operated leg, there is co-activation of the two muscles. Reprinted with permission from Gramsbergen et al., 2000.

The most extensive electrophysiologic study of nerve grafting was performed by Krarup and coworkers (Krarup et al., 2002) (Figure 7-9). As it involved monkey median nerve grafts followed for up to 4 years, it is also the most clinically relevant. CMAP amplitude returned to near-normal levels after end-to-end repair, but was reduced after grafting in a length-dependent manner; the amplitude restored through 50-mm grafts was only half that obtained with 20-mm grafts. The number of thenar motor units was drastically reduced after all transection injuries. The size of these units was increased in a compensatory manner after end-to-end repair and 20-mm grafts, but significantly less so after 50-mm grafts. CSAP amplitude was reduced by approximately 50% after all transection injuries, while SNCV was reduced by approximately 30% in all transection groups. CMAP amplitude and motor unit size were thus the best discriminators of graft length in this model.

Correlations

The search for correlations between electrophysiologic parameters and other outcome measures resembles that already described for axon counts and morphometry, except for greater disagreement as to whether the electrophysiologic characteristics of an axon population can predict voluntary function. The rat studies discussed above that found no correlation between morphologic and other parameters for whole axon populations similarly found that electrophysiologic measures either did

not predict axon morphometrics or voluntary function at all (Munro et al., 1998; Martins et al., 2006), or were at best weakly predictive; the ratio myelin thickness/axon diameter correlated somewhat with SFI (Kanaya et al., 1996; r = 0.53). Along similar lines, Kline and coworkers could demonstrate no correlation between mean fiber diameter and NCV after repair of the monkey tibial nerve (Kline et al., 1981), and Wolthers and coworkers (2005) found no correlation between myelinated axon count and the CMAP of reinnervated rat muscles. CMAP did, however, correlate with grip strength during the process of recovering from rat median nerve repair (Wang et al., 2008). In this instance there are few if any organizational issues, as the rat median-innervated muscles all contribute to grasp, and each increment of reinnervation would translate directly into an increment of grip strength. In addition to the previously cited correlations that relate electrophysiology to defined axon populations (Frey et al., 1990; Fugleholm et al., 2000), a correlation was found between a measure of the clustering of motor axons within the distal nerve stump, as determined by choline acetyltransferase (ChAT) staining of nerve cross-sections, and both gastrocnemius CMAP (r = 0.701) and SFI (r = 0.663), both p < 0.01 (Lago, Navarro, 2006). The topography of distal stump reinnervation, and thus the specificity with which axons are returned to appropriate targets, determined function in this model. In the context of other work from the same laboratory in which gross misalignment of sciatic nerve repair did not alter gastrocnemius CMAP (Valero-Cabré, Navarro, 2001;

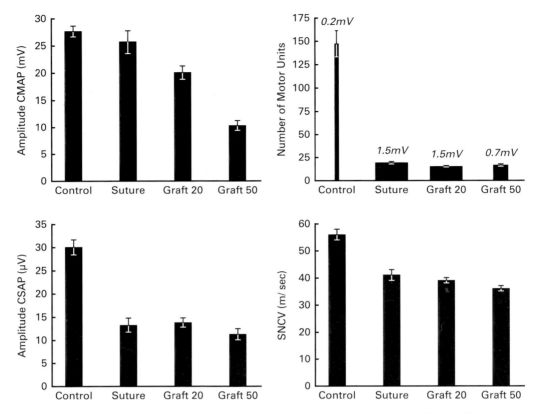

FIGURE 7-9   Electrophysiologic parameters at least 882 days after repair, 20-mm graft (Graft 20) or 50-mm graft (Graft 50) of the monkey median nerve. In the graph of motor unit number, the width of each bar represents the relative size of reinnervated motor units. CMAP amplitude after suture and 20-mm graft did not differ significantly from controls, while amplitude in the 50-mm grafts was significantly reduced ($p < 0.0005$). There was a dramatic decrease in the number of motor units after all types of repair with associated increase in motor unit size as indicated by the relative width of the bars. Whereas CMAP amplitude decreased progressively as the challenge to regeneration increased, CSAP amplitude was diminished substantially and to a similar degree in all operated groups ($p < 0.0005$). This difference could result from increased temporal dispersion of individual sensory action potentials. Conduction velocities were uniformly reduced after lesion, but to a lesser degree. Figure based on data from Krarup et al., 2002.

Valero-Cabré et al., 2004), these findings suggest that clustering of motor axons, rather than their location, determines functional outcome, an interesting possibility that awaits confirmation.

In contrast to much of the work cited above, a recent paper described significant correlations between gait parameters and the CMAP of reinnervated muscles (Valero-Cabré, Navarro, 2002). Print length correlated negatively with the CMAP of gastrocnemius, tibialis anterior, and plantar muscles, while toe spread, intermediate toe spread, and SFI correlated positively with these measures.

Correlations of the opposite sign were found between the various gait parameters and the CMAP obtained by stimulating misdirected axons. These findings highlight the need for caution in interpreting tests of correlation. The mean SFI was 3 in controls and varied only between –70 and –73 in the four experimental groups. SFI alone could thus differentiate clearly between control and repair, but not among repairs. In this data set, the lone control SFI value has undue leverage in determining the slope of the relationship. In his classic paper "Graphs in Statistical Analysis" Anscombe (1973) warned that "We are usually happier about asserting a regression relation if the relation is still apparent after a few observations (any ones) have been deleted. That is, we are happier if the regression relation seems to permeate all the observations and does not derive largely from one or two." This precise issue was addressed by Wolthers et al. (2005) in a study of rat sciatic crush and suture. Indices of amplitude and conduction velocity did not correlate with SFI within the two experimental groups, but correlated strongly when the groups were combined. The authors concluded that "due to the large differences in recovery reflected by the indices of the two lesion types, it was likely that the correlations were a reflection of these differences rather than true correlations between the evaluation methods"(p518).

Several correlations have been established between NCAC and other indices of recovery after rabbit peroneal nerve repair. In the proximal stump, NCAC amplitude correlated both with the number of large axons (10–15 μm) remaining (r = 0.85, p < 0.01) and the maximum diameter of these axons (r = 0.77, p < 0.05) (Walbeehm et al., 2003). Linear regression analysis of toe spread on a categorical scale of absent/poor/good against distal NCAC amplitude as a percentage of control demonstrated "strong correlation (p < 0.001)" (Kuypers et al., 1998). When the Mann-Whitney test was used to relate conduction velocity to toe spread in a similar model, a strong correlation was found between weeks 8 and 36 of the experiment, but not when earlier time points were included (Kuypers et al., 1999).

In summary, the majority of available evidence suggests that electrophysiologic parameters measured from reinnervated peripheral nerve do not correlate with the CMAP amplitude of reinnervated muscle or with indices of voluntary function. Correlations have been found between the morphology or location of specified axon subpopulations and both NCV and CMAP amplitude. One particularly relevant study has placed electrophysiologic measures of reinnervated monkey median nerve function in the context of time. The interval separating nerve repair and the earliest signs of peripheral reinnervation correlated with CMAP amplitude in reinnervated muscle ($r^2 = 0.8822$), the number of functioning motor units ($r^2 = 0.742$), and CSAP amplitude ($r^2 = 0.6351$) (Krarup et al., 2002). These primate experiments, followed for several years, imply that measures to speed the return of axons to the periphery should improve the results of clinical nerve repair.

ISOMETRIC MUSCLE STRENGTH

Isometric muscle strength can be characterized by either the maximum tetanic tension, a measure of the maximum force that can be produced by the muscle under any circumstances, or the twitch tension, the maximal response to a single stimulus. In the rat, the maximum tetanic tension generated by the soleus muscle after sciatic nerve repair recovered to 43% in 8 weeks, and to 70% in 32 weeks (Meyer et al., 1997). The rat tibialis anterior muscle recovered 55% of its contraction force 12 weeks after sciatic nerve repair in one study (Kanaya et al., 1992), and 83% in another (Zhao et al., 1992). A similar value of 85% was obtained after reinnervation of the peroneal nerve by the larger tibial nerve (Fu, Gordon, 1995a). In the monkey, tetanic tension generated by the triceps surae 1 year after tibial nerve repair returns to a mean of 78% of control values (range 57–100%; Kline et al., 1981). Repair of a nerve trunk in either rodents or mammals thus fails to restore normal muscle performance. This is likely to result from reinnervation of a given muscle by axons of inappropriate modality or that previously served other muscles with different functions. Repair of an individual muscle nerve, however, may result in the full recovery of tetanic strength, as the axon population is both functionally and topographically appropriate (Gordon, Stein, 1982). Twitch tension, which is approximately 1/3 of tetanic tension in the rat, may recover fully after rat nerve repair (Romano et al., 1991; Fu, Gordon, 1995).

Restoration of muscle force after nerve grafting has been examined in a range of species, in each case stimulating the nerve trunk or nerve that was grafted. In the rat, the tibialis anterior regained only 43% (+/−14%) of control force 12 weeks after grafting 2.5 cm of the sciatic nerve (Kanaya et al., 1992). The rat triceps surae muscles, reinnervated through a 3-cm graft for over a year, regained 88% of expected force after correction for growth during the experimental period (Evans et al., 1994). In the rabbit, FDS contraction force 62 weeks after 3-cm graft of the median nerve was 66% (+/−20%) of control when measured with the twitch-tension method, and 76% (+/−19%) when measured as maximal tetanic tension (Shibata et al., 1991). Two-stage grafting of the rabbit nerve to rectus femoris restored a normal quadriceps tetanic force of 27 N if the graft was 3 cm in length, but only 18 N if the graft was 7 cm long, a reduction of 29% (Koller et al., 1997). When a 7-cm graft was performed without delay, the resulting force was only 11 N (Rab et al., 2002). The greatest functional compromise is seen after grafting in the primate. One year after a 3 cm graft to the monkey tibial nerve, ankle plantar flexion force was only 19% of control (twitch tension) and 16% of control (tetanic tension) (Kim et al., 1991). The outcome of nerve grafting as measured by muscle force is thus inferior to that of end-to-end nerve repair. Ultimate recovery of force varies according to species, perhaps as a function of graft length, as well as by length within a given species; the length effect is discussed in detail later in this chapter.

Tetanic tension may also be used as a measure of nerve regeneration specificity (Zhao et al., 1992). After rat sciatic nerve repair, the tibial and peroneal fascicles are each stimulated both proximal and distal to the repair. For each muscle, the ratio of proximal force/distal force determines the relative contribution of the nerve being tested to the reinnervation of that muscle. Only 49–50% of gastrocnemius force was provided by the tibial nerve after either nerve suture or graft, indicating a marked lack of topographic specificity during regeneration. This finding is consistent with the relative reduction in muscle force after repair of a nerve trunk as opposed to a proper muscle nerve as discussed above.

Correlations

The force generated by reinnervated muscle has been correlated with several other outcome measures. Maximum tetanic tension generated by the rabbit rectus femoris muscle after staged nerve grafts of various lengths was found to correlate modestly with axon counts within the distal motor nerve (Koller et al., 1997; r = 0.53). The correlation became highly significant, however, in a similar 30 cm graft model in the sheep (Frey et al., 1990; r = 1.0 [p < 0.001]). No correlation was found between force and the higher axon counts within the graft in either case. When few axons are present, they all seem to contribute. In the monkey tibial nerve model, grouped data on repairs followed for various periods of time revealed a moderate correlation between tetanic force and mean myelinated axon diameter (Kline et al., 1981) (epineurial repair, r = 0.65; fascicular repair, r = 0.72). Most important, two studies that specifically examined the relationship between tetanic force and voluntary motor function, as measured by rat walking tracks, were unable to correlate the two (Kanaya et al., 1996; Urbanchek et al., 1999). Tetanic force obtained by

direct stimulation of a muscle nerve results from simultaneous firing of all motor units. It thus represents the maximum force that can be generated by that muscle under ideal circumstances. Voluntary contraction can generate similar force as long as coordinated firing of parent motoneurons is possible. However, reinnervation of muscle by incorrect motoneurons could degrade the ability to coordinate firing. Voluntary performance would thus represent the extent of muscle reinnervation (measured by tetanic force) as modified by the degree to which reinnervating motoneurons can be fired together (determined by regeneration specificity and central plasticity).

MUSCLE WEIGHT

Muscle weight has been used as an outcome measure in several models. Following rat sciatic nerve repair, soleus wet weight returned to 83% of control by 32 weeks (Meyer et al., 1997). Fourteen months after placement of a 3-cm sciatic nerve graft, rat gastrocnemius muscle weight returned to 1.1 grams, 47% of control weight (Evans et al., 1994). The return of gastrocnemius weight after tibial nerve repair was found to be age-dependent; approximately 80% was restored when the lesion was made at age 3 weeks, but only 50% if the injury was at 6 days of age (Watanabe et al., 1998). Grafting of the rabbit median nerve, in contrast, restored flexor digitorum sublimis weight slightly greater than the opposite, unoperated muscle (Shibata et al., 1991).

Several laboratories have examined the correlation between muscle weight and maximum tetanic tension. Were this correlation strong, it would be acceptable to weigh a muscle rather than to go through the process of strength determinations. The reinnervated rat gastrocnemius muscle has been examined with markedly divergent findings. Fourteen months after placement of a 3 cm sciatic graft, muscle weight and tension were strongly correlated (Evans et al., 1994; r = 0.9270), while 20 weeks after bridging a 5 mm sciatic gap with skin-derived graft they were not (Hie et al., 1982; r = 0.38). In the adjacent soleus muscle, these parameters correlated somewhat when a variety of sciatic lesions were considered (Bodine-Fowler et al., 1997; r = 0.82), yet the correlation for nerve repairs alone was poor (r = 0.12). In the case of the rat tibialis anterior muscle, the correlation was poor 12 weeks after sciatic nerve repair or grafting (Kanaya et al., 1996; r = 0.47) and moderate 1 year after reinnervation by the tibial nerve (Sulaiman, Gordon, 2000; r = 0.70). It is difficult to derive a clear explanation for this degree of variability. To some extent, it is consistent with the observation that outcome after more prolonged periods of denervation will be influenced by a decrease in the number of motoneurons regenerating and a reduction in pathway support for regeneration (Chapter 9). The muscles studied by Evans et al. (1994) had been reinnervated through 3-cm grafts, and were thus denervated longer than the others. The weight of reinnervated muscle should therefore not be used as a proxy for muscle function without first performing model-specific controls.

Muscle weight was included in a systematic search for correlations among outcome measures (Kanaya et al., 1996). Twelve weeks after sciatic nerve repair or grafting, no significant correlations were found between muscle weight and contraction force, various sciatic functional indices, electrophysiologic parameters, or axon morphology. The only positive finding was a weak negative correlation (r = −0.50) between muscle weight and axon count, consistent with the pruning of motor axon collaterals in response to muscle reinnervation (Redett et al., 2005).

CUTANEOUS END ORGAN REINNERVATION

Sweat gland reinnervation is nearly complete 75 days after crush of the mouse sciatic nerve, but only 79% of denervated glands are reinnervated after epineurial suture, and only 77% after isotopic grafting of a 4-mm sciatic nerve segment (Navarro, Kennedy, 1989). In this model, young mice recover pseudomotor function more rapidly and to a greater degree than do aged mice (Verdu et al., 1995). In the rat, sciatic nerve repair is followed by relatively complete reinnervation of the sural polymodal C-fiber population, while reinnervation of low-threshold mechanoreceptors is reduced substantially (Povlsen et al., 1993). Regeneration of type I fibers after cat femoral cutaneous nerve transection without formal repair reinnervates 60% of cutaneous touch domes, but without topographic specificity (Horch, 1979). In the monkey, digital Pacinian corpuscles display a wide range of morphologies after nerve grafting (Archibald et al., 1995). Fifty percent of Pacinian corpuscles are not reinnervated. In those that do receive axons, the central canal is never fully reoccupied, and many axonal branches are found ectopically among the lamellae.

The possibility of a correlation between cutaneous histology and nociceptive function has been explored in the mouse after sciatic nerve crush (Verdu, Navarro, 1997). The density of regenerated axons in the epidermis was correlated with the results of a pinprick test of nociception, yielding an r value of 0.63 (p < 0.01). Clearly, a great deal remains to be learned about the limitations imposed on function by the quantity and quality of end organ reinnervation.

RETROGRADE LABELING STUDIES

Single Labeling

Horseradish peroxidase was the first retrograde tracer applied to the study of nerve repair (Brushart, Mesulam, 1980). Intramuscular injection of the normal rat tibialis anterior muscle labeled a mean of 395 motoneurons (range: 368–434). Three months after sciatic nerve transection and repair, a mean of 273 motoneurons (69% of control; range: 245–291) was labeled. Reinnervating motoneurons were scattered among both tibial and peroneal motoneuron pools, and rarely met the size criteria for gamma neurons. The consequences of nerve injury and repair were thus shown to include defects in both the extent and specificity of alpha reinnervation as well as in the degree of gamma control.

The rat sciatic nerve was then used to compare the accuracy of muscle reinnervation after epineurial and individual fascicular suture (Brushart et al., 1983). A critical aspect of experiments in which one or more tracers are applied simultaneously is the criteria by which motoneurons are scored as in or out of a given motoneuron pool. In this instance, each pool labeled after surgery was compared to the normal pool on the other side of the spinal cord (Figure 7-10). This comparison is meaningful because of the high degree of side-to-side symmetry in normal animals (Chapter 6). Motoneurons were scored as "in" or "out" of the labeled pool based on either longitudinal or medial-lateral offset. Neurons that could not be assigned with confidence to either category were scored as "can't tell." In the rat sciatic model, individual fascicular suture improved the accuracy of muscle reinnervation over epineurial suture regardless of whether the indeterminate neurons were scored as in, out, or removed from the calculation (epineurial: 75% correct reinnervation; individual fascicular suture: 89% correct reinnervation). This technique of scoring location in

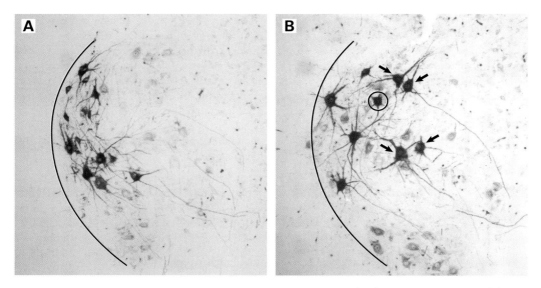

FIGURE 7-10   Motoneurons labeled by injection of the tibialis anterior (TA) muscle in normal rats (A) and after repair of the sciatic nerve (B). The normal motoneuron pool forms a crescent at the lateral margin of the anterior horn. After nerve repair, the TA has been reinnervated by appropriate motoneurons (no markings), as well as by those situated medially within the anterior horn in pools that activate muscles antagonistic to the TA (arrows indicate motoneurons clearly beyond the TA pool; the circled neuron cannot be assigned with certainty). Reprinted from Brushart et al., 1983.

comparison with a normal pool is thus sufficiently sensitive to differentiate two techniques of nerve repair that appear more similar when other, less precise techniques are used.

Horseradish peroxidase was also used as a single tracer to evaluate regeneration specificity after de Medinaceli's "reconnection" technique of nerve repair (Wikholm et al., 1988). This study included John Swett as an author and employed his meticulous technique of labeling and counting HRP-labeled motoneurons (Chapter 6). Transection and prolonged exposure of the peroneal nerve to HRP labeled a mean of 632 +/- 9 motoneurons in normal animals, a mean of 531 +/- 3 after "reconnection" (loss of 16%), and a mean of 497 +/- 79 after epineurial suture (loss of 21%). Although total reinnervation did not differ between repair techniques, the percentage of correct reinnervation, scored using the technique of Brushart et al. (1983), differed significantly; 66 +/- 7% correct after epineurial vs. 87 +/- 3% correct after "reconnection." Again, the side-to-side comparison was able to differentiate the accuracy of two repair techniques when only a single tracer was used.

The postoperative location of tibialis anterior (TA) motoneurons within the entire peroneal motoneuron pool was studied with HRP-WGA in the mouse (Wasserschaff, 1990). In this instance, since the TA pool lies laterally in the cord, and is totally contained within the peroneal pool, no measure of medial-lateral distribution is needed. Each motoneuron pool was characterized by a "weighted mean" position of labeled motoneurons, the point "from which the sum of distances to all cells located rostrally from it was equal to the sum of distances to all cells located caudally" (Wasserschaff, 1990). The mean control TA motoneuron pool contained 130 +/- 27 neurons, while the reinnervated pool contained 93 +/- 34 neurons, a reduction of 30%. On the longitudinal axis, the reinnervated pool was shifted caudally to a significant degree from normal, but still within the entire peroneal pool. By studying the motoneurons serving a single muscle within a larger motoneuron pool, rather than by comparing separate pools, these authors were able to differentiate a variety of postoperative changes to a degree sufficient to permit ready correlation with other outcome measures (see below). At the opposite extreme, using the "nearest neighbor distance" as a measure of specificity, with no reference to fixed landmarks, it was not possible to differentiate between repair of the rat median nerve to itself or to the ulnar nerve (Galtrey et al., 2007).

Simultaneous Double- and Triple-Labeling

The simultaneous application of tracers to two or three tributaries of a repaired nerve can identify the neurons projecting to each tributary. Additionally, however, this technique identifies a class of neuron that cannot be appreciated when only one tracer is used: the neuron that contains more than one label, and thus projects collaterals into more than one distal tributary (Figure 6-3). The controls and precautions needed for successful use of this technique were described in Chapter 6. The phenomenon of double-labeling proved to be particularly important in the rat femoral nerve model (Figure 7-11), which was developed to search for sensory/motor specificity during regeneration (Brushart, 1990; Brushart, 1993). The nerve is transected and repaired proximally, where motor and sensory axons intermingle. Regeneration specificity is then evaluated by applying HRP and Fluoro-Gold to the distal muscle (quadriceps) and cutaneous (saphenous, lower abdomen) nerve branches. Evaluation of regeneration at several time periods revealed that motoneurons initially reinnervated Schwann cell tubes leading to muscle or skin on a random basis, and many were double-labeled (Figure 7-12). Over time, the number of correct projections increased, the number of incorrect projections remained constant, and the number of double-labeled neurons decreased. These observations suggested the *Pruning Hypothesis*: motor axon collateral sprouts innervate cutaneous and muscle pathways on a random basis, then collaterals projecting incorrectly to skin are pruned, leaving only those projecting correctly to muscle. The tendency for motoneurons to project mostly to muscle rather than to skin was termed *Preferential Motor Reinnervation*.

Simultaneous multiple labeling contributed significantly to evaluation of the facial nerve, a model of the topographic specificity of motoneuron regeneration (Chapter 5; Figure 7-13). Application of multiple tracers in normal rats labeled 204 +/− 88 motoneurons from the zygomatic branch with DiI, 1324 +/− 29 motoneurons from the buccal branch with Fluoro-Gold, and 274 +/− 31 motoneurons from the marginal mandibular branch with Fast Blue (Guntinas-Lichius et al., 2001). After transection and repair of the proximal facial nerve, similar

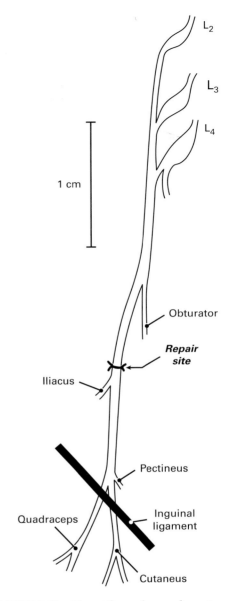

FIGURE 7-11   The rat femoral nerve drawn to scale. Most DRG neurons serving the femoral nerve are at the L3 level, with fewer at L2 and a highly variable contribution from L4. Repairs are performed as far proximally as possible to ensure the intermingling of axons destined to skin and muscle. The nerve bifurcates into a muscle branch to the quadriceps and a cutaneous branch that sends fibers to the lower abdomen and saphenous nerve.

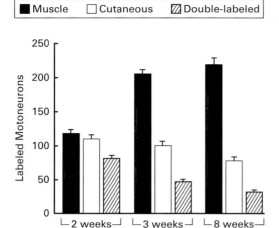

FIGURE 7-12   Motoneurons labeled by simultaneous double labeling of juvenile rat femoral cutaneous and muscle branches after proximal repair of the femoral nerve. Two weeks after repair, equal numbers of motoneurons project correctly to muscle and incorrectly to skin, and many project axons into both branches (double-labeled); pathfinding appears to be random. At 3 and 8 weeks, additional motoneurons project correctly to muscle, the number projecting to skin remains relatively constant, and the number of double-labeled neurons decreases. These findings are consistent with pruning of incorrectly projecting collaterals to generate correct projections. Reprinted from Brushart, 1990.

numbers of motoneurons were labeled, but a third of those projecting to the zygomatic branch also projected collaterals to the buccal branch. When the results of double labeling were analyzed by measuring the disruption of motoneuron pool somatotopy, 87% of motoneurons that reinnervated the temporal branch had grown in from other sources, confirming the absence of topographic specificity in the reinnervation of muscle (Choi, Raisman, 2002). Additionally, 17% of these motoneurons were still double-labeled after 10 months, suggesting that their collateral projections might persist indefinitely.

Our understanding of regeneration in the rat sciatic nerve (Figure 7-14) has also been enhanced through the use of multiple labels. In normal rats, exposure of the gastrocnemius nerve to Fast Blue, the tibialis anterior nerve to Fluoro-Gold, and the nerve serving the plantar muscles to DiI labeled a total of 1238 +/− 82 motoneurons (Valero-Cabré et al., 2004). Of these, 24% were from the gastrocnemius, 46% were from the tibialis anterior, and 30% were from the plantar muscles. A similar number of motoneurons was labeled after sciatic nerve repair, but their distribution was altered, with fewer in the gastrocnemius and more in the plantar. In these experiments the specificity of reinnervation was

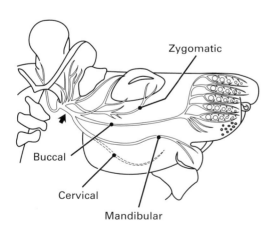

FIGURE 7-13   The rat facial nerve branches extensively to serve muscle throughout the face. The whiskers are innervated by the buccal branch. The arrow represents the site of experimental nerve transection and repair. Reprinted with permission from Guntinas-Lichius et al., 2002.

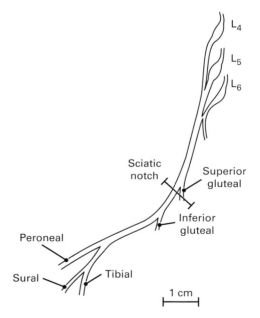

FIGURE 7-14   The rat sciatic nerve drawn to scale. Major contributions are from L4 and L5, with a variable contribution from L6. The nerve is readily accessible between the sciatic notch and its trifurcation in the popliteal fossa.

assessed by comparing the dimensions of each motoneuron pool along the three cardinal axes. Although this technique differentiated repair from normal and crush, it could not differentiate aligned from intentionally misaligned repairs, and is thus not sensitive enough to identify treatments that enhance regeneration specificity. English (2005) was able to extract more information from the sciatic system by comparing the relationship between tibial and peroneal motoneuron pools after sciatic nerve repair to that in normal animals. Normally, few peroneal motoneurons lie within the caudal 40% of the sciatic pool, and 91% of these are lateral to tibial motoneurons in the saggital plane; after sciatic nerve repair both of these relationships are disrupted significantly.

Sequential Double-Labeling

The most powerful evidence of regeneration specificity may be obtained through the careful use of sequential double-labeling. The stringent controls needed for this technique are described in Chapter 6. The neurons that innervate a structure of interest before a lesion can be identified individually at the end of the experiment, obviating the need for approximations based on contralateral normal anatomy or secondary calculations. This technique was applied initially to the femoral nerve model, prelabeling the sensory and motoneurons that projected to the quadriceps muscle nerve with DiI, then postlabeling the neurons that regenerated into this nerve after femoral nerve repair and regeneration with Fluoro-Gold (Madison et al., 1996). Sequential application of these tracers in normal controls double labeled 99 +/– 1% of motoneurons and 96 +/– 2% of DRG neurons, confirming the applicability of the technique. After transection and suture of the proximal femoral nerve, 59 +/– 3% of motoneurons reinnervating the quadriceps muscle had served this muscle previously, the others having innervated the iliacus or pectineus muscles. In the L3 DRG, 49 +/– 3% of afferent neurons that reinnervated the quadriceps muscle did so correctly. These numbers provide little evidence for native topographic specificity of either sensory or motor reinnervation. Sequential double labeling with DiI has not gained wide acceptance, probably due to the challenging nature of the technique. DiI is difficult to dissolve, travels slowly, thus taking several weeks to retrogradely label an entire motoneuron pool (Choi et al., 2002), and may result in sparse label within motoneurons (Madison et al., 1996). In the

course of routine screening with the paradigm described previously (Figure 6-4), we found that the DiI remaining at the injection site 3 weeks after application was sufficient to label over 100 motoneurons. This "depot effect" could inflate estimates of regeneration accuracy by labeling regenerating axons with the prelabel, creating the illusion that they were returning to their nerve of origin.

Rat femoral nerve repair was later reexamined using Fluoro-Gold as prelabel and Fluoro-Ruby as postlabel (Brushart et al., 2005). Were there an ideal model, in which prelabel persisted in 100% of neurons to which it was exposed, and in which both tracers labeled the exact same neurons, one could simply express reinnervation accuracy as the percentage of prelabeled neurons that also contained the postlabel (Figure 6-4). Since these ideal conditions have not been met, regeneration accuracy can be calculated directly with reference to the number of neurons in which prelabel persists (a subset of the original neuron pool) or with reference to the number of neurons regenerating. In controls for the Fluoro-Gold/Fluoro-Ruby experiments, 96 +/– 3% of neurons labeled by the first tracer were labeled by the second, while 95 +/– 4% labeled by the second tracer were also labeled by the first, an acceptable level of error (Figure 6-4). After femoral nerve repair, only 40 +/– 7% of the DRG neurons that regenerated to the muscle branch had returned to their original destination. The difference between the results of the first and second studies (49 +/– 3% vs. 40 +/– 7%), which does not appear to be significant, could be explained by the difference in the two models; in the first, only L3 DRG neurons were counted, while in the second all labeled neurons in L2, L3, and L4 were counted. In either case, there is little evidence for topographic specificity in sensory afferent reinnervation.

Sequential double labeling in the rat facial nerve model has confirmed the conclusions of simultaneous labeling studies. Prelabeling motoneurons that project through the buccal nerve by injecting the whiskerpad with Fluoro-Gold, then injecting the same area with Fast Blue, resulted in double labeling of 90% of normal motoneurons (Skouras et al., 2002). After buccal nerve repair, this figure dropped to 27 +/– 20%, even though the whiskerpad was reinnervated by normal numbers of motoneurons. These findings confirm the absence of topographic specificity in the reinnervation of muscle. Additionally, however, they present an even larger question: why did axons from other branches of the facial nerve sprout into the buccal branch? This type of redistribution is commonplace after repair of the entire facial nerve, when axons projecting to all of the facial tributary branches are injured, but would not be expected after isolated injury of the buccal nerve.

Unfortunately, no pair of labels both provides the accuracy of the HRP/Fluoro-Gold combination and remains stable for the two to three months needed to maximize recovery in rodent models of nerve repair. After performing a series of controls, Puigdellivol-Sánchez and colleagues (1998, 2000, 2002) chose the combination of diamidino yellow (DY) for prelabel and fast blue (FB) for postlabel, citing the following reasons for their choice: (1) DY can be taken up without axonal injury, (2) no histochemistry is required, (3) the two tracers are readily co-localized within a cell, and (4) only one filter is needed to visualize both tracers. Potential disadvantages of DY include secondary uptake from the injection site (Puigdellivol-Sánchez et al., 2003) and the failure to label all neurons to which it is exposed (Haase, Payne, 1990). Sequential double labeling of the tibial nerve with DY/FB before and after sciatic nerve repair resulted in the double labeling of 91% of DRG neurons and 87% of motoneurons, using the total number of cells that contain the prelabel at the end of the experiment as the basis for calculation ($FB\text{-}DY_{exp}/FB\text{-}DY_{exp} + DY$) (Puigdellivol-Sánchez et al., 2006). On the control side of these animals, sequential labeling without nerve repair, which defines the degree to which the two tracers label the same cells, double labeled a mean of 83% of DRG neurons and 76% of motoneurons. To take the control data into account, the authors proposed a second formula: $FB\text{-}DY_{exp}/FB\text{-}DY_{cont}$. Applying this to the same experimental data provides an estimate of 82% double labeling of the DRG, and 67% double labeling of motoneurons.

The DY/FB labeling pair was recently used by a second group to compare the accuracy of peroneal nerve reinnervation by motoneurons after crush, repair, or grafting of the sciatic nerve (de Ruiter et al., 2008). They found that 71% of peroneal motor neurons reinnervated the peroneal nerve after sciatic crush, 42% regenerated correctly after repair, and only 25% returned to the appropriate nerve branch after autografting. These estimates are somewhat pessimistic in the context of previous evaluations of nerve crush and repair. Substantial evidence that does not rely on double labeling indicates that fewer than 5% of motoneurons regenerate incorrectly after crush of the sciatic or other distal peripheral nerve

(Brown, Hardman, 1987; Horch, 1979; Nguyen et al., 2002). Similarly, previous studies of peroneal nerve reinnervation after epineurial repair of the sciatic nerve have estimated that 75–79% of motoneurons return to the correct fascicle (Brushart et al., 1983; Wilkholm et al., 1988). It will be important to determine the source of this variability and reach a consensus as to the baseline regeneration specificity that can be expected after common procedures.

Correlations

Correlation between the results of retrograde labeling and other outcome measures has received little attention, as evidenced by the exclusion of labeling from the three studies that focus on the interaction of outcome measures (Kanaya et al., 1996; Munro et al., 1998; Martins et al., 2006). The most convincing evidence for a direct relationship between regeneration specificity as determined by retrograde labeling and voluntary function comes from an evaluation of the accuracy of peroneal muscle reinnervation and SFI after a variety of rat sciatic lesions (Wikholm et al., 1988; Figure 7-15). Although the data presented do not permit direct analysis, the relationship between the mean percentages of correct regeneration and functional recovery is a straight line, suggesting a strong correlation. The accuracy of muscle reinnervation has been found to correlate directly with the degree of disruption of EMG patterns in walking mice (Wasserschaff, 1990; partial regression coefficient 0.0505, $p < 0.001$). Although SFI and EMG have been obtained in the same animals (Meek et al., 2003) their correlation has not been examined, so this evidence for a direct correlation between regeneration specificity and voluntary function is also incomplete. A substantial gap thus remains in our understanding of the significance of regeneration specificity as defined by retrograde labeling and the voluntary function regained after nerve repair.

VOLUNTARY MOTOR FUNCTION

Rat Walking Track Analysis

The sciatic functional index (SFI) was initially formulated by de Medinaceli to quantify recovery after rat sciatic nerve lesions (de Medinaceli et al., 1982). From a normal of 0% impairment, immediate postinjury function plummeted to a low of −110% to −120% on his scale. Following crush, function

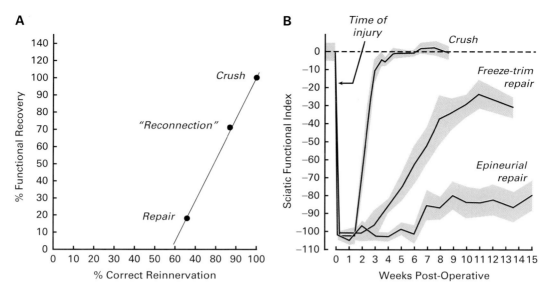

FIGURE 7-15   A: The relationship between functional recovery as measured by the mean SFI and the mean percentage of correct reinnervation assayed by retrograde labeling of the peroneal nerve. Although mathematical correlation is not possible without the original data, there is a linear relationship between mean functional recovery and mean percent correct reinnervation. Prepared using data from Wikholm et al., 1988. B: Recovery of the sciatic functional index (SFI) after crush, repair, and application of de Medinaceli's "reconnection" technique. There is little recovery after routine repair, but the near perfect anatomical alignment provided by "reconnection" results in a significant improvement in function. Reprinted with permission from Wikholm et al., 1988.

improved substantially to a final impairment of –21%, whereas following transection and suture it remained poor at –100%. When de Medinaceli used the SFI to evaluate his "reconnection" technique of nerve repair he found a reduction of impairment to 40%, a significant improvement over the results of nerve suture (de Medinaceli et al., 1983). Table 7-1 compares the SFI measurements recorded in several laboratories after nerve crush, repair, or grafting. Impairment after nerve transection and suture varies from 63 to 100% when the de Medinaceli equation (Chapter 6) is used, and between 55 and 82% when calculations are made with the Bain equation (Bain et al., 1989). The outcome of crush is uniformly superior at 0–21% impairment, de Medicaneli's "reconnection" technique provides results intermediate between those of crush and suture (Figure 7-15), and the impairment after nerve grafting is similar to that after suture. Although a broad pattern is easily discernible, the variation among laboratories is substantial, suggesting differences in either surgical technique or in walking track measurement. Although SFI measurements may be highly consistent within each

laboratory, their overall variability precludes comparison of results among different laboratories.

In several instances individual walking track parameters have been reported as discrete values. Navarro and coworkers found the recovery of print length (PL) to be full after crush, repair, or graft of the sciatic nerve (Valero-Cabré, Navarro, 2002; Lago, Navarro, 2006). Toe spread (from toes 1–5: TS) and intermediate toe spread (from toes 2–4: ITS) returned to normal after crush, confirming earlier findings (Walker et al., 1994). TS recovered only 52–53% after suture or graft, while ITS recovered 69–70% after both lesions. Mackinnon and coworkers calculated a print length factor [(experimental print length – normal print length)/normal print length], and found that this measure improved from an immediate postoperative value of 0.2 to a minimum of 0.022 after tibial nerve repair, and to between 0.061 and approximately 0.13 after tibial nerve grafting (Midha et al., 1993; Hertl et al., 1996; Watanabe et al., 1998).

In response to the inability of the SFI to differentiate among various forms of nerve repair,

Table 7-1 Rat Hindlimb Function after Sciatic Nerve Lesion as Measured by the Sciatic Functional Index (SFI).

Values obtained by applying the de Medinaceli formula (Chapter 6) after nerve transection and repair vary by as much as 37%, and values obtained after nerve grafting vary by up to 61%. These discrepancies could result from differences in repair technique, in footprint measurement, or in both.

Sciatic Function Index
(SFI)

Reference	Formula	Crush	Suture	Reconnection	Graft
DeMedinaceli et al, 1982	DeMedinaceli	−21	−100		
DeMedinaceli et al, 1983	DeMedinaceli		−100	−34	
Terzis & Smith 1987	DeMedinaceli	−5	−90	−60	
Wikholm et al, 1988	DeMedinaceli	0	−82	−29	
Zellem et al, 1989	DeMedinaceli		−63	−33	
Kanya et al, 1992	DeMedinaceli		−69		−99
Büttemeyer et al, 1995	DeMedinaceli				−38
Hare et al, 1992	Bain	approx. −15	approx. −82		
Maeda et al, 1999	Bain		−72		−73
Evans et al, 1999	Bain				approx. −75
Valero-Cabré & Navarro, 2002	Bain				−72
Wolthers et al, 2005	Bain	−3	−55		
Lago & Navarro 2006	Bain	+1	−79		

Bain et al. (1989) devised indices to quantify recovery of walking track patterns after isolated peroneal and tibial nerve injuries. Both factors return to normal after nerve crush (Hare et al., 1992). Their response to transection and repair, however, is quite different; the peroneal factor returns to normal, while the tibial factor never improves beyond 50%. This discrepancy could result from the differing functional characteristics of the muscles served by the peroneal and tibial nerves. The peroneal-innervated muscles are synergistic, so all reinnervation will enhance their function. The tibial-innervated muscles include synergists and antagonists; misdirected regeneration within the tibial territory would be expected to degrade function.

Recent interest in rat upper extremity nerve injury models has prompted evaluation of forepaw prints as an outcome measure. Both median and ulnar nerves must be injured to cause a decrease in toe spread (Bontioti et al., 2003; Galtrey, Fawcett, 2007). After transection and repair of both nerves, the 1–4 toe spread decreased to 48% of its preoperative value, eventually recovering to 74% (Bontioti et al., 2003). No recovery was seen after transection without repair or after crossed median/ulnar repair (Galtrey et al., 2007). The forepaw print thus reveals little about the recovery of isolated median or ulnar nerve injuries, but has proven useful in the analysis of CNS plasticity (Galtrey et al., 2007), and may prove useful in studies of the brachial plexus.

The parameters used to generate functional indices from rat walking tracks have also been measured on video images of the feet of stationary rats (Bervar, 2000). The three static video measurements—PL, TS, and ITS—were found to predict function to a degree different from that of their dynamic counterparts: TS was highly predictive, ITS was moderately so, and PL was minimally predictive. Further analysis revealed that TS could be used alone to predict function. Correspondence with other measures was confirmed by independent observers who found a strong correlation between static video TS and SFI ($r = 0.958$, $p < 0.001$; Smit et al., 2004). The TS factor, when calculated as toe spread–experimental/toe spread–control, dips to approximately 28% after sciatic injury, then returns to 60% after nerve transection and repair and 90% after nerve crush (Bervar, 2000).

Three laboratories have systematically correlated a wide variety of measures used to quantify the outcome of peripheral nerve repair. Kanaya et al. (1996) evaluated 24 rats 12 weeks after sciatic repair, autograft, or vascularized nerve graft (VNG), and found no correlation between SFI as calculated by Bain and a panel of morphologic and electrophysiologic measures. Munro et al. (1998) reviewed the results of tibial nerve grafting and allografting in 96 rats, and found no correlation between the tibial function index or print length factor and other outcome measures. In a similar analysis of 30 sciatic nerve repairs, Martins et al. (2006) were able to correlate SFI with the diameter of axons proximal to ($r = 0.57$) and distal to the repair ($r = 0.50$), though the exclusion of 46 additional rats because of autotomy or contractures suggests that only those animals with the best outcomes were evaluated. In more focused evaluations, Wolthers et al. (2005) found no correlation between SFI and indices of CMAP amplitude and conduction velocity, and Urbanchek et al. (1999) could not correlate toe spread factors with the force generated by the reinnervated EDL muscle.

In spite of the lack of correlation between SFI and other common outcome measures as described above, walking track parameters have been found to correlate with other outcome measures that are used less frequently. SFI correlated positively with a measure of motor axon localization distal to a nerve repair (Lago, Navarro, 2006; $r = 0.663$) and with histologic evaluation of nerve alignment (Keeley et al., 1993; $r = 0.76$). Additional correlation was found between SFI and an electrophysiologic measure of regeneration accuracy (Valero-Cabré, Navarro, 2002). As noted above, a strong association has been demonstrated between SFI and the percentage of correct muscle reinnervation as determined by retrograde labeling (Wikholm et al., 1988). SFI thus appears to relate most closely to measures of regeneration specificity, rather than to those that measure the function of individual neuromuscular components.

Video Gait Analysis

Gait parameters used to characterize function include the duration of the stance phase, the ankle angle at the end of stance, and the degree of lateral angulation of the foot (toe out angle). Gait stance duration in the injured leg as a percentage of normal decreases to approximately 60% after sciatic crush, returning to over 90% by 45 days, and correlates with contemporaneous SFI readings (Walker et al., 1994; $r = 0.797$, $p = 0.001$). After 1-cm sciatic autograft, the absolute value of the gait stance duration (115 ms) is paradoxically lower at 12 weeks than it is in the first weeks after the lesion, regaining only 65% of its normal value (Patel et al., 2006).

The terminal ankle angle, the angle formed by the axes of the foot and lower leg at the end of stance, was little altered by peroneal nerve transection, but reduced from 100° to 40° after tibial nerve section (Yu et al., 2001). When the entire sciatic nerve was transected, it dropped from 98° to 68°, returning to 80° after recovery from nerve grafting (Patel et al., 2006). In both this study ($r = 0.727$, $p = 0.041$) and one in which ankle angle was measured at midstance (Santos et al., 1995; $r = 0.84$), ankle angle correlated with gastrocnemius muscle weight, a finding consistent with the predominant role of the tibial nerve in determining ankle angle. The angular position of the ankle at various stages of recovery from sciatic crush injury is shown in Figure 6-6. Toe out angle, a relatively new measure (Varejão et al., 2003), increases from a normal of 6.4° to 23.5° after sciatic nerve injury, returning to 12.2° as the SFI improves from -93 to -43 (r = 0.99). Gait parameters can thus be measured with increasing precision and can be used to compare groups of experimental animals. It will, however, be necessary to correlate these findings with the reinnervation patterns of the muscles involved before any more general conclusions can be drawn.

Upper Extremity Grasping Test

The upper extremity grasping test is by nature subjective, as it relies on the day-to-day motivation of the rat to produce consistent results. The test is far easier to perform than walking track or gait analysis, however, and as a result is becoming increasingly popular. Bertelli and coworkers, measuring the break-away strength from a wire grid, found full recovery 1 month after median nerve crush (Bertelli, Mira, 1995), recovery to 98% after an 8-mm median nerve graft (Bertelli et al., 2005), and recovery to 85% after placement of a 20-mm median nerve graft (Bertelli et al., 2006). In a group of rats previously selected for their performance in the staircase test, the grasping test did not differentiate between rats with correct and crossed median and ulnar nerve repairs (Galtrey, Fawcett, 2007). In other studies performed at the completion of regeneration, the grasping test could not differentiate between nerve repair and graft, a distinction that could be established with measurements of CMAP (Werdin et al., 2009), or between nerve repair and controls (Tos et al., 2008). These findings are consistent with grip strength as a measure of the volume, rather than the specificity, of regeneration. This characteristic can be used to advantage in following the course of muscle reinnervation, a process during which grip strength correlates with the CMAP (Wang et al., 2008).

The Montoya Staircase Test

Performance in the staircase test was highly strain-dependent, with participation by 50% of Lewis rats, 70% of Sprague-Dawley rats, and 100% of Lister-Hooded rats (Galtrey, Fawcett, 2007). In animals selected for their performance during training,

skilled motor function (pellet retrieval) recovered fully after median nerve crush, 35% after correctly aligned median and ulnar nerve repairs, and only 7.5% after crossed median/ulnar repairs. Unskilled motor function, the ability to knock pellets out of wells and onto the floor, recovered to a similar degree regardless of repair technique. In additional studies, the severity of injury was found to correlate with the number of pellets retrieved (p < 0.001) (Galtrey et al., 2007). The Montoya test is thus capable of detecting both future improvements in the outcome of nerve repair and CNS compensation for misdirected regeneration.

REFLEX AND STEREOTYPICAL RESPONSES

Rabbit Toe Spread Test

As evaluated by Kuypers et al. (1998, 1999), rabbit toe spread is graded as absent, poor, or good. As measured with this scale, the functional outcome of peroneal nerve transection and suture is uniformly poor for the first 6 weeks, is a mixture of grades from 6 to 12 weeks, and is uniformly good thereafter. When animals from 6 to 26 weeks after repair are considered together, toe spread correlates with the amplitude of the NCAC during the reinnervation process (Kuypers et al., 1998; p <0.001). Given that toe spread returned to "good" in all animals with nerve repair in this series, it is unlikely that this test can be used to identify improvements in repair technique.

Extensor Postural Thrust

The extensor postural thrust (EPT) test is potentially subject to variables similar to those encountered during grip strength testing, because the rat is held by the waist as it is advanced toward a balance that it will push against. A percentage motor deficit is calculated as (normal EPT - experimental EPT)/normal EPT (Koka, Hadlock, 2001). Nerve crush lowers the motor deficit to approximately 90%, after which it recovers to near normal after 6 weeks (Hadlock et al., 1999). Nerve transection produces a similar initial deficit, but recovery is less with a residual deficit of approximately 50%. The recovery of EPT and SFI follow similar trajectories after both crush and transection injuries (Koka, Hadlock, 2001) though mathematical correlation has not been established.

Facial Nerve Function

Video analysis of whisking biometrics has provided a detailed description of whisker motion (Figure 6-9). In unoperated Lewis rats, the maximum protraction angle is 45°, the amplitude of the sweep is 69°, the angular velocity is 803°/second, and the angular acceleration is 25,485°/second² (Guntinas-Lichius et al., 2002). After recovery from facial nerve transection and suture, these values are all significantly different from those of normal controls (85°, 17°, 159°/second, 3308°/second² respectively). Addition of olfactory mucosa to repairs significantly altered the maximum angle and amplitude of protraction, but not the angular velocity or acceleration (Guntinas-Lichius et al., 2002); none of these parameters differed significantly between nerve suture and tubular repair with a 5-mm gap containing olfactory ensheathing cells (Guntinas-Lichius et al., 2001). The role of supranuclear factors in the functional outcome of facial nerve repair is shown dramatically by the return of near-normal whisking when nerve repair is performed in blind rats that rely more heavily on their whiskers for sensory input.

Sensory Function

The return of sensitivity to pain has been tested with pinprick and electric shock. Navarro and coworkers devised a "pinprick score" to quantify sensory recovery (Navarro et al., 1994; Verdu, Navarro, 1997; Lago, Navarro, 2006). Six areas are tested from the heel to the tip of the second toe; the response in each is graded as none (0), reduced or inconsistent (1), or normal (2), and the grades are added to form the pinprick score. This score returns to normal within 90 days of sciatic nerve crush or suture in both rats and mice, but the return of function in mice is more rapid after crush. The return of pinprick score has been correlated with the density of PGP-positive axons in the epidermis (r = 0.63). When the rat sciatic nerve territory in the foot is denervated, the threshold current needed to elicit a response rises from 0.1 mA to 1 mA (Meek et al., 1999). Reconstruction of the sciatic nerve with a 12-mm graft is followed by a gradual reduction of the threshold to approximately 0.4 mA over the next 12–15 weeks.

Semmes-Weinstein filaments have been used extensively to quantify allodynia (Chapter 6), but only occasionally to study the return of sensibility after nerve repair. One week after rat median and ulnar nerve injury, the force necessary to elicit a response increases from 20 grams to 80 grams, then gradually recovers to normal after crush and to approximately 35 grams after repair (Galtrey, Fawcett, 2007). Although these changes are substantial, the normal baseline of 20 grams is several orders of magnitude greater than physiologic threshold (Chapter 4), so this test cannot be measuring tactile acuity.

Sensitivity to heat and cold is measured as the time between application of stimulus to the paw and withdrawal of the limb (withdrawal latency). Normal rats withdraw from a 56° probe with a latency of 2 seconds. This is increased to at least 12 seconds after sciatic nerve crush, begins to improve by 4 weeks, and is back to normal by 8 weeks (Hadlock et al., 1999). Withdrawal of the rat upper extremity from an ice probe is normally brisk (0.27–0.29 seconds). Latency increases substantially after nerve crush (8 seconds), returning to normal within 4 weeks. After nerve repair, regardless of alignment, the residual latency is approximately 2 seconds (Galtrey, Fawcett, 2007)

EXPERIMENTAL OUTCOMES SCALE

Table 7-2 displays experimental outcome measures in a framework modeled on that used for clinical studies (Chapter 4, Table 4-4). Measures are assigned to one of four levels based on how much they reveal about functional outcome. To avoid confusion with the clinical outcomes scale and to minimize the appearance of relative value judgments, the groupings will be listed as categories; Category 4 (CAT 4) indicates that regeneration has occurred, Category 3 (CAT 3) that end organs have been reinnervated, Category 2 (CAT 2) that regeneration has been specific, and Category 1 (CAT 1) that voluntary function has been restored. In Table 7-2, correlations within each category and with higher categories are denoted by arrows accompanied by the r values derived from experiments mentioned in this chapter. Many of relationships are based on single experiments; those based on more than one experiment are characterized by a range of r values. Some of the observations appear to be species-specific; the relationship between mean myelinated axon diameter, for instance, was observed in monkeys but not in rats. Relationships that are contested, such as that between CMAP amplitude and walking track parameters, are not included.

Table 7-2 Experimental Outcome Scale. Arrows identify published correlations between the results of 2 techniques, and the accompanying numbers represent the published r or p values. Single r or p values are derived from a single study, whereas ranges are derived from 2 or more studies. Assn: association without statistical correlation. Category 4 measures, those that show that regeneration has occurred, can sometimes predict the results of category 3 tests, those that document end organ reinnervation, but do not predict results higher on the scale. Category 3 tests have not been found to predict results of category 2 tests, those that describe regeneration specificity, but can in some instances predict voluntary function, category 1. Category 2 tests uniformly predict voluntary function.

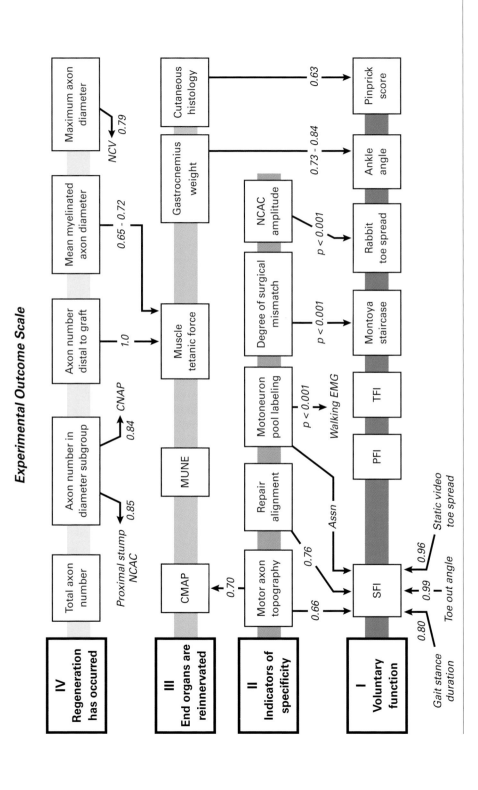

Experimental Outcome Scale

Many have observed that various measures used to characterize the quality of regeneration are assessing different aspects of the process (e.g., Kanaya et al., 1996; Munro et al., 1998; Martins et al., 2006), yet no unifying scheme has been advanced to relate these measures one to another. Table 7-2 represents a tentative view of this synthesis. It is meant to serve as the basis for discussion and further experimentation, and will doubtless be revised. Its most striking feature is the prediction of function by measures of regeneration specificity (or experiments in which specificity is manipulated surgically). In the repair of mixed nerve trunks such as the rat sciatic, restoration of appropriate connections, rather than the formation of individual neuromuscular or neuro-sensory units, emerges as the strongest predictor of functional outcome.

EXPERIMENTAL APPROACH TO CLINICAL QUESTIONS

Chapter 5 explored several aspects of the response to nerve repair and grafting in humans. Frequently, recognition of these clinical questions or challenges stimulated a course of experimentation. This section will summarize studies of the outcome of nerve repair or grafting that were designed to answer clinical questions. More basic experiments on the biology of the processes involved are discussed in later chapters.

The Effects of Age on Outcome

The positive effect of young age on recovery after nerve injury suggests that responsible factors could be manipulated to improve outcomes in adults. These factors could be peripheral—axons in young individuals might be better at growing and finding correct targets—or central—the juvenile brain and spinal cord might adapt more readily to peripheral miswiring. An early study comparing neonatal and adult rats demonstrated that facial nerve regeneration after transection was somatotopically appropriate in neonates, but not in adults, a finding attributed to peripheral factors (Aldskogius, Thomander, 1986). Unfortunately, it is difficult to isolate the role of axonal pathfinding in neonates, as axotomy results in substantial motoneuron death, potentially killing off neurons with inappropriate connections (e.g., Aldskogius, Thomander, 1986; Watanabe et al., 1998). A reexamination of the neonatal facial nerve model did not confirm somatotopically appropriate

reinnervation, and revealed incomplete cortical adaptation to the injury (Franchi et al., 2006). Similarly, neonatal rat tibial nerve injury compromised functional recovery when compared with injury at 22 days of age (Watanabe et al., 1998). These studies, focused on the neonatal period, are potentially relevant to the pathophysiology of human perinatal brachial plexus injuries. Direct comparison is not possible, however, since rodents are born at an earlier stage of their development than are primates.

Several aspects of nerve regeneration have been compared in juvenile and adult animals. An early study of peripheral axon morphology and electrophysiology found no differences after long-term follow-up of nerve injuries in juvenile and adult primates, leading to the conclusion that "central nervous system adaptation in young patients" was the responsible factor (Almquist et al., 1983). Central factors are also suggested by more recent work describing an age-related ability to compensate for severe disruption of EMG patterns after sciatic nerve injury and repair (Gramsbergen et al., 2001). In the periphery, the speed and extent of motor and pseudomotor reinnervation decrease with age in the mouse, with a prominent drop-off after 1 year of age (Verdú et al., 1995). The specificity of sensory/motor regeneration is also modified by age; juveniles generate sensory/motor specificity in fresh grafts of adult nerve, whereas adults cannot (Le et al., 2001). In the aged animal, facial motoneurons regenerate slowly and generate collateral sprouts in excess (Malessy et al., 1998). Both central and peripheral factors have thus been found to change with age, though none has been implicated specifically in the beneficial effect of young age on clinical outcome.

Delayed Repair

In the clinical setting, delay of nerve repair is accompanied by the evolution of changes to every component of the system, from neuron to end organ. The impact of these changes is readily apparent within a few weeks in experimental animals. Delay in repair of the rat sciatic nerve of 3 weeks reduces the final strength of foot flexion in response to both twitch and tetanic stimuli (Beek, Glover, 1975). Similarly, recovery of both muscle mass and integrated motor function are compromised if repair of the rat tibial nerve is delayed for more than 1 month (Kobayashi et al., 1997). In the rabbit, force generated by the

EDL after repair of its proper nerve is reduced significantly by delays of 3 weeks to 6 months (Bolesta et al., 1988). In the rat facial nerve, immediate repair is accompanied by hyperinnervation of target muscle, which is reduced by delay of 7 days, but not by longer delays of up to 56 days (Guntinas-Lichius et al., 1997).

The effects of delay on structures central to the repair site can be eliminated experimentally by reinnervating a previously denervated distal stump with a freshly cut proximal nerve. This has been achieved by transferring a predegenerated nerve graft from the opposite side of the animal, or by predegenerating a nerve, then reinnervating it from a nearby nerve that is newly transected. Contralateral grafting of fresh and predegenerated rat femoral nerve revealed that distal myelinated axon counts were higher when fresh grafts were used (Gordon et al., 1979). When fiber populations were isolated with retrograde tracing, in contrast, motoneurons were shown to reinnervate femoral nerve grafts predegenerated for 4 weeks in greater numbers and with greater specificity than they reinnervated fresh grafts (Brushart et al., 1998). In the sciatic nerve, freshly axotomized neurons responded to grafts predegenerated for 30 days with initial axon size and conduction properties superior to those of fresh grafts (Sorenson, Windebank, 1993). In small animal models, some aspects of regeneration may thus be enhanced by a short delay, the time during which potentially inhibitory debris is cleared from the distal stump and Schwann cell activity is maximized. This phenomenon is discussed in greater detail in Chapter 9, Part 3. After the experiments described above were performed, it was found that injuring a nerve on one side of an animal promotes subsequent regeneration on the other side (Yamaguchi et al., 1999; Ryoke et al., 2000), a factor that could influence results when attempting to isolate the effects of graft predegeneration. Transfer of grafts among members of a strain of inbred animals bypasses this problem.

The nerve transfer model was used by Fu and Gordon (1995a, 1995b) in an elegant series of experiments to separate the effects of prolonged neuronal axotomy from those of prolonged distal stump denervation. In the rat, the tibial nerve was axotomized for up to 12 months before transferring it to the freshly transected peroneal nerve. Conversely, the peroneal nerve and tibialis anterior muscle were denervated for up to 12 months before reinnervating them with the newly transected tibial nerve. Prolonged axotomy reduced the number of motoneurons regenerating by approximately 2/3; those reinnervating muscle were able to restore normal force with fewer, larger motor units. Prolonged denervation had more profound consequences by dramatically reducing the ability of the pathway to support regeneration; additionally, muscle that was reinnervated could not recover from denervation atrophy. Examination of the denervated nerve after reinnervation showed that even though the Schwann cells were unable to support regeneration, they could still myelinate effectively (Sulaiman, Gordon, 2000). This work helped focus attention on progressive deterioration of the distal pathway as a primary determinant of outcome. Previously, experimental attention had been focused on the CNS, the repair, and end organ reinnervation, with the tacit assumption that the pathway would function reliably.

Epineurial vs. Perineurial Repair

The matching and suture of fascicles, individually or as small groups, was first advocated by Langley and Hashimoto (1917). Sunderland revisited the concept in 1953, citing the potential of the technique to limit "the wasteful regeneration of axons into the epineurial tissue and functionally unrelated endoneurial tubes, and the erroneous cross-shunting of axons all of which combine to reduce and distort the original pattern of innervation" (Sunderland, 1953). Essentially, Sunderland believed that fascicular (funicular) suture could potentially increase both the volume and the specificity of regeneration.

Given the goals enumerated by Sunderland, it is appropriate to categorize the relevant experiments by evidence level. Five of six studies at Categories 3 or 4 found no significant differences between epineurial and fascicular suture. Conduction velocity and M wave area or amplitude revealed no differences between repair types in the rabbit sciatic (Orgel, Terzis, 1977), dog peroneal (Burke, O'Brien, 1978), or primate median and ulnar nerves (Grabb et al., 1970). Similarly, the force produced by reinnervated muscle after epineurial or fascicular repair was similar in both the rat sciatic (Lutz, 2004) and monkey tibial nerves (Kline et al., 1981); the latter study had too few animals at each time period to establish significance, but gave the overall impression that regeneration advanced more rapidly after epineurial suture. A difference was shown by one group that used more complex electrophysiologic techniques to evaluate conduction across the repair (Hentz et al., 1991). Although the proportion of proximal axons that crossed the repair did not differ between techniques, fascicular suture was found to reduce the conduction delay.

The few Category 1 and 2 studies that addressed this issue found fascicular suture to be superior to epineurial suture. In the cat sciatic nerve model, push-off in gait returned more rapidly after fascicular suture (Bora, 1967). In the rat, the specificity of muscle reinnervation at the fascicular level was significantly improved as assessed by both electrophysiologic and retrograde tracing criteria (Brushart et al., 1983; Zhao et al., 1992). We are thus left with the bulk of large animal data suggesting equality of technique, and a minority of experiments, none in the primate, suggesting that fascicular suture enhances regeneration specificity at the fascicular level. Viewing these results in the dual context of surgical goals and evidence levels helps to apportion their relative significance. The experiments designed to look for evidence of specificity all found it. It would thus be reasonable to recommend large animal experiments with category 1 and 2 outcomes measures, as these could demonstrate a clinically significant difference between repair techniques not demonstrated by the category 3 and 4 measures used on primates so far. An obvious limitation, however, is the paucifascicular nature of primate nerve trunks.

Proximal Steal Phenomenon

No experiments have been designed with the specific purpose of demonstrating reinnervation of proximal muscles at the expense of their distal counterparts. Evidence consistent with this possibility has been presented, however. In the rat sciatic model, the gastrocnemius and tibialis anterior muscles regain a higher percentage of their preoperative CMAP amplitude than do the more distal plantar muscles (Valero-Cabré, Navarro, 2002). Given that only a few weeks of regeneration separate the gastrocnemius from the foot, factors other than distance must contribute to this discrepancy.

At What Gap Size Should Nerve Be Grafted?

The gap length at which a nerve should be grafted rather than repaired primarily has been a subject of debate for the last century. During this time the pendulum has swung from severe tension to no tension and back to slight tension. Following the dismal experience with grafting in World War I (Platt, Bristow, 1924), every attempt was made to mobilize injured nerves and bring them together by flexing adjacent joints. The "critical resection length," the minimum gap that could be closed with this approach, was said to be 7 cm in the median nerve and 10 cm in the ulnar nerve (Brooks, 1955). The consequences of this approach soon became apparent. Highet and Holmes (1943) described poor results when gaps of over 4 cm were overcome with end-to-end suture. In the laboratory, Highet and Sanders (1943) found that nerve elongation of 12–42% resulted in severe intraneural damage. In spite of these findings and the progress reported by Seddon (1963), nerve grafting was not readily embraced for treatment of short and intermediate gaps.

The approach to nerve grafting experienced a paradigm shift in response to the work of Millesi. In the same year that he published his landmark clinical series (Millesi et al., 1972b), Millesi described the histopathology of nerve repair and grafting in the unrestrained rabbit (Millesi et al., 1972a). When compared with repair under tension, grafting resulted in a marked decrease in connective tissue proliferation and scar formation, and less dying back of axons that had already reinnervated the distal stump. Functional recovery was poor after repair under tension, and essentially equal after repair with minimal tension or grafting. Millesi also emphasized the distinction between the *defect*, the amount of nerve excised, and the resulting *gap*, the final distance between the nerve stumps (Millesi, 1986). In primary nerve grafting, elastic retraction makes the gap bigger than the defect. In secondary procedures, we are rarely aware of the true defect, and only the gap can be measured precisely.

Millesi's assertion that "intra-fascicular nerve grafting gives results which are at least as good as those with epineurial suture under ideal conditions" (Millesi et al., 1976, p209) stimulated further exploration of the indications for grafting. Excessive tension is clearly deleterious; for each nerve, there must be a gap length at which nerve graft is always superior to repair under tension. Conversely, avoidance of a second suture line is a theoretical goal that can be achieved easily at short gap distances.

When studying the effects of tension on nerve repair, It is probably inappropriate to generalize from rat to human (Millesi, 1985). A closer approximation is possible, however, in primate models.

Long-term follow up of direct repair or grafting of 5-mm monkey median nerve defects revealed no differences in CSAP amplitude, SNCV, or CMAP amplitude, though recovery was significantly more rapid after grafting (Archibald et al., 1995; Krarup et al., 2002). When a 1-cm monkey tibial nerve defect was repaired or grafted, muscle strength was superior after repair at 4 and 6 months, but equal after repair or grafting at 9 and 12 months (Bratton et al., 1979). In the primate median nerve, more proximal axons conducted into the distal stump after repair than after graft of a 15 mm defect at 21–31 weeks, with no significant differences in axon diameters (Hentz et al., 1993). The experimental evidence thus suggests that mild to moderate degrees of tension are tolerated without compromising outcome as characterized by Category 3 or 4 outcome measures. Although these experiments have not been translated into specific clinical guidelines, they have given surgeons the confidence to accept some tension at the repair site.

Is Graft Performance Length-Dependent?

The effect of graft length is best appreciated by comparing grafts of various lengths in the same neural defect. In the rabbit, 3 cm, 5 cm, and 7 cm saphenous nerve grafts attached to the vastus nerve convey 3–4 times the normal vastus fiber population after 8 months (Rab et al., 1998). If the distal graft is then sutured to the rectus nerve, the fiber population in the distal graft decreases by 30–40%, consistent with collateral pruning stimulated by muscle contact. The tetanic force generated by the rectus decreases with increasing graft length, but significance was not demonstrated with the small number of animals studied (Koller et al., 1997). When monkey tibial nerve defect and graft length are modified systematically, the length of the defect emerges as the primary determinant of outcome, though graft length is also significant (Kim et al., 1991).

The limits to graft function are demonstrated by experiments performed in sheep. Partial muscle function can be restored through a graft similar in length to the human sural nerve (30 cm) (Frey et al., 1990). Axon number and diameter decrease to various degrees in the distal portion of the graft, there is a sharp dropoff in fiber number across the distal juncture, and resulting muscle force is variable but never normal.

A long-term study of nerve grafting in the primate upper extremity provides the only modality-specific data on graft length (Krarup et al., 2002). As both gap and graft length were varied in these experiments, it is not possible to separate their effects. Comparison of 5-mm-, 20-mm-, and 50-mm-long grafts revealed that CSAP amplitude and SNCV were not affected significantly by graft length. In the motor system, CMAP amplitude dropped off approximately 50% between 20 and 50 mm, while the number of motor units dropped to a nonsignificant degree between 5 mm and 20 mm, with no additional change at 50 mm. Most dramatically, the time to first motor reinnervation increased progressively with increasing graft length (5 mm—57 days; 20 mm—84 days; 50 mm—177 days). This important paper established time to reinnervation as a primary determinant of outcome, so one would anticipate that outcomes would deteriorate with grafts of increasing length.

In aggregate, these studies suggest a modality-specific deterioration in function with increasing graft length. Five-cm-long cutaneous nerve grafts restore category 3 function well in the sensory system, but poorly in the motor system; this discrepancy could be defect-specific, or could reflect the differential ability of sensory nerve graft to promote sensory and motor axon regeneration (Hoke et al., 2006). Clinical series documenting the effects of graft length on recovery (Chapter 5) focused on only sensory or motor function; a differential effect should be sought in future studies.

Should the Distal Graft Juncture Be Delayed?

In the majority of clinical situations, nerve grafts are attached both proximally and distally during the same surgical procedure. This practice was questioned, however, when it became possible to provide a "fresh" muscle end organ through microvascular free muscle transfer. Two questions arose: (1) was the presence of a muscle end organ needed for regeneration *across* the graft, and (2) was regeneration across the distal juncture improved by performing a "fresh" repair once axons had reached this point. Mackinnon et al. (1988) addressed the first of these issues by examining regeneration through 10-cm-long grafts that routed monkey facial nerve axons to the contralateral side of the face. After 12 months, grafts with distal connections to the opposite facial nerve had larger axons and had undergone less atrophy than those left without distal connections. Animals with distal graft reconnection had regained facial function, however, providing ample evidence that regenerating axons had been trophically influenced by their muscle targets (Weiss et al., 1945; Sanders, Young, 1946; Aitken et al., 1947). As a result, these experiments shed no light on regeneration across the graft before muscle is reached. In experiments in which target contact was denied for 1–1.5 years, motor axons crossed 8-cm grafts in the rabbit (Koller et al., 1993) and 28-cm grafts in the sheep (Frey et al., 1992) in substantial numbers, confirming that regeneration may proceed through even the longest of grafts without need for support derived from end organs. Additionally, no known mechanism could account for retrograde transmission of information about end organ status in nerve that has previously undergone Wallerian degeneration and therefore has no retrograde transport.

The value of staged distal repair has proven more elusive. In early investigations, performance of dog homograft was improved subjectively by staged distal suture (Therkelsen, Pool, 1957). Recent studies, in contrast, have not confirmed these findings. Function was not improved by a 10-week delay in repairing the distal juncture of 3-cm rabbit median nerve grafts (Shibata et al., 1991). In this model, the short gap and brief delay may have been insufficient to elicit a difference. Delaying the distal repair of 30-cm grafts in the sheep also failed to improve outcome significantly (Frey et al., 1990), though marked interspecimen variability may have concealed a biologic difference between the groups. In related experiments, Rab et al. (2002) found that staged grafting to freshly denervated muscle was clearly superior to single-stage grafting, confirming the value of staged reinnervation of transplanted muscle. As the duration of muscle denervation was a prominent variable in these studies, they cannot isolate the effects of delay itself. When the duration of muscle denervation was eliminated as a variable in the rabbit crossfacial nerve graft model, tetanic tension was similar in immediate and delayed distal repair groups (Rab et al., 2006). Further work is clearly needed to define the evolution of the distal suture line and determine whether there is a time after which a staged approach is clearly superior.

Schwann Cell Phenotype and Nerve Grafting

Cutaneous nerve has long been the preferred source of graft material for both cutaneous and motor nerve defects. A potential difference between sensory and motor nerve was suggested, however, by experiments in which motor axons preferentially reinnervated motor nerve, even when they were unable to contact muscle (Brushart, 1993). Comparison of sensory and motor nerve as graft for motor axons, based on axon counts, has demonstrated that cutaneous nerve is superior to (Corte et al., 1984), equal to (Ghalib et al., 2001), or inferior to (Nichols et al., 2004; Brenner et al., 2006) motor nerve depending on the model. Since motor axons maintain more collaterals in cutaneous nerve than in muscle nerve (Redett et al., 2005), axon counts may not provide an accurate representation of the number of motoneurons regenerating in these experiments. A more precise comparison used pure populations of motor and sensory axons to reinnervate grafts of cutaneous nerve and ventral root, with retrograde labeling to identify neurons projecting to the middle of the grafts (Hoke et al., 2006). Under these conditions, sensory neuron regeneration was supported preferentially by grafts of cutaneous nerve, and motor neuron regeneration was supported preferentially by grafts of ventral root (Figure 7-16).

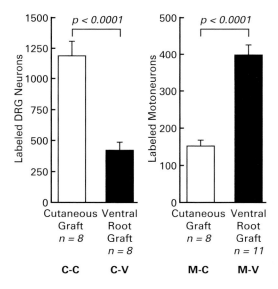

FIGURE 7-16 The numbers of DRG and motoneurons that have extended their axons 1 cm down nerve grafts after 2 weeks of regeneration. The support of regeneration is modality specific; graft of cutaneous nerve was a more effective pathway for sensory neurons, and graft of ventral root was a more effective pathway for motoneurons. Reprinted with permission from Hoke et al., 2006.

The differences in performance of cutaneous nerve and ventral root are associated with substantial differences in their production of a variety of growth factors (Hoke et al., 2006; Chapter 9). Work is currently under way in our laboratory to determine which of these differences influence axon behavior, with an ultimate goal of modifying graft Schwann cell phenotype to match the needs of a target axon population.

CONCLUSIONS

The overview of experimental outcomes presented in this chapter suggests several measures that could improve the effectiveness and clinical applicability of neural regeneration research. At the most basic level it is important to define what constitutes an acceptable nerve repair. Aside from the size of suture used, there is rarely discussion of what criteria are applied within each lab to deem a repair suitable for inclusion in an experimental group. It is critical that the mechanical aspects of repair be eliminated as a variable, especially when attempting to unmask the inherent behavior of regenerating axons. For example, similar nerve grafting experiments were recently performed in two laboratories with opposite results (Nichols et al., 2004; Neubauer et al., 2009). The difference must therefore reflect a variable that was not described by the authors, with repair technique a prominent candidate. As a general rule, if the outcome of an experimental nerve repair can be changed by intentional rotatory mal-alignment, the quality of the repair will affect the outcome, and should be controlled carefully.

Rodent peripheral nerve is currently the most popular setting for studies of the outcome of nerve repair and regeneration. It poses an adequate challenge in the realm of regeneration specificity and end-organ reinnervation, as evidenced by the consistently poor recovery of SFI after sciatic nerve repair. On the other hand, the ability of rat axons to surmount barriers such as rejected nerve allografts (Midha et al., 1993) and long unstructured gaps (Mackinnon et al., 1985), the short distances involved in these models, and the discrepancies in both complexity of function and neural control between rodents and humans limit the applicability of rat data to human nerve regeneration. To conclude that a new technique of nerve repair or treatment modality has clinical potential, it should be tested in higher primates before clinical trials are undertaken (Kline et al., 1964).

In the nerve regeneration literature, as is often seen in clinical reporting (Chapter 5), the potential usefulness of many experiments is limited by the presentation of data summaries rather than complete data sets. In the digital age, original data could be presented as supplemental material, available to those who wish to explore a given topic beyond the published summary. This minimal extra effort would allow data to be reevaluated from various points of view, or combined with data from other studies for meta-analysis.

Table 7-2 suggests that our investigations to date have provided information about two broad categories of function. The measures classified in categories 3 and 4 interact to describe the function of neuromuscular or neurosensory units, either singly or in bundles, but with little reference to their central connectivity. The measures in categories 1 and 2, in contrast, describe the consequences of systems organization. Great success in categories 3 and 4 may thus fail to predict voluntary function. A muscle that has regained full strength after reinnervation by large numbers of motoneurons that conduct through large-diameter axons will actually interfere with function if half of the reinnervating motoneurons are wired to fire during flexion, and the other half during extension. There will be, of course, some relationship between the volume of reinnervation and function, as there must be a level of reinnervation below which muscle contraction is not observed. Similarly, when a neuromuscular unit performs only one task, the volume of reinnervation will predict function until the muscle is fully innervated. Overall, the correlations among measures in categories 3 and 4, and especially their inability to predict voluntary function, are relatively well established. Category 3 and 4 measures provide meaningful answers to questions about the extent and the quality of regeneration and end organ reinnervation, but contribute little to the definition of functional outcome.

Measures in categories 1 and 2 are more useful in defining outcomes, yet require substantial further development. Neural connectivity is explored most often with techniques of retrograde axonal tracing, and these are far from perfect. There is a pressing need for new tracers that label all the neurons to which they are exposed, that persist in neurons without causing harm, and that do not interfere with each other's function or visibility. Once these tracers are available, it will be possible to better define the organizational consequences of imprecise nerve regeneration, and to correlate these with function.

Functional testing itself is undergoing constant refinement, with recent progress in detecting gait abnormalities that were not revealed by walking track analysis, and with the advent of upper extremity testing. In spite of these developments, however, the ability to generalize from many functional tests is compromised by their use of the rat paw or extremity as a "black box." There is no data on the central organization or number of motoneurons that are needed to innervate specific muscles in order to produce the function that is being measured. It is thus impossible to use the results of one functional test to predict outcomes of a specific treatment in another model or in humans. Similarly, all "function" is not of equal significance. The limited ability of the SFI to differentiate intermediate levels of recovery led to the development of tibial (TFI) and peroneal (PFI) indices (Chapter 6). After repair of the sciatic nerve, antagonistic muscles can be reinnervated from the same motoneuron pool, compromising the function of potentially well reinnervated muscle; after isolated tibial or peroneal nerve repair, these effects are reduced (tibial) or eliminated (peroneal). In these models, a given amount of axonal misdirection will thus have less impact by reinnervating synergists than it would by reinnervating antagonists in the sciatic model. Should a good SFI thus be given more weight than a good TFI? Similarly, there is no basis for comparing the recovery of strongly patterned activities such as gait to the recovery of more voluntary activities like those measured in the Montoya grasping test. In all of these models we are altering multijoint functions that are controlled by the coordinated firing of many motoneuron pools: in short, highly complex systems that we barely comprehend. To advance our understanding of motor control in complex situations we will need to step backward and develop new, simpler models in which detailed knowledge of the circuitry controlling each muscle can be correlated directly with the functional consequences of that circuitry; only then will we be able to generalize from the results of a given treatment in one model to its broad implications for nerve regeneration.

To be useful, a classification system must provide an overview of the topic on one hand and define roles for its component parts on the other. The key to applying the system described above for techniques of evaluating nerve regeneration is to understand that a category 1 test is not inherently more valuable than a category 4 test; what matters is that the tool be appropriate to the experimental question.

This cuts both ways—counting axons alone will rarely help one predict function, yet relying heavily on a functional test may conceal useful findings that the test cannot reveal. Questions regarding the presence or absence of regeneration can be answered with a category 4 test, confirmation of the volume and quality of end organ reinnervation requires a category 3 test, decoding the organization of reinnervation requires a category 2 test, and determining functional outcome requires a level 1 test, applied in the context of the model and its limitations.

Have experimental results modified our clinical behavior? So far, very little. Experiments have not superceded clinical experience in determining precise indications for epineurial vs. fascicular repair, or precisely how much nerve can be resected before grafting is preferable. They have, however, provided reassurance that some tension is tolerated. In the context of outcomes, the experimental approach has been most valuable in helping to define and analyze the pathophysiology that underlies clinical observations, such as the importance of patient age, graft length, and delay of treatment. The answers to clinical questions will ultimately be found in the clinic. The primary challenge to regeneration research going forward is thus not to model the clinic directly, but to identify biological variables that can be manipulated to enhance the regeneration process.

REFERENCES

Aitken JT, Sharman M, Young JZ (1947) Maturation of regenerating nerve fibers with various peripheral connexions. J Anat 81: 1–22.

Aguayo AJ, Attiwell M, Trecarten J, Perkins S, Bray GM (1977) Abnormal myelination in transplanted Trembler mouse Schwann cells. Nature 265: 73–75.

Aldskogius H, Thomander L (1986) Selective reinnervation of somatotopically appropriate muscles after facial nerve transection and regeneration in the neonatal rat. Brain Res 375: 126–134.

Almquist EE, Smith O, Fry L (1983) Nerve conduction velocity, microscopic, and electron microscopy studies comparing repaired adult and baby monkey median nerves. J Hand Surg 8: 406–410.

Anscombe FJ (1973) Graphs in statistical analysis. Amer Stat 27: 17–21.

Archibald SJ, Shefner J, Krarup C, Madison RD (1995) Monkey median nerve repaired by nerve graft or collagen nerve guide tube. Neurosci 15: 4109–4123.

Bain J, Mackinnon S, Hunter D (1989) Functional evaluation of complete sciatic, peroneal, and posterior tibial nerve lesions in the rat. PRS 83: 129–138.

Beek AV, Glover JL (1975) Primary versus delayed-primary neurorrhaphy in rat sciatic nerve. J Surg Res 18: 335–339.

Bertelli JA, Mira JC (1995) The grasping test: a simple behavioral method for objective quantitative assessment of peripheral nerve regeneration in the rat. J Neurosci Methods 58: 151–155.

Bertelli JA, Taleb M, Mira JC, Ghizoni MF (2005) Variation in nerve autograft length increases fibre misdirection and decreases pruning effectiveness: an experimental study in the rat median nerve. Neurol Res 27: 657–665.

Bertelli JA, Taleb M, Mira JC, Ghizoni MF (2006) Functional recovery improvement is related to aberrant reinnervation trimming: a comparative study using fresh or predegenerated nerve grafts. Acta Neuropathol (Berl) 111: 601–609.

Bervar M (2000) Video analysis of standing: an alternative footprint analysis to assess functional loss following injury to the rat sciatic nerve. J Neurosci Methods 102: 109–116.

Bodine-Fowler S, Meyer S, Moskovitz A, Abrams R, Botte MJ (1997) Inaccurate projection of rat soleus motoneurons: A comparison of nerve repair techniques. Muscle & Nerve 20: 29–37.

Bolesta MJ, Garrett WE Jr., Ribbeck BM, Glisson RR, Seaber AV, Goldner JL (1988) Immediate and delayed neurorrhaphy in a rabbit model: a functional, histologic, and biochemical comparison. J Hand Surg 13A: 364–369.

Bontioti EN, Kanje M, Dahlin LB (2003) Regeneration and functional recovery in the upper extremity of rats after various types of nerve injuries. JPNS 8: 159–168.

Bora FW (1967) Peripheral nerve repair in cats: the fascicular stitch. JBJS 49-A: 659–666.

Bratton BR, Kline DG, Coleman W, Hudson A (1979) Experimental interfascicular nerve grafting. J Neurosurg 51: 323–332.

Brenner MJ, Hess JR, Myckatyn TM, Hayashi A, Hunter D, Mackinnon SE (2006) Repair of motor nerve gaps with sensory nerve inhibits regeneration in rats. The Laryngoscope 116: 1685–1692.

Brooks D (1955) The place of nerve grafting in orthopaedic surgery. J Bone Joint Surg 37-A: 299–304.

Brown MC, Hardman V (1987) A reassessment of the accuracy of reinnervation by motoneurons following crushing or freezing of the sciatic or lumbar spinal nerves of rats. Brain 110: 695–705.

Brushart TM, Mesulam MM (1980) Alteration in connections between muscle and anterior horn motoneurons after peripheral nerve repair. Science 208: 603–605.

Brushart TM, Tarlov EC, Mesulam MM (1983) Specificity of muscle reinnervation after epineurial and individual fascicular suture of the rat sciatic nerve. J Hand Surg 8: 248–253.

Brushart TM (1990) Preferential motor reinnervation: a sequential double-labeling study. Restor Neuro Neurosci 1: 281–287.

Brushart TM (1993) Motor axons preferentially reinnervate motor pathways. J Neurosci 13: 2730–2738.

Brushart TM, Gerber J, Kessens P, Chen YG, Royall RM (1998) Contributions of pathway and neuron to preferential motor reinnervation. J Neurosci 18: 8674–8681.

Brushart TM, Jari R, Verge V, Rohde C, Gordon T (2005) Electrical stimulation restores the specificity of sensory axon regeneration. Exp Neurol 194: 221–229.

Burke PF, O'Brien BM (1978) A comparison of three techniques of micro nerve repairs in dogs. Hand 10: 135–143.

Buttemeyer R, Rao U, Jones NF (1995) Peripheral nerve allograft transplantation with FK506: Functional, histological, and immunological results before and after discontinuation of immunosuppression. Ann Plas Surg 35: 396–401.

Choi D, Raisman G (2002) Somatotopic organization of the facial nucleus is disrupted after lesioning and regeneration of the facial nerve: The histological representation of synkinesis. Neurosurgery 50: 355–362.

Corte MJ, Nieto CS, Ablanedo PA (1984) Motor and sensory facial nerve grafts. Arch Oto 110: 378–383.

de Medinaceli L, Freed WJ, Wyatt RJ (1982) An index of the functional condition of the rat sciatic nerve based on measurements made from walking tracks. Exp Neurol 77: 634–643.

de Medinaceli L, Freed W, Wyatt R (1983) Peripheral nerve reconnection: improvement of long-term functional effects under simulated clinical conditions in the rat. Exp Neurol 81: 488–496.

de Ruiter GC, Malessy MJ, Alaid AO, Spinner RJ, Engelstad JK, Sorenson EJ, Kaufman KR, Dyck PJ, Windebank AJ (2008) Misdirection of regenerating motor axons after nerve injury and repair in the rat sciatic nerve model. Exp Neurol 211: 339–350.

English AW (2005) Enhancing axon regeneration in peripheral nerves also increases functionally inappropriate reinnervation of targets. J Comp Neurol 490: 427–441.

English AW, Chen Y, Carp J, Wolpaw JR, Chen XY (2007) Recovery of electromyographic activity after transection and surgical repair of the rat sciatic nerve. J Neurophysiol 97: 1127–1134.

Evans PJ, Awerbuck DC, Mackinnon SE, Wade JA, McKee NH (1994) Isometric contractile function following nerve grafting: a study of graft storage. Muscle & Nerve 17: 1190–1200.

Evans PJ, MacKinnon SE, Midha R, Wade JA, Hunter DA, Nakao Y, Hare GM (1999) Regeneration across cold preserved peripheral nerve allografts. Microsurgery 19: 115–127.

Franchi G, Maggiolini E, Muzzioli V, Guandalini P (2006) The vibrissal motor output following severing and repair of the facial nerve in the newborn rat reorganises less than in the adult. Eur J Neurosci 23: 1547–1558.

Frey M, Gruber H, Happak W, Girsch W, Gruber I, Koller R (1990) Ipsilateral and cross-over elongation of the motor nerve by nerve grafting: an experimental study in sheep. Plast Reconstr Surg 85: 77–89.

Frey M, Koller R, Gruber I, Liegl C, Bittner R, Gruber H (1992) Time course of histomorphometric alterations in nerve grafts without connection to a muscle target organ: an experimental study in sheep. J Recon Micro 8: 345–357.

Fu SY, Gordon T (1995a) Contributing factors to poor functional recovery after delayed nerve repair: prolonged denervation. J Neurosci 15: 3886–3895.

Fu SY, Gordon T (1995b) Contributing factors to poor functional recovery after delayed nerve repair: prolonged axotomy. J Neurosci 15: 3876–3885.

Fugleholm K, Schmalbruch H, Krarup C (2000) Post reinnervation maturation of myelinated nerve fibers in the cat tibial nerve: chronic electrophysical and morphometric studies. JPNS 5: 82–95.

Galtrey CM, Asher RA, Nothais F, Fawcett J (2007) Promoting plasticity in the spinal cord with chondroitinase improves functional recovery after peripheral nerve repair. Brain 130: 926–939.

Galtrey CM, Fawcett J (2007) Characterization of tests of functional recovery after median and ulnar nerve injury and repair in the rat forelimb. JPNS 12: 11–27.

Ghalib N, Houstava L, Haninec P, Dubovy P (2001) Morphometric analysis of early regeneration of motor axons through motor and cutaneous nerve grafts. Ann Anat 183: 363–368.

Gillespie MJ, Stein RB (1983) The relationship between axon diameter, myelin thickness and conduction velocity during atrophy of mammalian peripheral nerves. Brain Res 259: 41–56.

Gordon L, Buncke H, Jewett DL, Muldowney B, Buncke G (1979) Predegenerated nerve autografts as compared with fresh nerve autografts in freshly cut and precut motor nerve defects in the rat. J Hand Surg 4: 42–47.

Gordon T, Stein R (1982) Time course and extent of recovery in reinnervated motor units of cat triceps surae muscles. J Physiol 323: 307–323.

Grabb WC, Bement S, Koepke GH, Green RA (1970) Comparison of methods of peripheral nerve suturing in monkeys. PRS 46: 31–38.

Gramsbergen A, Ijkema-Paassen J, Meek MF (2000) Sciatic nerve transection in the adult rat: abnormal EMG patterns during locomotion by aberrant innervation of hindleg muscles. Exp Neurol 161: 183–193.

Gramsbergen A, van Eykern LA, Meek MF (2001) Sciatic nerve transection in adult and young rats: abnormal EMG patterns during locomotion. Equine Vet J suppl 33: 36–40.

Guntinas-Lichius O, Streppel M, Angelov DN, Stennert E, Neiss WF (1997) Effect of delayed facial-facial nerve suture on facial nerve regeneration: a horseradish peroxidase tracing study in the rat. Acta Otolaryngol (Stockh) 117: 670–674.

Guntinas-Lichius O, Angelov DN, Tomov TL, Dramiga J, Neiss WF, Wewetzer K (2001) Transplantation of olfactory ensheathing cells stimulates the collateral sprouting from axotomized adult rat facial motoneurons. Exp Neurol 172: 70–80.

Guntinas-Lichius O, Wewetzer K, Tomov TL, Azzolin N, Kazemi S, Streppel M, Neiss WF, Angelov DN (2002) Transplantation of olfactory mucosa minimizes axonal branching and promotes the recovery of vibrissae motor performance after facial nerve repair in rats. J Neurosci 22: 7121–7131.

Gutmann E, Sanders FK (1943) Recovery of fiber numbers and diameters in the regeneration of peripheral nerves. J Physiol 101: 489–518.

Gómez N, Cuadras J, Butí M, Navarro X (1996) Histologic assessment of sciatic nerve regeneration following resection and graft or tube repair in the mouse. Restor Neurol Neurosci 10: 187–196.

Hadlock T, Koka R, Vacanti JP, Cheney ML (1999) A comparison of assessments of functional recovery in the rat. JPNS 4: 258–264.

Hare GM, Evans PJ, Mackinnon SE, Best TJ, Bain JR, Szalai JP, Hunter DA (1992) Walking track analysis: a long-term assessment of peripheral nerve recovery. Plast Reconstr Surg 89: 251–258.

Haase P, Payne JN (1990) Comparison of the efficiencies of true blue and diamidino yellow as retrograde tracers in the peripheral motor system. J Neurosci Methods 35: 175–183.

Hentz VR, Rosen J, Xiao S-J, McGill KC, Abraham G (1991) A comparison of suture and tubulization nerve repair techniques in a primate. J Hand Surg 16A: 251–261.

Hentz VR, Rosen J, Xiao SJ, McGill K, Abraham G (1993) The nerve gap dilemma: a comparison of nerves repaired end to end under tension with nerve grafts in a primate model. J Hand Surg 18A: 417–425.

Hertl MC, Strasberg SR, Mackinnon SE, Mohanakumar T, Hunter DA, Nyack LM, Miyasaka M (1996) The dose-related effect of monoclonal antibodies against adhesion molecules ICAM-1 and LFA-1 on peripheral nerve allograft rejection in a rat model. Restor Neurol Neurosci 10: 147–159.

Hie H, van Nie C, Vermeulen-van der Zee E (1982) Twitch tension, muscle weight, and fiber area of exercised reinnervating rat skeletal muscle. Arch Phys Med Rehabil 63: 608–612.

Highet WB, Holmes W (1943) Traction injuries to the lateral popliteal nerve and traction injuries to peripheral nerves after suture. Br J Surg 30: 212–233.

Highet WB, Sanders FK (1943) The effects of stretching nerves after suture. Brit J Surg 30: 355–369.

Hoke A, Redett R, Hameed H, Jari R, Li J-B, Griffin JW, Brushart TM (2006) Schwann cells express motor and sensory phenotypes that regulate axon regeneration. J Neurosci 26: 9646–9655.

Horch K (1979) Guidance of regrowing sensory axons after cutaneous nerve lesions in the cat. J Neurophysiol 42: 1437–1449.

Kanaya F, Firrell J, Tsai T-M, Breidenbach WC (1992) Functional results of vascularized versus nonvascularized nerve grafting. Plast Reconstr Surg 89: 924–930.

Kanaya F, Firrell JC, Breidenbach WC (1996) Sciatic function index, nerve conduction tests, muscle contraction, and axon morphometry as indicators of regeneration. Plast Reconstr Surg 98: 1264–1271.

Keeley R, Atagi T, Sabelman E, Padilla J, Kadlcik S, Keeley A, Nguyen K, Rosen J (1993) Peripheral nerve regeneration across 14-mm gaps: A comparison of autograft and entubulation repair methods in the rat. J Recon Micro 9: 349–358.

Kim DH, Connolly S, Gillespie JT, Voorhies RM, Kline D (1991) Electrophysiological studies of various graft lengths and lesion lengths in repair of nerve gaps in primates. J Neurosurg 75: 440–446.

Kline D, Hayes GJ, Morse AS (1964) A comparative study of response of species to peripheral-nerve injury. II. Crush and severance with primary suture. J Neurosurg 21: 980–988.

Kline DG, Hudson AR, Lassmann H (1981) Experimental study of fascicular nerve repair with and without epineurial closure. J Neurosurg 54: 513–520.

Kobayashi J, Mackinnon SE, Watanabe O, Ball D, Gu XM, Hunter DA, Kuzon WM (1997) The effect of duration of muscle denervation on functional recovery in the rat model. Muscle & Nerve 20: 858–866.

Koka R, Hadlock TA (2001) Quantification of functional recovery following rat sciatic nerve transection. Exp Neurol 168: 192–195.

Koller R, Frey M, Meier U, Liegel C, Gruber H, Meyer V (1993) Fiber regeneration in nerve grafts without connection to a target muscle: an experimental study in rabbits. Microsurgery 14: 516–526.

Koller R, Rab M, Todoroff BP, Neumayer C, Haslik W, Stohr HG, Frey M (1997) The influence of the graft length on the functional and morphological result after nerve grafting: an experimental study in rabbits. Brit J Plas Surg 50: 609–614.

Krarup C, Archibald SJ, Madison RD (2002) Factors that influence peripheral nerve regeneration: An electrophysiological study of the monkey median nerve. Ann Neurol 51: 69–81.

Kuypers PD, Walbeehm ET, Heel MD, Godschalk M, Hovius SE (1999) Changes in the compound action current amplitudes in relation to the conduction velocity and functional recovery in the reconstructed peripheral nerve. Muscle & Nerve 22: 1087–1093.

Kuypers PDL, Van Egeraat JM, Van Briemen LJ, Godschalk M, Hovius SER (1998) A magnetic evaluation of peripheral nerve regeneration: II. The signal amplitude in the distal segment in relation to functional recovery. Muscle & Nerve 21: 750–755.

Lago N, Navarro X (2006) Correlation between target reinnervation and distribution of motor axons in the injured rat sciatic nerve. J Neurotrauma 23: 227–240.

Langley JN, Hashimoto M (1917) On the suture of separate nerve bundles in a nerve trunk and on internal nerve plexuses. J Physiol 51: 318–345.

Le TB, Aszmann O, Chen YG, Royall RM, Brushart TM (2001) Effects of pathway and neuronal aging on the specificity of motor axon regeneration. Exp Neurol 167: 126–132.

Lutz BS (2004) The role of a barrier between two nerve fascicles in adjacency after transection and repair of a peripheral nerve trunk. Neurol Res 26: 363–370.

Mackinnon SE, Hudson A, Hunter D (1985) Histologic assessment of nerve regeneration in the rat. Plas Recon Surg 75: 384–388.

Mackinnon S, Dellon L, O'Brien J (1991) Changes in nerve fiber numbers distal to a nerve repair in the rat sciatic nerve model. Muscle & Nerve 14: 1116–1122.

Mackinnon SE, Dellon AL, Hunter DA (1988) Histological assessment of the effects of the distal nerve in determining regeneration across a nerve graft. Microsurgery 9: 46–51.

Madison RD, Archibald SJ, Brushart TM (1996) Reinnervation accuracy of the rat femoral nerve by motor and sensory neurons. J Neurosci 16: 5698–5703.

Maeda T, Hori S, Sasaki S, Maruo S (1999) Effects of tension at the site of coaptation on recovery of sciatic nerve function after neurorrhaphy: Evaluation by walking-track measurement, electrophysiology, histomorphometry, and electron probe X-ray microanalysis. Microsurgery 19: 200–207.

Malessy MJA, Van der Kamp W, Thomeer RTWM, Van Dijk JG (1998) Cortical excitability of the biceps muscle after intercostal-to-musculocutaneous nerve transfer. Neurosurgery 42: 787–794.

Martins RS, Siqueira MG, da Silva CF, Plese JP (2006) Correlation between parameters of electrophysiological, histomorphometric and sciatic functional index evaluations after sciatic nerve repair. Arq Neuropsiquiatr 64: 750–756.

Meek MF, Dijkstra JR, Den Dunnen WF, Ijkema-Paassen J, Schakenraad JM, Gramsbergen A, Robinson PH (1999) Functional assessment of sciatic nerve reconstruction: biodegradable poly (DLLA-e-CL) nerve guides versus autologous nerve grafts. Microsurgery 19: 381–388.

Meek MF, van der Werff JF, Klok F, Robinson PH, Nicolai J-P, Gramsbergen A (2003) Functional nerve recovery after bridging a 15mm gap in rat sciatic nerve with a biodegradable nerve guide. Scand J Plas Reconstr Hand Surg 37: 258–265.

Meyer RS, Abrams RA, Botte MJ, Davey JP, Bodine-Fowler SC (1997) Functional recovery following neurorrhaphy of the rat sciatic nerve by epineurial repair compared with tubulization. J Orthop Res 15: 664–669.

Midha R, Mackinnon SE, Evans PJ, Best TJ, Hare GMT, Hunter DA, Falk-Wade JA (1993) Comparison of regeneration across nerve allografts with temporary or continuous cyclosporin A immunosuppression. J Neurosurg 78: 90–100.

Millesi H, Berger A, Meissel G (1972a) Experimentelle Untersuchung zur Heilung durchtrennter peripheren Nerven. Chir Plastica (Berlin) 1: 174–206.

Millesi H, Meissl G, Berger A (1972b) The interfascicular nerve-grafting of the median and ulnar nerves. JBJS 54-A: 727–750.

Millesi H, Meissl G, Berger A (1976) Further experience with interfascicular grafting of the median, ulnar, and radial nerves. JBJS 58-A: 209–218.

Millesi H (1985) Discussion: when should nerve gaps be grafted? an experimental study in rats. Plast Reconstr Surg 75: 712–713.

Millesi H (1986) The nerve gap: theory and clinical practice. Hand Clinics 2: 651–663.

Munro CA, Szalai JP, Mackinnon SE, Midha R (1998) Lack of association between outcome measures of nerve regeneration. Muscle & Nerve 21: 1095–1097.

Navarro X, Kennedy WR (1989) Sweat gland reinnervation by sudomotor regeneration after different types of lesions and graft repairs. Exp Neurol 104: 229–234.

Navarro X, Verdu E, Buti M (1994) Comparison of regenerative and reinnervating capabilities of different functional types of nerve fibers. Exp Neurol 129: 217–224.

Neubauer D, Graham JB, Muir D (2009) Nerve grafts with various sensory and motor fiber compositions are equally effective for the repair of a mixed nerve defect. Exp Neurol 223: 203–206.

Nguyen QT, Sanes JR, Lichtman JW (2002) Pre-existing pathways promote precise projection patterns. Nat Neurosci 5:861–867.

Nichols CM, Brenner MJ, Fox IK, Tung TH, Hunter DA, Rickman SR, Mackinnon SE (2004) Effect of motor versus sensory nerve grafts on peripheral nerve regeneration. Exp Neurol 190: 347–355.

Orgel MG, Terzis JK (1977) Epineurial vs perineurial repair. PRS 60: 80–91.

Patel M, Vandevord PJ, Matthew H, Wu B, DeSilva S, Wooley PH (2006) Video-gait analysis of functional recovery of nerve repaired with chitosan nerve guides. Tissue Engineering 12: 3189–3199.

Platt H, Bristow R (1924) The remote results of operations for injuries of the peripheral nerves. Br J Surg 11: 535–567.

Pover C, Lisney SJ (1989) Influence of autograft size on peripheral nerve regeneration in cats. J Neurol Sci 90: 179–185.

Povlsen B, Hildebrand C, Wiesenfeld-Hallin Z, Stankovic N (1993) Functional projection of regenerated rat sural nerve axons to the hindpaw skin after sciatic nerve lesions. Exp Neurol 119: 99–106.

Puigdellívol-Sánchez A, Prats-Galino A, Ruano-Gil D, Molander C (1998) Efficacy of the fluorescent dyes fast blue, fluoro-gold, and diamidino yellow for retrograde tracing to dorsal root ganglia after subcutaneous injection. J Neurosci Methods 86: 7–16.

Puigdellívol-Sánchez A, Prats-Galino A, Ruano-Gil D, Molander C (2000) Fast blue and diamidino yellow as retrograde tracers in peripheral nerves: efficacy of combined nerve injection and capsule application to transected nerves in the adult rat. J Neurosci Methods 95: 103–110.

Puigdellívol-Sánchez A, Valero-Cabré A, Prats-Galino A, Navarro X, Molander C (2002) On the use of fast blue, fluoro-gold and diamidino yellow for retrograde tracing after peripheral nerve injury: uptake, fading, dye interactions, and toxicity. J Neurosci Methods 115: 115–127.

Puigdellívol-Sánchez A, Prats-Galino A, Ruano-Gil D, Molander C (2003) Persistence of tracer in the application site: a potential confounding factor in nerve regeneration studies. J Neurosci Methods 127: 105–110.

Puigdellívol-Sánchez A, Prats-Galino A, Molander C (2006) Estimations of topographically correct regeneration to nerve branches and skin after peripheral nerve injury and repair. Brain Res 1098: 49–60.

Rab M, Koller R, Haslik W, Neumayer C, Todoroff BP, Frey M, Gruber H (1998) The impact of a muscle target organ on nerve grafts with different lengths: a histomorphological analysis. Muscle & Nerve 21: 618–627.

Rab M, Koller R, Haslik W, Kamolz LP, Beck H, Meggeneder J, Frey M (2002) The influence of timing on the functional and morphological result after nerve grafting: an experimental study in rabbits. Br J Plast Surg 55: 628–634.

Rab M, Haslik W, Grunbeck M, Schmidt M, Gradl B, Giovanoli P, Frey M (2006) Free functional muscle transplantation for facial reanimation: experimental comparison between the one- and two-stage approach. J Plas Recon Aesth Surg 59: 797–806.

Redett R, Jari R, Crawford T, Chen Y-G, Rohde C, Brushart T (2005) Peripheral pathways regulate motoneuron collateral dynamics. J Neurosci 25: 9406–9412.

Romano VM, Blair SJ, Kerns JM, Wurster RD (1991) Comparison of fibrin glue, bioresorbable tubing and sutures in peripheral nerve repair. Restor Neurol Neurosci 3:75–80.

Ryoke K, Ochi M, Iwata A, Uchio Y, Yamamoto S, Yamaguchi H (2000) A conditioning lesion promotes *in vivo* nerve regeneration in the contralateral sciatic nerve of rats. Biochem Biophys Res Commun 267: 715–718.

Sanders FK, Young JZ (1944) The role of the peripheral stump in the control of fiber diameter in regenerating nerves. J Physiol 103: 119–136.

Sanders FK, Young JZ (1946) The influence of peripheral connection on the diameter of regenerating nerve fibers. J Exp Biol 22: 203–212.

Santos PM, Williams SL, Thomas SS (1995) Neuromuscular evaluation using rat gait analysis. J Neurosci Methods 61: 79–84.

Seddon H (1963) Nerve grafting. JBJS 45B: 447–461.

Shawe GDH (1955) On the number of branches formed by regenerating nerve-fibers. Brit 42: 474–488.

Shibata M, Tsai T-M, Firrell J, Breidenbach WC (1988) Experimental comparison of vascularized and nonvascularized nerve grafting. J Hand Surg 13A: 370–377.

Shibata M, Breidenbach W, Ogden L, Firrell J (1991) Comparison of one- and two-stage nerve grafting of the rabbit median nerve. J Hand Surg 16A: 262–268.

Skouras E, Popratiloff A, Guntinas-Lichius O, Streppel M, Rehm KE, Neiss W, Angelov DN (2002) Altered sensory input improves the accuracy of muscle reinnervation. Restor Neurol Neurosci 20: 1–14.

Smit X, Van Neck JW, Ebeli MJ, Hovius SE (2004) Static footprint analysis: a time-saving functional evaluation of nerve repair in rats. Scand J Plas Reconstr Hand Surg 38: 321–325.

Sorenson E, Windebank A (1993) Relative importance of basement membrane and soluble growth factors in delayed and immediate regeneration of rat sciatic nerve. J Neuropathology 52: 216–222.

Sulaiman OAR, Gordon T (2000) Effects of short- and long-term Schwann cell denervation on peripheral nerve regeneration, myelination, and size. Glia 32: 234–246.

Sunderland S (1953) Funicular suture and funicular exclusion in the repair of severed nerves. Brit 40: 580–587.

Terzis JK, Smith K (1987) Repair of severed peripheral nerves: comparison of the "de Medinaceli" and standard microsuture methods. Exp Neurol 96: 672–680.

Therkelsen J, Pool JL (1957) Stored nerve grafts for two-stage sciatic nerve repair in dogs. J Neuropath & Exp Neurol 16: 383–388.

Tos P, Ronchi G, Nicolino S, Audisio C, Raimondo S, Fornaro M, Battiston B, Graziani A, Perroteau I, Geuna S (2008) Employment of the mouse median nerve model for the experimental assessment of peripheral nerve regeneration. J Neurosci Methods 169: 119–127.

Urbanchek M, Chung K, Asato H, Washington L, Kuzon WM (1999) Rat walking tracks do not reflect maximal muscle force capacity. J Recon Micro 15: 143–149.

Valero-Cabré A, Navarro X (2001) H reflex restitution and facilitation after different types of peripheral nerve injury and repair. Brain Res 919: 302–312.

Valero-Cabré A, Tsironis K, Skouras E, Perego G, Navarro X, Neiss WF (2001) Superior muscle reinnervation after autologous nerve graft or poly-L-lactide-Œ-caprolactone (PLC) tube implantation in comparison to silicone tube repair. J Neurosci Res 63: 214–223.

Valero-Cabré A, Navarro X (2002) Functional impact of axonal misdirection after peripheral nerve injuries followed by graft or tube repair. J.Neurotrauma 19: 1475–1485.

Valero-Cabré A, Tsironis K, Skouras E, Navarro X, Neiss W (2004) Peripheral and spinal motor reorganization after nerve injury and repair. J Neurotrauma 21: 95–108.

Valero-Cabré A, Navarro X (2002) Functional impact of axonal misdirection after peripheral nerve injuries followed by graft or tube repair. J Neurotrauma 19: 1475–1485.

Varejão AS, Cabrita AM, Geuna S, Melo-Pinto P, Filipe VM, Gramsbergen A, Meek MF (2003) Toe out angle: a functional index for the evaluation of sciatic nerve recovery in the rat model. Exp Neurol 183: 695–699.

Verdú E, Butí M, Navarro X (1995) The effect of aging on efferent nerve fibers regeneration in mice. Brain Res 696: 76–82.

Verdú E, Navarro X (1997) Comparison of immunohistochemical and functional reinnervation of skin and muscle after peripheral nerve injury. Exp Neurol 146: 187–198.

Vleggeert-Lankamp CL, van den Berg RJ, Feirabend HK, Lakke EA, Thomeer TW (2004) Electrophysiology and morphometry of the Aa and Ab fiber populations in the normal and regenerating rat sciatic nerve. Exp Neurol 187: 337–349.

Walbeehm ET, Dudok van Heel EB, Kuypers PD, Terenghi G, Hovius SE (2003) Nerve compound action current (NCAC) measurements and morphometric analysis in the proximal segment after nerve transection and repair in a rabbit model. JPNS 8: 108–115.

Walker JL, Evans J, Meade P, Resig P, Sisken B (1994) Gait-stance duration as a measure of injury and recovery in the rat sciatic nerve model. J Neurosci Methods 52: 47–52.

Wang H, Sorenson EJ, Spinner RJ, Windebank AJ (2008) Electrophysiologic findings and grip strength after nerve injuries in the rat forelimb. Muscle & Nerve 38:1254–1265.

Wasserschaff M (1990) Coordination of reinnervated muscle and reorganization of spinal cord motoneurons after nerve transection in mice. Brain Res 515: 241–246.

Watanabe O, Mackinnon SE, Tarasidis G, Hunter DA, Ball DJ (1998) Long-term observation of the effect of peripheral nerve injury in neonatal and young rats. Plast Reconstr Surg 102: 2072–2081.

Weiss P, Edds MV, Cavanaugh M (1945) The effect of terminal connections on the caliber of nerve fibers. J Comp Neurol 92: 215–233.

Werdin F, Grussinger H, Jaminet P, Kraus A, Manoli T, Danker T, Guenther E, Haerlec M, Schaller HE, Sinis N (2009) An improved electrophysiological method to study peripheral nerve regeneration in rats. J Neurosci Methods 182: 71–77.

Wikholm R, Swett J, Torigoe Y, Blanks R (1988) Repair of severed peripheral nerve: A superior anatomic and functional recovery with a new "reconnection" technique. J Otol Head & Neck Surg 99: 353–361.

Wolthers M, Moldovan M, Binderup T, Schmalbruch H, Krarup C (2005) Comparative electrophysiological, functional, and histological studies of nerve lesions in rats. Microsurgery 25: 508–519.

Yamaguchi H, Ochi M, Mori R, Ryoke K, Yamamoto S, Iwata A, Uchio Y (1999) Unilateral sciatic nerve injury stimulates contralateral nerve regeneration. Neuroreport 10: 1359–1362.

Yu PR, Matloub HS, Sanger JR, Narini P (2001) Gait analysis in rats with peripheral nerve injury. Muscle & Nerve 24: 231–239.

Zellem R, Miller D, Kenning J, Hoenig E, Buchheit W (1989) Experimental peripheral nerve repair: Environmental control directed at the cellular level. Microsurgery 10: 290–301.

Zhao Q, Dahlin L, Kanje M, Lundborg G (1992) Specificity of muscle reinnervation following repair of the transected sciatic nerve. J Hand Surg 17B: 257–261.

8

THE NERVE GAP

BEYOND AUTOGRAFT

PERIPHERAL NERVE gaps may be bridged with a variety of structures, or circumvented with location-specific strategies. Surgically revascularized nerve grafts are most clearly indicated for use in scarred beds, and may also be helpful for long gaps or when a large caliber graft is needed. Cellular nerve allograft depends on a combination of reduced graft immunogenicity and diminished host response for its success; its current use is limited by the risks of immunosuppression. Grafts of acellular nerve and muscle basal lamina convey axons across short gaps, and may prove most useful as carriers for autologous Schwann cells. Vein graft has also been used as a graft substitute, but with variable success. A prospective, randomized trial of digital nerve grafting found the performance of permeable tubular prostheses to be equal to that of autologous nerve. A similar trial found gap repair of the median and ulnar nerves with a silicon tube to provide function equal to that

obtained after end-to-end nerve suture. Direct neurotization by implantation of motor nerve into denervated muscle can be an effective salvage procedure when multiple donor fascicles are used to distribute axons widely. Similarly, end-to-side nerve repair, which functions largely through terminal reinnervation from injured donor axons, is most effective at the level of distal sensory and motor nerves, but is ineffective at the nerve trunk level. Reimplantation of motor roots that have been avulsed from the spinal cord provides some motor reinnervation when performed soon after injury, but the topographic specificity of regeneration is lost. Distal nerve transfer is becoming an increasingly popular alternative to proximal nerve reconstruction, as it provides a functionally discrete, freshly axotomized axon population that can be directed to target muscle or skin over short distances, promoting rapid reinnervation and minimizing end organ atrophy.

NERVE GRAFT REVASCULARIZATION

Inosculation, Neovascularization, and Immediate Surgical Revascularization

The survival of a nerve graft, and thus its ability to convey regenerating axons across a nerve gap, requires that blood flow be restored to its cellular elements. The earliest evidence regarding graft revascularization was obtained indirectly through experimental observation of graft failure; the central portions of dog sciatic nerve grafts were found to be necrotic (Bielschowsky, Unger, 1917). This inability to restore central circulation was subsequently confirmed for both dog and cat sciatic grafts (Bunnell, Boyes, 1939; Tarlov, Epstein, 1945). In contrast to these large-caliber grafts, small grafts showed no signs of central degeneration (Maccabruni, 1911; Seddon, 1963). Early clinical experience was consistent with these findings. Thin grafts were found to support regeneration, and successfully restored function to the digital and facial nerves (Bunnell, 1927; Balance, Duel, 1932; Seddon et al., 1942), whereas thicker grafts of peroneal and radial nerve degenerated (Holmes, 1947; Seddon, 1963). Clearly, grafts of small diameter were revascularized more readily than those of large diameter.

The process of graft revascularization was evaluated directly by Tarlov and Epstein (1945), who performed intra-arterial injections of red lead to study the restoration of blood flow to 3-cm-long dog sciatic nerve grafts. They found that host vessels penetrated the proximal and distal ends of the graft within 3 days, then began to enter the lateral aspects of the graft from surrounding tissues after 6–8 days. This picture was incomplete, however, as small vessels and capillaries were not filled by the viscous lead. The most comprehensive early study was that of Almgren, who evaluated the perfusion of rabbit tibial nerve grafts by adding Evans blue-labeled albumin to the normal circulation (Almgren, 1974). Filling of graft endoneurial vessels was clearly established by 3 days in 32/35 grafts. During the first week, the majority of vessels entered through the ends of the graft to reconnect with existing circulation (the process of *inosculation*); thereafter, vessels were recruited to the lateral aspects of the graft from its bed (the process of *neovascularization*; Figure 8-1). In aggregate, these early studies suggest that graft revascularization begins by inosculation at the nerve ends, then continues by recruitment of vessels from the bed, possibly in a length-dependent fashion.

The process of graft revascularization became a topic of great interest when Taylor and Ham (1976) reported immediate microvascular restoration of circulation at the time of graft placement. Should this new technique become the standard, was it needed only in special circumstances, or was the natural process of revascularization uniformly adequate? These questions were addressed using a new method of measuring blood flow in tissues. Radioactive microspheres were injected in the systemic circulation and lodged in the capillary bed.

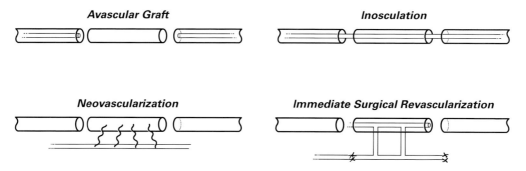

FIGURE 8-1   Routes of nerve graft revascularization. When a nerve graft is initially sewn in place it has no circulation; Schwann cell viability is maintained by diffusion from surrounding tissues. Circulation is initially restored through inosculation, the reconnection of preexisting vessels across the repair site. Neovascularization, the ingrowth of new vessels from the bed, occurs more slowly and to varying degrees. Surgical revascularization, in contrast, restores blood flow at the time of surgery, limiting the duration of relative graft ischemia.

Tissue blood flow could then be calculated from measurement of its radioactivity. Application of this technique to dog saphenous nerve grafts revealed that one-third of conventional grafts had regained adequate circulation by 3 days (Lind, Wood, 1986; Lux et al., 1988); by 4–6 days, both total blood flow and individual blood flow to the epineurium and endoneurium of conventional grafts exceed that of grafts with surgically restored circulation (Settergren, Wood, 1984; Daly, Wood, 1985). By this time it had also been demonstrated that Schwann cells within small-diameter conventional grafts not only survive, but undergo division within days of engraftment (Sanders, Young, 1942; Weiss, Taylor, 1946; Bray et al., 1981). There was thus no need for surgical revascularization of small-diameter grafts in normal tissue beds. There is still no consensus, however, regarding the primary route of graft revascularization. If anything, the debate has become polarized, with strong advocates for both the predominance of inosculation (Best et al., 1999; Chalfoun et al., 2003) and neovascularization (Penkert et al., 1988; Prpa et al., 2002).

Although revascularization is a necessary condition for graft success, the speed and degree of revascularization do not predict function (McCollough et al., 1984; Mani et al., 1992). Experimentation to define a role for surgical revascularization has proven inconclusive. Electrophysiologic and morphometric comparison of conventional and surgically revascularized grafts in rats and rabbits has demonstrated both the equality of the two types of graft (McCollough et al., 1984; Seckel et al., 1986; Kawai et al., 1990; Mani et al., 1992; Tark, Roh, 2001) and the superiority of surgically revascularized grafts (Shibata et al., 1988; Iwai et al., 2001). The results of functional testing are similarly inconclusive, with evidence that surgical revascularization does (Shibata et al., 1988; Kanaya et al., 1992) and does not (Bertelli et al., 1996b) improve the function of reinnervated muscle. It is difficult to reconcile these disparate findings. If one rejects studies performed in the rat because of their nonclinical scale, there is still no consensus, and no clear indication of the superiority of one rabbit model over another that could explain the conflicting findings.

Considerable effort has been focused on the effects of surgically manipulating graft blood supply. That this blood supply may also be manipulated biologically is just beginning to be recognized. Vascular endothelial growth factor (VEGF) is a potent stimulator of angiogenesis (Connolly et al., 1989). Application of VEGF to acellular nerve grafts promotes both neovascularization of the graft and invasion of the graft by Schwann cells (Sondell et al., 1999b). VEGF also stimulates axonal outgrowth from a subset of DRG neurons (Sondell et al., 1999a). When applied to conventional nerve grafts in avascular beds, VEGF promotes inosculation that allows these grafts to be revascularized to a degree similar to that of grafts placed in a healthy bed (Wongtrakul et al., 2002). Grafts that overexpress VEGF to promote rapid revascularization could potentially obviate the need for surgical revascularization altogether.

Clinical Experience

Clinically, two potential indications for maintaining or immediately restoring graft blood supply have been explored: the reconstruction of large gaps in the brachial plexus or extremity nerves, and grafting across a compromised bed. Severe brachial plexus injuries often result in extensive neural damage, requiring multiple long grafts to replace damaged neural elements. When the severity of injury precludes reinnervation of the ulnar nerve, it may be used as a graft, either based on existing circulation (pedicle graft) or surgically revascularized through the ulnar artery (so-called vascularized nerve graft, or VNG) (Terzis et al., 1995). Merle and Dautel, using both techniques, found that regeneration through VNG proceeded more rapidly than it did through conventional sural nerve grafts, yet outcomes were not improved (Merle, Dautel, 1991). Birch et al. (1988) studied 42 patients in whom ulnar nerve grafts to the brachial plexus had been revascularized surgically, and stated, "Although it cannot be proved that results are better than when conventional sural nerve grafts are performed, the authors believe that this is the case" (p96). In comparing the results of conventional nerve grafting with those of both pedicled and free vascularized grafts, Terzis and Kostopoulos (2009) found improved results when graft vascularity was maintained or restored, though the significance of the observed differences was not determined. The ulnar nerve, both as pedicled graft and as VNG, has also been used successfully to convey axons across the chest from the uninjured C7 root to reinnervate the contralateral plexus after nerve root avulsions (Gu et al., 1998; Waikakul et al., 1999a; Songcharoen et al, 2001; Terzis, Kostopoulos, 2009), and to reconstruct the proximal median and radial nerves (Kimata et al., 2005). Similarly, in the proximal arm, surgically revascularized sural nerve grafts were found in one series to restore function earlier, more reliably, and to a greater extent than did conventional sural grafts (Doi et al., 1992).

Surgical revascularization of nerve grafts that are to be placed in a compromised bed is clearly supported by clinical experience. Rose and Kowalski (1985) reported on 5 patients in whom conventional digital nerve grafts had failed and who could therefore serve as their own controls. Surgically revascularized deep peroneal nerve grafts restored an average two-point discrimination (2-PD) of 9.5 mm to these patients. A similar outcome was obtained with reversed venous arterialized grafts, a technique devised to avoid arterial sacrifice (Rose et al., 1989). In a comparison of conventional and surgically revascularized sural nerve grafts, Doi et al. (1992) found the latter to outperform the former in cases where flap coverage was needed to restore skin coverage. Reconstruction of the facial nerve with VNG has also been successful through scarred or poorly covered beds, although no comparison with conventional grafts was reported (Kimata et al., 2005).

CELLULAR NERVE ALLOGRAFT

The first reported nerve allograft procedure was performed by Albert (1885). It was not until the work of Sir Peter Medawar in the 1940s, however, that allograft performance was understood in the context of immune function (Medawar, 1944). Allogenic (between individuals of the same species) nerve graft is potentially the ideal substitute for autograft in the reconstruction of neural deficits, since living Schwann cells are able to enhance the regeneration environment. This assumption is borne out by performance of allografts protected by continuous immunosuppression (Bain et al., 1988). Allograft nerve transplantation without immunosuppression, however, usually results in rejection and loss of Schwann cells with subsequent graft failure (Pollard, McLeod, 1981; Tajima et al., 1991; Strasberg et al., 1996b). The severity of rejection depends primarily on the immunologic mismatch of graft and host (Mackinnon et al., 1985b), but may also be influenced to some extent by graft length. In rodents, axons grow around short (1- to 2-cm-long) allografts, eventually providing distal reinnervation equivalent to that seen with autograft (Midha et al., 1994b). Even in the primate, short nerve allografts (3 cm) may support regeneration in spite of mismatch sufficient to cause kidney rejection (Bain et al., 1992;

Fish et al., 1992). Only long allografts (5–8 cm) in the sheep and swine fail uniformly without immunosuppression (Strasberg et al., 1996b). The molecular interactions that lead to allograft failure are complex and beyond the scope of this chapter (pertinent reviews include Evans et al., 1994; Castejon et al., 1999; Doolabh, Mackinnon, 1999a; Trumble, Shon, 2000; Myckatyn, Mackinnon, 2004).

Reducing Graft Antigenicity

Allograft rejection can be modified by reducing either the antigenicity of the graft or the magnitude of the host response. Antigenicity is significantly reduced by subjecting the graft to a freeze/thaw cycle to kill its cellular elements (Zalewski, Gulati, 1982). This treatment preserves the laminin-rich basal lamina needed to promote axon regeneration (Hall, 1997), but nonetheless compromises the ability of these grafts to support regeneration (Mackinnon et al., 1984b; Gash et al., 1998). Alternatively, it is possible to reduce graft antigenicity without destroying Schwann cell function. Storing grafts at 5°C for 1 week in University of Washington solution decreases graft expression of ICAM-1 and class II MHC antigens (Atchabahian et al., 1999), graft markers that play key roles in the rejection process. Migration of lymphocytes into allografts treated in this manner is greatly reduced (Hare et al., 1993), yet storage of human nerve for 1 week has little impact on Schwann cell survival (Levi et al., 1994a); grafts stored for up to 3 weeks still contain some viable Schwann cells (Evans et al., 1998, 1999). Although cold storage alone does little to improve regeneration in the absence of immunosuppression (Strasberg et al., 1996b; Evans et al., 1999), it can enhance the effects of immunosuppressive treatments and reduce immunosuppression requirements (Hare et al., 1995; Strasberg et al, 1996a; Grand et al., 2002). When graft immunogenicity is reduced further by storage for 6–7 weeks, and host Schwann cells are replaced with cultured autologous Schwann cells, graft performance is superior to that of allograft alone, but is still inferior to that of autograft and even untreated allograft (Hess et al., 2007).

Blunting the Host Response

Allograft rejection may also be reduced by modifying the host response. Initial efforts involved nonspecific immunosuppression with cyclosporin A or FK506. Both bind to immunophilin receptors to block the action of calcineurin, and thus the activation of genes regulated by the NF-AT transcription factor (Ho et al., 1996). These include genes required for both B-cell helper function and T-cell proliferation. Regeneration across nerve allografts in rats immunosuppressed with cyclosporin A is similar to that across autograft by both histologic and functional criteria (Bain et al., 1988). When a 12-week course of cyclosporin treatment is terminated, however, the graft is rejected (Midha et al., 1993; Ishida et al., 1993). In the short allografts possible in the rat, this rejection does not preclude ultimate graft function. Destruction of allograft Schwann cells and regenerated axons during rejection is followed by repopulation of the graft with host Schwann cells and a second wave of axon regeneration (Midha et al., 1993; Ishida et al., 1993; Midha et al., 1994a; Zalewski et al., 1995). If the graft is then returned to a rat immunologically identical to its original donor, it will be rejected (Atchabahian et al., 1998). The degree to which allograft Schwann cells are eliminated may vary from complete obliteration (Midha et al., 1993) to only partial removal, with persistence of graft Schwann cells after the rejection response has subsided (Katsube et al., 1998). The severity of rejection is not diminished by previous reinnervation of end organs, but appears to vary by axon type, with somewhat better survival of sensory and small motor axons (Midha et al., 1997, 1998, 2001). When immunosuppression is maintained for longer periods, the transition from donor to host status occurs more slowly, allowing prolonged survival of the repopulated allograft once immunosuppression is discontinued (Frazier et al., 1993; Atchabahian et al., 1998).

In 1994, the immunosuppressant FK506 was found to enhance regeneration after nerve crush injury (Gold et al., 1994). This observation suggested the possibility that FK506 could be used in the setting of nerve allograft to provide immunosuppression and promote regeneration simultaneously. In subsequent autograft experiments, FK506 hastened the maturation of axons and return of function in the rat, restoring sensory and motor function after 12 weeks equal to that seen with autograft (Doolabh, Mackinnon, 1999b; Haisheng et al., 2008). In similar mouse allograft experiments, FK506 also enhanced the speed and degree of recovery (Navarro et al., 2001; Udina et al., 2004). Continuous FK506 administration at doses as low

as 1 mg/Kg/day prevents allograft rejection across major histocompatibility barriers (Buttemeyer et al., 1995; Weinzweig et al., 1996; Udina et al., 2004), whereas a dose of 0.2 mg/Kg/day appears to be ineffective (Udina et al., 2003). Withdrawal of FK506 is followed by varying degrees of allograft rejection (Buttemeyer et al., 1995; Udina et al., 2004; Auba et al., 2006), with excellent long-term recovery of nerve conduction after only temporary immunosuppression of rats grafted across a major histocompatibility barrier (Weinzweig et al., 1996). Immunosuppression with FK506 has also been used in conjunction with cold preservation of allograft material. In short-term rat studies, the number of neurons labeled retrogradely through the graft was similar with cold preservation, FK506, or both (Hontanilla et al., 2006a; Auba et al., 2006). In the mouse, the combination of FK506 and cold preservation improved footprint length when compared with either alone at 3 weeks, but not at subsequent time periods. The ultimate goal of combining these techniques—excellent outcome without the need for long-term immunosuppression—could not be achieved in the primate. Regeneration was sufficient to restore function, but evidence of rejection persisted for 8–9 months (Hontanilla et al., 2006a; Auba et al., 2006).

Systemic immunosuppression increases the risks of both infection and malignancy. The need to reduce these risks in the treatment of non-life-threatening disease has stimulated attempts to induce donor-specific tolerance of nerve antigen. Intercellular adhesion molecule-1 (ICAM-1) and leukocyte function-associated antigen-1 (LFA-1) are adhesion molecules that participate in the interaction between antigen-presenting cells and T-cells. Blocking their function with monoclonal antibodies can improve both the structure and function of allograft nerve while delaying the rejection of donor skin grafts (Nakao et al., 1995a, 1995b). In similar experiments, however, neither tolerance nor improved function was observed (Hertl et al., 1996; Ochi et al., 1998). Another, more aggressive approach is to induce alloantigen-specific immunosuppression by pretreating the graft recipient with donor antigens that have been altered by treatment with UV-B radiation. When injected into the portal venous circulation, these modified antigens undergo phagocytosis by Kupffer cells in the liver and present to circulating T-cells as self rather than as foreign (Liu et al., 1993). A single intraportal injection of UV-B-irradiated antigen 1 week before nerve allotransplantation in both the rat and pig induces prolonged tolerance to donor antigen and promotes regeneration and restoration of function (Genden et al., 2001; Tung et al., 2006). A third strategy involves blocking the CD40/CD40 ligand costimulatory pathway. In the mouse, this improved both histological and functional recovery; immune tolerance was enhanced as evidenced by reduced levels of interferon and interleukin and minimal response to a second allograft challenge after 60 days (Brown et al., 2006; Mungara et al., 2008), but was insufficient to protect allografts placed after the cessation of treatment (Brenner et al., 2004b). Similarly, regeneration through 5-cm primate allografts was robust when surgery and the beginning of treatment coincided, but not if graft placement was delayed (Brenner et al., 2004a).

Treatment Combinations

The failure of any single treatment to provide optimal long-term allograft survival has stimulated investigation of various treatment combinations. The dose of CSA needed for immunosuppression can be lowered significantly when it is used in conjunction with anti-ICAM and anti-LFA (Fox et al., 1999), and FK506 is effective at normally subtherapeutic levels when combined with anti-CD-40 antibodies (Brenner et al., 2005b). Similarly, CSA and anti-αβ T-cell receptor antibodies are synergistic in their effect, but still unable to induce immune tolerance (Scharpf et al., 2006). Other potentially useful combinations include donor antigen with anti-ICAM and anti-LFA (Genden et al., 1998) and multiple costimulation blockade with antibodies to LFA, CD40, and CTLA4lg (Kvist et al., 2007) or with antibodies to CD40, CD28/B7, and ICOS (Tai et al., 2009). The problem of Schwann cell rejection is skirted altogether by treating with donor antigen and injecting a cold-treated allograft with MHC-matched Schwann cells, a strategy that has been successful in promoting regeneration through long allografts in the pig (Brenner et al., 2005a). As techniques of culturing human Schwann cells improve, this approach to nerve grafting becomes more clinically feasible.

Clinical Experience

The clinical use of nerve allograft in a series of young patients was reported by Mackinnon et al. (2001). Cadaveric allografts were preserved for 7 days in University of Wisconsin solution before use; immunosuppression consisted of either cyclosporin or FK-506, azathioprine, and prednisone, and was discontinued 6 months after regenerating axons had crossed the grafts. Rejection of one allograft was the only complication reported. Nerves reconstructed with allograft alone regenerated sufficiently to restore proximal muscle function and varying degrees of sensory function, the best being two-point discrimination of 3 mm in a 2-year-old child. Significantly, none of the patients lost function after immunosuppression was discontinued. The use of allograft nerve to expand reconstructive options after severe injury in the young is thus clinically feasible. Extension of these indications will await further improvements in techniques of immunosuppression, induction of immune tolerance, and the repopulation of allograft nerve with patient-derived Schwann cells.

GRAFTS OF BASEMENT MEMBRANE

Nerve

The failure of nerve homograft and allograft experiments prior to the availability of immunosuppression suggested that highly antigenic cellular elements should be removed from the graft to prevent its rejection. Use of the remaining acellular basal lamina graft to support axon regeneration was first explored by Ide in the rat (Ide, 1983). Axons grew through the basal lamina scaffolds, bringing along Schwann cells from the proximal stump. The original basal lamina gradually disintegrated as regenerating axons increased in size, became myelinated, and were segregated into minifascicles by perineurial ensheathment. This process of "compartmentation" was initially conceptualized as a response to disturbance or total loss of perineurial function (Hall, 1986b; Chapter 9). Its persistence throughout the length of basal lamina grafts (Ide, 1983; McCollough et al., 1984) contrasts with the maintenance of normal architecture at the midportions of cellular autografts (Hudson et al., 1972).

Subsequent experiments focused on the relationship among axon, Schwann cell, and basal lamina during reinnervation of acellular grafts. Axons usually extend along the inner surface of the basal lamina, the side previously in contact with the parent Schwann cell (Ide et al., 1983; Hall, 1986b; Wang et al., 1992b). The presence of laminin in this location suggested its role as a permissive factor; by this time laminin was already known to promote neurite growth in vitro (Baron-Van Evercooren et al., 1982; Tohyama, Ide, 1984). The essential role of laminin was confirmed by experiments in which administration of antilaminin antibodies markedly perturbed axonal growth through basal lamina grafts whereas antifibronectin antibodies had no effect (Wang et al., 1992a, 1992b). Several observers have found that regenerating axons precede Schwann cells along the basal lamina surface (Ide et al., 1983; Sketelj et al., 1989; Wang et al., 1992b; Sondell et al., 1998), although two electronmicroscopic studies did not confirm this observation (Anderson et al., 1983; Hall, 1986b). Additional experiments showing that inhibition of Schwann cell migration from the proximal stump prevented reinnervation of acellular grafts were consistent with the need for Schwann cells to precede axons (Hall, 1986a). The relative requirements for Schwann cells and basal lamina during axon regeneration are discussed in more detail in Chapter 9.

Not surprisingly, acellular grafts impose limitations on axon regeneration that are not encountered when autograft is used. The speed of regeneration through nerve graft is reduced by 40% when cellular elements cannot contribute to the process (Bresjanac, Sketelj, 1989). The initial delay in reinnervating basal lamina graft (9.5 days) is significantly greater than that for reinnervation of fresh autograft (3.6 days), although graft predegeneration reduces this difference (Danielsen et al., 1995; Kerns et al., 2003). When one end of an acellular graft is connected and the other end is left free, axons can penetrate the graft to a depth of only 10–20 mm, a restriction imposed at least in part by the limited migratory ability of Schwann cells (Nadim et al., 1990; Anderson et al., 1991). This limitation may, in turn, result from the gradual degradation of laminin in grafts prepared by freezing, such that laminin-1 and -2 cannot be detected immunologically after 1 week in grafts that have been maintained in vivo but not reinnervated (Dubovy et al., 2001).

In most experimental trials, basal lamina graft has been prepared from allogenic nerve to duplicate most closely the clinical situation. Once the cellular elements have been removed, the remaining basal lamina is mildly immunogenic and can be transplanted without rejection (Gulati, Cole, 1994). Morphologic evidence of distal stump reinnervation through allogenic basal lamina has been obtained in the rat with grafts of 2 cm (Gulati, Cole, 1994) and 3 cm (Osawa et al., 1990); regeneration does not bridge 4-cm gaps in the rat, even through autograft basal lamina, unless the graft is pretreated with chondroitinase to remove inhibitory chondroitin sulfate proteoglycans (Gulati, 1988; Haase et al., 2003; Neubauer et al., 2007). In a recent comparison of treated nerve allografts with porous tubular prostheses, functional and histologic measures were similar and inferior to isograft when bridging a 14-mm gap; when the gap was increased to 28 mm, the distal stump was reinnervated more often through the allograft basal lamina than through a tubular prosthesis (Whitlock et al., 2009). Axons will cross basal lamina allografts of 3 cm in the monkey and 4 cm in the rabbit (Tajima et al., 1991; Gulati, Cole, 1994). A 5-cm gap in the beagle poses a serious challenge, however; myelinated axon counts 1.5 cm distal to the site of basal lamina engraftment 3 months previously were only 2.5% of those obtained at the same location when autograft was used (Ide et al., 1998).

The obvious limitations of neural basal lamina graft may be decreased by strategies to enhance axon regeneration through suboptimal terrain, or to improve the terrain by the addition of autologous Schwann cells. Treatment of 5-cm beagle basal lamina nerve grafts with fibroblast growth factor-2 (FGF-2) enhanced myelinated axon counts in the distal stump by 31.5% (Ide et al., 1998). In the rat, addition of Schwann cells to basal lamina grafts of 1 cm or 1.5 cm failed to improve morphological or functional outcomes (Dumont, Henz, 1997; Accioli-de-Vaconcellos et al., 1999); a difference was seen between acellular and seeded grafts when the gap was increased to 2 cm (Gulati et al., 1995). In a small series of 4-cm ulnar nerve grafts in monkeys, addition of either Schwann cells or mesenchymal stem cells improved CMAP and axon counts over values obtained with basal lamina alone (Hu et al., 2007). Ultimately, repopulation of acellular grafts with autologous Schwann cells has the potential to become a successful clinical strategy for the management of substantial nerve gaps. Providing a source of trophic and contact factors that is already programmed to respond to axonal contact is far more efficient than trying to replace a series of individual factors. The elective nature of nerve grafting provides time for culturing the patient's Schwann cells and repopulating stored allogenic basal lamina. Furthermore, there is no need for immunosuppression. The necessary techniques are

Muscle

Early studies of motor endplate specification and basal lamina function revealed that muscle basement membrane is an excellent substrate for axon elongation (Sanes et al., 1978; Ide, 1984). Axons prefer the inner surface of the basal lamina, much as they do when regenerating through peripheral nerve (Keynes et al., 1984). The realization of this similarity led to the experimental use of muscle basal lamina scaffolds as a substitute for autologous nerve graft (Fawcett, Keynes, 1986). The basis for the preliminary success of these grafts, the presence of laminin in the basal lamina, was later confirmed by immunolabeling and the reduction of graft function by 90% after treatment with antilaminin antibodies (Bryan et al., 1993; Hall, Kent, 1996).

Schwann cells are required for axonal progression through grafts of muscle basal lamina (Feneley et al., 1991; Enver, Hall, 1994). As regenerating axons mature, they are rigidly segregated into numerous minifascicles (Gschmeissner et al., 1990), a response to nonneural conditions similar to that described above. Regeneration proceeds more rapidly when basal lamina tubes are oriented in line with the nerve gap (Glasby et al., 1986a). Even so, gross misdirection of regenerating fibers within the graft has been described (Bertelli et al., 2005). Although the first grafts used in mammalian studies were purged of their cellular contents by a combination of chemical and mechanical treatment, the majority of studies have used a freeze-thaw cycle (Fawcett, Keynes, 1986; Glasby, 1990). Grafts prepared by killing myocytes with local anesthetic will also convey axons across a short gap in the rat after either delayed or immediate harvest, as will those subjected to heat treatment at 60° C (Hall, Enver, 1994; Santo Neto et al., 1998; Neto et al., 2004). In a comparative study of several techniques, chemical treatment with vacuum extraction resulted in the most open channels and the best early regeneration (Meek et al., 1999). Addition of Schwann cells to the construct enhances early regeneration (Fansa et al., 2001; Nishiura et al., 2004), but in one study had little impact on ultimate muscle function (Alluin et al., 2006).

Muscle basement membrane is a convenient source of nerve graft substitute, as it is readily available in the surgical wound and can be harvested in substantial quantities without compromise of neuromuscular function. Success in grafting 1-cm gaps (reviewed in Glasby, 1990) and this user-friendly quality stimulated trials in the grafting of longer gaps as a prelude to clinical application. When used to bridge a 5-cm gap in the rabbit peroneal nerve, muscle basal lamina was distinctly inferior to autologous nerve graft (Hems, Glasby, 1992). Distal fiber numbers were reduced sharply, muscle force was negligible, and sensory function could not be detected. When the gap was increased to 10 cm, basal lamina failed to support regeneration entirely (Hems, Glasby, 1993). Limitations at 5 cm were not seen in the sheep, where use of autologous nerve and muscle basal lamina grafts resulted in similar distal axon morphology 10 months after implantation (Glasby et al., 1990). Primate experiments were also encouraging, although axons were challenged with a shorter graft: 2-cm basal lamina grafts to the proximal median nerve of the marmoset supported detectable flexor carpi radialis function after 150 days (Norris et al., 1988), and 3-cm grafts to the radial or median nerves restored normal hand function, as judged by informal observation, by 6 months (Glasby et al., 1986b).

In spite of these mixed results, muscle basal lamina grafts were tried in humans. Grafting of 1–2.5 cm digital nerve gaps restored a mean 2-PD of 6 mm (range 4–12.5 mm) (Pereira et al., 1991). Grafts of median and ulnar nerves at the wrist and forearm levels fared less well: 5/12 patients regained S3+ sensibility, and none recovered S4 sensibility or motor function (Calder, Norris, 1993). Similarly, grafting of radial nerve gaps of 2.6–6 cm with muscle basal lamina failed to equal the performance of autologous nerve, with an inverse correlation between function and graft length (Roganovic et al., 2007).

The progression from rat experiments to human trials provides an interesting case study. When the issue is ability to convey axons over clinically relevant distances, success in the rodent model does not predict clinical success. In this case, even moving up to the scale of the rabbit was sufficient to detect significant limitations in basal lamina graft performance. On the basis of these findings, it would be difficult to recommend treating injuries to major human peripheral nerves with grafts of muscle basal lamina.

VEIN GRAFT

Vein graft has been used as a conduit for nerve regeneration, often in the setting of acute digital nerve injury. Although the best results of vein grafting short gaps are equal to those of grafting with autologous nerve, the technique is less reliable. In one prospective series of digital nerve reconstructions, patients achieved a mean 2-PD of only 11.1 +/- 3.4 mm (Chiu, Strauch, 1990); in other series, vein grafts failed to restore any 2pd in 7/15 and 6/18 patients, respectively (Walton et al., 1989; Tang et al., 1993), though 2-PD of 4–6mm was restored in 3 patients in one series (Lee and Shieh, 2008). More promising clinical results have been obtained by inserting muscle or segments of nerve within the graft (Battiston et al., 2000; Terzis, Kostas, 2007). Experimentally, functional outcomes of vein grafting have been improved by the addition of Schwann cells to the lumen of the graft (Foidart-Dessalle et al., 1997), although results are still inferior to those of grafting with autologous nerve (Zhang et al., 2002).

TUBES AND BIOENGINEERED NERVE GRAFT SUBSTITUTE

Over a century ago Forssman (1898) enclosed nerve gaps within straw tubes to investigate the mechanism of nerve regeneration. In similar studies a half century later, Weiss inserted nerve ends into segments of fresh artery (Weiss, 1944). As will be demonstrated in Chapter 10, Weiss's use of a bioactive tube led to erroneous conclusions about axon guidance. In the late 1950s, Bassett, Campbell and coworkers successfully bridged cat sciatic nerve gaps of 1–2.5 cm with Millipore filter, but were unable to translate this success to the clinic (Bassett et al., 1959; Campbell et al., 1961). Entubation of nerve gaps is thus another technique that has been with us nearly as long as nerve repair itself, and that has been revisited by several generations of investigators.

The Silicon Chamber Model

Lundborg and colleagues reintroduced the nerve gap as a model for the study of nerve regeneration in 1979. They demonstrated that nerve could regenerate across an enclosed gap, that the newly formed tissue contained all the structural components of normal nerve, and that its growth was dependent on contributions from the distal nerve stump that could not be provided by other tissues (Lundborg, Hansson, 1979; Lundborg et al., 1981; Lundborg et al., 1982a; Williams et al., 1984). Previously, the complex environment of intact peripheral nerve had discouraged analysis of individual cellular or

molecular contributions to regeneration. The "silicon chamber model," in contrast, facilitated the isolation and analysis of regeneration components by separating them along spatial and temporal gradients (Lundborg et al., 1982b).

The process by which peripheral nerve bridges a gap has been studied most extensively in the silicon chamber model. Lundborg chose this construct to minimize surgical trauma, to facilitate accumulation of neuroactive substances produced by the severed nerve ends, and to "increase the possibilities for neurotrophic and neurotropic mechanisms to act" (Lundborg, 2000, p400). The timing of events in this discussion is based on the findings in a 10-mm gap (Williams et al., 1983). During the hours following tube placement, the initial void fills with serum (Liu, 1992). Within 1–2 days a longitudinally oriented matrix condenses circumferentially, pulling away from the tube walls to form an hourglass-shaped bridge between nerve ends (Zhao et al., 1993) (Figure 8-2). The bridge is constructed of fibrin, fibrinogen, and fibronectin but does not contain laminin (Zhao et al., 1993; Dahlin et al., 1995), and is initially populated by blood-borne cells including red blood cells, macrophages, and polymorphonuclear leukocytes (Williams et al., 1983; Zhao et al., 1993; Dahlin et al., 1995). The fluid that collects in the gap between the bridge and the silicon wall supports the growth of neurons from the dorsal root ganglion, ciliary ganglion, and spinal cord (presumptive motoneurons) (Lundborg et al., 1982c; Longo et al., 1983a; Longo et al., 1984). It has subsequently been found to contain NGF, NT-3, NT-4/5, CNTF, and other uncharacterized factors (Bates et al., 1991, 1995; Danielsen, Varon, 1995; Ahmed et al., 2005).

By the end of the first week, Schwann cells and fibroblasts have begun to migrate into the bridge from both proximal and distal nerve stumps (Williams et al., 1983). During the second week, the fibrin matrix is replaced by collagen and Schwann cells expressing laminin (Longo et al., 1984; Liu, 1992), fibroblasts are approaching the middle of the bridge, and regenerating axons and blood vessels have entered the gap (Williams et al., 1983). Although vascular ingrowth proceeds from both ends of the tube, proximal-to-distal activity predominates (Podhajsky, Myers, 1994). Recent studies of the relationship between regenerating axons and Schwann cells, performed with gaps of 3–5mm, have emphasized the obligate partnership between these two elements (Chen et al., 2005;

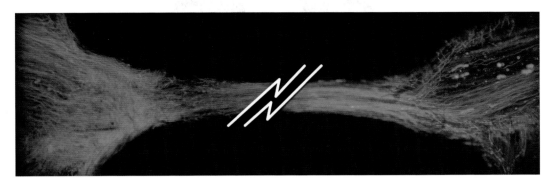

FIGURE 8-2   The hourglass shape of the regenerate within a Silastic tube used to bridge a 5-mm gap in the mouse sciatic nerve. Regenerating axons constitutively express green fluorescent protein. Six weeks after tube implantation, the axons still follow the contour established by the initial fibrin bridge that has pulled away from the tube walls and consolidated as a cable in the center of the tube. Axon trajectories within the tapering portion of the regenerate are grossly disordered.

McDonald et al., 2006). These authors found nearly all axons to be accompanied by Schwann cells, and noted "surprising and substantial hostility to local regrowth of axons into newly forming peripheral nerve bridges" (McDonald et al., 2006, p139). By the third week, the cellular bridge is completed, unmyelinated axons are approaching the distal stump, and myelination is proceeding near the center of the bridge. The initial fibronectin-rich bridge thus supports cellular ingrowth, but not axon regeneration; only modifications provided by ingrowing Schwann cells and fibroblasts render the terrain conducive to axonal penetration.

Axons mature within small bundles that are ensheathed by newly formed perineurium (Lundborg, Hansson, 1979). This physiologically active barrier is incompetent during at least the first month of regeneration, but by 6 months is able to exclude blood-borne horseradish peroxidase from reaching the axons (Azzam et al., 1991). By 9–10 months after surgery, all size classes of axon are represented in the regenerate in normal proportions, although none achieve normal diameter (Jenq, Coggeshall, 1985a; Fields, Ellisman, 1986b) (Figure 8-3). Similarly, the myelin sheath is thinner when compared with normal axons of similar size. These discrepancies lead to a permanent decrease in conduction velocity of 40% (Fields, Ellisman, 1986a).

The biology of the silicon chamber model was explored further by manipulating its components: the character of the distal insert, the dimensions of the chamber, and the chamber contents. A 10-mm gap was not bridged if the distal nerve stump was replaced with skin or tendon; if the distal end of a 6-mm tube was left open, granulation tissue bridged the gap but did not support regeneration (Williams et al., 1984). Even a 1-mm length of peripheral nerve, however, was sufficient to allow axons to bridge the gap (Zhang et al., 1997). The nature of the distal insert is thus critical, and the presence of a cellular bridge is not in itself sufficient to ensure axon growth. When the tube diameter is slightly larger than that of the rat sciatic nerve and both proximal and distal nerve stumps are present, regeneration is successful across 100% of 6-mm gaps, 40% of 10-mm gaps, but no 15-mm gaps (Lundborg et al., 1982a). Placing a small segment of nerve in the middle of the tube, however, allows a 15-mm gap to be bridged successfully (Francel et al., 1997). The relative width of the tube is also important, especially in the context of luminal contents; when the volume of a 10-mm gap is doubled by increasing tube diameter, myelinated axon counts are reduced if the tube is allowed to fill with fluid on its own, but increased substantially if the tube is prefilled with saline (Longo et al., 1983b). Prefilling also extends the length of gap that can be bridged, especially when plasma is used to fill the lumen (Williams et al., 1987). On the basis of these observations, the final success of an impermeable regeneration chamber appears to be determined predominantly by the size of the acellular bridge that forms in the early postoperative period (Longo et al., 1983b). Interestingly, an acellular bridge that is allowed to mature without axon ingrowth forms a "pseudo-nerve" that supports regeneration as if it were a nerve graft (Williams et al., 1993; Zhao et al., 1997).

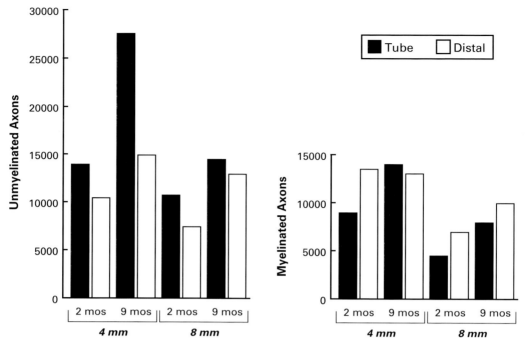

FIGURE 8-3   The population of myelinated and unmyelinated axons within and distal to Silicon tubes bridging 4-mm and 8-mm gaps in the rat sciatic nerve. At 2 months, myelinated axons appear to branch and increase in number as they enter the distal stump. At 9 months, myelinated axon counts within and distal to the tube have equalized across 4 mm gaps, but not across gaps of 8 mm. Unmyelinated axons increase in number within the tube between 2 and 9 months, but the additional axons fail to enter the distal stump. Based on data from Jenq, Coggeshall, 1985a.

A fully functional bridge can thus be constructed without the need for instructive cues from regenerating axons.

Two lines of evidence converged to limit the application of silicon tubing in nerve reconstruction. First, it was found that regeneration could be improved by reducing the isolation of tube contents from the wound environment. This effect was initially produced by cutting macroscopic holes in the tube wall (Jenq, Coggeshall, 1985b). In this construct, the holes needed to be large enough to admit migrating cells to have a significant effect (Jenq, Coggeshall, 1987). When the entire tube was made semipermeable, a 6-mm gap could be bridged successfully in the absence of a distal stump, a feat not accomplished with impermeable silicon tubes (Aebischer et al., 1988). Varying the pore size revealed that a molecular weight cutoff of 10^5 Da was significantly more effective than one of 10^6 Da (Aebischer et al., 1989). Subsequent direct comparison of silicon and permeable tubes confirmed the advantages of permeable material for nerve

grafting (e.g., Gomez et al., 1996; Valero-Cabré et al., 2001) (Figure 8-4). The second body of evidence suggested, but did not prove conclusively, that prolonged implantation of silicon tubes could compromise regeneration by compressing the regenerated nerve cable (Merle et al., 1989; Smahel et al., 1993), a risk that could be minimized by early removal of the tube (Gibson et al., 1991). This work coincided with the introduction of silicon tubulation as a model of nerve compression (Mackinnon et al., 1984a). Examination of human nerves intubated for more than 1 year, however, revealed minimal reaction when tubes were removed for an unrelated reason, local mechanical irritation of surrounding tissues (Dahlin et al., 2001).

Gap Nerve Repair

Impermeable silicon tubing has seen limited use in patients, primarily as an adjunct to nerve repair rather than as a substitute for nerve graft. In the course of basic experiments on nerve regeneration, Nageotte

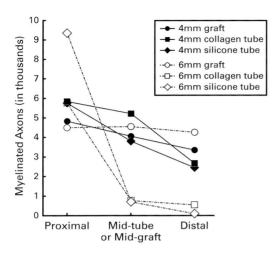

FIGURE 8-4   Counts of myelinated axons proximal, within, and distal to autografts, collagen tubes, and Silicon tubes used to bridge 4-mm and 6-mm gaps in the mouse sciatic nerve. The performance of all three materials is similar when bridging a 4-mm gap. At 6 mm, however, both collagen and silicon are inferior to autograft. The increased number of axons proximal to a 6-mm gap enclosed within a silicon tube probably reflects retrograde growth of axons along established basal lamina pathways. Data from Gomez et al., 1996.

discovered that the trajectory of axons across a nerve repair could be improved by leaving a slight gap between proximal and distal nerve stumps (Nageotte, 1922). This concept was investigated further by Weiss, who found that the fibrin clot between nerve ends would contract longitudinally, providing a longitudinal template for construction of the bridging tissue, and thus for axon regeneration (Weiss, Taylor, 1943; Weiss, 1944). In the modern era, Lundborg reintroduced the concept of tubular nerve repair as "a biologic approach to a nerve injury in which the role of the surgeon is limited and special emphasis is put on the role of intrinsic healing capacities of the nerve tissue" (Lundborg et al., 1997, p102). Enthusiasm for this approach was bolstered by the contemporaneous discovery of multiple new neurotrophic and neurotropic factors, and the assumption that "there is a high degree of specificity associated with . . . neurotropism" (Dellon, Mackinnon, 1988, p854) that would direct regenerating axons to functionally and topographically appropriate Schwann cell tubes in the distal nerve stump.

Experimental evaluation of the tubular, or "gap repair" technique (defined as a single nerve transection with little or no removal of tissue, followed by alignment of proximal and distal stumps within a tube, maintaining a short gap between them) revealed, however, that this technique produced results that were not superior to those of end-to-end nerve suture as measured by muscle reinnervation (Romano et al., 1991), improvement in SFI (Weber et al., 1996), and retrograde labeling (Valero-Cabré et al., 2004). Placement of a short gap at either the proximal or distal end of a nerve graft also failed to improve outcomes significantly (Papaloizos et al., 1997; Tomita et al., 2007). A prospective, randomized clinical trial that compared the results of end-to-end and gap repair similarly found little difference between outcomes 5 years after repair, although patients undergoing gap repair had less cold intolerance (Lundborg et al., 2004). Gap repair thus provides results that differ little from those of end-to-end suture, but greatly simplifies the technical aspects of the repair process. There is little evidence to suggest, however, that allowing neurotropic and neurotrophic factors to accumulate between nerve stumps improves either regeneration specificity or functional outcome.

Even before his introduction of the silicon chamber model, Lundborg was experimenting with regeneration in a more permeable tube. He fashioned "mesothelial" or "pseudosynovial" tubes by placing a silicon rod within a wire spring and embedding the construct subcutaneously for several weeks (Lundborg, Hansson, 1979). When the silicon rod was removed, the continuous layer of tissue that formed around the rod would be supported in tubular form by the embedded wire. The tube could then be used to bridge a gap between the ends of the transected rat sciatic nerve. The nerve cable that formed within the tube generated perineurium and epineurium, and supported the reinnervation of distal muscles (Lundborg et al., 1981) (Figure 8-5). Gaps of 10 mm in the rat sciatic nerve could be bridged reliably, but those of 15 mm could not be surmounted (Danielsen et al., 1983). A similar construct was subsequently used to bridge 3 cm gaps in the monkey ulnar nerve with category 3 and 4 results similar to those of conventional nerve grafting (Mackinnon et al., 1985a; Mackinnon, Dellon, 1988).

The first tubes developed for neural reconstruction in the United States have evolved along two similar pathways, and both have been subjected to evaluation in primate models. The Neurotube©, fashioned from polyglycolic mesh, and the NeuraGen©, a collagen-based construct, are both

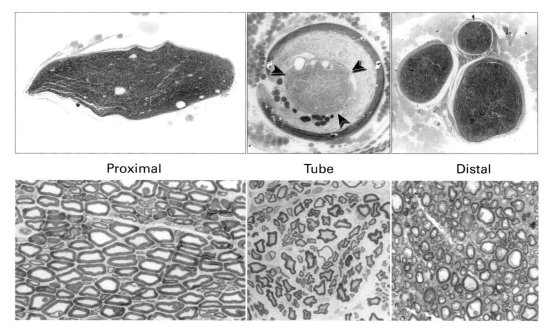

| Proximal | Tube | Distal |

FIGURE 8-5   Histology of the rat sciatic nerve proximal to, within, and distal to mesothelial chambers placed 18 months earlier across 10-mm gaps. Arrowheads delineate the neural cable that has formed within the center of the tube. Even after 18 months, distal axons are smaller and less well myelinated than their proximal counterparts.

permeable and resorbable. A precursor of the Neurotube© was used to bridge a 3-cm gap in the proximal ulnar nerve of 16 monkeys (Dellon, Mackinnon, 1988). Evaluation at 1 year revealed that performance of the tube was similar to that of sural nerve graft by category 3 and 4 criteria; conduction velocity and amplitude, and axonal morphometry (Dellon, Mackinnon, 1988). In similar experiments, regeneration was found to be poor across 5-cm gaps bridged by a variety of other synthetic conduits (Mackinnon, Dellon, 1990). In a landmark series, the performance of collagen tubes was compared with that of nerve graft in bridging gaps of 5, 20, and 50 mm in the monkey median nerve (Krarup et al., 2002). These preparations underwent serial electrophysiologic evaluation for 3–5 years after surgery. In comparison to nerves repaired after excision of a 5-mm nerve segment, CMAP amplitude was diminished significantly in 20-mm and 50-mm nerve guide groups, and in the 50-mm nerve graft group. CSAP amplitudes did not differ significantly between graft and tube preparations at 5 mm and 20 mm, but were lower than all other repairs with 50-mm tubes, and lower after 50-mm grafts than after 5-mm grafts. Analysis of the pooled results revealed that the final recovery of outcome measures correlated most directly with the time to end-organ reinnervation, which was significantly longer for tube grafts at both 20-mm and 50-mm (Figure 8-6). Overall, these results demonstrate that, in the primate, permeable tubes as short as 20 mm perform less well than do grafts of equivalent length by some criteria, and tubes of 50-mm length do quite poorly. Reliable grafting of gaps greater than 2–3 cm with permeable tubes will thus require modification of the substrate and/or the addition of growth factors.

Regeneration Specificity Within Tubes

The primate experiments cited above focused on the ability of particular tube constructs to promote axon regeneration across gaps of various dimensions. The specificity of reinnervation, in contrast, has been evaluated in only one primate study (Madison et al., 1999). Preferential reinnervation of thenar muscles by motor axons was found after repair or autografting of the median nerve, but not after enclosure of a 20-mm or 50-mm gap within a prosthetic tube.

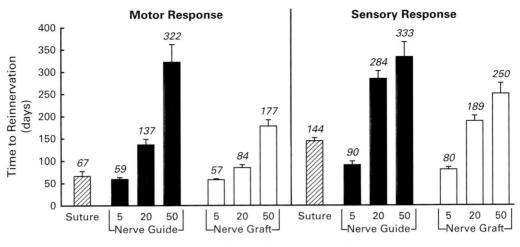

FIGURE 8-6   The time to end organ reinnervation across end-to-end nerve suture, and across gaps of
5 mm, 20 mm, and 50 mm that have been bridged with autografts or collagen tubes in the primate median nerve.
Significantly more time was required to bridge 20-mm and 50-mm gaps through collagen tubes as opposed to
nerve autograft (p < 0.005–0.01, ANOVA, post hoc). In these experiments, time to reinnervation was found to
be the most significant predictor of outcome as determined electrophysiologically. Reproduced with permission
from Krarup et al., 2002.

In the rat, application of retrograde tracing to quantify specificity demonstrated that axons regenerating across a 10-mm rat sciatic nerve gap reinnervated muscle on a random basis after 18 months (Brushart, 1990). Fully 53% of motoneurons that reinnervated the peroneal muscles lay outside of the normal confines of the peroneal motoneuron pool (Figure 8-7). Muscle bulk was restored but foot function was not, implicating the organization rather than the volume of regenerating axons as the source of dysfunction. The findings of subsequent investigations in the rat have varied according to the model used to evaluate specificity. A short-term sequential double labeling study found the tibialis anterior muscle to be reinnervated by only 30% of its original motoneurons after regeneration across a 10-mm gap enclosed within an impermeable tube (Rende et al., 1991). Electrophysiologic determination of specificity has variously identified 33% of gastrocnemius reinnervation across a 4-mm impermeable gap (Zhao et al., 1992) and 26% across an 8-mm impermeable gap to be inappropriate (Valero-Cabré, Navarro, 2002). When the location of peroneal axons was determined at the completion of reinnervation, they were found to be distributed randomly in the distal portion of the tube (Alzate et al., 2000).

Loss of regeneration specificity is thus an inescapable consequence of using an enclosed gap as a substitute for nerve graft. The degree to which this confusion degrades functional outcome will depend on the anatomical characteristics of the recipient nerve. If multiple functions are well localized within the nerve, imposition of a gap can be expected to degrade function. If there is little functional localization, such as in the digital nerve, randomizing axon location should have little effect. In the worst case scenario, when there is both localization of function within the nerve and mal-alignment of proximal and distal stumps, randomization will actually improve the quality of reinnervation (Hasegawa et al., 1996). In any case, the final result will depend on the capability for central reorganization to compensate for the peripheral miswiring.

Clinical Outcomes

The clinical use of tubular nerve graft substitutes in the repair and reconstruction of digital nerve injuries is now well documented. The initial case series reported by Mackinnon and Dellon described recovery after use of a PGA tube to bridge digital nerve gaps of 0.5–3.0 cm (mean 1.7 cm) (Mackinnon, Dellon,

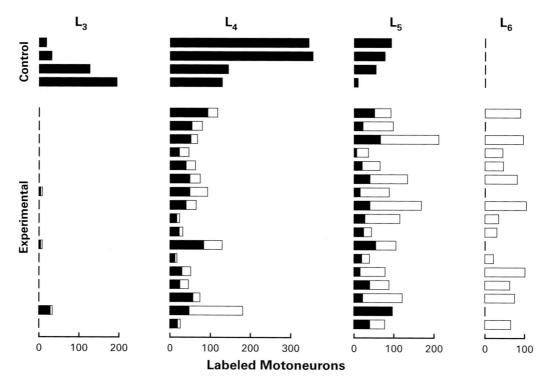

FIGURE 8-7   The spinal cord distribution of motoneurons serving the rat peroneal muscles normally (control: top 4 horizontal lines) and after regeneration across a 1-cm sciatic nerve gap bridged by a mesothelial chamber (shown in Figure 8-5). Data were obtained by injecting the peroneal muscles with HRP 18 months after tube placement to label reinnervating motoneurons. Each horizontal group of bars represents a single preparation. On the longitudinal axis of the spinal cord, the innervation of the peroneal muscles shifts caudally after entubation. On the medial/lateral axis, motoneurons lying within the confines of the normal peroneal motoneuron pool are represented in black; those within the tibial pool are in white. Taking both types of mismatch into account, 53% of the motoneurons that have reinnervated the peroneal muscles formerly served other, often antagonistic muscles. This mismatch degrades function even when muscles are innervated by adequate numbers of axons. Reproduced from Brushart, 1990.

1991). Static 2-PD of 6 mm or better was recovered in 33% of reconstructions, and static 2-PD of 7–15 mm in an additional 53%. A subsequent prospective, randomized trial employing the same tube material and postoperative sensory reeducation documented mean 2-PD of 8.3 mm with gaps of 4 mm or less, 9.6 mm with gaps of 5–7 mm, and 13.1 mm with gaps greater than 8 mm. (Weber et al., 2000). These results were significantly better than those of end-to-end repair of 4-mm gaps in control patients, and similar to those of end-to-end repair of 5–7 mm gaps and grafting of larger gaps. Three additional series of digital nerve repairs and reconstructions have been presented with sufficient detail to analyze the results of bridging gaps of 1–2 cm in adults (Table 8-1). In the series in which patients received postoperative

sensory reeducation, 45% achieved S4 recovery and the remainder recovered to S3+ (Bushnell et al., 2008). In two series without sensory reeducation, S4 was recovered in only 13–14%, with the majority of the patients (57–63%) recovering to S3+ (Battiston et al., 2007; Lohmeyer et al., 2009).

The outcomes of bridging more substantial gaps in mixed nerve are less promising. The only well-documented series of median and ulnar nerve reconstruction involved use of a permeable tube fashioned from expanded polytetrafluoroethylene (ePTFE) (Stanec, Stanec, 1998). Useful function, defined as M4 S3+, was obtained in 46% of patients with gaps of 1.5–4 cm, an outcome roughly comparable to that of nerve grafting (Figure 5-12). At longer gaps, however, only 7% of patients achieved this level of recovery.

Table 8-1 The Results of Digital Nerve Reconstruction with Tubular Prostheses in Adult Patients.
The percentage of patients that recover to S4 is enhanced substantially by sensory reeducation.

Authors	# of Patients ≥ 17 years old	% Recovery			Sensory Re-education
		S4	S3+	S3	
Weber *et al*	27	42	29	29	yes
Lohmeyer *et al*	08	13	63	24	no
Battison *et al*	14	14	57	21	no
Bushnell *et al*	11	45	55	00	yes

Recently, Moore et al. (2009) analyzed a group of patients in whom tubes had failed, and cautioned that gap volume rather than gap length should be considered as a limiting factor in large-diameter nerves.

Permeable tubes thus support regeneration similar to that obtained with standard techniques of repair and grafting when applied to short gaps in nerves that serve a single function such as the digital nerve. The digital nerve supplies a limited number of end organs in a well-circumscribed territory. In this setting, imposition of randomness on the formation of distal connections has a limited impact on outcome. Function conveyed through larger mixed nerves, however, is rapidly degraded by the progressive axonal disorganization imposed by longer gaps.

ENHANCING REGENERATION ACROSS NEURAL PROSTHESES

Over the past 20 years, attempts to enhance regeneration across tubular nerve graft substitutes have generated more publications than all other aspects of peripheral nerve repair combined. Modifications have included treatment with growth factors, manipulation of the tube wall, addition of various structures and substrates within the lumen, and placement of cellular elements within the construct. The details of engineering these modifications are beyond the scope of this work (many aspects are reviewed in Piotrowicz and Shoichet, 2006; Chang et al., 2008; Kemp et al., 2008; Chiono et al., 2009; de Ruiter et al., 2009; Hood et al., 2009; Yan et al., 2009).

Growth Factors

Nerve growth factor (NGF) and glial-derived growth factor (GDNF) have both been used extensively in attempts to promote axon growth across enclosed gaps. In early experiments with NGF, a single dose of the factor was placed within the tube at the time it was sewn into place. Short-term analysis of growth across gaps of 5–6 mm revealed that NGF increased the number and caliber of axons within the distal portions of the tube, and increased the conduction velocity of regenerating motor axons (Rich et al., 1989; He et al., 1992). At gaps of 10 mm, a single dose of NGF accelerated the growth of nonneuronal cells into the gap, resulting in higher counts of myelinated axons within the tube at early time periods and a greater overall success rate as defined by the proportion of tubes in which axons crossed the gap (Derby et al., 1993).

More recent experiments have used a variety of strategies to release NGF into the regeneration environment over a prolonged period. This approach has also resulted in an increase in the success rate with gaps of up to 15 mm, and an increase in the number and caliber of regenerating axons (Bloch et al., 2001; Lee et al., 2003; Xu et al., 2003). Even with these morphologic improvements, however, slow release of NGF failed to improve the sciatic functional index (SFI) after regeneration across gaps of 2 mm or 10 mm when compared with appropriate controls (Young et al., 2001; Chen et al., 2006). Currently, strategies to use soluble or immobilized gradients of NGF to guide regenerating axons across neural gaps are under development (Kapur, Shoichet, 2004; Kemp et al., 2007; Yu et al., 2008).

Several studies have documented the response to controlled release of GDNF within enclosed nerve gaps. Addition of GDNF facilitated bridging defects of 8 mm in the rat facial nerve and 15 mm in the rat sciatic nerve, gaps that were not bridged successfully in any control animals (Barras et al., 2002; Fine et al., 2002). The success rate with 13 mm rat sciatic gaps filled with fibrin was enhanced from 3/12 in controls to 6/12 by including a slow-release GDNF preparation (Wood et al., 2009). In spite of this anatomical success, motor function as evaluated by gait analysis was not improved over controls by releasing GDNF within gaps of 3 mm or 10 mm, even when there was a dramatic increase in axon numbers at the midtube level (Patel et al., 2007; Piquilloud et al., 2007). In one study that evaluated the withdrawal response to a series of Semmes-Weinstein monofilaments, GDNF enhanced sensitivity to a level above that of normal animals (Patel et al., 2007). Treatment of end-to-end nerve repair with GDNF increases signs of neuropathic pain (Jubran, Widenfalk, 2003), suggesting that the enhanced sensitivity after entubation with GDNF may result, at least in part, from a pain response rather than from useful sensibility (see Chapter 7). Overall, the experience with NGF and GDNF suggests that they enhance formation of the cellular bridge that conveys axons across the gap. It is difficult to ascertain whether the effects of these factors on axon morphology are proportional to the size and quality of the bridge, or are regulated independently. In either case, improvement in voluntary function is not commensurate with the observed morphologic enhancements.

Schwann Cells and Stem Cells

Early attempts to promote regeneration across entubated nerve gaps with cultured Schwann cells were limited by the need to use fetal or neonatal cells (Shine et al., 1985; Ikeda et al., 1995). Subsequently, however, a technique for culturing adult rat Schwann cells was developed as part of a program to treat spinal cord injury (Morrissey et al., 1991). When these cells were placed in an 8-mm rat sciatic nerve gap, they promoted regeneration in a dose-dependent manner, with cell concentrations of 120×10^6/ml generating axon counts at 3 weeks approaching those within nerve autograft controls (Guenard et al., 1992). Schwann cells derived from the nerves of adult human organ donors were also shown to promote regeneration across entubated gaps in immune-deficient rats (Levi et al., 1994b), confirming the clinical potential of the technique.

Schwann cells have been shown to survive within enclosed neural gaps and to promote regeneration across these gaps in a concentration-dependent

manner (Kim et al., 1994; Ansselin et al., 1997; Mosahebi et al., 2001). Including Schwann cells within the lumen of a tubular prosthesis supported regeneration across gaps of 2 cm in the rat median nerve (Sinis et al., 2005), 18 mm in the rat sciatic nerve (Ansselin et al., 1997), and 15 mm in the primate brachioradialis nerve (Levi et al., 1997), gaps that were not bridged in controls. Addition of Schwann cells improved the morphologic and electrophysiologic characteristics of the regenerate in a variety of rat gap models (Keeley et al., 1993; Kim et al., 1994; Sinis et al., 2005), though axon counts distal to reconstruction of a 15-mm gap in primate nerve were significantly lower than sural nerve graft controls when Schwann cell-filled tubes were used (Levi et al., 1997). Voluntary function as measured by the SFI was not improved in one study in which Schwann cells were added to an 18-mm rat sciatic nerve gap (Ansselin et al., 1997), but normal grasping strength was restored after bridging a 2-cm gap in the rat median nerve with a matrigel-Schwann cell construct (Sinis et al., 2005). Ongoing attempts to further enhance the performance of tubes seeded with Schwann cells have involved modification of the physical environment to encourage longitudinal cellular alignment (Kim et al., 2007; Lohmeyer et al., 2007; Wang et al., 2009) and viral transfection to enhance the expression of specific growth factors (Timmer et al., 2003; Li et al., 2006; Zhou et al., 2008).

With current technology, clinical use of artificial nerve grafts seeded with Schwann cells is not an appealing substitute for grafting with autologous nerve. Only autologous Schwann cells can be used without immunosuppression, so an additional operation is needed to harvest Schwann cells, followed by several weeks for expansion of the Schwann cell culture. Alternatively, it might be possible to harvest and expand autologous stem cells without the need to sacrifice peripheral nerve. This approach opens a range of possibilities, as stem cells derived from fat (Kingham et al., 2007; di Summa et al., 2009), bone marrow (Dezawa et al., 2001), embryonic neural tissue (Murakami et al., 2003), and skin (McKenzie et al., 2006) have all been manipulated to express elements of the Schwann cell phenotype.

Several studies have examined the promotion of regeneration across rat sciatic nerve gaps by stem cells that have been tagged to permit their identification at the end of the experiment. Skin-derived stem cells used to bridge a 16-mm gap did little to enhance

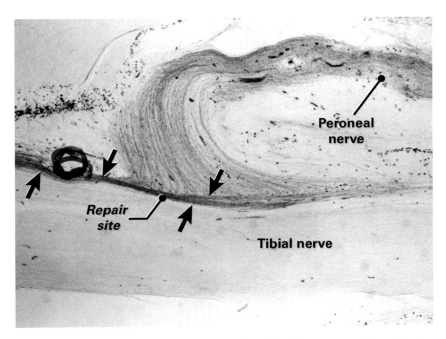

FIGURE 8-9   End-to-side nerve repair without perineurial window. The rat peroneal nerve has been transected, and the end of the distal stump sewn to the side of the adjacent tibial nerve; the proximal peroneal stump (not shown) has been tied off and reflected away from the repair. After allowing 6 weeks for regeneration, HRP-WGA has been used to trace axons that have reinnervated the distal peroneal stump. These are seen to originate not from axons within the tibial fascicle, but instead to travel along the outside of the tibial epineurium. Examination of the spinal cord confirmed that peroneal axons had escaped from the end of the tied-off proximal stump, and regenerated down the tibial epineurium to reenter the cut end of the peroneal nerve. The distal peroneal nerve was thus reinnervated, but with axons that would not be available in the clinical setting. These findings exemplify the need for caution in interpreting the results of experimental end-to-side nerve repair.

double labeling in the rat upper extremity model found that very little reinnervation occurred through collateral sprouting (Bontioti et al., 2005; Matsuda et al., 2005; Samal et al., 2006), while an additional study identified 10% of the reinnervating axons as collateral sprouts (Sananpanich et al., 2007). In aggregate, electrophysiologic and tracing techniques establish that limited collateral reinnervation occurs soon after end-to-side repair, but suggest that, if collaterals persist, they do not activate both targets. In any case, the dominant mode of reinnervation is terminal rather than collateral. The motoneurons that control most reinnervated muscle are thus distinct from those that control donor-innervated muscle, but within the same motoneuron pools, and subject to the same control problems that follow end-to-end repair of a nerve trunk; one set of inputs controls circuits that now serve two or more functions.

Substantial evidence indicates that the extent of end-to-side reinnervation is proportional to the trauma experienced by the donor nerve. At one extreme, suture to intact epineurium or atraumatic repair with fibrin glue may fail to elicit any response at all (Bertelli et al., 1996a; Al-Qattan, Al-Thunyan, 1998). Conversely, in a series of increasingly aggressive maneuvers, crush increased the response over simple repair (McCallister et al., 1999), and partial neurectomy provoked the most vigorous response of all (Noah et al., 1997b; Brenner et al., 2007). Recently, the ideal model for exploring this relationship became available in the form of mice that express fluorescent proteins in their neurons, allowing the configuration of axons at the end-to-side juncture to be imaged directly (Feng et al., 2000). Using this model, Hayashi et al. (2008) found that either compression or epineurectomy, which inevitably causes some axotomy, were necessary before axons would regenerate into the recipient nerve.

Formation of a perineurial window appears to be a reasonable compromise between donor injury and

Collateral Reinnervation

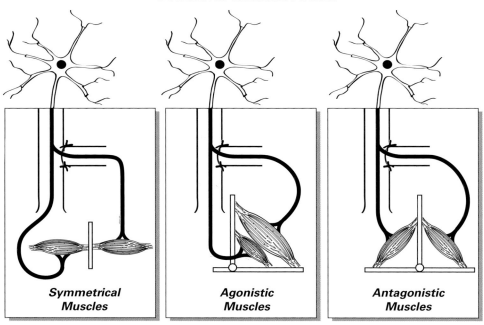

Symmetrical Muscles   **Agonistic Muscles**   **Antagonistic Muscles**

Terminal Reinnervation

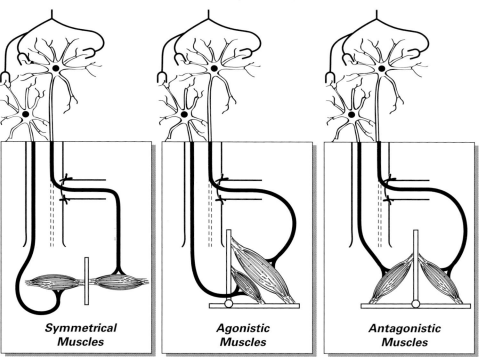

Symmetrical Muscles   **Agonistic Muscles**   **Antagonistic Muscles**

FIGURE 8-10   Collateral and terminal reinnervation. Collateral reinnervation may be useful when motoring a pair of symmetrical or agonistic muscles that normally contract together and perform the same or similar

(*Continues*)

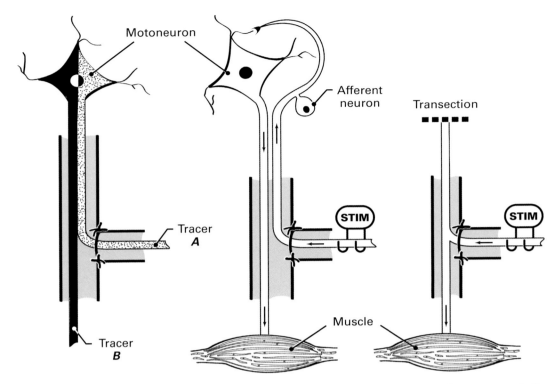

FIGURE 8-11   Differentiating between collateral and terminal reinnervation in end-to-side nerve repair. Left: After application of different retrograde tracers to donor (tracer B) and recipient (tracer A) nerves, the tracers will co-localize only within neurons that contribute collateral sprouts to the recipient nerve while maintaining their principal axon within the donor nerve. Middle: Muscle contraction in response to stimulation of a presumed axon collateral in an intact system may result from a reflex involving two separate axons. Contraction must persist after transection or blocking of the proximal donor nerve (Right) to prove that both stimulated axon and responding muscle are served by the same neuron.

target reinnervation (Rovak et al., 2001). The trauma of opening the perineurium results in Wallerian degeneration of 5–20% of axons within the donor nerve (Goheen-Robillard et al., 2002) and denervation of approximately 5% of fibers in a representative donor-innervated muscle (Cederna et al., 2001). In spite of this injury, neither individual muscle performance on physiologic testing (Giovanoli et al., 2000; Cederna et al., 2001; Sanapanich et al., 2002) nor coordinated function as assessed by walking track analysis (Noah et al., 1997a; Goheen-Robillard et al., 2002) are significantly degraded in the donor

system. Interestingly, in a study of baboon median and ulnar nerves, the best results were seen in those animals with the most severe degenerative changes in the distal donor nerve (Kelly et al., 2007), a finding consistent with terminal rather than collateral reinnervation.

The Volume of Reinnervation

The potential of end-to-side repair will depend on both the number and character of axons that reinnervate the target nerve. In the rat sciatic model,

FIGURE 8-10   (Continued)
functions. Control of antagonistic muscles by the same motoneuron, however, is likely to degrade rather than improve functional outcome. The degree to which antagonistic muscles can be controlled independently after terminal reinnervation will depend on the individual control of motoneurons within the same pool, which is normally minimal.

counts in the reinnervated nerve are approximately 60% of normal (Goheen-Robillard et al., 2002; Sanapanich et al., 2002), although in a cross-body rat model with 8-cm grafts (two 4-cm segments joined end-to-end) axon counts were supranormal (Goheen-Robillard et al., 2002). Reinnervation of the primate median nerve from the ulnar resulted in a mean of 62% of the normal ulnar myelinated population, but with tremendous variability (range 1.4 to 96%) (Kelly et al., 2007). There must be substantial collateral sprouting within the target nerve itself, as the number of parent neurons that support reinnervating axons is quite low. Estimates based on retrograde labeling range from 20 to 50% of the normal number of DRG neurons and from 1 to 15% of the normal number of motoneurons (Tarasidis et al., 1997; Bontioti et al., 2005). Other than one study in which motoneuron labeling was slightly more prominent (Sanapanich et al., 2007), labeled DRG neurons outnumbered their motor counterparts by as much as 10–20 to 1, indicating that the vast majority of fibers in reinnervated nerve are sensory (Tarasidis et al., 1997; Chen, Brushart, 1998; Bontioti et al., 2005).

Experimental Outcomes

The clinical applicability of end-to-side repair will be determined ultimately by its ability to restore function. The capabilities of muscle innervated through end-to-side repair have been assessed specifically by determination of tetanic force and muscle weight, and more generally by evaluation of voluntary activity. Where end-to-end and end-to-side repair have been compared, the former has proven to be superior (Cao et al., 1999; Kalliainen et al., 1999; Liu et al., 1999; Sanapanich et al., 2002; Sundine et al., 2003). In the majority of end-to-side experiments, the weight of reinnervated muscle was 50–75% that of the weight of the normal, contralateral muscle (Tham, Morrison, 1998; Kalliainen et al., 1999; Sanapanich et al., 2002; Bontioti et al., 2005). The force resulting from maximum tetanic contraction was often reduced to a similar extent, although in some instances near-normal force could be generated (Giovanoli et al., 2000). Voluntary function did not recover when there was negligible muscle reinnervation (Goheen-Robillard et al., 2002), or when muscle was reinnervated by motoneurons that previously served antagonistic muscles (Lutz et al., 2000a). In one instance, toe spread recovered to 60–70% of normal, but the

percentage recovery from the postinjury deficit (approximately 20–30%) was similar to that seen after transection without repair (Bontioti et al., 2005), and is thus of uncertain significance. These findings contrast with the restoration of function that follows reinnervation of one of a pair of symmetrical muscles from the other (Sundine et al., 2003). Modest functional restoration has also been noted when the digital flexors are reinnervated end-to-side from the nerve to the wrist extensors in the baboon (Schmidhammer et al., 2009). Although these muscle groups are nominally antagonists, wrist extension is synergistic with digital flexion, so co-contraction could actually be helpful.

Although there is too little information to support a firm conclusion, the findings to date emphasize the difficulty that may be encountered when motoneurons are asked to switch functions (Figure 8-10). If collaterals of a single motor axon reinnervate antagonistic muscles, discharge of the parent neuron will result in co-contraction and dysfunction as noted in a series of end-to-side repairs evaluated electrophysiologically (McCallister et al., 2001). A more common situation may arise after terminal regeneration through an end-to-side repair. The motoneurons that control a muscle or group of muscles are adjacent to one another within a discrete "pool" in the spinal cord, and are normally activated together to contract a muscle (Chapter 3). Activation of this pool will result in simultaneous contraction of all the muscles it serves, both original and newly reinnervated through end-to-side repair (Wikholm et al., 1988). When the original and reinnervated muscle are agonists or symmetrical muscles, useful function may result. If the muscles perform unrelated or antagonistic movements, co-contraction and dysfunction will be the norm. These possibilities are illustrated by the successful reinnervation of one orbicularis oculi muscle from the nerve to the other (Sundine et al., 2003) and by the poor outcome when the donor and recipient are antagonists (Lutz et al., 2000a). Function may deteriorate further when several muscles are reinnervated from a nerve that normally powers a single, unrelated muscle. Failure under these circumstances has been ascribed to reduction of the number of axons available for each muscle (Lutz et al., 2000b), but may also be an expression of the central connections of these axons. After all, Ballance was able to restore contraction by reinnervating several facial muscles from the nerve to the trapezius (Ballance, 1923); it was the poor coordination of these muscles that resulted in their dysfunction, and the consolidation of control by sectioning the donor nerve that unmasked their functional capabilities.

Enhancing Reinnervation

At a given level of injury, reinnervation through an end-to side repair can be improved by manipulating the local environment. Predegeneration of the recipient nerve to upregulate Schwann cell trophic factor production elicited end-to-side graft reinnervation by sensory axons in a minimal injury model, whereas use of fresh grafts did not (Lundborg et al., 1994). Nonetheless, predegeneration of the recipient nerve does not appear to alter long-term outcome (Zhang et al., 2000). With the more significant trauma of a perineurial window, products of locally grafted Schwann cells and degenerating muscle enhanced both sensory and motor reinnervation (Chen, Brushart, 1998). Application of growth factors to the repair site also enhanced reinnervation to varying degrees (Caplan et al., 1999; McCallister et al., 2001; Tiangco et al., 2001; Lykissas et al., 2007), although the mechanism of this effect remains to be determined.

Clinical Outcomes

Clinical outcomes of end-to-side repair are often disappointing. When used to reinnervate major peripheral nerves, usually through an epineurial window, this technique has resulted in either no improvement (Kayikcioglu et al., 2000; Bertelli, Ghizoni, 2003a) or recovery of only diminished protective sensibility in a substantial number of cases (Kostakoglu, 1999; Pienaar et al., 2004; Yuksel et al., 2004). In some series, promising outcomes cannot be attributed solely to the end-to-side repair because of alternative sources of innervation (Amr et al., 2006) or subsequent tendon transfers (Kostakoglu, 1999). The largest reported experience includes results of S3+ and/or M3+ in 7/33 ulnar-to-median procedures, but 0/7 median-to-ulnar operations achieved this level of recovery (Mennen, 2003). By far the best results have been obtained with terminal sensory or motor nerves. A mean two-point discrimination (2-PD) of 9-mm (range 6–12 mm) was restored in 10 patients in one series of end-to-side digital nerve reconstruction (Voche, Ouattara, 2005), while 2-PD of 12 mm or less was reached in 5/5 patients in another series

(Mennen, 2003). Similarly, Millesi has reported his best results when "a small denervated pure motor nerve is coapted to a functioning small pure motor nerve" (Millesi, Schmidhammer, 2008, p482). In a series of cases in which the thenar motor branch was reinnervated end-to-side from the motor branch of the ulnar nerve, M3+ or M4 function was achieved in 5 of 6 cases (Millesi, Schmidhammer, 2008).

From the neurobiological point of view, clinical assessment should improve our understanding of both the mechanism of reinnervation through end-to-side repair and the degree to which compensation for miswiring is possible. In the one clinical paper with substantial motor recovery, muscle function was said, on the basis of physical examination, to be individual without co-contraction (Mennen, 2003). In the two papers in which sensory localization was tested, it was found to be appropriate (Mennen, 2003; Voche, Ouattara, 2005). Overall, this implies that the majority of reinnervation is terminal rather than collateral, and that adequate central compensation for miswiring has occurred. These observations contrast with descriptions of sensibility after end-to-end nerve repair, where false sensory localization is a frequent occurrence (Chapter 5).

There is still much to learn from patients who have undergone end-to-side nerve repair. Detailed evaluation of the progress of postoperative sensory and motor function would shed light on the mechanisms of recovery and central plasticity. The robust reinnervation observed by Ballance is the consequence of intentional injury to the donor nerve in many of his patients (Ballance, 1923), as contrasted with the limited success achieved in modern patients when only the epineurium is breached (Mennen, 1998; Kostakoglu, 1999; Kayikcioglu et al., 2000; Ogun et al., 2003). To increase the number of axons in the recipient nerve, greater injury must be inflicted on the donor (Rovak et al., 2001). This process may be modified by the addition of growth factors or selective fascicular reunion (Lutz et al., 2000b). Success in the volume of reinnervation will be accompanied by progressive failure of motor control, however, unless donor and recipient are carefully matched. At its current level of development, end-to-side repair is most appropriate for salvage when protective sensibility is a reasonable goal, or when co-contraction of muscles served by donor and recipient nerves is desirable.

SPINAL IMPLANTATION OF AVULSED ROOTS

The study of peripheral nerve regeneration has benefited substantially from recent efforts to promote spinal cord repair. This is nowhere more apparent than in the treatment of root avulsions, injuries that occur at the interface between central and peripheral nervous systems. For many years, it was assumed that injury to the brain and spinal cord was permanent because CNS neurons could not regenerate. This dogma was challenged by Aguayo, Richardson, and coworkers at McGill University in the early 1980s (Richardson et al., 1980; Benfey, Aguayo, 1982). By inserting peripheral nerve grafts into the CNS, they showed that spinal cord and cortical neurons could regenerate over long distances when they were supported by peripheral Schwann cells. In an extension of this concept, others found that axons conveyed from the CNS within peripheral nerve grafts could in turn innervate muscle (Carlstedt et al., 1986; Horvat et al., 1989), and proved that motoneurons were responsible for the reinnervation that occurred (Cullheim et al., 1989).

Ventral Root

Until recently, ventral root avulsion from the spinal cord was seen as a hopeless lesion, amenable only to secondary reconstructive measures (Leffert, 1985). Experimental reinnervation of avulsed ventral roots by surgically inserting them into the spinal cord, however, suggested that clinical root avulsion could be treated (Carlstedt et al., 1993). In these experiments, insertion of the avulsed C5, C6, and C7 ventral roots of cynomologus monkeys improved shoulder and elbow function; injection of the neural tracer HRP into the reinnervated biceps muscle labeled between 97 and 137 innervating motoneurons in the C6 spinal cord segment.

The first 10 patients to undergo intraspinal repair of root avulsions were reported in 2000 (Carlstedt et al., 2000). Three of these recovered muscle function to at least M3, and none experienced serious neurologic complications from the surgery. Nonetheless, co-contractions of antagonistic muscles were a constant feature of recovery, indicating a lack of topographic specificity in muscle reinnervation. This finding is consistent with the primate labeling studies, in which the biceps was reinnervated by motoneurons that normally serve other

muscles (Carlstedt et al., 1993). In his discussion of this paper, Kline concluded that "The report . . . does show the possibility of some fiber growth, albeit not very functional, from cord to replanted roots or grafts to roots." (Kline, 2000, p337). With current techniques, the role of surgery to reestablish continuity between motoneurons and avulsed ventral roots is clearly limited, as was confirmed in subsequent clinical series (Bertelli, Ghizoni, 2003b; Hsu et al., 2004). Carlstedt and coworkers now consider the technique only for patients with at least four root avulsions, and only within a month of injury (Htut et al., 2007).

Ventral root avulsion both injures motoneurons and deprives them of peripherally derived growth factors, resulting in widespread motoneuron death (Chapter 11). In the adult rat, only 11–16% of motoneurons survive after avulsion of their ventral root (Gu et al., 2004; Hoang et al., 2006). If the avulsed root is inserted into the spinal cord, survival increases to 55–64%. The majority of surviving motoneurons project axons into the root, where they are exposed to Schwann cell–derived growth factors (Gu et al., 2004). The presumed neurotrophic effects of root insertion benefit not only the involved spinal segment, but also those above and below (Törnqvist, Aldskogius, 1994; Hoang, Havton, 2006). These effects are reduced but still prominent if root insertion is delayed for 2–3 weeks after injury (Wu et al., 2004; Gu et al., 2005).

Strategies to improve survival and outgrowth of motoneurons include the provision of growth factors and modification of the local environment. BDNF and/or CNTF applied to the site of spinal cord implantation reduce motoneuron loss by over 50% 3 weeks after injury, but this effect is lost by 6 months (Lang et al., 2005a, 2005b). In contrast, GDNF, when administered intrathecally with riluzole, maintains the positive effects of immediate root implantation and results in improved BBB scores at 3 months (Bergerot et al., 2004). Prolonged intraspinal overexpression of GDNF or BDNF by adeno-associated virus prolongs motoneuron survival, but promotes excessive sprouting without reinnervation of implanted roots (Blits et al., 2004). These results highlight the challenges of neurotrophin therapy—brief perioperative exposure is often insufficient, and concentration must be appropriate for the desired effect, as higher or lower doses may result in counterproductive neuronal behavior. Other successful strategies that avoid the risks of overexpressing growth factors include treatment with sialidase to decrease the inhibitory effects of MAG on axon outgrowth through the CNS (Yang et al., 2006), and the implantation of olfactory ensheathing cells along with the avulsed root (Li et al., 2007).

Dorsal Root

Promoting sensory axons to enter the spinal cord has proven to be a far greater challenge than promoting motor axons to leave it. Whereas injured motoneuron processes readily innervate a nerve graft, even crossing CNS terrain to do so (Risling et al., 1983), injured dorsal root axons normally regenerate only as far as the PNS/CNS border (Ramon y Cajal, 1928; Perkins et al., 1980). The transition from peripheral nerve to spinal cord, the dorsal root entry zone (DREZ), is characterized anatomically by extensions of central astrocytic processes among peripheral Schwann cells (Berthold, Carlstedt, 1977). These astrocytes may inhibit passage of dorsal root axons through the DREZ by a variety of mechanisms (reviewed in Golding et al., 1997).

CHANGING LOCAL TERRAIN

Early attempts to return dorsal root axons to their central terminations were based on two general strategies: change the DREZ and CNS terrain so that dorsal root axons will grow there, or restore the developmental relationship between DRG neurons and the dorsal horn. An obvious manipulation of the CNS environment was to bypass the DREZ by implanting avulsed dorsal roots directly within the spinal cord. This failed to promote central regeneration of dorsal root fibers (Carlstedt, 1985; Jamieson, Eames, 2003). Dorsal horn neurons projected axons peripherally into the root, however, and could conceivably mediate sensory function. This possibility was reinforced by recovery of some sensibility in patients who had undergone ventral root reimplantation (Carlstedt et al., 2000).

A second early strategy to modify the CNS terrain was derived from experimental attempts to enhance spinal cord regeneration. The spinal cords of neonatal animals were irradiated on the theory that reducing the population of astrocytes and oligodendrocytes would decrease the inhibition of subsequent regeneration (Gilmore, 1971). Irradiation was found to have a secondary benefit: exposed areas of the spinal cord were repopulated by Schwann cells, potentially rendering the environment conducive to axonal regeneration. This proved to be the case, as subsequent dorsal root injury was followed by regeneration of axons through the modified DREZ and into portions of the dorsal horn that had been repopulated with Schwann cells (Sims, Gilmore,1994). Environmental modification of such magnitude had other consequences as well: processes of dorsal horn neurons grew out the dorsal root (Sims, Gilmore, 1997), and synaptic density on central neurons was decreased when they were adjacent to Schwann cells (Sims, Gilmore, 2000). The altered terrain strategy has recently been modified by injecting the spinal cord with olfactory ensheathing cells. These unique glial cells normally serve as a pathway for regenerating olfactory axons to reenter the CNS (Graziadei, Monti Graziadei, 1980; Doucette, 1990). Reinnervation of the dorsal horn has been confirmed morphologically (Ramon-Cueto, Nieto-Sampedro, 1994; Li et al., 2004), and is sufficient to restore reflex pathways (Navarro et al., 1999). The ultimate extension of this strategy, redirecting injured dorsal root axons to reenter the spinal cord through an adjacent, uninjured root and DREZ, has also shown promise (Liu et al., 2009).

RECAPITULATING DEVELOPMENT

Dorsal root axons pass through the DREZ during development, and retrace this path if injured in the early neonatal period (Carlstedt et al., 1987). This relationship can be at least partially reproduced in the adult by replacement of native DRGs with fetal DRG tissue. Fetal rat DRGs grafted into adult rats restored peripheral connections (Rosario et al., 1995) but showed little evidence of central ingrowth (Rosario et al., 1993). However, when human fetal DRGs were grafted into rats, axons bypassed the DREZ, "grew around the transitional zone astrocytes in laminin-rich peripheral surroundings" (Kozlova et al., 1997, p881), and penetrated the CNS by following blood vessels (Kozlova, et al., 1995). These axons are able to mediate dorsal horn synaptic activity and ventral root reflexes, but are small in caliber, small in number, and lack access to significant dorsal horn circuitry (Levinsson et al., 2000). Interestingly, adult dorsal root axons will grow into transplants of fetal spinal cord (Tessler et al., 1988), confirming that the DREZ undergoes a significant developmental change from permissive to inhibitory terrain.

ENHANCING NEURONAL REGENERATION STATE

The current approach to crossing the PNS/CNS barrier is based on a new relativism. Inhibitory molecules form a potential barrier to regeneration that evolves after dorsal root injury; the effectiveness of this barrier can be decreased or eliminated by increasing the intrinsic growth state of the neuron. Axon growth will thus occur when the intrinsic growth state is sufficient to overcome the barriers confronted at that time. The afferent sensory system played a key role in elucidating this relationship. Sensory neurons in the dorsal root ganglion have two processes: a peripheral axon that reaches sense organs through peripheral nerve, and a central one that courses through the dorsal root, crosses the DREZ, and forms synapses on central neurons. When injured, the peripheral process regenerates more vigorously than does its central counterpart (Wujek, Lasek, 1983; Oblinger, Lasek, 1984) (Figure 8-12). This discrepancy can be minimized, however, by injuring the peripheral process first, and the central process a week later (Richardson, Verge, 1987). This "conditioning" effect is discussed extensively in Chapter 9. The potential for a neuron to regenerate has been correlated with its expression of the growth-associated protein GAP-43 (Skene, Willard, 1981). Not surprisingly, GAP-43 expression in the DRG is upregulated by injury to the peripheral but not the central processes of the neuron (Schreyer, Skene, 1993; Chong et al., 1994), and accurately reflects the relative "growth state" of the neuron after both types of injury. Other molecules such as laminin-associated integrins are also regulated differentially by injury to the central and peripheral process of the DRG neuron (Wallquist et al., 2004). Clearly, peripheral injury generates a conditioning signal that is not produced by central injury, and that enhances the regeneration state of the neuron.

The use of peripheral injury to promote central regeneration provided early clues to the importance of neuronal state, but is not a practical strategy for treating avulsion injury. Fortunately, parallel research focused on CNS regeneration has revealed other, atraumatic means of altering the regeneration state of the neuron. The myelin-associated glycoprotein, MAG, is a potent inhibitor of neurite elongation from a variety of brain-derived cells in culture (Mukhopadhyay et al., 1994; Tang et al., 1997), but also inhibits neurons contributing to peripheral nerve: adult DRGs (Mukhopadhyay et al., 1994),

xenopus motoneurons (Song et al., 1998), and a motoneuron-like cell line (McKerracher et al., 1994). In vivo, peripheral axon regeneration is inhibited by contact with MAG-bearing myelin (Schafer et al., 1996) and is enhanced by blocking MAG function with antibodies (Mears et al., 2003). The discovery that inhibition by MAG could be overcome by priming neurons with neurotrophins (Cai et al., 1999) and that this effect is mediated through a rise in intracellular cAMP (Song et al., 1998; Cai et al., 1999) suggested a new strategy for overcoming barriers to regeneration such as the DREZ. Treatment with NGF, NT-3, GDNF, artemin, or FGF-2 was subsequently found to promote regeneration of dorsal root axons into the CNS, in some cases restoring functional synapses and sensory function (Zhang et al., 1998; Ramer et al., 2000; Romero et al., 2001; Wang et al., 2008). Similarly, regeneration of dorsal root axons injured within the CNS was enhanced by treatment with cyclic AMP (Neumann et al., 2002; Qiu et al., 2002).

EVOLUTION OF THE DREZ AFTER INJURY

The nature and dynamic characteristics of the PNS/CNS interface have been appreciated only recently. The crucial event is axon growth from Schwann cell to astrocyte, a transition that can be encouraged by enhancing astrocytic expression of the adhesion molecule L1 or the growth-permissive substrate polysialic acid (PSA) (Adcock et al., 2004; Zhang et al., 2007). In the absence of dorsal root trauma, neurons transplanted into the DRG will grow through the normal interface without difficulty (McPhail et al., 2005). Once axon degeneration and regeneration are triggered, the early astrocytic barrier can be overcome by elevating neuronal GAP-43 with treatments such as NT-3. Delayed elevation of GAP-43, however, is not sufficient to promote axons across the evolving "degenerative" barrier (Ramer et al., 2001). This later boundary contains the chondroitin sulfate proteoglycans neurocan and brevican (Quaglia et al., 2008), and can be surmounted only by a combined approach of conditioning the neuron and removing these proteoglycans (Steinmetz et al., 2005; Quaglia et al., 2008). A combined therapy that includes both alteration of CNS terrain and increasing the intrinsic regeneration state of the neuron will thus be required to promote regenerating dorsal root axons to cross the DREZ and restore function after dorsal root avulsion injury.

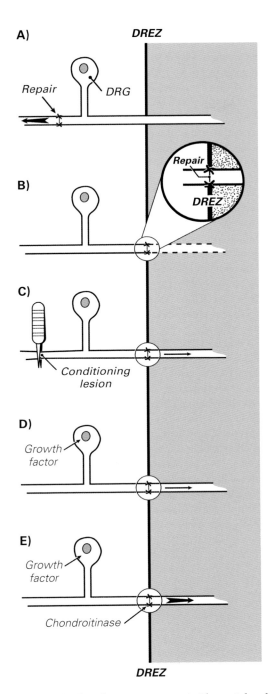

FIGURE 8-12   Regeneration across the dorsal root entry zone. A: The peripheral axons of DRG neurons regenerate readily when injured. B: Regeneration of fibers in the dorsal root is blocked at the dorsal root entry zone (DREZ). C, D: Some central regeneration occurs after a conditioning lesion is administered to the peripheral nerve before the test lesion is made, or when appropriate growth factors are applied during regeneration. E: The most robust regeneration is obtained by both increasing the neuronal growth state with growth factors and eliminating inhibitory molecules such as proteoglycans from the growth pathway.

NERVE TRANSFERS

Nerve transfer, like end-to-side repair, is a currently popular technique that was introduced in the early twentieth century. Tuttle described reinnervation of the brachial plexus with cervical roots in 1913 (Tuttle, 1913), and Harris reported the sacrifice of intact sensory nerves to reinnervate insensate areas of the hand in 1921 (Harris, 1921). Many of the early transfers, as exemplified by Seddon's experience with transfer of intercostal nerves to the musculocutaneous nerve to restore elbow flexion (Figure 8-13) (Seddon, 1963), were performed at proximal levels. Although these provided axons where none were available previously, they were still limited by long regeneration distances and loss of axons in tributary nerves such as the cutaneous branch of the musculocutaneous nerve. More recently, however, a variety of innovative transfers have been performed near their targets to provide rapid reinnervation with a freshly axotomized, functionally defined axon population, thereby minimizing end organ deterioration and speeding the return of function (reviewed in Brown, Mackinnon, 2008; Addas, Midha, 2009). In these transfers, one functional unit is substituted for another, leaving intact the relationship among first-order neurons. Although many transfers have been described, this section will focus on biceps reinnervation to restore elbow flexion. This has been accomplished with intercostal, cranial, and extremity nerves; comparison of the process of adaptation to these widely varied inputs should provide some insight into the pathways that are involved. Alterations in cortical function as a result of nerve transfer are described in Chapter 11.

Nerve Transfers for Elbow Flexion

INTERCOSTAL NERVES

Transfer of intercostal nerves to restore elbow function is the best studied of the nerve transfer procedures. Two large series reported outcomes when intercostal nerves had been coapted directly to the musculocutaneous nerve (ICM transfer), a total of 234 patients. Nagano was able to achieve MRC grade 4 biceps contraction in 26% of 159 cases and grade 3 in an additional 44% (Nagano et al., 1989). Of the 75 patients followed up by Waikakul (Waikakul et al., 1999b), 15% could lift a 2-Kg weight more than 30 times, and an additional 33%

could lift the weight, but fewer than 30 times. An additional large series included some patients in whom a nerve graft had been used to connect the intercostal and musculocutaneous nerves; 67% achieved at least grade 4 recovery (Chuang et al., 1992). When the transfer was performed in children under 5 years of age, 84% gained M4 function, an improvement over the results in adults (Kawabata et al., 2001). Motoneurons that normally innervate intercostal muscles are thus able to reinnervate biceps muscle and restore useful function to more than half of adult patients and more than three-quarters of children.

The functions of respiration and elbow flexion are seemingly quite different, yet patients gradually recover voluntary biceps flexion after intercostal transfer. The process through which this occurs has been the subject of several investigations. Chuang et al. (1992) have analyzed the clinical course of patients who have undergone ICM transfer. The 5 stages of recovery illustrate the gradual shift in control of biceps activity: (1) biceps squeeze elicits chest pain (intercostal sensory axons have regenerated into biceps muscle); (2) contraction of the proximal biceps is noted with deep respiration, usually 3–6 months after transfer; (3) visible contraction progresses to the distal biceps, but still without elbow motion; a Tinel's sign is present over the lateral antebrachial cutaneous nerve, the cutaneous component of the musculocutaneous nerve (12 months postoperatively); (4) by 12–18 months elbow flexion is possible, but only during forced respiration; (5) 2–3 years after surgery voluntary elbow flexion is no longer linked to respiration; sensation has returned to the lateral forearm. These clinical events have been correlated with electrical activity in the biceps muscle as determined by electromyography (EMG). Spontaneous discharges from the relaxed biceps are synchronized with respiration for 2–3 years after ICM transfer, and can be enhanced by coughing, deep breathing, or postural changes such as trunk flexion (Takahashi, 1983; Chalidapong et al., 2006). Each intercostal nerve innervates muscles of both inspiration and expiration. In some patients the greatest EMG activity can be elicited by inspiration, and in others by expiration, although voluntary biceps strength is not determined by this variable. Respiratory changes in the biceps EMG persist after voluntary function is regained, providing evidence that at least some connections with the respiratory control centers are maintained (Malessy et al., 1993).

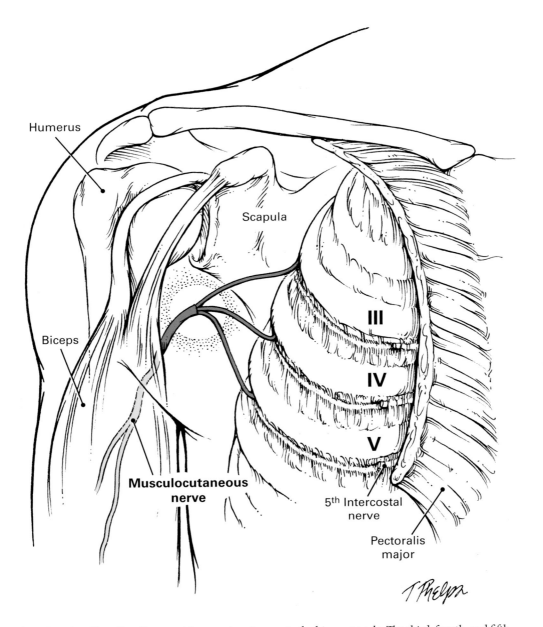

Humerus

Scapula

Biceps

III

IV

V

**Musculocutaneous
nerve**

5th Intercostal
nerve

Pectoralis
major

T Phelps

FIGURE 8-13   Transfer of intercostal nerves to reinnervate the biceps muscle. The third, fourth, and fifth intercostal nerves have been transected anteriorly and elevated to the midlateral line, then sutured to the musculocutaneous nerve. Transecting the intercostal nerves distally eliminates the need for a graft, but also limits the number of motor axons that can be transferred. In either case, motor axons may be lost to the cutaneous branch of the musculocutaneous nerve. These problems are circumvented by direct transfer of an ulnar nerve fascicle to the nerve to biceps.

The changes in afferent function after ICM transfer are also of interest. In 4 of 14 ICM patients, Kanamauru et al. (1993) were able to detect mechanoreceptor function that generated a classic stretch reflex. Reviewing a series of 159 patients (Nagano et al., 1989), Nagano found that sensation over the biceps was referred to the area of the chest wall served previously by the transferred nerves. Although this situation was maintained indefinitely in adults, appropriate localization of touch was regained in three young children 3–8 years after the transfer was performed. The results of ICM transfer have thus demonstrated that CNS plasticity can restore voluntary function after transfer of a relatively discrete motor function (a portion of the intercostal mechanism), but perception of a transferred block of sensory function (2–4 sensory dermatomes) as native to its new location is rare, and occurs in only a few children. This observation is consistent with the differences in organization of the sensory and motor systems. The former is designed to localize and characterize incoming stimuli, a task that requires maintenance of narrowly focused communications channels from skin to cortex. The motor system, in contrast, coordinates the function of groups of muscles through a variety of overlapping programs, and is characterized by wide peripheral distribution of cortical inputs. One would suspect on the basis of this structure that of the two systems, the motor is more likely to be flexible.

ULNAR AND MEDIAN NERVE FASCICLES

Transfer of a single ulnar nerve fascicle to the adjacent nerve to biceps was one of the first "second generation" transfers. The procedure avoids loss of motor axons into the cutaneous branch of the musculocutaneous nerve, and minimizes the distance from repair site to motor endplate. As a result, biceps reinnervation is noted between 3 and 6 months after surgery (Sungpet et al., 2000; Mackinnon et al., 2005; Nath et al., 2006; Venkatramani et al., 2008), a dramatic improvement over ICM transfer. In two large series that included measurements of patient strength, 63–94% of patients achieved M4 function, with mean elbow flexion of 2.8 Kg in one series (Leechavengvongs et al., 1998) and 4.1 Kg in the other (Teboul et al., 2004). Maximum strength was 7 and 9 Kg, respectively. Postoperative ulnar nerve function, as evaluated by pinch and grip strength measurements, was not compromised by redirection of a single, carefully chosen fascicle (Leechavengvongs et al., 1998; Mackinnon et al., 2005). Although patients seem to adapt to the transfer quite readily, there have been no EMG studies of biceps and FCU co-contractions, nor has there been analysis of FCU control during elbow flexion. It is unlikely that all fibers to the FCU have been transferred; the degree to which the remaining fibers respond to either central commands for elbow flexion or stimulation of afferents that have reinnervated the biceps would provide

unique insights into the organizational plasticity of the motor pool. The persistent biceps weakness after transfer of a single ulnar fascicle led to modifications in which both biceps and brachialis were reinnervated. This was done by using single fascicle transfers from both median and ulnar nerves to restore Grade 4 function in 6/6 patients (Mackinnon et al., 2005), and by using two median nerve fascicles to restore Grade 4 function in 36/40 patients (Nath et al., 2006).

PHRENIC, ACCESSORY, PECTORALIS MINOR, AND THORACODORSAL NERVES

The phrenic, accessory, pectoralis minor, and thoracodorsal nerves have also been used to restore elbow flexion. Although over 200 cases of phrenic transfer have been reported, only one publication addresses the independence of resulting elbow flexion, noting "the involuntary movement of the neurotized biceps gradually changes to a voluntary movement after 2 years" (Songcharoen et al., 2005, p86). A prospective, randomized comparison of accessory and intercostal transfers in 205 patients revealed the former to require longer for muscle reinnervation, but to provide excellent function (the ability to lift a 2 Kg weight from 0 to 90 degrees of elbow flexion 30 times) in 43% of cases as opposed to 20% after intercostal transfer (Waikakul et al., 1999b). Function was also more independent two years after accessory transfer; no patients had uncontrolled elbow flexion in the accessory group, whereas 7 patients in the intercostal group continued to have involuntary flexion with coughing or yawning. Although a meta-analysis of nerve transfers concluded that intercostal transfer was superior (Merrell et al., 2001), a large, prospective trial in which the evaluation criteria and procedures were the same throughout is likely to provide the most meaningful comparison of the two procedures.

Transfer of the thoracodorsal nerve has been performed infrequently, but has provided muscle strength at the M4 or M5 level in 80–85% of patients in two small series (Novak et al., 2002; Samardzic et al., 2005). Medial pectoral transfer has also been relatively effective in adults, resulting in recovery to at least M4 in 60% of patients (Brandt, Mackinnon, 1993; Samardzic et al., 2002). Apparently no difficulty was experienced in transferring control of biceps function in these patients.

The relative facility with which patients learn to use their reinnervated biceps after transfer of other extremity nerves probably results from inclusion of the donor nerves in an upper extremity flexion program (Chapter 3). One would expect this relationship to be much closer than that of biceps and intercostals or phrenic, where the transition must be made from a primary respiration program to a primary flexion program. It will thus be important to study patients with extremity nerve transfers so that their central response to rewiring the biceps can be compared with the now well documented response to intercostal nerve transfer.

Sensory Nerve Transfer

Sensory nerve transfer is a fairly reliable means of restoring sensibility to digits that have been denervated by proximal or extended nerve injury. Two-point discrimination of less than 10 mm can be expected in at least 85% of patients (Ozkan et al., 2001; Ducic et al., 2006). There is widespread agreement that sensation is initially referred to the donor area (Stocks et al., 1991; Ozkan et al., 2001; Ducic et al., 2006); in some cases this pattern may persist (Stocks et al., 1991), although others state that sensation is normal by 12–18 months after transfer (Ozkan et al., 2001; Ducic et al., 2006). In neither instance, however, was false sensory localization sought out and scored on a grid as described in Chapter 4. In comparing these results with those of ICM transfer, restoration of accurate sensory localization appears to occur more readily between digits than between chest wall and anterior arm.

CONCLUSIONS

The various manipulations discussed in Chapter 8 illustrate the plastic nature of nerve as a tissue, and their outcomes demonstrate the relative flexibility of control mechanisms within the CNS. Nerve can be formed de novo across gaps approaching 1 cm in the rat and 3 cm in the primate. These distances have been increased by providing a more organized substrate for regeneration, and/or by adding cellular elements that elaborate both contact and diffusible factors supportive of the bridging process. Restoration of peripheral continuity, however, is not in itself sufficient to restore function. Neurons that give rise to regenerated axons in the periphery must also have central connections appropriate to their coordinated activity. Were these central connections as plastic as their peripheral counterparts, normal function would be expected whenever peripheral

targets are reinnervated by adequate numbers of axons. The degree to which the outcomes of procedures discussed above are able to approximate this ideal provides insight into the limits imposed by the CNS.

At one extreme of the range of CNS plasticity is the well-coordinated function that often results from nerve transfer. In this case, discrete afferent and efferent circuits are transferred together as a relatively intact functional module (Chapter 11). The circuitry required for these neurons to assume a new function is robust within the motor system, but less prominent in the sensory system. Altering the effectiveness of established central connections is thus well within the capability of the mature CNS. The middle ground is exemplified by end-to-side nerve repair, which occurs predominantly through terminal reinnervation (Figure 8–10). The majority of circuits remain intact, while a subset of neurons is redirected to innervate the recipient muscle and/or skin. End-to-side repair is most effective when applied to distal nerves serving symmetrical or synergistic functions (Figure 8-10). It is unclear, however, whether this success is based on the organizational relationship between donor and recipient nerves, or the relative ease with which sprouting can be elicited from a small terminal nerve. Similarly, the poor results at the nerve trunk level could reflect confused reinnervation of the diverse functions represented in the median and ulnar nerves, or the difficulty in eliciting a sprouting response from a large, multifascicular nerve. The vivid descriptions of Ballance, based on reinnervation of the small yet complex facial nerve, suggest that little compensation is possible when a motorneuron pool is forced to serve disparate functions.

Maximum disorganization is represented by tubular substitutes for nerve graft. An enclosed gap between nerve ends imposes topographic disorganization on the regenerate that becomes progressively severe as the gap increases. The consequences of using such a device will thus be determined by the relative need for topographically and functionally appropriate end organ reinnervation. In the digital nerve, axons serve a small number of receptor types in a topographically defined area, so axonal disorganization is relatively well tolerated; the performance of nerve autograft and of tubular prostheses are similar, though cost and risk of graft extrusion are both reduced by using autograft. As the nerve increases in complexity, the organizational challenge increases proportionally. A critical factor that limits the success of tubes in larger, complex nerves is also a factor that limits the success of nerve repair and grafting: regenerating axons enter functionally and topographically inappropriate Schwann cell tubes in the distal nerve stump. The ultimate success of prosthetic nerve graft will thus depend on solving the universal problem of regeneration specificity. Nerve substitutes cannot bypass this problem, but they do present a unique opportunity that could lead to its solution. Whereas axon trajectory is constrained by Schwann cell tubes within graft and/or the distal nerve stump, it is initially unconstrained when a gap is imposed between nerve ends. Within this gap, axons are free to respond to contact and diffusible factors, and could potentially be sorted into appropriate tributary subpopulations.

REFERENCES

Abe I, Tsujino A, Hara Y, Ochiai N (2008) Effect of the rate of prestretching a peripheral nerve on regeneration potential after transection and repair. Ortho Sci 8: 693–699.

Addas BM, Midha R (2009) Nerve transfers for severe nerve injury. Neurosurg Clin N Am 20: 27–38, vi.

Accioli-de-Vaconcellos ZA, Kassar-Duchossoy L, Mira JC (1999) Long term evaluation of experimental median nerve repair by frozen and fresh nerve autografts, allografts and allografts repopulated by autologous Schwann cells. Restor Neurol Neurosci 15: 17–24.

Adcock KH, Brown DJ, Shearer MC, Shewan D, Schachner M, Smith GM, Geller HM, Fawcett JW (2004) Axon behaviour at Schwann cell astrocyte boundaries: manipulation of axon signalling pathways and the neural adhesion molecule L1 can enable axons to cross. Eur J Neurosci 20: 1425–1435.

Aebischer P, Guenard V, Winn SR, Valentini RF, Galletti PM (1988) Blind-ended semipermeable guidance channels support peripheral nerve regeneration in the absence of a distal nerve stump. Brain Res 454: 179–187.

Aebischer P, Guenard V, Brace S (1989) Peripheral nerve regeneration through blind-ended semipermeable guidance channels: Effect of the molecular weight cutoff. J Neurosci 9: 3590–3595.

Ahmed MR, Basha SH, Gopinath D, Muthusamy R, Jayakumar R (2005) Initial upregulation of growth factors and inflammatory mediators during nerve regeneration in the presence of cell adhesive peptide-incorporated collagen tubes. JPNS 10: 17–30.

Aitken JT (1950) Growth of nerve implants in voluntary muscle. J Anat 84: 38–49.

Al-Qattan MM, Al-Thunyan A (1998) Variables affecting axonal regeneration following end-to-side neurorrhaphy. Br J Plast Surg 51: 238–242.

Alzate LH, Sutachan JJ, Hurtado H (2000) An anterograde degeneration study of the distribution of regenerating rat myelinated fibers in the silicone chamber model. Neurosci Lett 286: 17–20.

Albert E (1885) Einige operationen an nerven. Wied Med Presse 26: 1285–1288.

Alluin O, Feron F, Desouches C, Dousset E, Pellissier JF, Magalon G, Decherchi P (2006) Metabosensitive afferent fiber responses after peripheral nerve injury and transplantation of an acellular muscle graft in association with Schwann cells. J Neurotrauma 23: 1883–1894.

Almgren KG (1974) Revascularization of free peripheral nerve grafts. Acta Orthop Scand Suppl 154: 1–104.

Amr SM, Moharram AN, Abdel-Meguid KM (2006) Augmentation of partially regenerated nerves by end-to-side side-to-side grafting neurotization: experience based on eight late obstetric brachial plexus cases. J Brach Plex P N Injury 1: 6.

Anderson PN, Mitchell J, Mayor D, Stauber VV (1983) An ultrastructural study of the early stages of axonal regeneration through rat nerve grafts. Neuropathol Appl Neurobiol 9: 455–466.

Anderson PN, Nadim W, Turmaine M (1991) Schwann cell migration through freeze-killed peripheral nerve grafts without accompanying axons. Acta Neuropath (Berl) 82: 193–199.

Ansselin AD, Fink T, Davey DF (1997) Peripheral nerve regeneration through nerve guides seeded with adult Schwann cells. Neuropathol Appl Neurobiol 23: 387–398.

Askar I, Sabuncuoglu BT (2002) Superficial or deep implantation of motor nerve after denervation: an experimental study—superficial or deep implantation of motor nerve. Microsurgery 22: 242–248.

Atchabahian A, Doolabh VB, Mackinnon SE, Yu S, Hunter DA, Flye MW (1998) Indefinite survival of peripheral nerve allografts after temporary cyclosporine A immunosuppression. Restor Neurol Neurosci 13: 129–139.

Atchabahian A, Mackinnon SE, Hunter DA (1999) Cold preservation of nerve grafts decreases expression of ICAM-1 and class II MHC antigens. J Recon Micro 15: 307–311.

Auba C, Hontanilla B, Arcocha J, Gorria O (2006) Peripheral nerve regeneration through allografts compared with autografts in FK506-treated monkeys. J Neurosurg 105: 602–609.

Azzam NA, Zalewski AA, Williams LR, Azzam R (1991) Nerve cables formed in silicon chambers reconstitute a perineurial but not a vascular endoneurial permeability barrier. J Comp Neurol 314: 807–819.

Bain JR, Mackinnon SE, Hudson AR, Falk RE, Falk JA, Hunter DA (1988) The peripheral nerve allograft: an assessment of regeneration across nerve allografts in rats immunosuppressed with cyclosporin A. Plast Reconstr Surg 82: 1052–1064.

Bain JR, Mackinnon SE, Hudson AR, Wade J, Evans P, Makino A, Hunter D (1992) The peripheral nerve allograft in the primate immunosuppressed with cyclosporin A. I. Histologic and electrophysiologic assessment. Plast Reconstr Surg 90: 1036–1046.

Ballance C (1923) Some results of nerve anastomosis. Brit J Surg 11: 327–346.

Ballance C, Duel AB (1932) the operative treatment of facial palsy. Arch Oto 15: 1–70.

Baron-Van Evercooren A, Kleinman HK, Ohno S, Marangos P, Schwartz JP, Dubois-Dalcq ME (1982) Nerve growth factor, laminin, and fibronectin promote neurite outgrowth in human fetal sensory ganglia cultures. J Neurosci Res 8: 179–182.

Barras FM, Pasche P, Bouche N, Aebischer P, Zurn AD (2002) Glial cell line-derived neurotrophic factor released by synthetic guidance channels promotes facial nerve regeneration in the rat. J Neurosci Res 70: 746–755.

Bassett CA, Campbell JB, Husby J (1959) Peripheral nerve and spinal cord regeneration: Factors leading to success of a tubulation technique employing millipore. Exp Neurol 1: 386–406.

Bates DJ, Ranford JA, Mangelsdorf DC (1991) Blot and culture analysis of neuronotrophic factors in nerve regeneration chamber fluids. Neurochem Res 16: 621–628.

Bates DJ, Mangelsdorf DC, Ridings JA (1995) Multiple neurotrophic factors including NGF-like activity in nerve regeneration chamber fluids. Neurochem Int 26: 281–293.

Battiston B, Tos P, Cushway T, Geuna S (2000) Nerve repair by means of vein filled with muscle grafts I. Clinical results. Microsurgery 20: 32–36.

Battiston B, Tos P, Conforti LG, Geuna S (2007) Alternative techniques for peripheral nerve repair: conduits and end-to-side neurorrhaphy. Acta Neurochir Suppl 100: 43–50.

Becker M, Lassner F, Fansa H, Mawrin C, Pallua N (2002) Refinements in nerve to muscle neurotization. Muscle Nerve 26: 362–366.

Benfey M, Aguayo AJ (1982) Extensive elongation of axons from rat brain into peripheral nerve grafts. Nature 296: 150–152.

Bergerot A, Shortland PJ, Anand P, Hunt SP, Carlstedt T (2004) Co-treatment with riluzole and GDNF is necessary for functional recovery after ventral root avulsion injury. Exp Neurol 187: 359–366.

Bertelli JA, Soares dos Santos AR, Calixto JB (1996a) Is axonal sprouting able to traverse the conjunctival layers of the peripheral nerve? A behavioral, motor, and sensory study of end-to-side nerve anastomosis. J Recon Micro 12: 559–563.

Bertelli JA, Taleb M, Mira JC, Calixto JB (1996b) Muscle fiber type reorganization and behavioral functional recovery of rat median nerve repair with vascularized or conventional nerve grafts. Restor Neurol Neurosci 10: 5–12.

Bertelli JA, Ghizoni MF (2003a) Nerve repair by end-to-side coaptation or fascicular transfer: a clinical study. J Recon Micro 19: 313–318.

Bertelli JA, Ghizoni MF (2003b) Brachial plexus avulsion injury repairs with nerve transfers and nerve grafts directly implanted into the spinal cord yield partial recovery of shoulder and elbow movements. Neurosurgery 52: 1385–1389.

Bertelli JA, Taleb M, Mira J-C, Ghizoni MF (2005) The course of aberrant reinnervation following nerve repair with fresh or denatured muscle autografts. JPNS 10: 359–368.

Berthold C-H, Carlstedt T (1977) Observations on the morphology at the transition between the peripheral and the central nervous system in the cat. II. General organization of the transitional region in S1 dorsal rootlets. Acta Physiol Scand Suppl. 446: 23–42.

Best TJ, Mackinnon SE, Midha R, Hunter DA, Evans PJ (1999) Revascularization of peripheral nerve autografts and allografts. Plast Reconstr Surg 104: 152–160.

Bielschowsky M, Unger E (1917) Die uberbruckung grossser nervenlucken. J Psychol Neurol, Leipz 22: 267–318.

Birch R, Dunkerton M, Bonney G, Jamieson AM (1988) Experience with the free vascularized ulnar nerve graft in repair of supraclavicular lesions of the brachial plexus. Clin Orthop 237: 96–104.

Blits B, Carlstedt TP, Ruitenberg MJ, De Winter F, Hermens WTJMC, Dijkhuizen PA, Claasens JWC, Eggers R, Van der Sluis R, Tenenbaum L, Boer GJ, Verhaagen J (2004) Rescue and sprouting of motoneurons following ventral root avulsion and reimplantation combined with intraspinal adeno-associated viral vector-mediated expression of glial cell line-derived neurotrophic factor or brain-derived neurotrophic factor. Exp Neurol 189: 303–316.

Bloch J, Fine EG, Bouche N, Zurn AD, Aebischer P (2001) Nerve growth factor- and neurotrophin-3-releasing guidance channels promote regeneration of the transected rat dorsal root. Exp Neurol 172: 425–432.

Bontioti E, Kajne M, Lundborg G, Dahlin LB (2005) End-to-side nerve repair in the upper extremity of rat. JPNS 10: 58–68.

Brandt KE, Mackinnon SE (1993) A technique for maximizing biceps recovery in brachial plexus reconstruction. J Hand Surg Am 18: 726–733.

Bray GM, Rasminsky M, Aguayo AJ (1981) Interactions between axons and their sheaths. Annu Rev Neurosci 4: 127–162.

Brenner MJ, Jensen JN, Lowe JB, Myckatyn TM, Fox IK, Hunter DA, Mohanakumar T, Mackinnon SE (2004a) Anti-CD40 ligand antibody permits regeneration through peripheral nerve allografts in a nonhuman primate model. PRS 114: 1802–1814.

Brenner MJ, Tung THH, Mackinnon SE, Myckatyn TM, Hunter DA, Mohanakumar T (2004b) Anti-CD40 ligand monoclonal antibody induces a permissive state, but not tolerance, for murine peripheral nerve allografts. Exp Neurol 186: 59–69.

Brenner MJ, Lowe JB, Fox IK, Mackinnon SE, Hunter D, Darcy MD, Duncan JR, Wood P, Mohanakumar T (2005a) Effects of Schwann cells and donor antigen on long-nerve allograft regeneration. Microsurgery 25: 61–70.

Brenner MJ, Mackinnon SE, Rickman SR, Jaramillo A, Tung TH, Hunter D, Mohanakumar T (2005b) FK506 and anti-CD40 ligand in peripheral nerve allotransplantation. Rest Neuro Neurosci 23: 237–249.

Brenner MJ, Dvali L, Hunter D, Myckatyn TM, Mackinnon SE (2007) Motor neuron regeneration through end-to-side repairs is a function of donor nerve axotomy. PRS 120: 215–223.

Bresjanac M, Sketelj J (1989) Neurite-promoting influences of proliferating Schwann cells and target-tissues are not prerequisite for rapid axonal elongation after nerve crush. J Neurosci Res 24: 501–507.

Brown DL, Bishop DK, Wood SY, Cederna PS (2006) Short-term anti-CD40 ligand costimulatory blockade induces tolerance to peripheral nerve allografts, resulting in improved skeletal muscle function. PRS 117: 2250–2258.

Brown JM, Mackinnon SE (2008) Nerve transfers in the forearm and hand. Hand Clin 24: 319–340.

Brunelli, G. (1981) Direct neurotisation of denervated muscles. In: *Posttraumatic Peripheral Nerve Regeneration: Experimental Basis and Clinical Implications*, Vol. 10, A. Gorio, H. Millesi and S. Mingrino, eds., pp. 523–526, New York: Raven Press.

Brunelli G (1982) Direct neurotization of severely damaged muscles. J Hand Surg 7: 572–579.

Brunelli GA, Brunelli GR (1993) Direct muscle neurotization. J Recon Micro 9: 81–89.

Brushart TM (1990) Topographic specificity of peripheral axon regeneration across enclosed gaps. Soc Neurosc Abstr 16: 806. (Abstract)

Bryan DJ, Miller RA, Costas PD, Wang K-K, Seckel BR (1993) Immunocytochemistry of skeletal muscle basal lamina grafts in nerve regeneration. Plast Reconstr Surg 92: 927–940.

Bunnell S (1927) Surgery of the nerves of the hand. S G &O 44: 145–152.

Bunnell S, Boyes JH (1939) Nerve grafts. Am J Surg 44: 64–75.

Bushnell BD, McWilliams AD, Whitener GB, Messer TM (2008) Early clinical experience with collagen nerve tubes in digital nerve repair. J Hand Surg Am 33: 1081–1087.

Buttemeyer R, Rao U, Jones NF (1995) Peripheral nerve allograft transplantation with FK506: Functional, histological, and immunological results before and after discontinuation of immunosuppression. Ann Plas Surg 35: 396–401.

Cai DM, Shen YJ, De Bellard M, Tang S, Filbin MT (1999) Prior exposure to neurotrophins blocks inhibition of axonal regeneration by MAG and myelin via a cAMP-dependent mechanism. Neuron 22: 89–101.

Calder JS, Norris RW (1993) Repair of mixed peripheral nerves using muscle autografts: A preliminary communication. Br J Plast Surg 46: 557–564.

Campbell JB, Bassett CA, Husby J, Thulin C-A, Feringa ER (1961) Microfilter sheaths in peripheral nerve surgery: a laboratory report and preliminary clinical study. J Trauma 1: 139–158.

Cao X, Tamai M, Kizaki K, Akahane M, Ono H, Ohgushi H, Yajima H, Tamai S (1999) Choline acetyltransferase activity in collateral sprouting of peripheral nerve after surgical intervention: experimental study in rats. J Recon Micro 15: 443–448.

Caplan J, Tiangco DA, Terzis J (1999) Effects of IGF-II in a new end-to-side model. J Recon Micro 15: 351–358.

Carlstedt T (1985) Dorsal root innervation of spinal cord neurons after dorsal root implantation into the spinal cord of adult rats. Neurosci Lett 55: 343–348.

Carlstedt T, Linda H, Cullheim S, Risling M (1986) Reinnervation of hind limb muscles after ventral root avulsion and implantation in the lumbar spinal cord of the adult rat. Acta Physiol Scand 128: 645–646.

Carlstedt T, Dalsgaard C-J, Molander C (1987) Regrowth of lesioned dorsal root nerve fibers into the spinal cord of neonatal rats. Neurosci Lett 74: 14–18.

Carlstedt T, Anand P, Hallin R, Misra PV, Norén G, Seferlis T (2000) Spinal nerve root repair and reimplantation of avulsed ventral roots into the spinal cord after brachial plexus injury. J Neurosurg 93 Suppl: 237–247.

Carlstedt TP, Hallin R, Hedstrom KG, Nilsson-Remahl IA (1993) Functional recovery in primates with brachial plexus injury after spinal cord implantation of avulsed ventral roots. J Neurol Neurosurg Psychiatry 56: 649–654.

Castejon MS, Culver DG, Glass JD (1999) Generation of spectrin breakdown products in peripheral nerves by addition of m-calpain. Muscle Nerve 22: 905–909.

Cederna PS, Kalliainen LK, Urbanchek MG, Rovak JM, Kuzon WM (2001) "Donor" muscle structure and function after end-to-side neurorrhaphy. Plast Reconstr Surg 107: 789–2001.

Chalfoun C, Scholz T, Cole M, Steward E, Vanderkam V, Evans G (2003) Primary nerve grafting: a study of revascularization. Microsurgery 23: 60–65.

Chalidapong P, Sananpanich K, Klaphajone J (2006) Electromyographic comparison of various exercises to improve elbow flexion following intercostal nerve transfer. JBJS 88-B: 620–622.

Chang WC, Kliot M, Sretavan DW (2008) Microtechnology and nanotechnology in nerve repair. Neurol Res 30: 1053–1062.

Chen MH, Chen PR, Chen MH, Hsieh ST, Lin FH (2006) Gelatin-tricalcium phosphate membranes immobilized with NGF, BDNF, or IGF-1 for peripheral nerve repair: an in vitro and in vivo study. J Biomed Mater Res A 79: 846–857.

Chen YG, Brushart TM (1998) The effect of denervated muscle and Schwann cells on axon collateral sprouting. J Hand Surg [Am] 23A: 1025–1033.

Chen YY, McDonald D, Cheng C, Magnowski B, Durand J, Zochodne DW (2005) Axon and Schwann cell partnership during nerve regrowth. J Neuropathol Exp Neurol 64: 613–622.

Chiono V, Tonda-Turo C, Ciardelli G (2009) Chapter 9: artificial scaffolds for peripheral nerve reconstruction. Int Rev Neurobiol 87: 173–198.

Chiu DT, Strauch B (1990) A prospective clinical evaluation of autogenous vein grafts used as a nerve conduit for distal sensory nerve defects of 3cm or less. Plast Reconstr Surg 86: 928–934.

Chiu DT, Chen L, Spielholtz N, Beasley RW (1991) A comparative electrophysiological study on neurotisation in rats. J Hand Surg 16B: 505–510.

Chong M, Reynolds M, Irwin N, Coggeshall R, Emson P, Benowitz L, Woolf C (1994) GAP-43 expression in primary sensory neurons following central axotomy. J Neurosci 14: 4375–4384.

Chuang DC-C, Yeh M-C, Wei F-C (1992) Intercostal nerve transfer of the musculocutaneous nerve in avulsed brachial plexus injuries: evaluation of 66 patients. J Hand Surg 17A: 822–828.

Connolly DT, Heuvelman DM, Nerson R, Olander JV, Eppley BL (1989) Tumor vascular permeability factor stimulates endothelial cell growth and angiogenesis. JCI 84: 1478–1489.

Cui L, Jiang J, Wei L, Zhou X, Fraser JL, Snider BJ, Yu SP (2008) Transplantation of embryonic stem cells improves nerve repair and functional recovery after severe sciatic nerve axotomy in rats. Stem Cells 26: 1356–1365.

Cullheim S, Carlstedt T, Linda H, Risling M, Ulfhake B (1989) Motoneurons reinnervate skeletal muscle after ventral root implantation into the spinal cord of the cat. Neuroscience 29: 725–733.

Dahlin LB, Zhao Q, Bjursten LM (1995) Nerve regeneration in silicone tubes: distribution of macrophages and interleukin-1b in the formed fibrin matrix. Restor Neurol Neurosci 8: 199–203.

Dahlin LB, Anagnostaki L, Lundborg G (2001) Tissue response to silicone tubes used to repair human median and ulnar nerves. Scand J Plast Reconstr Surg Hand Surg 35: 29–34.

Daly PJ, Wood MB (1985) Endoneural and epineural blood flow evaluation with free vascularized and conventional nerve grafts in the canine. J Recon Micro 2: 45–49.

Danielsen N, Dahlin L, Lee YF, Lundborg G (1983) Axonal growth in mesothelial chambers. Scand J Plas Reconstr Surg 17: 119–125.

Danielsen N, Kerns JM, Holmquist B, Zhao Q, Lundborg G, Kanje M (1995) Predegeneration enhances regeneration into acellular nerve grafts. Brain Res 681: 105–108.

Danielsen N, Varon S (1995) Characterization of neurotrophic activity in the silicon-chamber model for nerve regeneration. Recon Micro 11: 231–235.

Dellon L, Mackinnon S (1988) An alternative to the classical nerve graft for the management of the short nerve gap. PRS 82: 849–856.

de Ruiter GC, Spinner RJ, Yaszemski MJ, Windebank AJ, Malessy MJ (2009) Nerve tubes for peripheral nerve repair. Neurosurg Clin N Am 20: 91–105, vii.

Derby A, Engleman VW, Frierdich GE, Neises G, Rapp SR, Roufa DG (1993) Nerve growth factor facilitates regeneration across nerve gaps: morphological and behavioral studies in rat sciatic nerve. Exp Neurol 119: 176–191.

Dezawa M, Takahashi I, Esaki M, Takano M, Sawada H (2001) Sciatic nerve regeneration in rats induced by transplantation of in vitro differentiated bone-marrow stromal cells. Eur J Neurosci 14: 1771–1776.

di Summa PG, Kingham PJ, Raffoul W, Wiberg M, Terenghi G, Kalbermatten DF (2009) Adipose-derived stem cells enhance peripheral nerve regeneration. J Plast Reconstr Aesthet Surg. Doi:10. 1016/j.bjps.2009.09.012.

Doi K, Tamaru K, Sakai K, Kuwata N, Kurafuji Y, Kawai S (1992) A comparison of vascularized and conventional sural nerve grafts. J Hand Surg 17-A: 670–676.

Doolabh, V.B. and S.E. Mackinnon (1999a) Transplantation of the peripheral nerve allograft. In: *Composite Tissue Transplantation*, C.W. Hewitt and K.S. Black, eds., pp. 87–105, Austin, TX: R.G. Landes.

Doolabh VB, Mackinnon SE (1999b) FK506 accelerates functional recovery following nerve grafting in a rat model. Plast Reconstr Surg 103: 1928–1936.

Doucette R (1990) Glial influences on axonal growth in the primary olfactory system. Glia 3: 433–449.

Dubovy P, Svizenská I, Klusáková I, Zitkova A, Houst'ava L, Haninec P (2001) Laminin molecules in freeze-treated nerve segments are associated with migrating Schwann cells that display the corresponding a6b1 integrin receptor. Glia 33: 36–44.

Dubovy P (2004) Schwann cells and endoneurial extracellular matrix molecules as potential cues for sorting of regenerated axons: a review. Anat Sci Int 79: 198–208.

Ducic I, Dellon AL, Bogue DP (2006) Radial sensory neurotization of the thumb and index finger for prehension after proximal median and ulnar nerve injuries. J Recon Micro 22: 73–77.

Dumont CE, Hentz VR (1997) Enhancement of axon growth by detergent-extracted nerve grafts. Transplantation 63: 1210–1215.

El-Kashlan HK, Carroll WR, Hogikyan ND, Chepeha DB, Kileny PR, Esclamado RM (2001) Selective cricothyroid muscle reinnervation by muscle-nerve-muscle neurotization. Arch Otolaryngol Head Neck Surg 127: 1211–1215.

Enver MK, Hall SM (1994) Are Schwann cells essential for axonal regeneration into muscle autografts? Neuropathol Appl Neurobiol 20: 587–598.

Erlacher P (1915) Direct and muscular neurotization of paralyzed muscles. Am J Ortho Surg 13: 22–32.

Evans PJ, Midha R, Mackinnon SE (1994) The peripheral nerve allograft: a comprehensive review of regeneration and neuroimmunology. Prog Neurobiol 43: 187–201.

Evans PJ, Mackinnon SE, Levi ADO, Wade JA, Hunter DA, Nakao Y, Midha R (1998) Cold preserved nerve allografts: changes in basement membrane, viability, immunogenicity, and regeneration. Muscle Nerve 21: 1507–1522.

Evans PJ, Mackinnon SE, Midha R, Wade JA, Hunter DA, Nakao Y, Hare GM (1999) Regeneration across cold preserved peripheral nerve allografts. Microsurgery 19: 115–127.

Fansa H, Keilhoff G, Wolf G, Schneider W (2001) Tissue engineering of peripheral nerves: a comparison of venous and acellular muscle grafts with cultured Schwann cells. Plast Reconstr Surg 107: 485–494.

Fawcett JW, Keynes RJ (1986) Muscle basal lamina: a new graft material for peripheral nerve repair. J Neurosurg 65: 354–363.

Feneley MR, Fawcett JW, Keynes RJ (1991) The role of Schwann cells in the regeneration of peripheral nerve axons through muscle basal lamina grafts. Exp Neurol 114: 275–285.

Feng G, Mellor R, Bernstein M, Keller-Peck C, Nguyen QT, Wallace M, Nerbonne J, Lichtman J, Sanes J (2000) Imaging neuronal subsets in transgenic mice expressing multiple spectral variants of GFP. Neuron 28: 41–51.

Fields RD, Ellisman MH (1986a) Axons regenerated through silicone tube splices. I. Conduction Properties. Exp Neurol 92: 48–60.

Fields RD, Ellisman MH (1986b) Axons regenerated through silicone tube splices. II. Functional Morphology. Exp Neurol 92: 61–74.

Fine EG, Decosterd I, Papaloãzos M, Zurn AD, Aebischer P (2002) GDNF and NGF released by synthetic guidance channels support sciatic nerve regeneration across a long gap. Eur J Neurosci 15: 589–601.

Fish JS, Bain JR, McKee N, Mackinnon SE (1992) The peripheral nerve allograft in the primate immunosuppressed with cyclosporin A: II. Functional evaluation of reinnervated muscle. Plast Reconstr Surg 90: 1047–1052.

Foidart-Dessalle M, Dubuisson A, Lejeune A, Severyns A, Manassis Y, Delree P, Crielaard JM, Bassleer R, Lejeune G (1997) Sciatic nerve regeneration through venous or nervous grafts in the rat. Exp Neurol 148: 236–246.

Forssman J (1898) Ueber die Ursachen, welche die Wachstumsrichtung der peripheren Nervenfasern bei der Regeneration bestimmen. Beitr z pathol Anat 24: 56–100.

Fox DJ, Doolabh VB, Mackinnon SE, Genden EM, Hunter DA (1999) Decreased cyclosporin A requirement with anti-ICAM-1 and anti-LFA-1a in a peripheral nerve allotransplantation model. Restor Neurol Neurosci 15: 319–326.

Francel PC, Francel TJ, Mackinnon SE, Hertl C (1997) Enhancing nerve regeneration across a silicone tube conduit by using interposed short-segment nerve grafts. J Neurosurg 87: 887–892.

Frazier J, Yu L, Rhee E, Shaw L, LaRossa D, Rostami A (1993) Extended survival and function of peripheral nerve allografts after cessation of long-term cyclosporin administration in rats. J Hand Surg [Am] 18A: 100–106.

Frey M, Gruber H, Holle J, Freilinger G (1982) An experimental comparison of the different kinds of muscle reinnervation: nerve suture, nerve implantation, and muscular neurotization. Plast Reconstr Surg 69: 656–667.

Fukuda A, Hirata H, Akeda K, Morita A, Nagakura T, Tsujii M, Uchida A (2005) Enhanced reinnervation after neurotization with Schwann cell transplantation. Muscle Nerve 31: 229–234.

Gash DM, Zhang ZM, Gerhardt G (1998) Neuroprotective and neurorestorative properties of GDNF. Ann Neurol 44 Suppl. 1: S121–S125.

Genden EM, Mackinnon SE, Yu S, Flye MW (1998) Induction of donor-specific tolerance to rat nerve allografts with portal venous donor alloantigen and anti-ICAM-1/LFA-1 monoclonal antibodies. Surgery 124: 448–456.

Genden EM, Mackinnon SE, Yu S, Hunter D, Flye MW (2001) Pretreatment with portal venous ultraviolet B irradiated donor alloantigen promotes donor-specific tolerance to rat nerve allografts. The Laryngoscope 111: 439–447.

Gibson KL, Remson L, Smith A, Satterlee N, Strain GM, Daniloff JK (1991) Comparison

of nerve regeneration through different types of neural prostheses. Microsurgery 12: 80–85.

Gilmore SA (1971) Autoradiographic studies of intramedullary Schwann cells in irradiated spinal cords of immature rats. Anat Rec 171: 517–528.

Giovanoli P, Koller R, Meuli-Simmen C, Rab M, Haslik W, Mittlböck M, Meyer VE, Frey M (2000) Functional and morphometric evaluation of end-to-side neurorrhaphy for muscle reinnervation. Plast Reconstr Surg 106: 383–392.

Glasby MA, Gschmeissner G, Hitchcock RJ, Huang CL (1986a) The dependence of nerve regeneration through muscle grafts in the rat on the availability and orientation of basement membrane. J Neurocytol 15: 497–510.

Glasby MA, Gschmeissner SE, Huang C, de Souza BA (1986b) Degenerated muscle grafts used for peripheral nerve repair in primates. JBJS 11-B: 347–351.

Glasby MA (1990) Nerve growth in matrices of oriented muscle basement membrane: developing a new method of nerve repair. Clin Anat 3: 161–182.

Glasby MA, Gilmour JA, Gschmeissner SE, Hems TE, Myles LM (1990) The repair of large peripheral nerves using skeletal muscle autografts: a comparison with cable grafts in the sheep femoral nerve. Brit J Plas Surg 43: 169–178.

Goheen-Robillard B, Myckatyn TM, Mackinnon SE, Hunter DA (2002) End-to-side neurorrhaphy and lateral axonal sprouting in a long graft rat model. Laryngoscope 112: 899–905.

Gold BG, Storm-Dickerson T, Austin DR (1994) The immunosuppressant FK506 increases functional recovery and nerve regeneration following peripheral nerve injury. Restor Neurol and Neurosci 6: 287–296.

Golding J, Shewan D, Cohen J (1997) Maturation of the mammalian dorsal root entry zone: from entry to no entry. Trends Neurosci 20: 303–308.

Gomez N, Cuadras J, Butí M, Navarro X (1996) Histologic assessment of sciatic nerve regeneration following resection and graft or tube repair in the mouse. Restor Neurol Neurosci 10: 187–196.

Grand AG, Myckatyn TM, Mackinnon SE, Hunter DA (2002) Axonal regeneration after cold preservation of nerve allografts and immunosuppression with tacrolimus in mice. J Neurosurg 96: 924–932.

Graziadei P, Monti Graziadei G (1980) Neurogenesis and neuron regeneration in the olfactory system of mammals. III. Deafferentation and reinnervation of the olfactory bulb following section of the filia olfactoria in rat. J Neurocytol 9: 145–162.

Gschmeissner SE, Gattuso JM, Glasby MA (1990) Morphology of nerve fibers regenerating through freeze-thawed autogenous skeletal muscle grafts in rats. Clin Anat 3: 107–119.

Gu H-Y, Chai H, Yao Z-B, Zhou L-H, Wong W-M, Bruce I, Wu W-T (2004) Survival, regeneration and functional recovery of motoneurons in adult rats by reimplantation of ventral spinal root following spinal root avulsion. Eur J Neurosci 19: 2123–2131.

Gu HY, Chai H, Zhang JY, Yao ZB, Zhou LH, Wong WM, Bruce IC, Wu WT (2005) Survival, regeneration and functional recovery of motoneurons after delayed reimplantation of avulsed spinal root in adult rat. Exp Neurol 192: 89–99.

Gu YD, Chen DS, Zhang GM (1998) Long term functional results of contralateral C7 transfer. J Recon Micro 14: 57–59.

Guenard V, Kleitman N, Morrissey T, Bunge R, Aebischer P (1992) Syngeneic Schwann cells derived from adult nerves seeded in semipermeable guidance channels enhance peripheral nerve regeneration. J Neurosci 12: 3310–3320.

Gulati AK (1988) Evaluation of acellular and cellular nerve grafts in repair of rat peripheral nerve. J Neurosurg 68: 117–123.

Gulati AK, Cole GP (1994) Immunogenicity and regenerative potential of acellular nerve allografts to repair peripheral nerves in rats and rabbits. Acta Neurochir 126: 158–164.

Gulati AK, Rai DR, Ali AM (1995) The influence of cultured Schwann cells on regeneration through acellular basal lamina grafts. Brain Res 705: 118–124.

Guth L, Zalewski AA (1963) Disposition of cholinesterase following implantation of nerve into innervated and denervated muscle. Exp Neurol 7: 316–326.

Haase SC, Rovak JM, Dennis RG, Kuzon WM, Cederna PS (2003) Recovery of muscle contractile function following nerve gap repair with chemically acellularized peripheral nerve grafts. J Recon Micro 19: 241–248.

Haisheng H, Songjie Z, Xin L (2008) Assessment of nerve regeneration across nerve allografts treated with tacrolimus. Artif Cells Blood Substit Immobil Biotechnol 36: 465–474.

Hall S (1997) Axonal regeneration through acellular muscle grafts. J Anat 190: 57–71.

Hall SM (1986a) The effect of inhibiting Schwann cell mitosis on the reinnervation of acellular autografts in the peripheral nervous system of the mouse. Neuropathol Appl Neurobiol 12: 401–414.

Hall SM (1986b) Regeneration in cellular and acellular autografts in the peripheral nervous system. Neuropathol Appl Neurobiol 12: 27–46.

Hall SM, Enver K (1994) Axonal regeneration through heat pretreated muscle autografts. An immunohistochemical and electron microscopic study. J Hand Surg [Br] 19B: 444–451.

Hall SM, Kent AP (1996) An immuno-electronmicroscopical study of the distribution of laminin within autografts of denatured muscle. J Neurocytol 25: 209–217.

Hare GM, Evans PJ, Mackinnon SE, Nakao Y, Midha R, Wade JA, Hunter DA, Hay JB (1993) Effect of cold preservation on lymphocyte migration into peripheral nerve allografts in sheep. Transplantation 56: 154–162.

Hare GM, Evans PJ, Mackinnon SE, Wade JA, Young JA, Hay JB (1995) Phenotypic analysis of migrant, efferent lymphocytes after implantation of cold, preserved, peripheral nerve allografts. J Neuroimmunol 56: 9–16.

Harris R (1921) The treatment of irreparable nerve injuries. Can Med Assn J 11: 833–841.

Hasegawa J, Shibata M, Takahashi H (1996) Nerve coaptation studies with and without a gap in rabbits. J Hand Surg Am 21(2): 259–265.

Hayashi A, Yanai A, Komuro Y, Nishida M, Inoue M, Seki T (2004) Collateral sprouting occurs following end-to-side neurorrhaphy. Plast Reconstr Surg 114: 129–137.

Hayashi A, Pannucci C, Moradzadeh A, Kawamura D, Magill C, Hunter DA, Tong AY, Parsadanian A, Mackinnon SE, Myckatyn TM (2008) Axotomy or compression is required for axonal sprouting following end-to-side neurorrhaphy. Exp Neurol 211: 539–550.

He C, Chen Z, Chen Z (1992) Enhancement of motor nerve regeneration by nerve growth factor. Microsurgery 13: 151–154.

Heineke D (1914) Die directe enipflanzung des nerven in den muskel. Zentralbl Chir 41: 465–466.

Hems TE, Glasby MA (1992) Comparison of different methods of repair of long peripheral nerve defects: an experimental study. Brit J Plas Surg 45: 497–502.

Hems TEJ, Glasby MA (1993) The limit of graft length in the experimental use of muscle grafts for nerve repair. J Hand Surg [Br] 18B: 165–170.

Hertl MC, Strasberg SR, Mackinnon SE, Mohanakumar T, Hunter DA, Nyack LM, Miyasaka M (1996) The dose-related effect of monoclonal antibodies against adhesion molecules ICAM-1 and LFA-1 on peripheral nerve allograft rejection in a rat model. Restor Neurol Neurosci 10: 147–159.

Hess JR, Brenner MJ, Fox IK, Nichols CM, Myckatyn TM, Hunter D, Rickman SR, Mackinnon SE (2007) Use of cold-preserved allografts seeded with autologous Schwann cells in the treatment of a long-gap peripheral nerve injury. PRS 119: 246–259.

Ho S, Clipstone N, Timmermann L, Northrop J, Graef I, Fiorentino D, Nourse J, Crabtree GR (1996) The mechanism of action of cyclosporin A and FK506. Clin Immunol Immunopath 80: S40–S45.

Hoang TX, Havton LA (2006) A single re-implanted ventral root exerts neurotropic effects over multiple spinal cord segments in the adult rat. Exp Brain Res 169: 208–217.

Hoang TX, Nieto JH, Dobkin BH, Tillakaratne NJ, Havton LA (2006) Acute implantation of an avulsed lumbosacral ventral root into the rat conus medullaris promotes neuroprotection and graft reinnervation by autonomic and motor neurons. Neuroscience 138: 1149–1160.

Hoffman H (1951) A study of factors influencing innervation of muscles by implanted nerves. Aust NZ J Exp Biol Med 29: 289–307.

Hogikyan ND, Johns MM, Kileny PR, Urbanchek M, Carroll WR, Kuzon WM, Jr. (2001) Motion-specific laryngeal reinnervation using muscle-nerve-muscle neurotization. Ann Otol Rhinol Laryngol 110: 801–810.

Holmes W (1947) Histological observations on the repair of nerves by autografts. Brit J Surg 35: 167–173.

Hontanilla B, Auba C, Arcocha J, Gorria O (2006a) Nerve regeneration through nerve autografts and cold preserved allografts using tacrolimus (FK506) in a facial paralysis model: a topographical and neurophysiological study in monkeys. Neurosurgery 58: 768–779.

Hontanilla B, Yeste L, Auba C, Gorria O (2006b) Neuronal quantification in cold-preserved nerve allografts and treatment with FK-506 through osmotic pumps compared to nerve autografts. J Recon Micro 22: 363–374.

Hood B, Levene HB, Levi AD (2009) Transplantation of autologous Schwann cells for the repair of segmental peripheral nerve defects. Neurosurg Focus 26. DOI:10.3171/FOC.2009.26.2.E4.

Horvat JC, Pecot-Dechavassine M, Mira JC, Davarpanah Y (1989) Formation of functional endplates by spinal axons regenerating through a peripheral nerve graft: a study in the adult rat. Brain Res Bull 22: 103–114.

Hsu SP, Shih Y-H, Huang M-C, Chuang T-Y, Huang W-C, Wu H-M, Lin P-H, Lee L-S, Cheng H (2004) Repair of multiple cervical root avulsion with sural nerve graft. Injury 35: 896–907.

Htut M, Misra VP, Anand P, Birch R, Carlstedt T (2007) Motor recovery and the breathing arm after brachial plexus surgical repairs, including re-implantation of avulsed spinal roots into the spinal cord. J Hand Surg 32E: 170–178.

Hu J, Zhu Q-T, Liu X-L, Xu Y-B, Zhu J-K (2007) Repair of extended peripheral nerve lesions in rhesus monkeys using acellular allogenic nerve grafts implanted with autologous mesenchymal stem cells. Exp Neurol 204: 658–666.

Hudson AR, Morris J, Weddell G, Drury A (1972) Peripheral nerve autografts. J Surg Res 12: 267–274.

Ide C (1983) Nerve regeneration and Schwann cell basal lamina: Observations of the long-term regeneration. Arch Histol Jap 46: 243–257.

Ide C, Tohyama K, Yokota R, Nitatori T, Onodepa H (1983) Schwann cell basal lamina and nerve regeneration. Brain Res 288: 61–65.

Ide C (1984) Nerve regeneration through the basal lamina scaffold of the skeletal muscle. Nsci Res 1: 379–391.

Ide C, Tohyama K, Tajima K, Endoh K, Sano K, Tamura M, Mizoguchi A, Kitada M, Morihara T, Shirasu M (1998) Long acellular nerve transplants for allogeneic grafting and the effects of basic fibroblast growth factor on the growth of regenerating axons in dogs: a preliminary report. Exp Neurol 154: 99–112.

Ikeda K, Oda Y, Nakanishi I, Tomita K, Nomura S (1995) Cultured Schwann cells transplanted between nerve gaps promote nerve regeneration. Neuro Orthopaedics 11: 7–16.

Ishida O, Daves J, Tsai T-M, Breidenbach WC, Firrell J (1993) Regeneration following rejection of peripheral nerve allografts of rats on withdrawal of cyclosporine. Plast Reconstr Surg 92: 916–926.

Iwai M, Tamai S, Yajima H, Kawanishi K (2001) Experimental study of vascularized nerve graft: evaluation of nerve regeneration using choline acetyltransferase activity. Microsurgery 21: 43–51.

Jamieson AM, Eames RA (2003) Reimplantation of avulsed brachial plexus roots: an experimental study in dogs. Int J Microsurg 2: 75–85.

Jenq C-B, Coggeshall RE (1985a) Long-term patterns of axon regeneration in the sciatic nerve and its tributaries. Brain Res 345: 34–44.

Jenq C-B, Coggeshall RE (1985b) Nerve regeneration through holey silicone tubes. Brain Res 361: 233–241.

Jenq C-B, Coggeshall RE (1987) Nerve regeneration changes with filters of different pore size. Exp Neurol 97: 662–671.

Jerregård H, Nyberg T, Hildebrand C (2001) Sorting of regenerating rat sciatic nerve fibers with target-derived molecules. Exp Neurol 169: 298–306.

Jubran M, Widenfalk J (2003) Repair of peripheral nerve transections with fibrin sealant containing neurotrophic factors. Exp Neurol 181: 204–212.

Kalliainen LK, Cederna PS, Kuzon WM, Jr. (1999) Mechanical function of muscle reinnervated by end-to-side neurorrhaphy. Plast Reconstr Surg 103: 1919–1927.

Kanamaru A, Suzuki S, Sibuya M, Homma I, Sai K, Hara T (1993) Sensory reinnervation of muscle receptor in human. Neurosci Lett 161: 27–29.

Kanaya F, Firrell J, Tsai T-M, Breidenbach WC (1992) Functional results of vascularized versus nonvascularized nerve grafting. Plast Reconstr Surg 89: 924–930.

Kanje M, Arai T, Lundborg G (2000) Collateral sprouting from sensory and motor axons into an end to side attached nerve segment. Neuroreport 11: 2455–2459.

Kapur TA, Shoichet MS (2004) Immobilized concentration gradients of nerve growth factor guide neurite outgrowth. J Biomed Mater Res A 68: 235–243.

Katsube K, Doi K, Fukumoto T, Fujikura Y, Shigetomi M, Kawai S (1998) Successful nerve regeneration and persistence of donor cells after a limited course of immunosuppression in rat peripheral nerve allografts. Transplantation 66: 772–777.

Katz B, Miledi R (1964) The development of acetylcholine sensitivity in nerve-free segments of skeletal muscle. J Physiol 170: 389–396.

Kawabata H, Shibata T, Matsui Y, Yasui N (2001) Use of intercostal nerves for neurotization of the musculocutaneous nerve in infants with birth-related brachial plexus palsy. J Neurosurg 94: 386–391.

Kawai H, Baudrimont M, Travers V, Sedel L (1990) A comparative experimental study of vascularized and nonvascularized nerve grafts. J Recon Micro 6: 255–259.

Kayikcioglu A, Karamursel S, Agaoglu G, Kecik A, Celiker R, Cetin A (2000) End-to-side neurorrhaphies of the ulnar and median nerves at the wrist: Report of two cases without sensory or motor improvement. Ann Plas Surg 45: 641–643.

Keeley R, Atagi T, Sabelman E, Padilla J, Kadlcik P, Agras J, Eng L, Wiedman TW, Nguyen K, Sudekum A, Rosen J (1993) Synthetic nerve graft containing collagen and synthetic Schwann cells improves functional, electrophysiological, and histological parameters of peripheral nerve regeneration. Restor Neurol Neurosci 5: 353–366.

Keilhoff G, Fansa H (2005) Successful intramuscular neurotization is dependent on the denervation period. A histomorphological study of the gracilis muscle in rats. Muscle & Nerve 31: 221–228.

Kelly EJ, Jacoby C, Terenghi G, Mennen U, Ljungberg C, Wiberg M (2007) End-to-side nerve coaptation: a qualitative and quantitative assessment in the primate. J Plas Recon Aesth Surg 60: 1–12.

Kemp SW, Walsh SK, Zochodne DW, Midha R (2007) A novel method for establishing daily in vivo concentration gradients of soluble nerve growth factor (NGF). J Neurosci Methods 165: 83–88.

Kemp SW, Walsh SK, Midha R (2008) Growth factor and stem cell enhanced conduits in peripheral nerve regeneration and repair. Neurol Res 30: 1030–1038.

Kermer C, Millesi H, Paternostro T, Nuhr M, Sabbas A (2000) Experimental study of muscle-nerve-muscle neurotization. J Recon Micro 16: 569–572.

Kermer C, Millesi W, Paternostro T, Nuhr M (2001) Muscle-nerve-muscle neurotization of the orbicularis oris muscle. J Cranio Maxill Surg 29: 302–306.

Kerns JM, Danielsen N, Zhao Q, Lundborg G, Kanje M (2003) A comparison of peripheral nerve regeneration in acellular muscle and nerve autografts. Scand J Plas Reconstr Hand Surg 37: 193–200.

Keynes RJ, Hopkins WG, Huang C (1984) Regeneration of mouse peripheral nerves in degenerating skeletal muscle: guidance by residual muscle fibre basement membrane. Brain Res 295: 275–281.

Kim DH, Connolly SE, Kline DG, Voorhies RM, Smith A, Powell M, Yoes T, Daniloff JK (1994) Labeled Schwann cell transplants versus sural nerve grafts in nerve repair. J Neurosurg 80: 254–260.

Kim SM, Lee SK, Lee JH (2007) Peripheral nerve regeneration using a three dimensionally cultured schwann cell conduit. J Craniofac Surg 18: 475–488.

Kimata Y, Sakuraba M, Hishinuma S, Ebihara S, Hayashi R, Asakage T (2005) Free vascularized nerve grafting for immediate facial nerve reconstruction. Laryngoscope 115: 331–336.

Kingham PJ, Kalbermatten DF, Mahay D, Armstrong SJ, Wiberg M, Terenghi G (2007) Adipose-derived stem cells differentiate into a Schwann cell phenotype and promote neurite outgrowth in vitro. Exp Neurol 207: 267–274.

Kline DG (2000) Letter to the editor: spinal nerve root repair after brachial plexus injury. J Neurosurg Spine 93: 336–337.

Kostakoglu N (1999) Motor and sensory reinnervation in the hand after an end-to-side median to ulnar nerve coaptation in the forearm. Br J Plast Surg 52: 404–407.

Kozlova EN, Strömberg I, Bygdeman M, Aldskogius H (1995) Peripherally grafted human foetal dorsal root ganglion cells extend axons into the spinal cord of adult host rats by circumventing dorsal root entry zone astrocytes. Neuroreport 6: 269–272.

Kozlova EN, Seiger A, Aldskogius H (1997) Human dorsal root ganglion neurons from embryonic donors extend axons into the host rat spinal cord along laminin-rich peripheral surroundings of the dorsal root transitional zone. J Neurocytol 26: 811–822.

Krarup C, Archibald SJ, Madison RD (2002) Factors that influence peripheral nerve regeneration: an electrophysiological study of the monkey median nerve. Ann Neurol 51: 69–81.

Kvist M, Lemplesis V, Kanje M, Ekberg H, Corbascio M, Dahlin M (2007) Immunomodulation by costimulation blockade inhibits rejection of nerve allografts. JPNS 12: 83–90.

Lang EM, Asan E, Plesnila N, Hofmann GO, Sendtner M (2005a) Motoneuron survival after C7 nerve root avulsion and replantation in the adult rabbit: effects of local ciliary neurotrophic factor and brain-derived neurotrophic factor application. Plast Reconstr Surg 115: 2042–2050.

Lang EM, Schlegel N, Sendtner M, Asan E (2005b) Effects of root replantation and neurotrophic factor treatment on long-term motoneuron survival and axonal regeneration after C7 spinal root avulsion. Exp Neurol 194: 341–354.

Leechavengvongs S, Witoonchart K, Uerpairojkit C, Thuvasethakul P, Ketmalasiri W (1998) Nerve transfer to biceps muscle using a part of the ulnar nerve in brachial plexus injury (upper arm type): a report of 32 cases. J Hand Surg [Am] 23A: 711–716.

Lee AC, Yu VM, Lowe JB, III, Brenner MJ, Hunter DA, Mackinnon SE, Sakiyama-Elbert SE (2003) Controlled release of nerve growth factor enhances sciatic nerve regeneration. Exp Neurol 184: 295–303.

Lee YH, Shieh SJ (2008) Secondary nerve reconstruction using vein conduit grafts for neglected digital nerve injuries. Microsurgery 28: 436–440.

Leffert, R.D. (1985) Brachial Plexus Injuries, New York: Churchill Livingston.

Leong J, Hayes A, Austin L, Morrison W (1999) Muscle protection following motor nerve repair in combination with leukemia inhibitory factor. J Hand Surg [Am] 24A: 37–45.

Levi ADO, Evans PJ, Mackinnon SE, Bunge RP (1994a) Cold storage of peripheral nerves: an in vitro assay of cell viability and function. Glia 10: 121–131.

Levi ADO, Guenard V, Aebischer P, Bunge RP (1994b) The functional characteristics of Schwann cells cultured from human peripheral nerve after transplantation into a gap within the rat sciatic nerve. J Neurosci 14: 1309–1319.

Levi ADO, Sonntag VKH, Dickman C, Mather J, Li RH, Cordoba SC, Bichard B, Berens M (1997) The role of cultured Schwann cell grafts in the repair of gaps within the peripheral nervous system of primates. Exp Neurol 143: 25–36.

Levinsson A, Holmberg H, Schouenborg J, Seiger Å, Aldskogius H, Kozlova EN (2000) Functional connections are established in the deafferented rat spinal cord by peripherally transplanted human embryonic sensory neurons. Eur J Neurosci 12: 3589–3595.

Li Q, Ping P, Jiang H, Liu K (2006) Nerve conduit filled with GDNF gene-modified Schwann cells enhances regeneration of the peripheral nerve. Microsurgery 26: 116–121.

Li Y, Carlstedt T, Berthold CH, Raisman G (2004) Interaction of transplanted olfactory-ensheathing cells and host astrocytic processes provides a bridge for axons to regenerate across the dorsal root entry zone. Exp Neurol 188: 300–308.

Li Y, Yamamoto M, Raisman G, Choi D, Carlstedt T (2007) An experimental model of ventral root repair showing the beneficial effect of transplanting olfactory ensheathing cells. Neurosurgery 60: 734–741.

Lind R, Wood M (1986) Comparison of the pattern of early revascularization of conventional versus vascularized nerve grafts in the canine. Recon Micro 2: 229–232.

Liu HM (1992) The role of extracellular matrix in peripheral nerve regeneration: a wound chamber study. Acta Neuropathol (Berl) 83: 469–474.

Liu K, Chen LE, Seaber AV, Goldner RV, Urbaniak JR (1999) Motor functional and morphological findings following end-to-side neurorrhaphy in the rat model. J Orthop Res 17: 293–300.

Liu S, Bohl D, Blanchard S, Bacci J, Said G, Heard JM (2009) Combination of microsurgery and gene therapy for spinal dorsal root injury repair. Mol Ther 17: 992–1002.

Liu Z, Sun YK, Xi YP, Maffei A, Reed E, Harris P, Suciu-Foca N (1993) Contribution of direct and indirect recognition pathways to T cell alloreactivity. J Exp Med 177: 1643–1650.

Lohmeyer JA, Shen ZL, Walter GF, Berger A (2007) Bridging extended nerve defects with an artificial nerve graft containing Schwann cells pre-seeded on polyglactin filaments. Int J Artif Organs 30: 64–74.

Lohmeyer JA, Siemers F, Machens HG, Mailander P (2009) The clinical use of artificial nerve conduits for digital nerve repair: a prospective cohort study and literature review. J Reconstr Microsurg 25: 55–61.

Lomo T, Slater CR (1980) Acetylcholine sensitivity of developing ectopic nerve-muscle junctions in adult rat soleus muscles. J Physiol 303: 173–189.

Longo FM, Manthorpe M, Skaper SD, Lundborg G, Varon S (1983a) Neuronotrophic activities accumulate in vivo within silicone nerve regeneration chambers. Brain Res 261: 109–117.

Longo FM, Skaper SD, Manthorpe M, Williams LR, Lundborg G, Varon S (1983b) Temporal changes in neuronotrophic activities accumulating in vivo within nerve regeneration chambers. Exp Neurol 81: 756–769.

Longo FM, Hayman EG, Davis GE, Ruoslahti E, Engvall E, Manthorpe M, Varon S (1984) Neurite-promoting factors and extracellular matrix components accumulating in vivo within nerve regeneration chambers. Brain Res 309: 105–117.

Lundborg G, Rydevik B (1973) Effects of stretching the tibial nerve of the rabbit: a preliminary study of the intraneural circulation and the barrier function of the perineurium. JBJS 5B: 390–401.

Lundborg G, Hansson H-H (1979) Regeneration of peripheral nerve through a preformed tissue space: preliminary observations on the reorganization of regenerating nerve fibers and perineurium. Brain Res 178: 573–576.

Lundborg G, Dahlin L, Danielsen N, Hansson H, Larsson K (1981) Reorganization and orientation of regenerating nerve fibers, perineurium, and epineurium in preformed mesothelial tubes: an experimental study on the sciatic nerve of rats. J Neurosci Res 6: 265–281.

Lundborg G, Dahlin L, Danielsen N, Gelberman R, Longo F, Powell H, Varon S (1982a) Nerve regeneration in silicon chambers: influence of gap length and of distal stump components. Exp Neurol 76: 361–375.

Lundborg G, Gelberman R, Longo F, Powell H, Varon S (1982b) In vivo regeneration of cut nerve encased in silicon tubes. J Neuropath & Exp Neurol 41: 412–422.

Lundborg G, Longo FM, Varon S (1982c) Nerve regeneration model and trophic factors in vivo. Brain Res 232: 157–161.

Lundborg G, Zhao Q, Kanje M, Danielsen N, Kerns JM (1994) Can sensory and motor collateral sprouting be induced from intact peripheral nerve by end-to-side anastomosis? J Hand Surg [Br] 19B: 277–282.

Lundborg G, Rosén B, Dahlin L, Danielsen N, Holmberg J (1997) Tubular versus conventional repair of median and ulnar nerves in the human forearm: early results from a prospective, randomized, clinical study. J Hand Surg [Am] 22A: 99–106.

Lundborg G (2000) A 25-year perspective of peripheral nerve surgery: evolving neuroscientific concepts and clinical significance. J Hand Surg [Am] 25A: 391–414.

Lundborg G, Rosén B, Dahlin L, Holmberg J, Rosén I (2004) Tubular repair of the median or ulnar nerve in the human forearm: a 5-year follow-up. J Hand Surg [Br Eur] 29B: 100–107.

Lutz BS, Chuang DCC, Hsu JC, Ma SF, Wei FC (2000a) Selection of donor nerves: an important factor in end-to-side neurorrhaphy. Br J Plast Surg 53: 149–154.

Lutz BS, Ma S-F, Chuang D, Wei F-C (2000b) Role of the target in end-to-side neurorrhaphy: reinnervation of a single muscle vs. multiple muscles. J Recon Micro 16: 443–448.

Lux P, Breidenbach W, Firrell J (1988) Determination of temporal changes in blood flow in vascularized and nonvascularized nerve grafts in the dog. PRS 82: 133–142.

Lykissas MG, Sakellariou E, Vekris MD, Kontogeorgakos VA, Batistatou AK, Mitsionis GI, Beris AE (2007) Axonal regeneration stimulated by erythropoietin: an experimental study in rats. J Neurosci Methods 164: 107–115.

Maccabruni F (1911) Der degenerationsprogress der nerven bei homoplastischen und heteroplastischen pfropfungen. Folia Neurobiol, Leipz 5: 598–601.

Mackinnon SE, Dellon AL, Hudson AR, Hunter DA (1984a) Chronic nerve compression-an experimental model in the rat. Ann Plas Surg 13: 112–120.

Mackinnon SE, Hudson AR, Falk RE, Kline D, Hunter DA (1984b) Peripheral nerve allograft: an assessment of regeneration across pretreated nerve allografts. Neurosurgery 15: 690–693.

Mackinnon SE, Dellon AL, Hudson AR, Hunter DA (1985a) Nerve regeneration through a pseudosynovial sheath in a primate model. PRS 75: 833–839.

Mackinnon SE, Hudson AR, Falk RE, Hunter DA (1985b) The nerve allograft response-an experimental model in the rat. Ann Plas Surg 14: 334–339.

Mackinnon SE, Dellon AL (1988) A comparison of nerve regeneration across a sural nerve graft and a vascularized pseudosheath. J Hand Surg 13A: 935–942.

Mackinnon SE, Dellon AL (1990) A study of nerve regeneration across synthetic (Maxon) and biologic (collagen) nerve conduits for nerve gaps up to 5cm in the primate. J Recon Micro 6: 117–121.

Mackinnon SE, Dellon AL (1991) Clinical nerve reconstruction with a bioabsorbable polyglycolic acid tube. Plast Reconstr Surg 85: 419–424.

Mackinnon SE, Doolabh VB, Novak C, Trulock EP (2001) Clinical outcome following nerve allograft transplantation. Plast Reconstr Surg 107: 1419–1429.

Mackinnon SE, Novak CB, Myckatyn TM, Tung TH (2005) Results of reinnervation of the biceps and brachialis muscles with a double fascicular transfer for elbow flexion. J Hand Surg [Am] 30A: 978–985.

Madison RD, Archibald SJ, Lacin R, Krarup C (1999) Factors contributing to preferential motor reinnervation in the primate peripheral nervous system. J Neurosci 19: 11007–11016.

Malessy MJA, Van Dijk JG, Thomeer RT (1993) Respiration-related activity in the biceps brachii muscle after intercostal-musculocutaneous nerve transfer. Clin Neurol Nsurg 95(Suppl.): S95–S102.

Mani GV, Shurey C, Green CJ (1992) Is early vascularization of nerve grafts necessary? J Hand Surg 17B: 536–543.

Marchesi C, Pluderi M, Colleoni F, Belicchi M, Meregalli M, Farini A, Parolini D, Draghi L, Fruguglietti ME, Gavina M, Porretti L, Cattaneo A, Battistelli M, Prelle A, Moggio M, Borsa S, Bello L, Spagnoli D, Gaini SM, Tanzi MC, Bresolin N, Grimoldi N, Torrente Y (2007) Skin-derived stem cells transplanted into resorbable guides provide functional nerve regeneration after sciatic nerve resection. Glia 55: 425–438.

Matsuda K, Kakibuchi M, Fukuda K, Kubo T, Madura T, Kawai K, Yano K, Hosokawa K (2005) End-to-side nerve grafts: experimental study in rats. J Reconstr Microsurg 21: 581–591.

McCallister WV, Tang P, Trumble T (1999) Is end-to-side neurorrhaphy effective? A study of axonal sprouting stimulated from intact nerves. J Recon Micro 15: 597–604.

McCallister WV, Tang P, Smith J, Trumble TE (2001) Axonal regeneration stimulated by the combination of nerve growth factor and ciliary neurotrophic factor in an end-to-side model. J Hand Surg [Am] 26A: 478–488.

McCollough CJ, Gagey O, Higginson DW, Sandin BM, Crow JC, Sebille A (1984) Axon regeneration and vascularization of nerve grafts: an experimental study. J Hand Surg 9-B: 323–327.

McDonald D, Cheng C, Chen Y, Zochodne D (2006) Early events of peripheral nerve regeneration. Neuron Glia Biol 2: 139–147.

McKenzie IA, Biernaskie J, Toma JG, Midha R, Miller FD (2006) Skin-derived precursors generate myelinating Schwann cells for the injured and dysmyelinated nervous system. J Neurosci 26: 6651–6660.

McKerracher L, David S, Jackson DL, Kottis V, Dunn RJ, Braun PE (1994) Identification of myelin-associated glycoprotein as a major myelin-derived inhibitor of neurite growth. Neuron 13: 805–811.

McNamara MJ, Garrett WE, Seaber AV, Goldner JL (1987) Neurorrhaphy, nerve grafting, and neurotization: a functional comparison of nerve reconstruction techniques. J Hand Surg 12A: 354–360.

McPhail LT, Plunet WT, Das P, Ramer MS (2005) The astrocytic barrier to axonal regeneration at the dorsal root entry zone is induced by rhizotomy. Eur J Neurosci 21: 267–270.

Meals R, Nelissen RG (1995) The origin and meaning of "neurotization." J Hand Surg 20A: 144–146.

Mears S, Schachner M, Brushart TM (2003) Antibodies to myelin-associated glycoprotein accelerate preferential motor reinnervation. JPNS 8: 91–99.

Medawar PB (1944) The behavior and fate of skin autografts and skin homografts in rabbits. J Anat 78: 176.

Meek MF, Den Dunnen WFA, Schakenraad JM, Robinson PH (1999) Evaluation of several techniques to modify denatured muscle tissue to obtain a scaffold for peripheral nerve regeneration. Biomaterials 20: 401–408.

Menderes A, Yilmaz M, Vayvada H, Ozer E, Barutcu A (2002) Effects of nerve growth factor on the neurotization of denervated muscles. Ann Plas Surg 48: 415–422.

Mennen U (1998) End-to-side nerve suture in the human patient. Hand Surgery 3: 7–15.

Mennen U (2003) End-to-side nerve suture in clinical practice. Hand Surgery 8: 33–42.

Merle M, Dellon AL, Campbell JN, Chang PS (1989) Complications from silicon-polymer intubulation of nerves. Microsurgery 10: 130–133.

Merle M, Dautel G (1991) Vascularized nerve grafts. J Hand Surg 16B: 483–488.

Merrell GA, Barrie KA, Katz DL, Wolfe SW (2001) Results of nerve transfer techniques for restoration of shoulder and elbow function in the context of a meta-analysis of the English literature. J Hand Surg[Am] 26A:303–314.

Midha R, Mackinnon SE, Evans PJ, Best TJ, Hare GMT, Hunter DA, Falk-Wade JA (1993) Comparison of regeneration across nerve allografts with temporary or continuous cyclosporin A immunosuppression. J Neurosurg 78: 90–100.

Midha R, Mackinnon SE, Becker LE (1994a) The fate of Schwann cells in peripheral nerve allografts. J Neuropathol Exp Neurol 53: 316–322.

Midha R, Mackinnon SE, Evans PJ, Hunter DA, Becker LE (1994b) Rejection and regeneration through peripheral nerve allografts: immu-noperoxidase studies with laminin, S100 protein and neurofilament antisera. Restor Neurol Neurosci 7: 45–57.

Midha R, Munro CA, Mackinnon SE, Ang LC (1997) Motor and sensory specificity of host nerve axons influence nerve allograft rejection. J Neuropathol Exp Neurol 56: 421–434.

Midha R, Munro CA, Ang LC (1998) End-organ reinnervation does not prevent axonal degeneration in nerve allografts following immunosuppression withdrawal. Restor Neurol Neurosci 13: 163–172.

Midha R, Nag S, Munro CA, Ang LC (2001) Differential response of sensory and motor axons in nerve allografts after withdrawal of immuno-suppressive therapy. J Neurosurg 94: 102–110.

Miledi R (1960) The acetylcholine sensitivity of frog muscle after complete or partial denervation. J Physiol 151: 1–23.

Miledi R (1962) Induced innervation of end plate-free muscle segments. Nature 193: 281–282.

Millesi, H. and L.R. Walzer (1985) Muscular neurotization. In: 2nd Vienna Muscle Symposium, G. Freilinger, ed., pp. 149–154, Vienna: Facultas Wien.

Millesi H, Schmidhammer R (2008) Nerve fiber transfer by end-to-side coaptation. Hand Clin 24: 461–483, vii.

Moore AM, Kasukurthi R, Magill CK, Farhadi HF, Borschel GH, Mackinnon SE (2009) Limitations of conduits in peripheral nerve repairs. Hand (NY) 4: 180–186.

Morrissey T, Kleitman N, Bunge R (1991) Isolation and functional characterization of Schwann cells derived from adult peripheral nerve. J Neurosci 11: 3398–3411.

Mosahebi A, Woodward B, Wiberg M, Martin R, Terenghi G (2001) Retroviral labeling of Schwann cells: In vitro characterization and in vivo transplantation to improve peripheral nerve regeneration. Glia 34: 8–17.

Mukhopadhyay G, Doherty P, Walsh FS, Crocker PR, Filbin MT (1994) A novel role for myelin-associated glycoprotein as an inhibitor of axonal regeneration. Neuron 13: 757–767.

Mungara AK, Brown DL, Bishop DK, Wood SY, Cederna PS (2008) Anti-CD40L monoclonal antibody treatment induces long-term, tissue-specific, immunologic hyporesponsiveness to peripheral nerve allografts. J Reconstr Microsurg 24: 189–195.

Murakami T, Fujimoto Y, Yasunaga Y, Ishida O, Tanaka N, Ikuta Y, Ochi M (2003) Transplanted neuronal progenitor cells in a peripheral nerve gap promote nerve repair. Brain Res 974: 17–24.

Myckatyn TM, Mackinnon SE (2004) A review of research endeavors to optimize peripheral nerve reconstruction. Neurol Res 26: 124–138.

Nadim W, Anderson PN, Turmaine M (1990) The role of Schwann cells and basal lamina tubes in the regeneration of axons through long lengths of freeze-killed nerve grafts. Neuropathol Appl Neurobiol 16: 411–421.

Nagano A, Tsuyama N, Ochiai N, Hara T, Takahashi M (1989) Direct nerve crossing with the intercostal nerve to treat avulsion injuries of the brachial plexus. J Hand Surg 14A: 980–985.

Nageotte, J. (1922) L'organisation de la matiere dans ses rapports avec la vie, Paris: Felix Alcan.

Nakao Y, Mackinnon S, Strasberg SR, Hertl MC, Isobe M, Susskind BM, Mohanakumar T, Hunter D (1995a) Immunosuppressive effect of monoclonal antibodies to ICAM-1 and LFA-1 on peripheral nerve allograft in mice. Microsurgery 16: 612–620.

Nakao Y, Mackinnon SE, Hertl MC, Miyasaka M, Hunter DA, Mohanakumar T (1995b) Monoclonal antibodies against ICAM-1 and LFA-1 prolong nerve allograft survival. Muscle & Nerve 18: 93–102.

Nath RK, Lyons AB, Bietz G (2006) Physiological and clinical advantages of median nerve fascicle transfer to the musculocutaneous nerve following brachial plexus root avulsion injury. J Neurosurg 105: 830–834.

Navarro X, Valero A, Gudiño G, Forés J, Rodríguez FJ, Verdú E, Pascual R, Cuadras J, Nieto-Sampedro M (1999) Ensheathing glia transplants promote dorsal root regeneration and spinal reflex restitution after multiple lumbar rhizotomy. Ann Neurol 45: 207–215.

Navarro X, Udina E, Ceballos D, Gold BG (2001) Effects of FK506 on nerve regeneration and reinnervation after graft or tube repair of long nerve gaps. Muscle & Nerve 24: 905–915.

Neto HS, Pertille A, Teodori RM, Somazz MC, Marques MJ (2004) Primary nerve repair by muscle autografts prepared with local anesthetic. Microsurgery 188–193.

Neubauer D, Graham JB, Muir D (2007) Chondroitinase treatment increases the effective length of acellular nerve grafts. Exp Neurol 207: 163–170.

Neumann S, Bradke F, Tessier-Lavigne M, Basbaum AI (2002) Regeneration of sensory axons within the injured spinal cord induced by intraganglionic cAMP elevation. Neuron 34: 885–893.

Nie X, Zhang YJ, Tian WD, Jiang M, Dong R, Chen JW, Jin Y (2007) Improvement of peripheral nerve regeneration by a tissue-engineered nerve filled with ectomesenchymal stem cells. Int J Oral Maxillofac Surg 36: 32–38.

Nishiura Y, Brandt J, Nilsson A, Kanje M, Dahlin LB (2004) Addition of cultured Schwann cells to tendon autografts and freeze-thawed muscle grafts improves peripheral nerve regeneration. Tissue Eng 10: 157–164.

Noah EM, Williams A, Fortes W, Terzis JK (1997a) A new animal model to investigate axonal sprouting after end-to-side neurorrhaphy. J Recon Micro 13: 317–325.

Noah EM, Williams A, Jorgenson C, Skoulis TG, Terzis J (1997b) End-to-side neurorrhaphy: a histologic and morphometric study of axonal sprouting into an end-to-side nerve graft. J Recon Micro 13: 99–106.

Nogueira MP, Paley D, Bhave A, Herbert A, Nocente C, Herzenberg JF (2003) Nerve lesions associated with limb-lengthening. JBJS 85: 1502–1510.

Norris RW, Glasby MA, Gattuso JM, Bowden RE (1988) Peripheral nerve repair in humans using muscle autografts. JBJS 70-B: 530–533.

Novak CB, Mackinnon SE, Tung THH (2002) Patient outcome following a thoracodorsal to musculocutaneous nerve transfer for reconstruction of elbow flexion. Br J Plast Surg 55: 416–419.

Oblinger MM, Lasek RJ (1984) A conditioning lesion of the peripheral axons of dorsal root ganglion cells accelerates regeneration of only their peripheral axons. J Neurosci 4: 1736–1744.

Ochi M, Adachi N, Dohi D, Amano K, Masuda Y, Sawai T, Bashuda H, Okumura K (1998) Improvement in nerve regeneration by monoclonal antibodies to ICAM-1 and LFA-1 in allogeneic mice. Scand J Plast Reconstr Surg Hand Surg 32: 373–380.

Ogun TC, Ozdemir M, Senaran H, Ustun M (2003) End-to-side neurorrhaphy as a salvage procedure for irreparable nerve injuries. J Neurosurg 99: 180–185.

Osawa T, Tohyama K, Ide C (1990) Allogenic nerve grafts in the rat, with special reference to the role of Schwann cell basal laminae in nerve regeneration. J Neurocytol 19: 833–849.

Ozkan T, Ozer K, Gulgonen A (2001) Restoration of sensibility in irreparable ulnar and median nerve lesions with use of sensory nerve transfer: long-term follow-up of 20 cases. J Hand Surg 26A: 44–51.

Papakonstantinou KC, Terzis JK, Kamin E, Luka J (2005) Early effect of gene therapy on a direct muscle neurotization model. J Recon Micro 21: 383–389.

Papaloïzos MY, Holmquist B, Lundborg G (1997) An experimental study of nerve grafting combined with silicone tubes in the rat model: functional outcome and specificity of muscle reinnervation. Restor Neurol Neurosci 11: 161–168.

Patel M, Mao L, Wu B, Vandevord PJ (2007) GDNF-chitosan blended nerve guides: a functional study. J Tissue Eng Regen Med 1: 360–367.

Payne SH, Brushart TM (1997) Neurotization of the rat soleus muscle: a quantitative analysis of reinnervation. J Hand Surg 22A: 640–643.

Penkert G, Bini W, Samii M (1988) Revascularization of nerve grafts: an experimental study. J Recon Micro 4: 319–325.

Pereira JH, Bowden RE, Gattuso JM, Norris RW (1991) Comparison of results of repair of digital nerves by denatured muscle grafts and end-to-end sutures. JBJS 16B: 519–523.

Perkins CS, Carlstedt T, Mizuno K, Aguayo AJ (1980) Failure of regenerating dorsal root axons to regrow into the spinal cord. Can J Neurol Sci 7: 323.

Pfister BJ, Iwata A, Meaney DF, Smith DH (2004) Extreme stretch growth of integrated axons. J Neurosci 24: 7978–7983.

Pfister BJ, Bonislawski DP, Smith DH, Cohen AS (2006a) Stretch-grown axons retain the ability to transmit active electrical signals. FEBS Letters 580: 3525–3531.

Pfister BJ, Iwata A, Taylor AG, Wolf JA, Meaney DF, Smith DH (2006b) Development of transplantable nervous tissue constructs comprised of stretch-grown axons. J Neurosci Methods 153: 95–103.

Pfister BJ, Huang JH, Kameswaran N, Zager E, Smith DH (2007) Neural engineering to produce in vitro nerve constructs and neurointerface. Neurosurgery 60: 137–141.

Pienaar C, Swan MC, De Jager W, Solomons M (2004) Clinical experience with end-to-side nerve transfer. J Hand Surg 5: 438–443.

Piotrowicz A, Shoichet MS (2006) Nerve guidance channels as drug delivery vehicles. Biomaterials 27: 2018–2027.

Piquilloud G, Christen T, Pfister LA, Gander B, Papaloizos MY (2007) Variations in glial cell line-derived neurotrophic factor release from biodegradable nerve conduits modify the rate of functional motor recovery after rat primary nerve repairs. Eur J Neurosci 26: 1109–1117.

Podhajsky RJ, Myers RR (1994) The vascular response to nerve transection: neovascularization in the silicone nerve regeneration chamber. Brain Res 662: 88–94.

Pollard JD, McLeod JG (1981) Fresh and predegenerate nerve allografts and isografts in trembler mice. Muscle & Nerve 4: 274–281.

Prpa B, Huddleston PM, An K-N, Wood M (2002) Revascularization of nerve grafts: a qualitative and quantitative study of the soft tissue bed contributions to blood flow in canine nerve grafts. J Hand Surg 27A: 1041–1047.

Qiu J, Cai CM, Dai HN, McAtee M, Hoffman PN, Bregman BS, Filbin MT (2002) Spinal axon regeneration induced by elevation of cyclic AMP. Neuron 34: 895–903.

Quaglia X, Beggah AT, Seidenbecher C, Zurn AD (2008) Delayed priming promotes CNS regeneration post-rhizotomy in neurocan and brevican-deficient mice. Brain 131: 240–249.

Ramer MS, Priestley JV, McMahon SB (2000) Functional regeneration of sensory axone into the adult spinal cord. Nature 403: 312–316.

Ramer MS, Duraisingam I, Priestley JV, McMahon SB (2001) Two-tiered inhibition of axon regeneration at the dorsal root entry zone. J Neurosci 21: 2651–2660.

Ramon y Cajal, S. (1928) *Degeneration and Regeneration of the Nervous System*, London: Oxford University Press.

Ramon-Cueto A, Nieto-Sampedro M (1994) Regeneration into the spinal cord of transected dorsal root axons is promoted by ensheathing glia. Exp Neurol 127: 232–244.

Rende M, Granato A, Lo Monaco M, Zelano G, Toesca A (1991) Accuracy of reinnervation by peripheral nerve axons regenerating across a 10-mm gap within an impermeable chamber. Exp Neurol 111: 332–339.

Rich K, Alexander T, Pryor J, Hollowell J (1989) Nerve growth factor enhances regeneration through silicon chambers. Exp Neurol 105: 162–170.

Richardson PM, McGuiness UM, Aguayo AJ (1980) Axons from CNS neurones regenerate into PNS grafts. Nature 284: 264–265.

Richardson PM, Verge VMK (1987) Axonal regeneration in dorsal spinal roots is accelerated by peripheral axonal transection. Brain Res 411: 406–408.

Risling M, Cullheim S, Hildebrand C (1983) Reinnervation of the ventral root L7 from ventral horn neurons following intramedullary axotomy in adult cats. Brain Res 280: 15–23.

Roganovic Z, Ilic S, Savic M (2007) Radial nerve repair using autologous denatured muscle graft: comparison with outcomes of nerve graft repair. Acta Neurochir 149: 1033–1039.

Romano VM, Blair SJ, Kerns JM, Wurster RD (1991) Comparison of fibrin glue, bioresorbable tubing and sutures in peripheral nerve repair. Restor Neurol Neurosci 3: 75–80.

Romero MI, Rangappa N, Garry MG, Smith GM (2001) Functional regeneration of chronically injured sensory afferents into adult spinal cord after neurotrophin gene therapy. J Neurosci 21: 8408–8416.

Rosario CM, Aldskogius H, Carlstedt T, Sidman RL (1993) Differentiation and axonal outgrowth pattern of fetal dorsal root ganglion cells orthotopically allografted into adult rats. Exp Neurol 120: 16–31.

Rosario CM, Dubovy P, Sidman RL, Aldskogius H (1995) Peripheral target reinnervation following orthotopic grafting of fetal allogeneic and xenogeneic dorsal root ganglia. Exp Neurol 132: 251–261.

Rose, EH, Kowalski TA (1985) Restoration of sensibility to anaesthetic scarred digits with free vascularized nerve grafts from the dorsum of the foot. J Hand Surg 10A:514–512.

Rose EH, Kowalski TA, Norris MS (1989) The reversed venous arterialized nerve graft in digital nerve reconstruction across scarred beds. PRS 83: 593–602.

Rovak JM, Cederna PS, Macionis V, Urbanchek MS, Van der Meulen JH, Kuzon WM (2000) Termino-lateral neurorrhaphy: the functional axonal anatomy. Microsurgery 20: 6–14.

Rovak JM, Cederna PS, Kuzon W (2001) Terminolateral neurorrhaphy: A review of the literature. J Recon Micro 17: 615–624.

Samal F, Haninec P, Raska O, Dubovy P (2006) Quantitative assessment of the ability of collateral sprouting of the motor and primary sensory neurons after the end-to-side neurorrhaphy of the rat musculocutaneous nerve with the ulnar nerve. Ann Anat 188: 337–344.

Samardzic M, Grujicic D, Rasulic L, Bacetic D (2002) Transfer of the medial pectoral nerve: myth or reality? Neurosurgery 50: 1277–1282.

Samardzic MM, Grujicic DM, Rasulic LG, Milicic BR (2005) The use of thoracodorsal nerve transfer in restoration of irreparable C5 and C6 spinal nerve lesions. Br J Plast Surg 58: 541–546.

Sananpanich K, Morrison W, Messina A (2002) Physiologic and morphologic aspects of nerve regeneration after end-to-side coaptation in a rat model of brachial plexus injury. J Hand Surg 27A: 133–142.

Sananpanich K, Galea M, Morrison W, Messina A (2007) Quantitative characterization of regenerating axons after end-to-side and end-to-end coaptation in a rat brachial plexus model: a retrograde tracer study. J Neurotrauma 24: 864–875.

Sanders FK, Young JZ (1942) The degeneration and re-innervation of grafted nerves. J Anat 76: 143–170.

Sanes JR, Marshall LM, McMahan UJ (1978) Reinnervation of muscle fiber basal lamina after removal of myofibers. J Cell Biol 78: 176–198.

Santo Neto H, Teodori RM, Somazz MC, Marques MJ (1998) Axonal regeneration through muscle autografts submitted to local anaesthetic pretreatment. Br J Plast Surg 51: 555–560.

Schafer M, Fruttiger M, Montag D, Schachner M, Martini R (1996) Disruption of the gene for the myelin-associated glycoprotein improves axonal regrowth along myelin in C57BL/Wld mice. Neuron 16: 1107–1113.

Scharpf J, Strome M, Siemionow M (2006) Immunomodulation with anti-∂b T-cell receptor monoclonal antibodies in combination with cyclosporine A improves regeneration in nerve allografts. Microsurgery 26: 599–607.

Schmidhammer R, Nogradi A, Szabo A, Redl H, Hausner T, van der Nest DG, Millesi H (2009) Synergistic motor nerve fiber transfer between different nerves through the use of end-to-side coaptation. Exp Neurol 217: 388–394.

Schreyer DJ, Pate Skene JH (1993) Injury-associated induction of GAP-43 expression displays axon branch specificity in rat dorsal root ganglion neurons. J Neurobiol 24: 959–970.

Seckel BR, Ryan S, Simons J, Gagne R, Watkins E (1986) Vascularized versus nonvascularized nerve grafts: an experimental structural comparison. PRS 78: 211–220.

Seddon H (1963) Nerve grafting. JBJS 45B: 447–461.

Seddon HJ, Young JZ, Holmes W (1942) The histological condition of a nerve autograft in man. Brit J Surg 29: 378–384.

Settergren CR, Wood MB (1984) Comparison of blood flow in free vascularized versus nonvascularized nerve grafts. J Recon Micro 1: 95–101.

Shibata M, Tsai T-M, Firrell J, Breidenbach WC (1988) Experimental comparison of vascularized and nonvascularized nerve grafting. J Hand Surg 13A: 370–377.

Shine HD, Harcourt PG, Sidman R (1985) Cultured peripheral nervous system cells support peripheral nerve regeneration through tubes in the absence of a distal nerve stump. J Neurosci Res 14: 393–401.

Sims TJ, Gilmore SA (1994) Regeneration of dorsal root axons into experimentally altered glial environments in the rat spinal cord. Exp Brain Res 99: 25–33.

Sims TJ, Gilmore SA (1997) Schwann cells can misdirect regrowing neuronal processes. Brain Res 763: 141–144.

Sims TJ, Gilmore SA (2000) Schwann cell-induced loss of synapses in the central nervous system. Brain Res 882: 221–225.

Sinis N, Schaller HE, Schulte-Eversum C, Schlosshauer B, Doser M, Dietz K, Risner H, Muller HW, Haerle M (2005) Nerve regeneration across a 2-cm gap in the rat median nerve using a resorbable nerve conduit filled with Schwann cells. J Neurosurg 103: 1067–1076.

Skene JP, Willard M (1981) Axonally transported proteins associated with axon growth in rabbit central and peripheral nervous systems. J Cell Biol 89: 96–103.

Sketelj J, Bresjanac M, Popovic M (1989) Rapid growth of regenerating axons across the segments of sciatic nerve devoid of Schwann cells. J Neurosci Res 24: 153–162.

Smahel J, Meyer V, Morgenthaler W (1993) Silicon cuffs for peripheral nerve repair: experimental findings. J Recon Micro 9: 293–297.

Sondell M, Lundborg G, Kanje M (1998) Regeneration of the rat sciatic nerve into allografts made acellular through chemical extraction. Brain Res 795: 44–54.

Sondell M, Lundborg G, Kanje M (1999a) Vascular endothelial growth factor has neurotrophic activity and stimulates axonal outgrowth, enhancing cell survival and Schwann cell proliferation in the peripheral nervous system. J Neurosci 19: 5731–5740.

Sondell M, Lundborg G, Kanje M (1999b) Vascular endothelial growth factor stimulates Schwann cell invasion and neovascularization of acellular nerve grafts. Brain Res 846: 219–228.

Song HJ, Ming GL, He ZG, Lehmann M, McKerracher L, Tessier-Lavigne M, Poo MM (1998) Conversion of neuronal growth cone responses from repulsion to attraction by cyclic nucleotides. Science 281: 1515–1518.

Songcharoen P, Wongtrakul S, Mahaisavariya B, Spinner RJ (2001) Hemi-contralateral C7 transfer to median nerve in the treatment of root avulsion brachial plexus injury. J Hand Surg [Am] 26A: 1058–1064.

Songcharoen P, Wongtrakul S, Spinner RJ (2005) Brachial plexus injuries in the adult: nerve transfers; the Siriraj Hospital experience. Hand Clin 21: 83–89.

Sorbie C, Porter TL (1969) Reinnervation of paralysed muscles by direct motor nerve implantation. J Bone Joint Surg 51B: 156–164.

Stanec S, Stanec Z (1998) Reconstruction of upper-extremity peripheral nerve injuries with ePTFE conduits. J Recon Micro 14: 227–232.

Steindler A (1915) The method of direct neurotization of paralyzed muscles. Am J Ortho Surg 13: 33–45.

Steinmetz MP, Horn KP, Tom VJ, Miller JH, Busch SA, Nair D, Silver DJ, Silver J (2005) Chronic enhancement of the intrinsic growth capacity of sensory neurons combined with the degradation of inhibitory proteoglycans allows functional regeneration of sensory axons through the dorsal root entry zone in the mammalian spinal cord. J Neurosci 25: 8066–8076.

Stocks G, Cobb T, Lewis R (1991) Transfer of sensibility in the hand: a new method to restore sensibility in ulnar nerve palsy with use of microsurgical digital nerve translocation. J Hand Surg 16A: 219–226.

Strasberg SR, Hertl MC, Mackinnon SE, Lee CK, Watanabe O, Tarasidis G, Hunter DA, Wong PY (1996a) Peripheral nerve allograft preservation improves regeneration and decreases systemic cyclosporin A requirements. Exp Neurol 139: 306–316.

Strasberg SR, Mackinnon SE, Genden EM, Bain JR, Purcell CM, Hunter D, Hay JB (1996b) Long-segment nerve allograft regeneration in the sheep model: experimental study and review of the literature. J Recon Micro 12: 529–537.

Sundine MJ, Quan EE, Saglam O, Dhawan V, Quesada PM, Ogden L, Harralson T, Gossman MD, Maldonado CJ, Barker JH (2003) The use of end-to-side nerve grafts to reinnervate the paralyzed orbicularis oculi muscle. PRS 111: 2255–2003.

Sungpet A, Suphachatwong C, Kawinwonggowit V, Patradul A (2000) Transfer of a single fascicle from the ulnar nerve to the biceps muscle after avulsions of upper roots of the brachial plexus. J Hand Surg [Br Eur] 25B: 325–328.

Swanson AN, Wolfe SW, Khazzam M, Feinberg J, Ehteshami J, Doty S (2008) Comparison of neurotization versus nerve repair in an animal model of chronically denervated muscle. J Hand Surg Am 33: 1093–1099.

Tai CY, Weber RV, Mackinnon SE, Tung TH (2009) Multiple costimulatory blockade in the peripheral nerve allograft. Neurol Res 32: 332.

Tajima K, Tohyama K, Ide C, Abe M (1991) Regeneration through nerve allografts in the cynomolgus monkey (Macaca fascicularis). JBJS 73-A: 172–185.

Takahashi M (1983) Studies on conversion of motor function in intercostal nerves crossing for complete brachial plexus injuries of root avulsion type. J Jpn Orthop Ass 57: 1799–1807.

Tang JB, Gu YQ, Song YS (1993) Repair of digital nerve defect with autogenous vein graft during flexor tendon surgery in zone 2. J Hand Surg [Br] 18B: 449–453.

Tang S, Woodhall RW, Shen YJ, DeBellard ME, Saffell J, Doherty P, Walsh FS, Filbin M (1997) Soluble myelin-associated glycoprotein (MAG) found in vivo inhibits axonal regeneration. Mol Cell Neurosci 9: 333–346.

Tarasidis G, Watanabe O, Mackinnon SE, Strasberg SR, Haughey BH, Hunter DA (1997) End-to-side neurorrhaphy resulting in limited sensory axonal regeneration in a rat model. Ann Otol Rhinol Laryngol 106: 506–512.

Tark KC, Roh TS (2001) Morphometric study of regeneration through vascularized nerve graft in a rabbit sciatic nerve model. J Recon Micro 17: 109–114.

Tarlov IM, Epstein JA (1945) Nerve grafts: the importance of an adequate blood supply. J Neurosurg 2: 49–71.

Taylor I, Ham FJ (1976) The free vascularized nerve graft. PRS 57: 413–426.

Teboul F, Kakkar R, Ameur N, Beaulieu JY, Oberlin C (2004) Transfer of fascicles from the ulnar nerve to the nerve to the biceps in the treatment of upper brachial plexus palsy. J Bone Joint Surg [Am] 86A: 1485–1490.

Terzis J, Kostas I (2007) Vein grafts used as nerve conduits for obstetrical brachial plexus palsy reconstruction. Plast Reconstr Surg 120: 1930–1941.

Terzis JK, Skoulis TG, Soucacos PN (1995) Vascularized nerve grafts. Int Angio 14: 264–277.

Terzis JK, Kostopoulos VK (2009) Vascularized ulnar nerve graft: 151 reconstructions for posttraumatic brachial plexus palsy. Plast Reconstr Surg 123: 1276–1291.

Tessler A, Himes BT, Houle J, Reier PJ (1988) Regeneration of adult dorsal root axons into transplants of embryonic spinal cord. J Comp Neurol 270: 537–548.

Tham SK, Morrison W (1998) Motor collateral sprouting through an end-to-side nerve repair. J Hand Surg 23A: 844–851.

Tiangco DA, Papakonstantinou KC, Mullinax KA, Terzis JK (2001) IGF-1 and end-to-side nerve repair: a dose-response study. J Recon Micro 17: 247–256.

Timmer M, Robben S, Muller-Ostermeyer F, Nikkhah G, Grothe C (2003) Axonal regeneration across long gaps in silicone chambers filled with Schwann cells overexpressing high molecular weight FGF-2. Cell Transplant 12: 265–277.

Tohill M, Mantovani C, Wiberg M, Terenghi G (2004) Rat bone marrow mesenchymal stem cells express glial markers and stimulate nerve regeneration. Neurosci Lett 362: 200–203.

Tohyama K, Ide C (1984) The localization of laminin and fibronectin of the Schwann cell basal lamina. Arch Hist Jap 47: 519–532.

Tomita K, Kubo T, Matsuda K, Hattori R, Fujiwara T, Yano K, Hosokawa K (2007) Effect of conduit repair on aberrant motor axon growth within the nerve graft in rats. Microsurgery 27: 500–509.

Törnqvist E, Aldskogius H (1994) Motoneuron survival is not affected by the proximo-distal level of axotomy but by the possibility of regenerating axons to gain access to the distal nerve stump. J Neurosci Res 39: 159–165.

Trumble, T.E. and F.G. Shon (2000) The physiology of nerve transplantation. In: Hand Clinics, T.E. Trumble and C. Allan, eds., pp. 105–122, Philadelphia: Saunders.

Tung TH, Doolabh V, Mackinnon S, Mohanakumar T, Hicks ME (2006) Survival of long nerve allografts following donor antigen pretreatment: a pilot study. J Recon Micro 22: 443–450.

Tuttle HK (1913) Exposure of the brachial plexus with nerve transplantation. JAMA 61: 15–17.

Udina E, Voda J, Gold B, Navarro X (2003) Comparative dose-dependence study of FK506 0n transected mouse sciatic nerve repaired by allograft or xenograft. JPNS 8: 145–154.

Udina E, Gold BG, Navarro X (2004) Comparison of continuous and discontinuous FK506 administration on autograft or allograft repair of sciatic nerve resection. Muscle & Nerve 29: 812–822.

Urbanchek MG, Ganz DE, Aydin MA, Van der Meulen JH, Kuzon WM, Jr. (2004) Muscle-nerve-muscle neurotization for the reinnervation of denervated somatic muscle. Neurol Res 26: 388–394.

Valero-Cabre A, Tsironis K, Skouras E, Perego G, Navarro X, Neiss WF (2001) Superior muscle reinnervation after autologous nerve graft or

poly-L-lactide-Œ-caprolactone (PLC) tube implantation in comparison to silicone tube repair. J Neurosci Res 63: 214–223.

Valero-Cabré A, Tsironis K, Skouras E, Navarro X, Neiss W (2004) Peripheral and spinal motor reorganization after nerve injury and repair. J Neurotrauma 21: 95–108.

Valero-Cabré A, Navarro X (2002) Functional impact of axonal misdirection after peripheral nerve injuries followed by graft or tube repair. J Neurotrauma 19: 1475–1485.

Van der Wey LP, Gabreëls-Festen AAWM, Merks MHJH, Polder TW, Stegeman DF, Spauwen PHM, Gabreëls FJM (1995) Peripheral nerve elongation by laser Doppler flowmetry controlled expansion: morphological aspects. Acta Neuropathol (Berl) 89: 166–171.

Venkatramani H, Bhardwaj P, Faruquee SR, Sabapathy SR (2008) Functional outcome of nerve transfer for restoration of shoulder and elbow function in upper brachial plexus injury. J Brachial Plex Peripher Nerve Inj 3: 15.

Viterbo F, Trindade JC, Hoshino K, Mazzoni A (1992) Latero-terminal neurorrhaphy without removal of the epineurial sheath: experimental study in rats. Rev Paul Med 110: 267–275.

Voche P, Ouattara D (2005) End-to-side neurorrhaphy for defects of palmar sensory digital nerves. Br J Plast Surg 58: 239–244.

Waikakul S, Orapin S, Vanadurongwan V (1999a) Clinical results of contralateral C7 root neurotization to the median nerve in brachial plexus injuries with total root avulsions. J Hand Surg [Br Eur] 24B: 556–560.

Waikakul S, Wongtragul S, Vanadurongwan V (1999b) Restoration of elbow flexion in brachial plexus avulsion injury: comparing spinal accessory nerve transfer with intercostal nerve transfer. J Hand Surg [Am] 24: 571–577.

Wallquist W, Zelano J, Plantman S, Kaufman SJ, Cullheim S, Hammarberg H (2004) Dorsal root ganglion neurons up-regulate the expression of laminin-associated integrins after peripheral but not central axotomy. J Comp Neurol 480: 162–169.

Walton RL, Brown R, Matory E, Borah GL, Dolph JL (1989) Autogenous vein graft repair of digital nerve defects in the finger: A retrospective clinical study. PRS 84: 944–949.

Wang G-Y, Hirai K-I, Shimada H (1992a) The role of laminin, a component of Schwann cell basal lamina, in rat sciatic nerve regeneration within antiserum-treated nerve grafts. Brain Res 570: 116–125.

Wang G-Y, Hirai K-I, Shimada H, Taji S, Zhong S-Z (1992b) Behavior of axons, Schwann cells and perineurial cells in nerve regeneration within transplanted nerve grafts: effects of anti-laminin and anti-fibronectin antisera. Brain Res 583: 216–226.

Wang R, King T, Ossipov MH, Rossomando AJ, Vanderah TW, Harvey P, Cariani P, Sah DW, Porreca F (2008) Persistent restoration of sensory function by immediate or delayed systemic artemin after dorsal root injury. Nat Neurosci 11: 488–496.

Wang W, Itoh S, Konno K, Kikkawa T, Ichinose S, Sakai K, Ohkuma T, Watabe K (2009) Effects of Schwann cell alignment along the oriented electrospun chitosan nanofibers on nerve regeneration. J Biomed Mater Res A 91: 994–1005.

Watrous WG (1940) Axon branching after nerve regeneration. Proc Soc Exp Biol Med 44: 541–542.

Weber RA, Warner MR, Verheyden CN, Proctor WH (1996) Functional evaluation of gap vs. abutment repair of peripheral nerves in the rat. J Recon Micro 12: 159–163.

Weber RA, Breidenbach WC, Brown RE, Jabaley ME, Mass DP (2000) A randomized prospective study of polyglycolic acid conduits for digital nerve reconstruction in humans. Plast Reconstr Surg 106: 1036–1045.

Weinzweig N, Grindel S, Gonzalez M, Kuy D, Fang J, Shahani B (1996) Peripheral nerve allotransplantation in rats immunosuppressed with transient or long-term FK506. J Recon Micro 12: 451–459.

Weiss P, Taylor AC (1943) Histomechanical analysis of nerve reunion in the rat after tubular splicing. Arch Surg 47: 419–447.

Weiss P (1944) The technology of nerve regeneration: a review; sutureless tubulation and related methods of nerve repair. J Neurosurg 1: 400–450.

Weiss P, Taylor C (1946) The viability of isolated nerve fragments and its modification by methylene blue. J Cell Comp Physiol 27: 87–103.

Whitlock EL, Tuffaha SH, Luciano JP, Yan Y, Hunter DA, Magill CK, Moore AM, Tong AY, Mackinnon SE, Borschel GH (2009) Processed allografts and type I collagen conduits for repair of peripheral nerve gaps. Muscle & Nerve 39: 787–799.

Wikholm R, Swett J, Torigoe Y, Blanks R (1988) Repair of severed peripheral nerve: a superior anatomic and functional recovery with a new "reconnection" technique. J Otol Head & Neck Surg 99: 353–361.

Williams L, Longo F, Powell H, Lundborg G, Varon S (1983) Spatial-temporal progress of peripheral nerve regeneration within a silicon chamber: parameters for bioassay. J Comp Neurol 218: 460–470.

Williams LR, Powell HC, Lundborg G, Varon S (1984) Competence of nerve tissue as distal insert promoting nerve regeneration in a silicon chamber. Brain Res 293: 201–211.

Williams LR, Danielsen N, Muller H, Varon S (1987) Exogenous matrix precursors promote functional nerve regeneration across a 15-mm gap within a silicon chamber in the rat. J Comp Neurol 264: 284–290.

Williams LR, Azzam NA, Zalewski AA, Azzam RN (1993) Regenerating axons are not required to induce the formation of a Schwann cell cable in a silicone chamber. Exp Neurol 120: 49–59.

Wongtrakul S, Bishop A, Friedrich PF (2002) Vascular endothelial growth factor promotion of neoangiogenesis in conventional nerve grafts. J Hand Surg 27A: 277–285.

Wood MD, Moore AM, Hunter DA, Tuffaha S, Borschel GH, Mackinnon SE, Sakiyama-Elbert SE (2009) Affinity-based release of glial-derived neurotrophic factor from fibrin matrices enhances sciatic nerve regeneration. Acta Biomater 5: 959–968.

Wu WT, Chai H, Zhang JY, Gu HY, Xie YY, Zhou LH (2004) Delayed implantation of a peripheral nerve graft reduces motoneuron survival but does not affect regeneration following spinal root avulsion in adult rats. J Neurotrauma 21: 1050–1058.

Wujek JR, Lasek RJ (1983) Correlation of axonal regeneration and slow component b in two branches of a single axon. J Neurosci 3: 243–251.

Xu XY, Yee WC, Hwang PYK, Yu H, Wan ACA, Gao SJ, Boon KL, Mao HQ, Leong KW, Wang S (2003) Peripheral nerve regeneration with sustained release of poly(phosphoester) microencapsulated nerve growth factor within nerve guide conduits. Biomaterials 24: 2405–2412.

Yan H, Zhang F, Chen MB, Lineaweaver WC (2009) Chapter 10: conduit luminal additives for peripheral nerve repair. Int Rev Neurobiol 87: 199–225.

Yang LJ, Lorenzini I, Vajn K, Mountney A, Schramm L, Schnaar RL (2006) Sialidase enhances spinal axon outgrowth in vivo. PNAS 103: 11057–11062.

Yuksel F, Peker F, Celikoz B (2004) Two applications of end-to-side nerve neurorrhaphy in severe upper-extremity nerve injuries. Microsurgery 24: 363–368.

Young C, Miller E, Nicklous DM, Hoffman JR (2001) Nerve growth factor and neurotrophin-3 affect functional recovery following peripheral nerve injury differently. Restor Neurol Neurosci 18: 167–175.

Yu LM, Wosnick JH, Shoichet MS (2008) Miniaturized system of neurotrophin patterning for guided regeneration. J Neurosci Methods 171: 253–263.

Zalewski AA, Gulati AK (1982) Evaluation of histocompatibility as a factor in the repair of nerve with a frozen nerve allograft. J Neurosurg 56: 550–554.

Zalewski AA, Azzam NA, Azzam RN (1995) The loss of regenerated host axons in nerve allografts after stopping immunosuppression with cyclosporin A is related to immune effects on allogeneic Schwann cells. Exp Neurol 133: 189–197.

Zhang F, Blain B, Beck J, Zhang J, Chen Z, Chen Z-W, Lineweaver WC (2002) Autogenous venous graft with one-stage prepared Schwann cells as a conduit for repair of long segmental nerve defects. J Recon Micro 18: 295–300.

Zhang WG, Ochi M, Takata H, Ikuta Y (1997) Influence of distal nerve segment volume on nerve regeneration in silicone tubes. Exp Neurol 146: 600–603.

Zhang Y, Dijkhuizen PA, Anderson PN, Lieberman AR, Verhaagen J (1998) NT-3 delivered by an adenoviral vector induces injured dorsal root axons to regenerate into the spinal cord of adult rats. J Neurosci Res 54: 554–562.

Zhang Y, Zhang X, Wu D, Verhaagen J, Richardson P, Yeh J, Bo X (2007) Lentiviral-mediated expression of polysialic acid in spinal cord and conditioning lesion promote regeneration of sensory axons into spinal cord. Mol Ther 15: 1796–1804.

Zhang Z, Soucacos P, Bo J, Beris AE (1999) Evaluation of collateral sprouting after end-to-side nerve coaptation using a fluorescent double-labeling technique. Microsurgery 19: 281–286.

Zhang Z, Soucacos P, Beris A, Bo J, Ioachim E, Johnson E (2000) Long-term evaluation of rat peripheral nerve repair with end-to-side neurorrhaphy. J Recon Micro 16: 303–311.

Zhao Q, Dahlin L, Kanje M, Lundborg G (1992) Specificity of muscle reinnervation following repair of the transected sciatic nerve. J Hand Surg 17B: 257–261.

Zhao Q, Dahlin L, Kanje M, Lundborg G (1993) Repair of the transected rat sciatic nerve: matrix formation within implanted silicon tubes. Restorative Neurology and Neuroscience 5: 197–204.

Zhao Q, Lundborg G, Danielsen N, Bjursten LM, Dahlin LB (1997) Nerve regeneration in a "pseudo-nerve" graft created in a silicone tube. Brain Res 769: 125–134.

Zheng H, Zhou S, Chen S, Li Z, Cuan Y (1998) An experimental comparison of different types of laryngeal muscle reinnervation. Otolaryngol Head Neck Surg 119: 540–547.

Zhou L, Du HD, Tian HB, Li C, Tian J, Jiang JJ (2008) Experimental study on repair of the facial nerve with Schwann cells transfected with GDNF genes and PLGA conduits. Acta Otolaryngol 128: 1266–1272.

9

NERVE REGENERATION

INTRODUCTION

INTEREST IN the broad topic of neural regeneration has been stimulated by the search for techniques of CNS repair, a quest that has recently gained considerable momentum. The more focused study of peripheral regeneration has benefited from these efforts, both through conceptual advances and through development of new techniques. As a result, knowledge of the factors that determine the outcome of peripheral nerve repair has increased exponentially in recent years. Regeneration has come to be viewed as the summation of positive and negative external influences in the context of the intrinsic "growth state" of the neuron.

The results of clinical and experimental nerve repair presented earlier suggest that important intrinsic factors must be regulated by patient age, whereas critical environmental factors are found at the repair site where integrity of the basal lamina is lost. Regeneration is dramatically more effective in children than in adults (Chapter 5), and after nerve

crush, which preserves the integrity of the basal lamina, than after nerve transection (Chapter 7). This chapter will provide several examples of regeneration components that are more concentrated or more effective in the young or when the basal lamina remains intact. A primary example of the former is the second messenger cyclic adenosine monophosphate (cAMP), which is present in higher concentrations in young neurons and is responsible for their ability to grow on substrates that are inhibitory for adult neurons (Cai et al., 2001; Qiu et al., 2002). Similarly, activation of integrin receptors by laminin (LN) within the basal lamina is critical for regeneration to proceed normally (Werner et al., 2000; Chen, Strickland, 2003).

An example of the interdependence of intrinsic and extrinsic factors is provided by the age-dependent response of regenerating dorsal root ganglion (DRG) neurites to a gradient of nerve growth factor (NGF). Embryonic DRG neurites turn briskly in a gradient of NGF without the need for interaction with laminin, whereas adult DRG neurites require

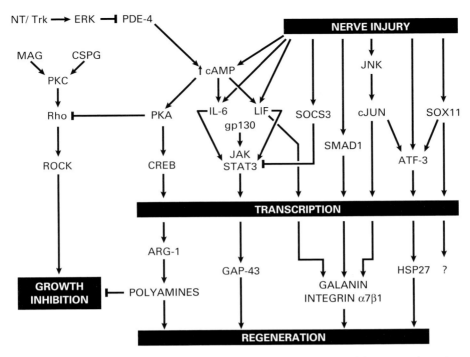

FIGURE 9-1   Signaling pathways that influence the intrinsic growth capacity of the neuron through activation of transcription factors.

Overcoming Inhibition

In addition to promoting regeneration by phosphorylating CREB, PKA blocks the inhibitory effects of the regeneration inhibitors MAG and chondroitin sulfate proteoglycans (CSPGs), both of which may be present at the site of peripheral nerve repair and in the distal nerve stump (Figure 9-1). One form of MAG signaling requires the NOGO receptor and LINGO-1, a leucine-rich repeat protein, to form a complex with either the p75NTR or TROY, a member of the TNF receptor family (Hannila, Filbin, 2008). Binding of MAG to one of these receptor complexes activates protein kinase C (PKC), which in turn promotes the small GTPase Rho to its active, GTP-bound state (Yamashita et al., 2002; Yamashita, Tohyama, 2003). While this pathway has been found to predominate in the DRG, MAG may also signal in other tissues by binding to the gangliosides GD1a and GT1b (Mehta et al., 2007), as well as to the recently discovered paired immunoglobulin-like receptor B (PirB) (Atwal et al., 2008). Chondroitin sulfate proteoglycans also signal through PKC and Rho, although their specific receptor has

not been identified (Dergham et al., 2002; Sivasankaran et al., 2004). Once activated, Rho initiates a series of downstream effectors including the Rho-activated kinase (ROCK), ultimately leading to actin polymerization and growth cone collapse (Dergham et al., 2002). Although much of this work has been done in vitro, inhibition of the PKC pathway in vivo has been found to enhance the regeneration of central DRG projections within the dorsal columns of the spinal cord (Sivasankaran et al., 2004).

The Role of Neuropoietic Cytokines

The neuropoietic cytokines IL-6 and LIF provide alternative pathways through which cAMP may enhance the neural growth state without activation of PKA (Figure 9-1). IL-6 is upregulated within DRG neurons after either a conditioning lesion or treatment with dibutyryl cAMP (Cao et al., 2006; Wu et al., 2007). Treatment of DRG neurons in vivo with IL-6 enhances their regeneration state when they are cultured subsequently, as they gain the ability to overcome MAG inhibition. Elimination of the direct IL-6 pathway by knocking out the IL-6 gene, however, does not prevent DRG neurons from responding to a conditioning lesion as assayed by growth on MAG substrates in vitro, suggesting that IL-6 is sufficient but not necessary for conditioning as defined by growth on MAG (Cao et al., 2006). These observations contributed to the hypothesis of Deng et al. (2009) described above. Signaling downstream from IL-6 involves interaction with the signal transducing receptor component gp130, leading to phosphorylation of STAT3 (Qiu et al., 2005; Wu et al., 2007).

The role of IL-6 in peripheral nerve regeneration has been evaluated most extensively in IL-6 knockout mice. When the sciatic nerves of these animals were crushed, regeneration distance was reduced 4 days after injury, and recovery of sciatic functional index (SFI) was delayed (Inserra et al., 2000; Galiano et al., 2001). Longer-term studies have shown incomplete recovery of SFI and impaired recovery of sensory function after nerve crush (Zhong et al., 1999); after transection and repair, axon counts and morphometry were similar and return of SFI was equally poor in knockouts and controls (Inserra et al., 2000). In normal animals, the gp130 receptor can be activated by administration of a combination of IL-6 and its receptor or a chimera of the two (Hirota et al., 1996; Haggiag et al., 2001). In either case, regeneration is accelerated, demonstrating a clear role for IL-6 in the regeneration process.

LIF is also upregulated by DRG neurons in response to cAMP, and signals through the same gp130 receptor as IL-6 to activate STAT3 (Qiu et al., 2005; Wu et al., 2007). It has also been shown to be a fundamental component of the conditioning response in vitro and in vivo (Cafferty et al., 2001). Regeneration is impaired after sciatic nerve crush in LIF knockout mice (Cafferty et al., 2001) and is enhanced when LIF is placed in sciatic nerve gaps (Tham et al., 1997; Dowsing et al., 2000; Brown et al., 2002; McKay Hart et al., 2003). The role of LIF in the recovery from end-to-end nerve repair has not been determined.

STAT3, the transcription factor downstream from LIF and IL-6, is upregulated after peripheral but not after central DRG axotomy (Schwaiger et al., 2000). It plays a critical role in promoting regeneration, as blocking the STAT3 pathway also blocks upregulation of the growth cone protein GAP-43 (Cafferty et al., 2004; Qiu et al., 2005). GAP-43 was one of the earliest growth-associated proteins to be

identified, and was also among the first to be characterized by a differential response to central and peripheral axotomy (Skene, Willard, 1981; Chong et al., 1994). STAT3 activity is suppressed within DRG neurons in vitro by suppressor of cytokine signaling-3 (SOCS3), a protein that is upregulated by nerve injury and that is thought to regulate cytokine signaling during Wallerian degeneration (Nilsson et al., 2005; Miao et al., 2006; Girolami et al., 2009).

Additional Transcription Factors

The pathways influenced by the second messenger cAMP were among the first to undergo extensive scrutiny, and as a result are relatively well understood (Figure 9-1). These pathways control gene expression by activating the transcription factors CREB and STAT3. Subsequently, however, other transcription factors have been shown to respond to peripheral axotomy through as yet incompletely defined pathways. These include c-Jun, activating transcription factor-3 (ATF-3), SRY box-containing factor-11 (Sox11), and Smad-1 (Leah et al., 1991; Tsujino et al., 2000; Tanabe et al., 2003; Zou et al., 2009). The c-Jun terminal kinase (JNK), which activates c-Jun through phosphorylation, is upregulated within the DRG soon after nerve injury (Kenney and Kocsis, 1998; Lindwall et al., 2004). This activity appears to be a hallmark of PNS regeneration, as cJun is not upregulated by either axotomized CNS neurons or developing PNS neurons (Broude et al., 1997; Raivich et al., 2004). Expressed and activated in response to peripheral but not central axotomy, cJun persists at elevated levels until axons reinnervate their target (Broude et al., 1997; Herdegen et al., 1998). Inhibitors of c-Jun activation reduce axonal outgrowth from cultured DRG neurons (Lindwall et al., 2004). In c-Jun knockout animals, facial nerve regeneration is impaired significantly, and the production of the neuropeptide galanin, the neural adhesion molecule $\alpha 7\beta 1$ integrin (a laminin receptor), and the hyaluronic acid receptor CD44 are all reduced (Raivich et al., 2004). Activation of c-Jun is thus a key step in switching on the neuronal regeneration program.

Galanin and the $\alpha 7\beta 1$ integrin, both downstream from transcription induced by cJun, have also been shown to play important roles in regeneration. Galanin is upregulated in both sensory and motor neurons in response to axotomy (Saika et al., 1991;

Wiesenfeld-Hallin et al., 1992). In galanin knockout mice, the speed of early sensory axon regeneration is reduced by 30–40% after sciatic nerve crush as determined by the pinch test, and the return of toe spread is delayed (Holmes et al., 2005). Neuronal galanin may also be upregulated in response to LIF transported from the axotomy site, although the pathway responsible for this interaction has not been elucidated (Sun, Zigmond, 1996; Kerekes et al., 1999; Ozturk, Tonge, 2001). Function of the α7β1 integrin will be discussed below in the context of axon-substrate interactions.

The transcription factor ATF-3 is expressed by many of the same neurons that upregulate cJun after injury, and can enhance neurite growth in culture both alone and when dimerized with cJun (Pearson et al., 2003; Seijffers et al., 2006). Overexpression of ATF-3 in DRG neurons is sufficient to enhance early reinnervation of the distal nerve stump after crush, but is not sufficient to promote regeneration after dorsal column injury (Seijffers et al., 2007). ATF-3 is differentially regulated within subpopulations of DRG neurons, and its expression correlates with the relative ability of these neurons to regenerate (Averill et al., 2004; Reid et al., 2010). Heat shock protein 27 (Hsp-27) is upregulated in response to ATF-3, and has been shown to promote the regeneration of adult DRG neurons in vitro in addition to its role in promoting neuronal survival (Williams et al., 2005; Williams et al., 2006). ATF-3 is also upregulated by expression of Sox11, a transcription factor that influences regeneration as evidenced by a reduction in the speed of axon regeneration in vivo in response to Sox11 knockdown (Jankowski et al., 2006; Jankowski et al., 2009). Recently Smad1, a transcription factor that mediates intracellular TGFβ/BMP signaling, has also been found to enhance the growth of adult DRG neurons in vitro (Zou et al., 2009). Preliminary results also suggest that blocking action of the phosphatase and tensin homolog (PTEN), a tumor suppressor, enhances signaling through the mammalian target of rapamycin (mTOR) to enhance the growth of DRG neurons in vitro (Park et al., 2010). As this pathway promotes the regeneration of retinal ganglion neurons (Park et al., 2008), it may also prove to be relevant in the PNS.

A Possible Role for BDNF

A growing body of evidence has linked BDNF signaling to neuronal growth state. The expression of brain-derived neurotrophic factor (BDNF) and its receptor TrkB by adult neurons suggest that BDNF may act through autocrine and/or paracrine mechanisms rather than as a target-derived growth factor. Postnatal motoneurons express BDNF and respond briskly to nerve transection or excitotoxic stimuli with additional gene expression; the concentration of BDNF protein resulting from this activity is greatest at 1 week, normalizing at 3–4 weeks (Kobayashi et al., 1996; Scarisbrick et al., 1999; Buck et al., 2000). Motoneurons normally express the TrkB receptor at low levels, but respond to nerve transection with enhanced expression for 3–4 weeks (Piehl et al., 1994; Kobayashi et al., 1996; Hammarberg et al., 2000a).

In the adult DRG, BDNF is expressed by a subpopulation of small-to-medium neurons, from which it undergoes anterograde transport both to the periphery and to nerve terminals in Lamina I and II of the dorsal horn, where it may contribute to central sensitization and chronic pain (Zhou, Rush, 1996; Woolf, Salter, 2000; Luo et al., 2001; Lu et al., 2009). TrkB is expressed by 33% of DRG neurons; 35% of these, in turn, also express BDNF, so that 10–20% of DRG neurons normally express both (Apfel et al., 1996; Karchewski et al., 1999). After axotomy, BDNF messenger RNA and protein are increased within 24 hours within both DRG neurons and satellite cells, and remain elevated for 2–3 weeks, a process that depends on the presence of endogenous IL-6 (Murphy et al., 2000). Additionally, many large neurons that do not express BDNF at rest initiate expression in response to axotomy, increasing the population that express both TrkB and DBNF (Michael et al., 1999; Karchewski et al., 2002).

Initial evidence relating BDNF to neuronal growth state was obtained from experiments in knockout mice and during investigation of the effects of electrical stimulation on nerve regeneration. In mice with reduced expression of the TrkB receptor, the number of motoneurons that reinnervated muscle after nerve repair was reduced by 25% and coordinated muscle function was impaired (Irintchev et al., 2005; Eberhardt et al., 2006). In wild-type rodents, electrical stimulation at the time of nerve repair was found to enhance early motor axon regeneration and to speed the onset and magnitude of BDNF and TrkB expression by motoneurons (Al-Majed et al., 2000, 2004). Subsequent work established that enhanced BDNF expression correlated temporally with increased expression of the growth-related proteins tubulin and GAP-43

(Al-Majed et al., 2004) and that DRG neurons responded to stimulation in a similar fashion (Brushart et al., 2005; English et al., 2007; Geremia et al., 2007). The strongest evidence linking BDNF expression to neuronal growth state was obtained in recent experiments in which function-blocking antibodies or small interfering RNAs (siRNAs) were used to minimize BDNF signaling in axotomized DRG neurons in vivo (Geremia et al., 2010). Under these circumstances, axotomy-induced expression of tubulin and GAP-43 were reduced in concert with the capacity of the neurons to regenerate when cultured, implicating BDNF in the activation of the regeneration program. The mechanism through which neuronal BDNF influences regeneration has yet to be determined (Gordon, 2009; Geremia et al., 2010).

Conditioning in Context

When characterizing the modification of axon growth by a particular factor or manipulation, it is often difficult to separate the effects that occur in the cell body, the focus of the above discussion, from those that are more prominent in the growth cone. Much of the work discussed above was carried out in the DRG model, and shares transcription, the majority of which occurs in the cell body, as its endpoint. The pathway linking cAMP to the overcoming of inhibition by MAG and CSPGs, however, bridges the two compartments. Interactions that are known to occur predominantly within the growth cone are discussed in Part 2 of this chapter.

As the experience with ATF-3 amply illustrates, all potential manifestations of conditioning do not necessarily follow every type of "conditioning" stimulus; overexpression of ATF-3 enhances the response to peripheral nerve crush, but does not promote regeneration after dorsal column injury (Seijffers et al., 2007). This is also true in the case of IL-6, which is required for regeneration after dorsal column injuries, but not for growth of cultured DRG neurons on MAG substrates (Cafferty et al., 2004; Cao et al., 2006). Similarly, a single injection of dibutyryl cAMP into the DRG conditions neurons as evidenced by the regeneration of their central projections in vivo and by their ability to overcome MAG in vitro (Neumann et al., 2002; Qiu et al., 2002), yet similar treatment was not found to increase the rate of peripheral nerve regeneration after crush in vivo (Han et al., 2004). Finally, conclusions derived from the results of experiments in the single treatment ex vivo DRG model may not

apply to motoneurons, or to situations in which treatment is prolonged: elevation of cAMP with systemic application of the phosphodiesterase rolipram hastens motor reinnervation of the distal nerve stump after peripheral nerve transection and repair (Udina et al., 2010), yet treatment of the DRG with dibutyryl cAMP does not (Han et al., 2004). Clearly, many of these manipulations allow central DRG projections to regenerate more like their peripheral counterparts, but whether or not they actually speed peripheral nerve regeneration, the classical conditioning effect, remains to be determined in many instances. Greater precision could thus be achieved by describing "central conditioning" and "peripheral conditioning" as separate entities.

The degree to which conditioning may enhance human peripheral nerve regeneration has not been determined. As mentioned previously, the outcomes of nerve repairs delayed for 2–3 weeks have not been compared to those of immediate repair. The effects of conditioning have been examined in small animal models, predominantly after nerve crush rather than transection, and usually in the early days after the test lesion. Two important questions cannot be asked until conditioning is evaluated in large-scale models: do the axons of conditioned neurons continue to extend at increased rates over long distances, and do the axons of unconditioned neurons speed up 2 weeks after they have been injured, so that conditioning would confer only a clinically insignificant 2 week advantage?

NEURONAL SIGNALING

Baseline neuronal activity, the summation and transmission of electrical impulses, is the tip of the functional iceberg. This activity is supported by a complex web of intraneuronal signaling pathways that provide information about the environment of the neuron and maintain the apparatus needed for electrical transmission. Signaling takes on an even more prominent role when the configuration of the nervous system is undergoing modification. During development, retrograde signaling determines which neurons will prosper and which will die. When an injured axon is regenerating, signaling to preserve homeostasis is replaced by signaling to promote and guide regeneration and to provide the necessary raw materials. An ongoing challenge in regeneration research is thus to characterize and manipulate pathways that contribute to regeneration in an attempt to enhance the process.

As our knowledge of signaling pathways matures it becomes progressively clear that we are actually dealing with a signaling "web": the recognized pathways have the potential to interact with one another, often at several levels, so that the consequences of a growth factor-receptor interaction can be highly context-dependent. The context of a signaling event encompasses the cell type in which it occurs, the developmental stage of the organism from which the cell is taken, and coincident interactions at the cell surface including those that trigger other signaling events in response to the local environment. This section will describe signaling initiated by the neurotrophins, the prototypical diffusible growth factors, by the p75NTR, a neurotrophin receptor with unique properties, and by GDNF, a multifunctional factor with the potential to promote regeneration. These examples will provide an overview of the complexity and interrelatedness of neuronal signaling. Much of this work is done in immortalized cell lines, so that it defines a range of possibilities rather than pathways specific to peripheral axon regeneration. The section "Signaling to Promote Regeneration" below will focus on specific pathways that have actually been shown to influence the regeneration of adult mammalian neurons.

The Neurotrophins and Their Receptors

NGF was discovered by Levi-Montalcini and Hamburger more than half a century ago (Levi-Montalcini, Hamburger, 1951). It was identified as a diffusible factor that was transported within axons from the periphery to central neurons, where it promoted their survival (Levi-Montalcini, Hamburger, 1951; Thoenen, Barde, 1980; Levi-Montalcini, 1987). Dependence on NGF was confirmed by the loss of target neuronal populations when NGF activity was prevented with blocking antibodies (Levi-Montalcini, Booker, 1960). These observations led to the formulation of the Neurotrophic Hypothesis: developing neurons compete for a limited supply of a neurotrophic factor that is provided by their target tissues. Successful competitors survive and mature, while unsuccessful competitors die (Oppenheim, 1996b; Yuen et al., 1996). These observations established that axons signal the cell body about specific features of the peripheral environment.

The second neurotrophin to be discovered, BDNF, was isolated from pig brain on the basis of its ability to support neurons that did not respond to

NGF (Barde et al., 1982). Once the structural similarities of NGF and BDNF were appreciated (Leibrock et al., 1989), a homology cloning approach led to the identification of the other two neurotrophins, neurotrophin-3 (NT-3) and neurotrophin 4/5 (NT-4/5) (Hohn et al., 1990; Berkemeier et al., 1991).

The neurotrophins are approximately 120 amino acids in length, with 28 invariant residues. The protein product of each neurotrophin gene, or proneurotrophin, consists of a signal sequence, a prodomain, and the "mature" neurotrophin sequence (Hempstead, 2006). The proneurotrophin is cleaved to release the mature C-terminal peptide, long thought to be the only source of biological activity. Recently, however, proneurotrophins have been found to exert significant effects that often oppose the actions of their mature counterparts (reviewed in Hempstead, 2006; Barker, 2009; see below).

Neurotrophins signal through three classes of receptor. The Trk family of receptor tyrosine kinases are transmembrane receptors that interact with the neurotrophins with a high degree of specificity (reviewed in Neet, Campenot, 2001; Arevalo, Wu, 2006; Skaper, 2008). NGF binds to TrkA, BDNF and NT4/5 bind to TrkB, and NT-3 binds to TrkC (Figure 9-2). NT-3 can also bind to TrkA and TrkB, but with reduced efficiency. The extracellular portion of the Trk receptor includes two immunoglobulin-like domains; the intracellular portion ends in a tyrosine kinase flanked by tyrosine residues that, when activated, initiate the signaling process. Interaction with an appropriate neurotrophin dimerizes the Trk receptor, leading to its phosphorylation and subsequent activation of the intracellular tyrosine kinase. This kinase then phosphorylates the adjacent tyrosine residues, which serve as docking sites for a variety of adaptor proteins and enzymes that determine which signaling pathways will be activated. Trk receptors are not spread uniformly across the cell membrane, but are concentrated within lipid rafts, microdomains that increase their interaction with adaptor and signaling proteins (Suzuki et al., 2004). Blocking the aggregation of Trk receptors within these areas has been shown to interfere with their function (Pereira, Chao, 2007).

Once activated, the Trk receptor is internalized to an endosomal compartment (Shao et al., 2002). From this reservoir, the neurotrophin-Trk complex is recycled, degraded, or transported in retrograde fashion (Arevalo et al., 2006); neurotrophin-Trk complexes that are destined for transport appear to

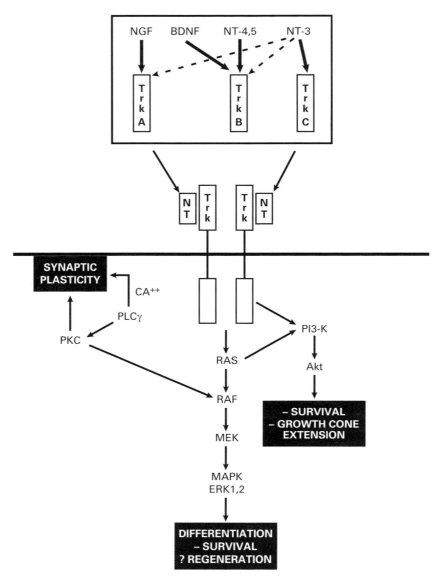

FIGURE 9-2   Neurotrophin signaling through tyrosine kinase receptors. The upper box demonstrates the possible neurotrophin/receptor combinations. The receptor dimerizes at the cell membrane (horizontal line), then activates a variety of signaling intermediates.

remain intact throughout their journey (Ginty, Segal, 2002). Transport of activated Trk receptors is microtubule-dependent, and is required for nuclear signaling responses (Watson et al., 1999). Regulating the traffic of neurotrophin-Trk complexes within the endosome has emerged as an additional means of modulating neurotrophin signaling, and has been the subject of recent interest (reviewed in Reichardt, 2006; Moises et al., 2007).

Downstream signaling from neurotrophin receptors involves multiple interacting pathways, each of which can be modulated by other cellular events. The most thoroughly studied of these are characterized by activation of the MAPK, PI3-K, or PLC-γ pathways (Figure 9-2). Recent reviews have described current knowledge of these pathways in detail (Arevalo, Wu, 2006; Cui, 2006; Reichardt, 2006; Skaper, 2008).

The MAPK/ERK pathway is initiated by activation of the small guanosine triphosphate hydrolase (GTPase) Ras (Stephens et al., 1994). Activated Ras then signals through one of several protein kinases, including Raf and the p38 MAP kinase, leading to the phosphorylation of the MAPK isoforms ERK-1 and ERK-2 (Thomas et al., 1992). Signaling downstream from these kinases supports neuronal differentiation, survival, and possibly regeneration (Skaper, 2008). PI3-K, which can be activated directly by Trk activation and indirectly by Ras, generates 3-phosphoinositides that in turn trigger activation of the serine-threonine kinase Akt, known also as protein kinase B (Kauffmann-Zeh et al., 1997; Marte, Downward, 1997). Akt promotes neuronal survival by blocking the pro-apoptotic protein BAD, by interfering with the pro-apoptotic transcription factor forkhead, and by enhancing retrograde signaling (Kuruvilla et al., 2000; Brunet et al., 2001; Yuan et al., 2003). It also plays a critical role in the growth cone, where it promotes microtubule assembly and axon growth by inactivating glycogen synthase kinase 3β (GSK-3β) (Zhou et al., 2004). Docking of PLC-γ on dimerized Trk receptors initiates pathways that trigger release of calcium stores and activate PKC. These interactions result in synaptic plasticity, and modify other cellular activities by influencing the MAPK pathway through activation of RAF (summarized in Reichardt, 2006).

The p75NTR is the sole member of the second type of neurotrophin receptor family. It is a transmembrane glycoprotein that was first recognized as a low-affinity receptor for NGF (Radeke et al., 1987). As other neurotrophins were studied, the p75NTR was found to bind them all with similar affinity (Hallbook et al., 1991). The receptor lacks intracellular catalytic activity, and signals by interacting with intracellular proteins that are either constitutively present or are recruited by receptor activation. Whereas the critical aspects of Trk receptor function were elucidated soon after their discovery, the role of the p75NTR remained an enigma for many years, and is only now being clarified. In contrast with the Trk receptors, p75NTR can exert both positive and negative effects on both cell survival and axon guidance.

Activation of the p75NTR can enhance neuronal survival through both direct and indirect means (Figure 9-3). A direct consequence of binding NGF to the p75NTR is activation of the pro-survival transcription factor nuclear factor kappa B (NF-κB) (Carter et al., 1996), a process that is enhanced when cells are stressed (Bhakar et al., 1999). The p75NTR also enhances the function of the Trk receptors, and thus cell survival, by inhibiting their activation by inappropriate neurotrophins (Bibel et al., 1999), by augmenting the activation of TrkA by low concentrations of NGF (Davies et al., 1993), by joining with TrkA to bind NGF with high affinity (Esposito et al., 2001), and by promoting retrograde transport of the neurotrophins (Curtis et al., 1995).

The apoptotic effects of p75NTR activation can also be obtained through several pathways, as exemplified by its interaction with intracellular proteins. TNF receptor-associated factor 6 (TRAF-6), neurotrophin receptor interacting factor (NRIF), and neurotrophin receptor-interacting MAGE homolog (NRAGE) are all activated by binding of neurotrophins to the p75NTR, and signal apoptosis through the c-Jun-N-terminal kinase (JNK) (Casademunt et al., 1999; Salehi et al., 2000; Gentry et al., 2004; Yeiser et al., 2004). NRAGE blocks the association of the p75NTR with TrkA, and its effect can be overcome by overexpressing TrkA (Salehi et al., 2000). The apoptotic effects of p75NTR were not fully understood until the discovery that p75NTR could bind the NGF precursor pro-NGF and the BDNF precursor pro-BDNF with relatively high affinity and trigger cell death at low concentrations (Lee et al., 2001; Fan et al., 2008). This interaction is enhanced by binding of the pro-neurotrophins to sortilin, which acts as a p75NTR coreceptor (Nykjaer et al., 2004). In the hippocampus, pro-neurotrophin signaling occurs through NRIF (Volosin et al., 2008).

The p75NTR exerts a similarly dichotomous influence on growth cone dynamics. Neurotrophin binding to p75NTR inactivates the small GTPase RhoA, blocking its inhibitory influence on the actin cytoskeleton and thus promoting axonal growth (Yamashita et al., 1999; Jaffe, Hall, 2005). This effect is potentiated by laminin, which downregulates p75NTR expression by regenerating neurites (Rankin et al., 2008). Growth is inhibited, in contrast, when p75NTR and the Nogo receptor (NgR) act as coreceptors with the LRR and Ig domain containing Nogo receptor-interacting protein (LINGO) to signal the binding of inhibitory molecules such as Nogo or MAG (Wang et al., 2002; Wong et al., 2002; Yamashita, Tohyama, 2003; Yamashita et al., 2005). Under these circumstances PKC promotes the small GTPase Rho to its active, GTP-bound state (Yamashita et al., 2002; Yamashita, Tohyama, 2003), leading to actin polymerization and growth cone collapse.

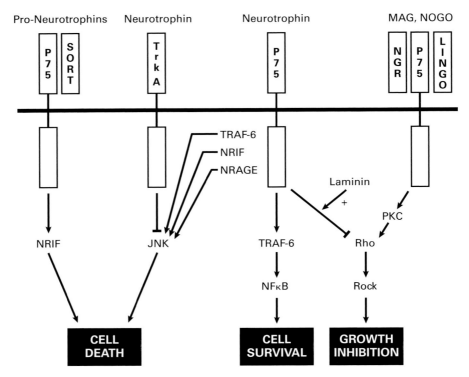

FIGURE 9-3 Signaling pathways activated by the low-affinity neurotrophin receptor p75NTR, often described as the "death receptor." Details are described in the text.

Recently, a third class of NGF receptor has been identified. The α9β1 integrin, known to be a receptor for osteopontin and tenascin C, also binds NGF, BDNF and NT-3 with low affinity to activate the MAPK/Erk pathway and promote cell survival and proliferation (Staniszewska et al., 2008).

GDNF

GDNF is a member of the TGF-β superfamily, a group of homodimers characterized by the similar spacing of 7 cysteine residues (Airaksinen, Saarma, 2002). It is the prototype of a family of growth factors that includes artemin, neurturin, and persephin. GDNF family signaling can be initiated in at least five ways, and may proceed through many of the known neuronal pathways (Runeberg-Roos, Saarma, 2007). Each family member binds to a distinctive receptor; GDNF to GDNF family receptor α-1 (GFRα-1), neurturin to GFRα-2, artemin to GFRα-3, and persephin to GFRα-4 (Figure 9-4). The transport of these receptors to the cell membrane, except in motoneurons, requires TGF-β itself (Krieglstein

et al., 1998; Peterziel et al., 2002). GDNF signaling is promoted by spatially concentrating the necessary components: GFRs are linked to the membrane by glycosyl phosphatidylinositol (GPI) anchors that congregate within lipid rafts (Poteryaev et al., 1999b), and membrane-bound heparin sulfate proteoglycans concentrate GDNF in the vicinity of GFRs and RET (Barnett et al., 2002). Strategies of promoting peripheral nerve regeneration by blocking or removing local proteoglycans could thus interfere with GDNF signaling at the site of nerve repair.

In the first GDNF signaling pathway to be identified, binding of the GDNF family members to their cognate GFRα receptors recruits two molecules of the tyrosine kinase RET to the lipid raft, where they are joined to initiate downstream signaling (Tansey et al., 2000). RET and the alpha receptors may interact "in cis," when both receptors are in the same cell, or "in trans," when RET interacts with alpha receptors in target neurons (Yu et al., 1998). RET signaling through the adaptor protein SHC activates both the PI3-K and MEK/ERK pathways, resulting,

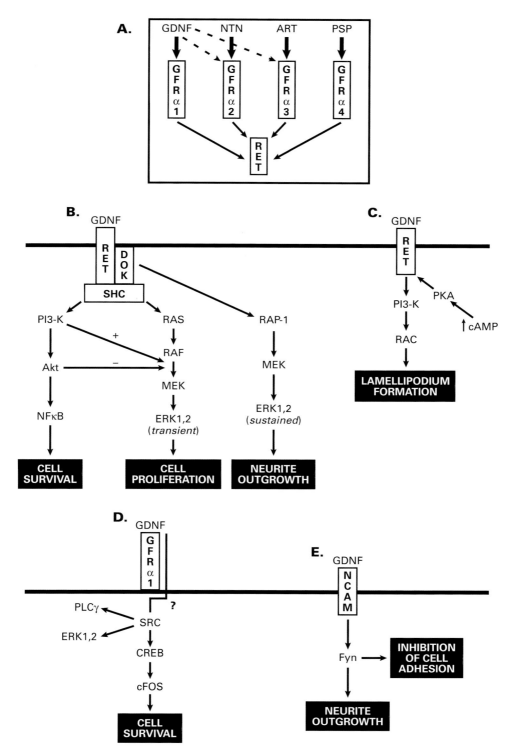

FIGURE 9-4   GDNF family signaling pathways. GDNF, neurturin (NTN), artemin (ART), and persephin (PSP) bind to GDNF family receptors α1 to α4 to activate RET as shown in the upper box. Signaling through RET, as well as through a variety of other pathways is diagrammed below. Details are found in the text.

respectively, in cell survival and cell proliferation (Besset et al., 2000; Hayashi et al., 2000). These pathways interact, as the level of ERK can be increased by PI3-K and decreased by Akt, providing a mechanism for fine-tuning the MEK/ERK pathway (Mograbi et al., 2001). RET may also signal through the adaptor protein downstream of kinase-4 (Dok-4), providing an alternative means of activating the MEK/ERK pathway through the small GTPase RAS-proximal-1 (RAP-1) (Uchida et al., 2006). Activation of ERK through SHC/RAS is only transient, leading to cell proliferation, whereas activation by Dok-4/RAP is longer-lasting, and results in neurite outgrowth. A third method of initiating GDNF signaling through RET requires elevation of cAMP to activate PKA, leading to phosphorylation of RET and direct activation of the PI-3 K pathway, resulting ultimately in the formation of lamellipodia (Fukuda et al., 2002). Alternatively, NGF can activate a long isoform of RET without the participation of either GDNF or the alpha receptors (Tsui-Pierchala et al., 2002).

GDNF may also signal without RET. Binding of GDNF to GFR-1 can activate the sarcoma kinase (SRC), promoting cell survival through CREB and the immediate early gene product cFOS (Poteryaev et al., 1999a; Trupp et al., 1999). The ERK1/2 and PLCγ pathways may also be activated through this interaction. In a related mechanism, GDNF can bind to the neural cell adhesion molecule (NCAM) to activate the SRC family kinase FYN and both promote neurite outgrowth and inhibit NCAM-mediated cell adhesion (Paratcha et al., 2003; Nielsen et al., 2009).

SIGNALING IN RESPONSE TO INJURY

Peripheral neurons are unique in the human body in that they may be injured inches, or even feet, from their cell bodies. If they are to respond to injury, and to adjust the neural regeneration state in a fashion that reflects the environment where regeneration must occur, the fact of injury must be communicated to the cell body as rapidly as possible. The signals that initiate regeneration have been studied in a variety of models, some of which may be relevant to peripheral nerve. These signals include immediate axotomy-induced electrical activity, deprivation of signals conveyed normally by retrograde transport, and retrograde transport of newly generated injury signals (Figure 9-5).

An immediate consequence of transecting the axons of cultured rodent cortical and sympathetic axons is vigorous electrical activity that leads to an increase in intracellular calcium, both at the site of injury and in the cell body (Mandolesi et al., 2004). When this discharge is blocked by inactivating sodium channels, regeneration cannot proceed. Axotomy also deprives the neuron of homeostatic signals from the periphery; retrograde transport of NGF in the rat sciatic nerve drops off rapidly after axotomy (Raivich et al., 1991). A potential role for this sudden decrease in NGF within DRG neurons is suggested by activation of some components of the axotomy response by treating uninjured animals with NGF antiserum, or, conversely, by blunting the injury response by treating with NGF after axotomy (Verge et al., 1995; Shadiack et al., 2001; Hirata et al., 2002). Nerve injury also precipitates local events that result in long-distance signaling via axonal transport. The trauma of axotomy releases the cytokines LIF, IL-6, and ciliary neuronotrophic factor (CNTF) into the wound environment. These bind to the gp130 receptor on the proximal nerve and together activate members of the janus kinase (JAK) family (Heinrich et al., 2003) (Figure 9-1). The function of these cytokines is tissue-specific: IL-6 is the only one to activate STAT3 in Schwann cells, while CNTF and LIF, but not IL-6, activate STAT3 in DRG neurons (Wang et al., 2009).

The contributions of LIF and IL-6 to regeneration have been discussed previously in the context of conditioning and the neuronal regeneration state. A third neuropoietic cytokine, CNTF, is transported proximally from a site of nerve injury and functions primarily as an injury factor. Significant quantities of CNTF have been found in the extracellular milieu of injured nerve; transport from this area to the neuron results in early activation of STAT3 (Sendtner et al., 1992; Kirsch et al., 2003). Within the distal stump, in contrast, the concentration of both CNTF mRNA and protein decreases during Wallerian degeneration, recovering only as Schwann cells are reinnervated (Rabinovsky et al., 1992; Seniuk et al., 1992). Consistent with this concept, injection of CNTF into the DRG conditions sensory neurons as judged by enhanced regeneration of crushed dorsal roots (Wu et al., 2007). CNTF null mice do not recover fully from nerve crush; the relative contributions of axon regeneration and muscle reinnervation to this deficit are still a matter of controversy (Yao et al., 1999; Siegel et al., 2000; Wright, Son, 2007). When CNTF is pumped onto the site of

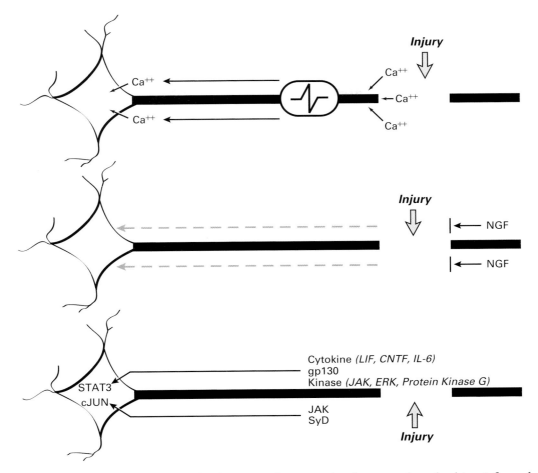

FIGURE 9-5   The occurrence of peripheral injury may be conveyed to the neuron through calcium influx and the generation of electrical impulses (top), through interruption of the flow of homeostatic retrograde signals such as NGF (middle), or through proximal transport of positive injury signals (bottom). Adapted from Abe and Cavalli, 2008.

sciatic nerve repair, the slope of SFI improvement is increased significantly, yet the outcome is still poor (Newman et al., 1996). Systemic delivery of CNTF enhances early distal stump reinnervation in mice, whereas pumping CNTF into the CSF of sheep has no significant impact on muscle reinnervation (Sahenk et al., 1994; Kelleher et al., 2006). The role of CNTF in nerve repair thus appears to be consistent with its mode of action: it accelerates the early phases of axon regeneration. It is quite possible that this is due to a reduction in regeneration stagger (see below) rather than an actual acceleration of regeneration per se.

A common theme in transport-mediated injury signaling is the activation of kinases at the site of nerve injury. In compartmentalized cultures of sympathetic neurons, a complex of one of the cytokines mentioned above with the gp130 receptor and activated JAK is transported centrally where it activates the transcription factor STAT3 (Figures 9-1, 9-5) (Schwaiger et al., 2000; O'Brien, Nathanson, 2007). In a similar fashion, the kinases Erk and protein kinase G may also be activated in the proximal stump of injured nerve and transported proximally (Perlson et al., 2005; Sung et al., 2006). Maintaining the integrity of these messages during transport poses a significant challenge, as their phosphorylation is easily reversible (Abe, Cavalli, 2008). A mechanism to protect the phosphorylated kinases with scaffolding proteins en route has evolved as a solution to this problem (Hanz et al., 2003; Perlson et al., 2005; Perlson et al., 2006; Hanz, Fainzilber, 2006). A similar transport process may occur in the mouse sciatic nerve when the protein Sunday driver (SYD) forms a complex with JNK and the molecular motors kinesin-1 and dynein (Cavalli et al., 2005). Once in the nucleus, JNK phosphorylates c-Jun, influencing regeneration as described above.

CHRONIC NEURONAL AXOTOMY

By the beginning of the twentieth century it was already apparent that clinical outcomes deteriorated as the interval from injury to nerve repair increased (Sherren, 1908). This problem was first approached experimentally by Kilvington, who performed nerve transfers in the forelimb of the dog to isolate the effects of chronic neuronal axotomy from those of chronic pathway denervation (Kilvington, 1912). The effects of axotomy were examined by uniting a chronically transected proximal nerve to a fresh distal stump, and the effects of pathway denervation by joining a fresh proximal stump to a previously denervated distal stump. In the four dogs that underwent these procedures, chronic neuronal axotomy appeared to be the primary determinant of outcome. As a result, Kilvington suggested nerve transfer, thereby using fresh neurons to reinnervate chronically denervated muscle. In similar nerve-crossing experiments in the forelimbs of rabbits, Holmes and Young (1942) found early reinnervation of the distal stump to be robust after up to a year of axotomy, and concluded that chronic axotomy was well tolerated. It is possible that they failed to account for microscopic reinnervation across the gap separating proximal and distal stumps. Soon after, Gutmann and Young provided histological evidence that prolonged denervation caused significant motor endplate abnormalities (Gutmann, Young, 1944). Together, these studies indicated to the investigators that end organ deterioration was responsible for the poor outcomes of delayed surgery, a view that persisted for half a century. Ironically, Holmes and Young described markedly increased outgrowth from nerves that had been injured 1 week previously, but did not recognize this conditioning effect as a discrete phenomenon.

The relative roles of neuronal and pathway deterioration were reexamined in elegant nerve-crossing experiments by using the tibial and peroneal branches of the rat sciatic nerve (Fu, Gordon, 1995a, 1995b). The number of motoneurons that were able to reestablish functional connections with denervated muscle fibers decreased by over 50% after only 2 months of axotomy, with slight further decline up to 1 year. Muscle force was restored in all groups, however, due to progressive increase in the size of the remaining motor units. Further experiments in this model confirmed that chronic peripheral axotomy does not result in significant motoneuron death, suggesting that a substantial number of motoneurons must survive but lose their ability to regenerate (Xu et al., 2009). The loss of regenerative capacity occurs irrespective of whether the axotomized nerve is blocked off or permitted to regenerate into a cutaneous nerve with no muscle end organs, is accompanied by progressive decrease in the expression of ATF-3 (Figure 9-1) in neurons and Schwann cells, and may be partially overcome by administration of BDNF or GDNF (Boyd, Gordon, 2003b; Furey et al., 2007; Saito, Dahlin, 2008). In the facial nerve model, re-injury after 10 weeks of axotomy upregulates GAP-43 and tubulin, indicating some resilience of these motoneurons, yet there is still a substantial reduction in the number of motoneurons that regenerate. Enhancement of the intrinsic regeneration state of chronically denervated motoneurons is thus a potentially fruitful therapeutic goal.

PART 2: THE REPAIR SITE

The growth cone, located at the tip of the axon, guides axonal elongation during development and probably during peripheral axon regeneration. Growth cone extension results when longitudinally oriented actin bundles anchor to the substrate and are lengthened by polymerization at their distal tips. Microtubules, the longitudinal skeleton of the axon, explore the advancing edge of the growth cone and collect where adhesive interactions occur between actin and the substrate, biasing the direction of growth cone advance and consolidating to form new axon as the growth cone progresses. Growth cones may be directed by adhesion and antiadhesion molecules on cell surfaces or the extracellular matrix (ECM) and by diffusible growth factors, neurotransmitters, and secreted morphogens. Experiments performed with the Campenot dual-chamber culture system established that local signaling at the growth cone is required for axon elongation. The Rho GTPases RhoA, Rac1, and Cdc42 link upstream guidance cues, mediated through PI3-K signaling, to downstream cytoskeletal

actin bundles with new axon shaft structure (Suter, Forscher, 2000; Buck, Zheng, 2002). Both of these activities are, in turn, influenced by actin. Peripherally, the rate at which actin couples and uncouples from dynamic microtubules influences their exploratory activity (Lee, Suter, 2008). Centrally, consolidation requires that actin arcs in the T zone limit the incursion of microtubules into trailing filopodia along the sides of the growth cone, thereby facilitating the bundling of these microtubules to form new axon shaft (Burnette et al., 2008; Schaefer et al., 2008).

Growth Cone Guidance

Growth in a straight line requires symmetrical protrusion of the leading filopodia and a reduction of lateral activity. To turn, growth cones modify filopodial protrusion asymmetrically. The same turning response can be elicited by interacting with positive signals to enhance extension on one side of the growth cone or by interacting with negative signals to reduce extension on the other side (Lowery, Van Vactor, 2009). Growth cones can be influenced by three classes of molecules: (1) adhesion molecules displayed by other cells or anchored within the extracellular matrix, the primary example being laminin (McKerracher et al., 1996); (2) antiadhesion molecules that prevent the growth cone from advancing, such as Ephrins (Chilton, 2006); and (3) a variety of diffusible neurotropic molecules, including growth factors (Gunderson, Barrett, 1979), neurotransmitters (Zheng et al., 1994), and secreted morphogens (Brunet et al., 2005). Parenthetically, it is important to note that growth factors such as NGF may have both trophic (nourishing) and tropic (guidance) functions. Receptors present on the growth cone signal through a variety of kinases, phosphatases, and GTPases, as well as through calcium ions (Ensslen-Craig, Brady-Kalnay, 2004; Govek et al., 2005; Gomez, Zheng, 2006; Robles, Gomez, 2006). An aspect of growth cone guidance that has been appreciated only recently is that the response to a given stimulus is context-dependent. Examples of this phenomenon are the conversion of growth cone attraction by BDNF to repulsion by interfering with cAMP signaling (Song et al., 1997), and the reversal of MAG-mediated repulsion by elevating intracellular cAMP (Song et al., 1998).

Neurotrophins were among the earliest molecules found to interact with the growth cone to modify axon behavior (Gunderson, Barrett, 1979). Determining the role of individual growth factors in promoting axon elongation and localizing their source are, however, complex tasks in the living animal. Growth factors may be produced by the neuron itself, by neurons with which it forms synapses, by central and/or peripheral glia, by infiltrating cells such as macrophages, or by target organs (Korsching, 1993; Oppenheim, 1996a). To simplify the analysis of growth factor effects, Campenot devised a culture system that physically separates the neuronal cell body from the elongating axon, allowing the environment of each component to be manipulated individually (Campenot, 1977) (Figure 9-9). Using NGF-sensitive sympathetic neurons, Campenot found the effects of NGF to be dependent on the site of application; neurite outgrowth was promoted when NGF was applied to the growing axon tip, but not when it was applied to the cell body (Campenot, 1982a). Axon collaterals that had elongated with initial NGF support were later pruned soon after NGF deprivation, but the neuron remained healthy as long as NGF was provided to the remaining collaterals (Campenot, 1982b). When adult DRG neurons were substituted for sympathetic neurons, in contrast, collaterals that had extended with NGF support survived after NGF depletion, as they were no longer dependent on NGF for survival (Kimpinski et al., 1997). In both sympathetic and DRG neurons, these experiments

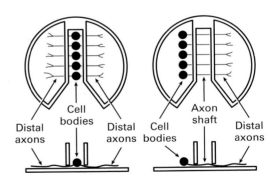

FIGURE 9-9 Two configurations of the Campenot chamber viewed from above (top) and from the side (below). On the left, collateral axons from individual neurons grow into two separate chambers where they can be exposed to various combinations of growth factors. On the right, single axons grow through two chambers, permitting separate control of the growth factor environment of the axon shaft and growth cone. Adapted from Zweifel et al., 2005.

established that local signaling at the growth cone is required for axon elongation. For this growth to proceed, however, there must also be a supply of raw materials provided by activation of a genetic program centrally (Zhou, Snider, 2006).

SIGNALING TO PROMOTE REGENERATION IN ADULT MAMMALIAN NEURONS

The signaling that links receptor activation to axonal growth has been studied most frequently in embryonic and nonneural cells. For the reasons discussed at the beginning of this chapter, the relevance of this information to adult regeneration is uncertain. A growing body of pathway studies, however, has used the regeneration of adult mammalian neurons, both in vitro and in vivo, as their outcome measure. The majority of these have been performed in vitro on adult DRG neurons, as these are no longer dependent on neurotrophins for their survival and can be cultured readily. Additional approaches have included the use of mice genetically engineered to over- or underexpress a specific pathway intermediate, or manipulation of the concentration of a specific intermediate in normal neurons through RNAi interference or viral vector-mediated overexpression.

Many of the experiments mentioned previously in the discussion of neuronal growth state used regeneration of adult DRG neurons as their endpoint, including those that established the role of the cAMP-PKA pathway in overcoming growth inhibition (e.g., Qiu et al., 2002). Several transcription factors were also shown to play a critical role in the regeneration of cultured adult DRG neurons: STAT3 (Qiu et al., 2005), cJun (Lindwall et al., 2004), ATF-3 (Seijffers et al., 2006), and Smad1 (Zou et al., 2009), or in regeneration in vivo: Sox11 (Jankowski et al., 2009).

Recent additional work has explored the roles of the MAPK pathways (JNK, ERK1,2, p38) and the PI3-K pathway in the regeneration of adult neurons.

JNKs phosphorylate the transcription factor cJun, a process that is necessary for effective regeneration both in vitro and in vivo (Lindwall et al., 2004; Raivich et al., 2004). Activated cJun influences regeneration through upregulation of galanin and the α 7β1 integrin (Raivich et al., 2004) (Figure 9-1), as well as by upregulating expression of the transcription factor ATF3 (Lindwall et al., 2004). The kinase ERK1,2 is activated by axotomy in vivo within axons in the proximal nerve stump and within Schwann cells in the distal stump (Agthong et al., 2006). ERK is required for neuronal conditioning in the ex vivo DRG model (Wiklund et al., 2002) and is required for initiation of growth cone formation when cultured adult DRG neurites are transected (Chierzi et al., 2005). Systemic blockade of ERK1,2 function impairs regeneration after nerve crush, but whether this results from impaired activity within Schwann cells or axons has not been determined. Given the diversity of neurons within the DRG, it is no surprise that activation of ERK1,2 and its downstream effects are neuronal type-specific. Not only have NGF, GDNF, and NT-3 been found to activate ERK1,2 in discrete subsets of DRG neurons, but also the effects of this activation are factor-dependent (Wiklund et al., 2002). NGF and GDNF promote neurite growth in their sensitive populations, whereas NT-3 upregulates ERK1,2 to promote regeneration in TrkC-positive neurons and downregulates it to inhibit regeneration in TrkA-positive neurons (Wilson-Gerwing et al., 2009). In contradistinction to growth that is stimulated by growth factors, unstimulated outgrowth from Trk-A-positive DRG neurons does not require ERK1,2 activity but utilizes the PI3-K pathway (Tucker et al., 2006).

Substantial evidence confirms participation of the PI3-K pathway in adult regeneration. Blocking PI3-K signaling in cultures of adult rodent DRG neurons reduces spontaneous neurite outgrowth (Edstrom, Ekstrom, 2003), and blocks the promotion of outgrowth by NGF, IGF, and GDNF (Kimpinski, Mearow, 2001; Edstrom, Ekstrom, 2003; Jones et al., 2003). Inactivation of PI3-K in vivo inhibits regeneration and compromises functional recovery after sciatic nerve crush in the mouse (Eickholt et al., 2007). The role of these pathways in the conditioning effect remains controversial. Once the conditioning has taken place in vivo, enhanced neurite outgrowth from conditioned DRG neurons in vitro has variously been found to depend on MAPK signaling (Wiklund et al., 2002), or to be independent of both MAPK and PI3-K activation (Liu, Snider, 2001).

PI3-K signaling may influence the axonal cytoskeleton through a variety of intermediate pathways (reviewed in Zhou, Snider, 2006; Tucker, Mearow, 2008). Neurite outgrowth stimulated by NGF requires activation of the signaling intermediates focal adhesion kinase (FAK) and the kinase Src, both upstream of PI3-K activation (Tucker et al.,

2008). An immediate downstream target of PI3-K in DRG neurons is the serine/threonine kinase Akt, also known as protein kinase B (PKB) (Edstrom, Ekstrom, 2003; Jones et al., 2003; Tucker et al., 2005). Once activated, Akt phosphorylates and thereby inactivates GSK-3β, triggering cytoskeletal assembly and axon growth (Jones et al., 2003; Zhou et al., 2004; Zhou, Snider, 2006). Overexpression of Akt in hypoglossal motoneurons results in accelerated regeneration after axotomy (Namikawa et al., 2000). The protein kinase target of rapamycin (TOR) is also downstream of PI3-K, and controls local protein synthesis needed for the genesis of growth cones on injured DRG neurons (Verma et al., 2005).

Currently, the majority of evidence thus links the PI3-K and ERK1,2 pathways to regeneration in adults. Nearly all of this work has been done on DRG neurons because of their ease of culture relative to motoneurons. In response to this shortcoming we have recently introduced an organotypic model of nerve repair in vitro to evaluate growth factor and pathway effects on motoneurons as they regenerate in a three-dimensional peripheral nerve environment (Vyas et al., 2010) (Figure 9-10).

LOCAL PROTEIN SYNTHESIS

Cultured adult DRG neurons are able to regenerate new growth cones as soon as 20 minutes after their axons are transected, long before axoplasmic transport could supply structural material from the cell body (Verma et al., 2005). Evaluation of the transition from cut axon to growth cone revealed that local translation of RNA into protein plays a critical role in this process, forcing a revision of the entrenched belief that all protein synthesis occurs within the cell body (Zheng et al., 2001; Verma et al., 2005). Similarly, a conditioning lesion was found to increase the immunostaining for several components of the protein synthetic machinery within axons. Although this machinery is not morphologically obvious, elements of the Golgi apparatus and endoplasmic reticulum have been identified within axons, and intermittent "plaques" of ribosomes have been localized to the periphery of the axoplasm near the axon-myelin border (Koenig et al., 2000; Merianda et al., 2009). Recent work has also shown that axonal ribosomes can be supplied by adjacent Schwann cells, revealing previously unappreciated avenues of communication between axons and glia (Court et al., 2008). Intra-axonal protein synthesis is modulated by RNA binding proteins that control both the transport and localization of specific mRNAs in response to axonal stimuli (Vuppalanchi et al., 2009; Yoo et al., 2009). These stimuli include the neurotrophins, which function in this context to localize individual mRNAs within the axon, and MAG and semaphorin 3A (SEMA 3A), both of which exert the opposite effect (Willis et al., 2007). The proteins synthesized within the axonal compartment include those used for injury signaling (described above), β-actin, β-tubulin, molecules involved in the control of actin dynamics, and calcitonin gene-related peptide (CGRP), a stimulus to

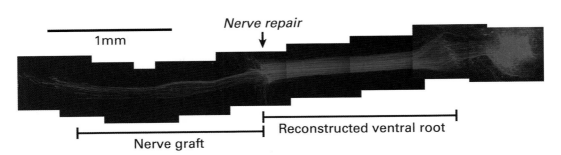

FIGURE 9-10   Nerve repair in vitro. A transverse section of spinal cord from a mouse that expresses YFP in its motoneurons (extreme right) is co-cultured with a three-dimensional segment of peripheral nerve to reconstruct a ventral root. One week after the co-culture is established, the newly reinnervated ventral root is transected and joined to a fresh nerve graft. Motor axons cross the repair site and reinnervate the graft. Their progress can be followed sequentially by fluorescence microscopy. This model was designed to investigate the signaling pathways and growth factors involved in motor axon regeneration. From Vyas et al., 2010.

Schwann cell proliferation (Toth et al., 2009; Vogelaar et al., 2009).

BRIDGING THE GAP

The process of bridging the gap between nerve ends has been modeled within silicon chambers, making the assumption that the steps involved in bridging a large, silicon-enclosed gap are the same as those involved in closing the microscopic gap between proximal and distal stumps of a nerve repair (Figure 9-11) (Chen et al., 2005; McDonald et al., 2006). The degree to which these assumptions are warranted is still under discussion. The steps have been described in detail in Chapter 8. In brief, the gap fills with serum in the first 2–3 hours after surgery. Over the following 1–2 days this is replaced by a solid matrix of fibrin, fibrinogen, and fibronectin that is infiltrated by macrophages and polymorphonuclear leukocytes and contains soluble growth factors. Fibroblasts migrate into the matrix, replacing fibrin with collagen, and Schwann cells invade and lay down laminin. Within enclosed gaps, nearly all axons invade in partnership with Schwann cells rather than as naked axons.

Schwann cells and their basal lamina play pivotal roles during early regeneration. Comparison of the clinical sequelae of nerve crush and nerve transection reveals that continuity of the basal lamina is equal to, and in some cases surpasses, age as a

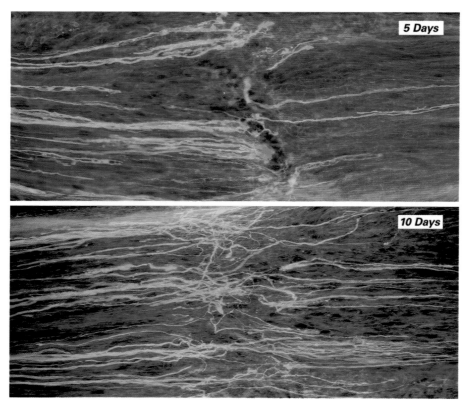

FIGURE 9-11   Evolution of the site of nerve repair. Nerve grafts from nonexpressing littermates were used to bridge gaps in the sciatic nerves of mice that express YFP in a subset of sensory and motor axons. Sections cut at 100 μm, counterstained for laminin (red), fluorescent image at 20x. The host-graft juncture site passes vertically through the midportion of each image; the proximal stump is on the left. Five days after repair, a small gap separates the proximal and distal stumps. The few axons that have crossed have penetrated far into the distal stump. Ten days after repair, the gap has been obliterated. Axonal trajectories are grossly distorted, yet many axons have penetrated the distal stump, where they resume a straight trajectory in response to the Schwann cell basal lamina. From Witzel et al., 2005.

primary determinant of outcome (Brushart, 1998). Nerve crush, which disrupts basal lamina integrity only occasionally (Haftek, Thomas, 1968), hastens the onset of regeneration and increases its subsequent speed relative to nerve transection (Forman, Berenberg, 1978; Forman et al., 1979). Axons that must bridge a gap in the basal lamina eventually regain their initial spatial relationship with Schwann cells and basal lamina as they reinnervate the distal stump. Nonetheless, their regeneration speed will never be restored to that of axons that were crushed but never lost contact with basal lamina to begin with. A critical interaction thus occurs in the first days after injury that modifies the entire future course of regeneration. This interaction, in analogy to the conditioning effect, results in what could be termed "de-conditioning."

De-conditioning could result from the absence of a critical interaction with basal lamina, and/or from the addition of wound components that interfere with injury and/or regenerative signaling. It is also conceivable that propagation of axons through distal basal lamina tubes containing phenotypically mismatched Schwann cells could slow regeneration. Two molecules that are known to guide axons in the developing CNS could potentially serve as indicators of basal lamina status after nerve injury. Slit2, which is upregulated by Schwann cells after nerve transection but not after nerve crush, is a potent stimulus to axon collateral sprouting (Wang et al., 1999; Tanno et al., 2005). Netrin-1 is also upregulated after transection but not after crush, and is a potent inhibitor of growth from adult DRG explants (Madison et al., 2000; Park et al., 2007). A further indication that discontinuity of the laminin surface may influence regeneration through mechanisms beyond a lack of local guidance is the observation that contact with laminin in vitro activates the phosphatidylinositol-3 kinase (PI3-K) pathway in regenerating neurites (Menager et al., 2004). Since this pathway is critical for the regeneration of adult neurons (see below), it is conceivable that its inactivation by a laminin gap may alter the regeneration state of the neuron.

Disruption of the basal lamina by nerve transection will expose regenerating axons to potentially negative influences emanating from both the wound environment and the distal nerve stump. An example of the former is plasma-derived fibrinogen, which leads to deposition of fibrin, a known inhibitor of regeneration (Zou et al., 2006). Two components of normal nerve, MAG and CSPGs, are usually discussed in the context of the distal stump, but may also influence axons as they cross the interstump gap (Udina et al., 2009). Both are reviewed in more detail in Part 3 of this chapter. The inhibitory effects of MAG are overcome by laminin in vitro (David et al., 1995); as long as axons are traveling along a laminin-containing surface they can overcome MAG inhibition, but at a site of basal lamina discontinuity, where the presence of soluble MAG has been confirmed in vivo (Torigoe, Lundborg, 1998), this "rescue" would be lacking. Similarly, CSPGs are normal components of the endoneurium that are upregulated after nerve injury by both Schwann cells and fibroblasts (Morgenstern et al., 2003; Muir, 2010). Eliminating the inhibitory function of CSPGs with Chondroitinase ABC enhances distal stump reinnervation after nerve transection but not after nerve crush (Zuo et al., 2002), suggesting that loss of contact with laminin is required for CSPGs to exert their effects. The finding that chondroitinase treatment strongly enhances the reinnervation of nerve grafts as soon as 4 days after surgery (Krekoski et al., 2001) is consistent with a role for CSPG inhibition within the interstump gap or directly at the entrance to the distal Schwann cell tube.

Experiments that modify the nature of the lesion and/or the distal pathway have helped clarify the relative contributions of the Schwann cell and basal lamina to early regeneration. Mutual attraction of proliferating Schwann cells in proximal and distal stumps helps bridge the repair gap (Abernethy et al., 1994), yet the contribution from the distal stump is sufficient to promote brisk reinnervation by itself (Hall, 1986). Schwann cells are able to migrate for 6–8 mm through basal lamina grafts without accompanying axons (Anderson et al., 1991); even in the company of axons, they require interaction with inflammatory infiltrates to migrate over longer distances (Sorensen et al., 2001). The process of regeneration through basal lamina devoid of Schwann cells is particularly revealing. When basal lamina is presented as a graft, and thus is not continuous with basal lamina in the proximal stump, axons can only enter in the company of Schwann cells, similar to their behavior when confronted with an experimental gap (Anderson et al., 1983; Hall, 1986; McDonald et al., 2006). Freezing a segment of nerve to kill the Schwann cells distal to a crush lesion, in contrast, presents regenerating axons with a continuous basal lamina surface. These axons enter the basal lamina ahead of Schwann cells, and still regenerate more rapidly than they would if the basal lamina had been transected, resembling their growth on artificial surfaces (Sketelj et al., 1989; Fugleholm et al., 1994; Torigoe et al., 1996). In one instance, crushed rat sciatic axons regenerated through a 25-mm-long acellular segment to restore skin sensitivity to pinch and the toe spread reflex (Bajrovic et al., 1994). The integrity of the basal lamina thus influences not only the onset and speed of regeneration, but also the growth requirements of regenerating axons.

MORPHOLOGIC RESPONSES TO NERVE TRANSECTION AND REPAIR

Axon Branching

It is no exaggeration to suppose that from a simple axonic collateral there arise, through successive divisions within the central stump, scar, and peripheral stump, dozens of branches.
—Ramon y Cajal, 1928, p172

The production of multiple sprouts by regenerating axons was readily apparent when the Golgi stain was applied to peripheral nerve (discussed in Ramon y Cajal, 1928). In the subsequent half-century, regenerative axon branching was investigated as a potential solution to the denervation of otherwise healthy muscle in polio patients. Determining the extent of branching under various circumstances and the limits to the ability of branched axons to support muscle became an important experimental goal (Thomas, Davenport, 1949). Comparing axon counts in the proximal and distal stumps after nerve repair by light microscopy, early investigators estimated that each proximal axon generated three to five branches in the distal stump (Thomas, Davenport, 1949; Shawe, 1955; Evans, Murray, 1956). Although the advent of electron microscopy facilitated more precise quantification of both myelinated and unmyelinated axons (Jenq, Coggeshall, 1984), studies based on distal axon counts, no matter how precise the counting, can only provide estimates of the extent of neuronal branching. This imprecision results from the failure to quantify

(1) proximal axons that do not regenerate after nerve repair, and (2) the variable degree of branching by axons that do cross the nerve repair. The comparison of two hypothetical constructs illustrates this problem. If five axons in the proximal stump each regenerate successfully without branching, there will be five axons in the distal stump, leading to the assumption that branching has not occurred. If only one axon regenerates, but branches four times, there will also be five axons distally, again resulting in an estimate of no branching. Clearly, quantification of axons that do not regenerate will increase the precision of these calculations.

Both electrophysiological and tracing techniques have been combined with axon counts to increase the accuracy of branching estimates. Single fiber recordings from regenerated cat sural nerve revealed that 87% of proximal axons crossed the repair, resulting in a mean of 1.7 branches per axon (Horch, Lisney, 1981). The number of branches maintained by motor neurons in the muscle and cutaneous tributaries of the rat femoral nerve was estimated by excising the L2, L3, and L4 DRGs at the time of nerve repair, so that only motor axons would regenerate across the repair site (Redett et al., 2005). Comparing the number of myelinated axons in the distal nerves after 8 weeks with the number of motoneurons retrogradely labeled from each nerve revealed that motoneurons maintained a mean of 5.66 branches in cutaneous nerve but a mean of only 2.84 branches in muscle nerve (Figure 7-2). In spite of the refinements offered by these techniques, the results describe the mean branching behavior of an entire population of neurons. Only direct observation of a series of individual axons can provide an accurate view of the variability in branch formation within and among axon populations (Figure 9-12).

REGENERATIVE AXON BRANCHING

Axon branching during the early stages of nerve regeneration was analyzed at the ultrastructural level in the landmark studies of Morris, Hudson, and

---

FIGURE 9-12 (Continued from page 277) provide access to a large area and thus Schwann cell tubes that lead to a variety of destinations. D. Longitudinal section similar to A. The regenerating axon has generated several collateral sprouts as it contacts the distal stump. E. Diagram similar to B. In this case the sampling circle is defined by the diameter of the surface contacted by the collaterals. Presumably, collaterals could contact Schwann cell tubes anywhere within this circle. F. The sampling circle for the axon in D is more constrained than that of the axon in A, as the axon defines the full diameter of the circle rather than the radius.

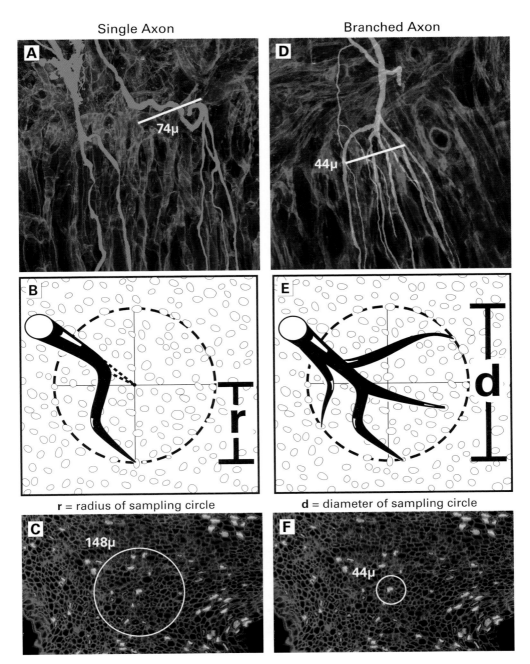

Single Axon

A 74µ

B r = radius of sampling circle

C 148µ

Branched Axon

D 44µ

E d = diameter of sampling circle

F 44µ

FIGURE 9-12 The consequences of axon branching at the repair site. Confocal images of peripheral nerve in mice expressing YFP in a subset of neurons, laminin counterstained red, original magnification 40x. A. Longitudinal section of a nerve repair. The axon on the right encounters the cut surface of the distal stump, defined by the scale bar, and travels laterally 74 µm before sending collateral sprouts distally (downward) into Schwann cell tubes of the distal stump. B. Diagram of the cut surface of the distal stump after transection of a peripheral nerve perpendicular to its long axis. Multiple Schwann cell tubes are seen in cross section. By defining a "sampling circle" centered on the point of initial contact with the distal stump and of a radius equal to the lateral excursion of the axon, it is possible to calculate the number of Schwann cell tubes that could theoretically be contacted by that axon. C. The sampling circle for the axon in A, demonstrating that lateral movement can

(Continues on page 276)

Weddell (Morris et al., 1972a, 1972b, 1972c, 1972d). They described the "regenerating unit," the progeny of a single axon contained within its original Schwann cell basal lamina. Regenerating units were further classified into two types: those with a single myelinated axon associated with unmyelinated axons, and those with only unmyelinated axons. Morris and colleagues examined only the proximal stump, so their term "regenerating unit" was not meant to apply to a group of axons within a single basal lamina tube in the distal stump (see below). The organizational unit of the distal stump is the Schwann cell tube, the cylindrical basal lamina made by Schwann cells that previously served a single myelinated axon. Distal Schwann cell tubes are likely to contain the progeny of more than one proximal axon, and are more appropriately termed "regenerating bundles." The early ultrastructural events in the proximal stump were further illuminated by the painstaking reconstructions of ordered electronmicroscopic sections performed by Friede and Bischhausen (1980). Because of their high magnification, these provide the most detailed view of early (72 hours post-transection) axon regeneration available. Multiple sprouts are seen arising from the site of injury as well as from the first node of Ranvier proximal to this, and travel both proximally and distally along the remaining axon. In specimens in which sprouting did not occur, the distal nerve was swollen with a volume of axoplasm equivalent to that within the sprouts in other specimens, suggesting a uniform production of axoplasm by the injured neuron.

Ramon y Cajal noted intermittent branching in the scar between nerve ends, but found most branches to be generated as the axon encountered the distal stump (Ramon y Cajal, 1928). A recent study of the morphology of individual regenerating axons confirmed this observation (Witzel et al., 2005) (Figure 9-12). The direct consequence of distal branching is the reinnervation of multiple Schwann cell tubes by branches of a single axon. As a result, each parent axon is able to sample a variety of distal environments. Although the actual number of tubes sampled is limited by the number of branches, the width of the entire arborization defines a "sampling circle," within which any Schwann cell tube could conceivably be sampled. Seven days after nerve repair in mice that express YFP in their axons, branched axons had a mean sampling circle diameter of 40 μ (Witzel et al., 2005). A similar analysis can be made for axons that travel along the surface of the distal stump before they branch and reinnervate Schwann cell tubes. In this case, the length of the lateral movement defines a radius that could pivot in any direction around the axis of the parent axon. In mice expressing a variant of yellow fluorescent protein in their neurons (YFP mice), axons that displayed lateral movement 7 days after nerve repair had a mean sampling circle radius of 28 μm (Witzel et al., 2005). With this degree of lateral motion, an axon would probably pass directly over the entrance to 5–10 Schwann cell tubes before making a right angle turn into the distal stump. Taking into account all possible radii from the same starting point, this axon could theoretically access a total population of 142 Schwann cell tubes, depending on the direction of outgrowth from the initial point of contact. Many regenerating axons thus have the capability of sampling multiple Schwann cell tubes before they are committed to a distal pathway. Failures of regeneration specificity are thus more likely to result from inability to detect appropriate pathways than from inability to reach them.

In addition to its implications for pathway sampling, regenerative axon branching might also influence regeneration by reducing its speed. As noted above, axon regeneration after nerve transection is slower than that after nerve crush. Transection also increases the number of axon branches relative to crush (Chapter 7). When axons branch the total microtubule mass in the daughter branches is greater than that in the parent axon (Watson et al., 1989). As a result, the speed of axoplasmic transport, and thus of regeneration, should be slower in the branches than it would be for a single parent axon (Miller, Samuels, 1997). The need for a pure population of branched peripheral axons with long tributaries makes this hypothesis difficult to test.

MODULATION OF BRANCHING

Several factors have recently been identified that modulate axon branching during regeneration of mammalian peripheral nerve. The rat facial nerve is an ideal in vivo model for the study of regenerative branching, as reinnervation of more than one distal tributary by branches of a single neuron is readily identified by retrograde double- or triple-labeling. Whereas 85% of motoneurons regenerating after routine facial nerve repair contribute branches to at least two tributary nerves, blocking BDNF signaling with antibodies reduces this to only 18% (Streppel et al., 2002). The effects of blocking NGF and IGF-1 are similar, but less pronounced. In the same model, local addition of extracellular matrix proteins had no significant effect (Dohm et al., 2000).

Experiments on cultured DRG neurons have also implicated microtubule-associated protein 1B (MAP1B), the chemorepellant Slit 2, and fibroblast growth factor-2 (FGF-2) as potential mediators of regenerative branching. MAP1B is a scaffold protein that regulates the interaction between actin and microtubules in the growth cone (Riederer, 2007). DRG neurons cultured from MAP1B homozygous knockout animals branch twice as often as do those from controls, often from the axonal shaft rather than from the growth cone. Slit 2, originally identified as a chemorepellant in *Drosophila*, is produced by denervated Schwann cells in vivo and promotes the branching of embryonic DRG neurites in vitro (Wang et al., 1999; Tanno et al., 2005). As noted previously, Slit 2 is upregulated when the basal lamina is disrupted, a situation in which frequent branching occurs, but not after nerve crush, an injury that leaves the basal lamina intact and is associated with little branching. The effects of FGF-2 on branching of cultured DRG neurons are context-dependent: in cultures from control rats FGF-2 promotes branching, whereas in cultures from previously conditioned neurons it enhances axon elongation (Klimaschewski et al., 2004). In the context of observed axon morphology, it appears that axons that branch at the face of the distal nerve stump could either be responding positively to growth factors that diffuse from reactive Schwann cells, or negatively to chemorepellants such as Slit2 that are also upregulated in the same area. The striking differences in motoneuron branching during reinnervation of the femoral sensory and muscle nerves, which differ markedly in growth factor expression, suggests the former (Witzel et al., 2005; Hoke et al., 2006).

Staggered Regeneration

As all the sprouts are not equally vigorous, and as they are formed at different times, the invasion of the foreign tissues occurs progressively as if by shifts.
—Ramon y Cajal, 1928, p167

The return of function after nerve repair is a gradual process. Months may separate the first evidence of end organ reinnervation from the restoration of substantial function. In the clinic, it is difficult to ascertain whether the repair, the pathway, or the end organ is responsible for this time course. In the laboratory, however, it is possible to examine these factors individually. When regeneration of the rat femoral nerve is evaluated by retrograde labeling at several intervals after nerve repair, motoneurons are shown to arrive at their destinations intermittently over a period of 8 weeks (Brushart, 1990). There is thus no need to invoke end organ factors to explain the clinical findings. To determine whether this process, later termed "staggered regeneration" (Al-Majed et al., 2000), was generated at the repair site or within the distal pathway, a technique of proximal labeling was developed to identify motoneurons as soon as they crossed the repair and entered the distal nerve stump (Brushart et al., 2002) (Figure 9-13). This technique revealed that the rate of distal stump reinnervation in the rat increases to a maximum between 1 and 2 weeks after repair, diminishes between 2 and 3 weeks, then rises again between 3 and 4 weeks. Surprisingly, after routine nerve repair under ideal conditions, a significant number of motor axons do not cross the repair for at least 3 weeks.

STAGGERED REGENERATION IN YFP MICE

The timing of distal stump reinnervation was also investigated in mice expressing YFP in their neurons (Witzel et al., 2005) (Figures 9-11, 9-14). The sciatic nerves of these mice were reconstructed with grafts from animals not expressing YFP so that the progress of YFP+ axons through the grafts could be assessed without the interference of background fluorescence. Regeneration stagger was already apparent immediately distal to the repair, consistent with a critical role for the repair site in its generation. Additionally, however, survivorship analysis of axon extension revealed that axons were progressing at different speeds once they entered the distal stump (Figure 9-14). This potential contribution to regeneration stagger would not be identified by very proximal labeling studies, but should become progressively more apparent as axons extend through the distal pathway.

Further evaluation of the repairs in the YFP mice revealed a population of axons that were unsuccessful in crossing the repair in the first 10 days, and thus contributed to regeneration stagger (Figure 9-15). These axons exhibited a wide range of morphologies, ranging from those that had done little more

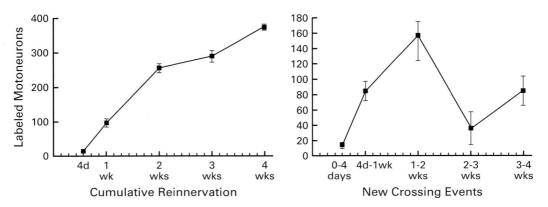

FIGURE 9-13   Staggered regeneration after peripheral nerve transection and repair. Motoneurons have been identified as soon as they reinnervate the distal nerve stump by applying Fluoro-Ruby to a crush site 3 mm distal to the repair. Left. The cumulative total of motoneurons that have crossed the repair from 4 days to 4 weeks, demonstrating progressive reinnervation. Right. Crossing events that occur in defined time intervals. The greatest number of motoneurons cross between 1 and 2 weeks with a lull between 2 and 3 weeks. A second wave of crossings then occurs between 3 and 4 weeks. Because of the progress of Wallerian degeneration, the distal stump environment encountered by the late-crossing motoneurons will be very different from that encountered by their swifter counterparts. From Brushart et al., 2002.

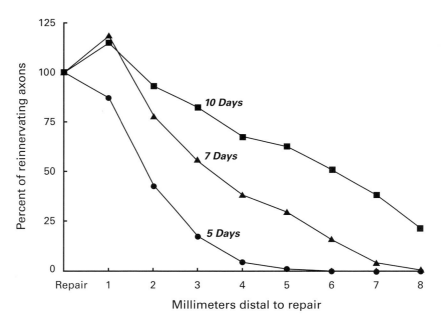

FIGURE 9-14   Survival analysis of YFP-expressing axons elongating within nonexpressing nerve grafts. Regenerating axons were counted at the repair site and at 1 mm intervals distally. Each segment was characterized by the percentage of reinnervating axons that penetrated to that level. A Poisson regression equivalent grouped survival analysis demonstrated that the survival curve at each time period differed significantly from that at the other times (p < 0.001). The distribution of axons within the distal stump is thus affected not only by the staggered nature of reinnervation but also by differential progress within the stump itself. From Witzel et al., 2005.

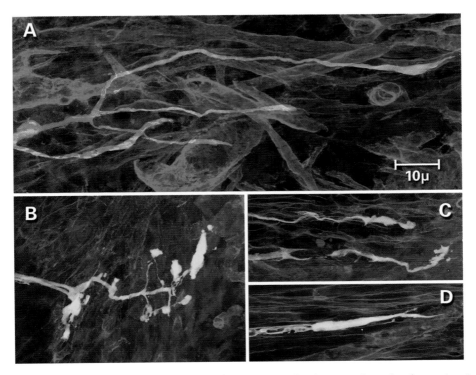

FIGURE 9-15   Axons that have failed to cross a nerve repair. Confocal images of peripheral nerve in mice expressing YFP in a subset of neurons, laminin counterstained red, original magnification 40x. Axons are regenerating from left to right. A. Regenerative axon collaterals penetrating a maze of disordered laminin in the gap between nerve ends. The relatively sharp tips on the axon branches suggest that they still represent viable collaterals. B. Multiple collaterals have explored various pathways through the interstump environment, but apparently all have regressed and are represented only by amorphous pools of axoplasm. C. The cut ends of axons that appear to have died back one internode, but show no signs of regenerating. D. Same as C, except a minute retrograde sprout is growing proximally from the upper surface of the penultimate node.

than die back one or two nodes of Ranvier to those that appear to have moved ahead through a series of adjacent microenvironments, only to be repulsed from each in turn. The end structures on axons that had penetrated but not crossed the repair site include the "terminal clubs" and "balls of retraction" described by Ramon y Cajal (1928). He believed that the former were precursors to further growth or branching, whereas the latter were accumulations of axoplasm from previous failed attempts at axon extension. Many of these endbulbs contain high concentrations of neuroactive peptides (Zochodne et al., 2001). Failure to reinnervate the distal stump could result from an inadequate neuronal intrinsic regeneration state or a preponderance of negative factors in the repair environment. In the YFP mouse model, nerve crush is followed by uniform and nearly simultaneous regeneration (Brushart, unpublished data),

indicating that most neurons are able to regenerate briskly under ideal circumstances. The repair environment must therefore play a substantial role in staggered regeneration. The possibility that motoneurons themselves might contribute to staggered regeneration by differing intrinsically in their regeneration state, and thus in their response to more challenging environments, remains untested.

Scar Formation

Early descriptions of the repair site emphasized postoperative scar formation (Young, 1949). Scar was viewed as a purely physical barrier, leading to the observation that "The process of nerve regeneration can be viewed as a race at the site of nerve repair involving the sprouting axons creeping toward the distal endoneurial tubes and the ingrowing fibrous tissue derived from the epineurium" (Bucko et al., 1981, p23). The potentially deleterious role of scarring at the site of nerve repair has been addressed both surgically and pharmacologically. Attempts to minimize scarring by excising the epineurium, a prominent source of fibroblasts, did not improve functional outcome in primates (Kline et al., 1981). Wrapping the repair with impermeable or permeable barriers to prevent fibroblast ingrowth enjoyed brief clinical popularity, but was found to enhance cellular reaction as the wraps fragmented (Guth, 1956; Campbell et al., 1961). Pharmacological interference with collagen synthesis by using the proline analog cis-hydroxyproline enhanced distal myelination in initial studies (Pleasure et al., 1974). Subsequently, more critical evaluations revealed no significant benefit to this treatment, nor to induction of experimental lathyrism with D-penicillamine or local application of collagenase (Bucko et al., 1981; Nachemson et al., 1985; Rydevik et al., 2002). Recently, however, mice with increased scarring as a result of knockout of the anti-inflammatory cytokine interleukin-10 (IL-10) were found to have impaired return of electrophysiological parameters when compared with mice that made less scar because they lacked the receptor for transforming growth factor-β (TGF-β) (Atkins et al., 2006). In subsequent experiments, local application of IL-10 to the repair site reduced collagen deposition and enhanced electrophysiological evidence of muscle reinnervation, confirming the relevance of collagen deposition to regeneration and opening a potential therapeutic avenue (Atkins et al., 2007).

Evolution of the Repair Environment

The nerve repair environment presents an evolving menu of positive and negative cues that are likely to influence the process of staggered regeneration; conversely, staggered regeneration assures that regenerating axons will encounter a distal stump environment that is constantly changing during the early weeks of regeneration. This is illustrated by experiments that unite freshly cut proximal stumps with grafts in which Wallerian degeneration has progressed for varying periods. The delay between nerve transection and the arrival of axons in the distal stump must, to a substantial degree, be a reflection of the repair environment. This delay varies according to the duration of graft predegeneration; the shortest delay, 0.6 day, was seen after a predegeneration period of 3 days (Kerns et al., 1993;

Danielsen et al., 1994). Interestingly, predegeneration before freezing also dramatically reduces the delay in the reinnervation of basal lamina grafts, indicating that the predegeneration process modifies the basal lamina as well as the cellular elements (Danielsen et al., 1995). Soluble extracts of distal stump tissue, presumably representative of the fluid environment between nerve ends, also vary in their ability to support regeneration depending on the length of predegeneration (Marcol et al., 2003).

The positive and negative factors responsible for the evolution of the repair environment largely reflect the progress of Wallerian degeneration in the distal stump, although CGRP and some growth factors have been localized to the proximal stump in experimental neuromas (Zochodne, Cheng, 2000; Zochodne et al., 2001). Early experiments with the silicon chamber model demonstrated the accumulation of growth factors within enclosed neural gaps, and these were thought to have a positive influence on regeneration (Longo et al., 1983a, 1983b). Production of soluble growth factors and cytokines by Schwann cells in the distal stump varies widely over the hours, days, and weeks after nerve transection (Hoke et al., 2006; temporal sequence reviewed by Boyd, Gordon, 2003a), and they may serve a variety of functions. Cytokines are released into the wound environment soon after injury and participate in nerve injury signaling (Sendtner et al., 1992; Heinrich et al., 2003). Growth factors may guide and support regeneration, but in a context-dependent fashion. The outgrowth of both sensory and motor neurons can be guided by growth factors at the population level in vitro (Gu et al., 1995; Mi et al., 2007). When the neurotropic (directional guidance) influence of NGF on cultured adult DRG neurons was evaluated, however, it was found that a laminin substrate and preconditioning, both of which may be lacking during early regeneration, were needed for a positive directional response (Webber et al., 2008). Currently there is no evidence to suggest that an individual axon can be guided to a specific Schwann cell tube in vivo. The overall support of regeneration by NGF is also context-dependent. NGF-responsive adult DRG neurons only require a laminin substrate and activation of the PI3-K pathway to promote their regeneration in vitro, whereas IB4+ neurons require both laminin and GDNF and activation of both PI3-K and MEK/ERK pathways (Tucker et al., 2006).

Negative influences from the distal stump include MAG, CSPGs, and nitric oxide (NO).

Soluble MAG inhibits early regeneration in vivo in a time-dependent fashion, and may be responsible for limiting the branching response of regenerating neurons (Torigoe, Lundborg, 1998; Tomita et al., 2007a). CSPGs inhibit regeneration locally in the distal stump (Zuo et al., 2002), and are probably also present in debris in the intraneural gap. Similarly, NO may be present transiently, and could potentially exert either positive or negative effects on regeneration (Levy et al., 2001; McDonald et al., 2007).

Retrograde Regeneration

Postoperative increase in the number of myelinated fibers proximal to the site of nerve transection and repair was revealed by early attempts to quantify axon regeneration (Gutmann, Sanders, 1943). Counts determined at several intervals by modern counting techniques have confirmed this phenomenon, and have shown the highest counts to be reached 6 months after repair in the rat model (Mackinnon et al., 1991). Proximal axon counts are elevated even further when the transected nerve ends in a neuroma (Carter, Lisney, 1991). Retrograde growth of axons is clearly illustrated in the drawings of Ramon y Cajal (1928) and the reconstruction performed by Friede and Bischhausen (1980). In the YFP mouse, retrograde growth is a common event (Figure 9-6). Similar growth along pathways that have not yet undergone Wallerian degeneration has been described in the C57Bl6/Ola (currently termed C57Bl6/wlds) mouse (Brown et al., 1992). These observations confirm the vital role played by the basal lamina: for many axons it is presumably easier to grow backward along basal lamina, even when the accompanying Schwann cells are not engaged in Wallerian degeneration, than it is to cross a void without basal lamina.

PART 3: THE DISTAL PATHWAY

Schwann cells denervated by axotomy downregulate genes involved in myelin maintenance and upregulate those needed for Wallerian degeneration, the process of clearing axoplasm and myelin from the Schwann cell tube. They proliferate within 3–4 days of axotomy and increase their migratory activity, both in response to growth factors. After a latent period of 1–2 days, axonal cytoskeleton is broken down by calpains and the ubiquitin-proteasome system. Axon debris then initiates signaling to

activate a network of cytokines and transcription factors that stimulate myelin breakdown, promote macrophage invasion, and target myelin for phagocytosis by macrophages and Schwann cells. Axon regeneration in rodents and rabbits proceeds at 3–4 mm/day after nerve crush and 2.5–3 mm/day after transection and repair; in humans, clinical observation suggests a regeneration speed for transected axons of 1–2 mm/day. The collaterals of multiple parent axons that regenerate together within a single Schwann cell tube in the distal stump are called a "regenerating bundle" to distinguish them from a "regenerating unit," the progeny of a single axon that remain within the parent Schwann cell tube in the proximal stump. Distal stump Schwann cell tubes provide initial direction and receptor-mediated interactions to the regenerating bundle, then fragment as the Schwann cells that ensheath constituent axons form new basal lamina tubes within the old framework. Myelination of regenerating axons proceeds under the control of the transcription factor SCIP in response to growth factors and the extracellular matrix. The endoneurium responds to injury by subdividing into multiple small perineurial compartments, the functions of which remain unclear. Soon after peripheral nerve transection the blood-brain barrier ceases to function at and distal to the site of injury. Barrier function is recovered only after several months, and progresses from proximal to distal behind the front of regenerating axons. Denervated Schwann cells upregulate expression of several growth factors that could potentially support regeneration, including the neurotrophins (NGF, BDNF, NT-3, NT-4/5), members of the TGF-β superfamily including GDNF, TGF-β, and the bone morphogenic proteins (BMPs), as well as hepatocyte growth factor (HGF), vascular endothelial growth factor (VEGF), pleiotrophin (PT), the insulin-like growth factors (IGF-I, IGF-II), and fibroblast growth factors (FGF-1,2). Contact with the extracellular matrix will expose regenerating axons to its constituents, including laminin, fibronectin, and tenascin-C. Additionally, axons will encounter a variety of proteins and glycoproteins that act as recognition molecules, including Galectin-1, Netrin-1, the neuropilins, NCAM, L1, and the potential regeneration inhibitors MAG and the CSPGs. The net effect of this complex environment is positive, as axons pass through myelin debris containing MAG and confront newly synthesized CSPGs yet proceed rapidly once they have entered the distal stump. This initial permissiveness is transient, however, so that support for regeneration in the rodent model is poor after only 2–3 months of denervation.

THE DENERVATED SCHWANN CELL

Myelinating Schwann cells in stable, one-to-one relationships with axons express a phenotype that reflects their support of myelination, with expression of myelin components such as MBP, P0, and MAG (Chapter 1; Trapp et al., 1988; LeBlanc, Poduslo, 1990). When Schwann cells are denervated by axotomy their function is altered radically: they reenter the cell division cycle, they migrate, and they participate in the process of clearing myelin and axonal debris from the denervated pathway. Eventually, they may also support axon regeneration. Denervated Schwann cells downregulate genes needed for their homeostatic function and upregulate genes related to cellular division, signaling, growth factor production, protein and myelin destruction, and reconfiguration of the extracellular matrix. These include transcription factors, neurotrophic factors, neuropoetic cytokines, cell-surface receptors, cell adhesion molecules, basement membrane components, gap junction proteins, and matrix metalloproteinases (reviewed by Fu, Gordon, 1997; Hall, 2001). Recently, activation of the transcription factors cJun and Notch has been found to play a prominent role in the de-differentiation of Schwann cells from the myelinating to a more primitive phenotype (Parkinson et al., 2008; Woodhoo et al., 2009).

Denervated Schwann cells proliferate soon after axotomy, and again when they are contacted by regenerating axons. The first wave of proliferation begins 3 days after axotomy in the cat and rat, and lasts an additional 2–3 days (Pellegrino et al., 1986; Oaklander et al., 1987; Griffin, Hoffman, 1993). Entering the cell division cycle is not necessary for regeneration after nerve crush (Kim et al., 2000; Yang et al., 2008), but is probably required for bridging proximal and distal stumps after nerve transection, and is most certainly required for regeneration into environments that do not contain Schwann cells (Hall, 1986). The control of Schwann cell proliferation during development has been studied extensively (reviewed by Jessen, Mirsky, 2005; Ogata et al., 2006), yet less is known about what stimulates the proliferation of denervated adult Schwann cells. For many years elevation of intracellular cAMP has been known to be a potent stimulus to the proliferation of cultured neonatal Schwann cells (Raff et al.,

1978; Ridley et al., 1989). In cultured segments of adult peripheral nerve, however, conditions that increase intracellular cAMP levels actually block Schwann cell proliferation (Svenningsen, Kanje, 1998), demonstrating yet again the critical roles played by cell age and environment in determining the response to a particular stimulus.

Recent in vivo studies of early Schwann cell proliferation have implicated growth factor signaling. The hematopoetic cytokine erythropoietin (Epo) stimulated Schwann cell division when applied to a site of chronic nerve constriction and promoted return of sensory and motor function after sciatic nerve crush (Li et al., 2005; Toth et al., 2008). Similarly, mice overexpressing basic fibroblast growth factor (FGF-2) were characterized by increased Schwann proliferation just distal to a crush site (Jungnickel et al., 2006). The role of neuregulin signaling through Erb receptors to stimulate the first wave of Schwann cell proliferation is less clear. In one set of experiments the neuregulin receptor ErbB2 was found to be activated on Schwann cell microvilli soon after injury of the adjacent axon; blocking this activation inhibited the Schwann cell response to axotomy (Guertin et al., 2005). In conditional ErbB2 knockouts, in contrast, neuregulin signaling was not required for Schwann cell proliferation (Atanasoski et al., 2006).

Although Schwann cell migration goes hand-in-hand with proliferation during development (Jessen, Mirsky, 2005), its role in nerve repair is less clear. The propensity for Schwann cells to travel into a void is well documented. They will migrate into a contiguous segment of acellular nerve (Dubový et al., 2001), into a basal lamina graft (Hall, 1986), out onto the surface of a denervated muscle (Dubový, Svízenská, 1994) into an enclosed nerve gap (Lundborg, Hansson, 1979; Lundborg et al., 1981), and even onto a plastic sheet (Torigoe et al., 1996). Whereas identification of migrating Schwann cells in environments that did not previously contain them is straightforward, identification of Schwann cells that have been exchanged between a fresh nerve graft and the contiguous recipient nerve requires a marker of their origin. Early experiments in which graft Schwann cells were radiolabeled indicated little exchange of Schwann cells between graft and host (Aguayo et al., 1976). More recently, grafting between sexes and using a Y chromosome-specific probe, Symons et al. (2001) found that after 3 months of regeneration adult mouse Schwann cells had migrated 2 mm from nerve graft into recipient nerve.

WALLERIAN DEGENERATION

Not long after Theodore Schwann discovered the cell that bears his name, the English physician Augustus Waller observed the degeneration of transected cranial nerves in the frog (Waller, 1850). He described a "coagulation or curdling" of the myelin that occurred 5–6 days after transection, fragmentation and partial absorption between days 7 and 9, and an amorphous granular structure thereafter. He was awarded the Medal of the Royal Society for his efforts (Waller, 1850). Waller's observations were made on unfixed tissue immersed in distilled water, and were probably facilitated by the contrasting refraction of myelin lipids with their surrounding fluid. Waller realized the dependence of the axon on the cell body for its survival, establishing a concept that would later mature into the Neurotrophic Hypothesis (Ochs, 1975). By the end of the nineteenth century, Ramon y Cajal was able to apply osmic acid stain to delineate myelin and silver nitrate to define other axonal structures within teased axons, allowing him to further delineate the morphology of Wallerian degeneration, which he also called "trophic degeneration" (Ramon y Cajal, 1928). He described the clumping and fragmentation of myelin in great detail, confirmed the proliferation of Schwann cells detected earlier by von Bungner (Bungner, 1891), and made numerous observations on the fine structure of the axon and axon sheath.

Axonal Breakdown

Wallerian degeneration is a complex sequence of events that results in the breakdown and recycling of both axon and myelin and stimulates the upregulation of growth factors that are presumed to enhance axonal regeneration (reviewed by Stoll, Müller, 1999; Stoll et al., 2002; Ehlers, 2004; Chen et al., 2007; Martini et al., 2008). The immediate sequelae of axonal transection have been observed by imaging the central processes of DRG neurons in mice that express GFP in their axons (Kerschensteiner et al., 2005). Ten to twenty minutes after an axon is transected, 200–300 µm of both proximal and distal stumps fragment suddenly, a process termed acute axonal degeneration (AAD). Retrograde axonal transport continues in the distal stump for several hours, so axonal organelles accumulate near the site of transection, and local breakdown of the blood-nerve barrier results in focal edema (Griffin, et al.,

1977; Bouldin et al., 1991). The more distal portions of the nerve remain relatively unchanged for a variable period of time. Ultrastructure may appear normal except for accumulation of organelles near nodes of Ranvier, and electrical conduction is still possible (Ballin, Thomas, 1969; Miledi, Slater, 1970; Gilliatt, Hjorth, 1972). The duration of this latent period depends on the size of the axon, varying between 25.6 and 45 hours in the rat phrenic nerve (Lubinska, 1977), as well as on the species, length of distal stump, and temperature (reviewed in Griffin et al., 1995).

The end of the latent period is defined by the onset of cytoskeletal breakdown. Once this process starts it proceeds very rapidly from the site of injury, with measured speeds of 46 mm/day for large axons and 250 mm/day for small axons (Lubinska, 1977). The disassembly of cytoskeletal proteins is triggered by the influx of calcium, which activates members of the calpain family of cysteine proteases and the ubiquitin-proteasome system (Schlaepfer, Micko, 1979; George et al., 1995; Zhai et al., 2003). The caspase family of cysteine proteases, the mediators of apoptosis, are not involved (Finn et al., 2000). Calpains are highly sensitive to intracellular calcium concentrations and are regulated by the inhibitor calpastatin (Cottin et al., 1981). Activated calpains disassemble neurofilament proteins (Zimmerman, Schlaepfer, 1982): inhibiting calpain activity by removing calcium or by adding specific inhibitors can prevent breakdown of neurofilaments (Glass et al., 1994; George et al., 1995). Evidence that calpain levels drop rapidly after nerve injury, before the onset of neurofilament breakdown, suggests that it may function at the onset of a proteolytic cascade rather than as the direct agent of protein destruction (Glass et al., 2002).

Involvement of the ubiquitin-proteasome system in Wallerian degeneration was detected through analysis of the C57Bl/Wlds mouse. In this mouse mutant, initially identified as C57Bl6/Ola, the onset of Wallerian degeneration is delayed for several weeks (Lunn et al., 1989). Localization of the defect to the axon, rather than to glia or infiltrating cells, indicated that axonal degeneration was not the inescapable consequence of separation from the cell body, but was instead an active process that might be manipulated (Glass et al., 1993; Finn et al., 2000). Further analysis of the C57Bl/Wld[s] mouse revealed that a chimeric gene encoded an N-terminal fragment of ubiquitination factor E4B (Ube4b) fused to nicotinamide mononucleotide adenyltransferase

(Nmat), and that this conferred a dose-dependent block of Wallerian degeneration (Mack et al., 2001). The 76 amino acid polypeptide ubiquitin is added to proteins to target them for destruction by the proteasome (Glickman, Ciechanover, 2002). Several sets of enzymes are needed for this process, including the E4 protein that forms part of the Wld^s fusion protein, suggesting involvement of the ubiquitin system in Wallerian degeneration. This involvement was confirmed by experiments on cervical ganglion neurons from young rats that showed marked delay of Wallerian degeneration when activity of the ubiquitin-proteasome system was blocked (Zhai et al., 2003).

Myelin Breakdown and Clearance

The products of axon disassembly initiate the next step in Wallerian degeneration, the breakdown and

clearance of myelin from the Schwann cell tube. Recent studies have indicated that the Toll-like receptors (TLRs), in conjunction with the adaptor protein MyD88, are activated by axonal debris in vitro (Lee et al., 2006). Signaling through the TLRs activates the chemokine monocyte chemotactic protein-1 (MCP-1) and the pro-inflammatory cytokine interleukin 1β (IL-1β), both in vitro and in vivo (Karanth et al., 2006; Boivin et al., 2007) (Figure 9-16). TLR signaling also stimulates production of the pro-inflammatory cytokine tumor necrosis factor α (TNFα) in vitro (Lee et al., 2006). TNFα further amplifies the injury effect by enhancing expression of MCP-1 and IL-1β (Subang, Richardson, 2001; Shamash et al., 2002). Additional experiments in vitro have demonstrated that TLR activation stimulates production of iNOS, an enzyme responsible for production of nitric oxide that is upregulated by Schwann cells and macrophages

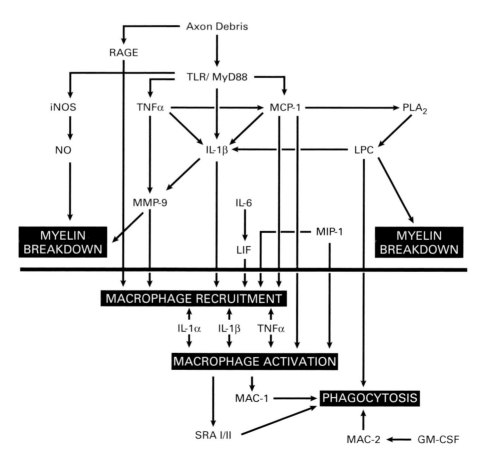

FIGURE 9-16   A schematic summary of pathways involved in Wallerian degeneration. Details are provided in the text. Modified from Martini et al., 2008.

soon after nerve injury (Levy et al., 1999; Lee et al., 2006). Nitric oxide participates in the breakdown of myelin, and is necessary for the normal progression of Wallerian degeneration and subsequent nerve regeneration (van der Veen, Roberts, 1999; Levy et al., 2001).

Breakdown of myelin is initiated before macrophages invade the nerve, implicating an intrinsic Schwann cell mechanism (Martini et al., 2008). The participation of the enzyme phospholipase A_2 (PLA_2) in this process has been demonstrated in vivo by blocking myelin breakdown with a PLA_2 inhibitor (De et al., 2003). PLA_2 is upregulated in response to MCP-1 (Carnevale, Cathcart, 2001), and hydrolyzes membrane phospholipids to lysophospholipids such as lysophosphatidylcholine (LPC), long known to initiate demyelination within minutes of intraneural injection (Hall, Gregson, 1971; Gregson, Hall, 1973). Injection of LPC into CNS white matter tracts upregulates MCP-1, IL-1β, and the pro-inflammatory chemokine monocyte chemoattractant protein-1α (MIP-1α) (Ousman, David, 2001). Myelin breakdown can also result from upregulation of matrix metalloproteinase-9 (MMP-9) by TNFα and IL-1β (Chattopadhyay et al., 2007).

Macrophages, both resident and hematogenous, play a central role in the phagocytosis and breakdown of myelin debris (Beuche, Friede, 1984; Beuche, Friede, 1986) (Figure 9-17). Peripheral nerve normally hosts a population of resident macrophages that may constitute up to 9% of the cells within the endoneurium (Griffin et al., 1992; Monaco et al., 1992). Recently, participation of these macrophages in Wallerian degeneration has been confirmed by using chimeric mice with GFP-positive hematogenous macrophages and GFP-negative resident macrophages (Mueller et al., 2003). Resident Schwann cells may also contribute to myelin breakdown to a limited degree, as demonstrated by teased fiber and in vitro studies (Stoll et al., 1989; Fernandez-Valle et al., 1995).

The invasion of hematogenous macrophages begins 24–48 hours after nerve injury, reaching a peak after 2 weeks by which time the population has increased 150-fold (Mueller et al., 2003; Bendszus, Stoll, 2003; Omura et al., 2005a). Degenerating nerve recruits hematogenous macrophages through a variety of mechanisms. Among the more robust macrophage attractants are the chemokines MCP-1 and MIP-1α (Adams, Lloyd, 1997; Ousman, David, 2001). Expression of these factors increases rapidly

and peaks 1–3 days after peripheral nerve injury, appropriate timing for macrophage attractants (Toews et al., 1998; Perrin et al., 2005). Blocking MCP-1 and MIP-1α function in vivo with antibodies results in a 78% drop in the number of macrophages recruited, and also reduces the phagocytic ability of those that enter the nerve (Perrin et al., 2005). IL-1β is also a strong macrophage attractant. The concentration of IL-1β in denervated nerve reaches a peak at 1 day and then again at 2 weeks (Perrin et al., 2005); the former is thought to result from Schwann cell activity and the latter from production by macrophages (Martini et al., 2008). Additional recruitment may result from expression of MMP-9 in response to TNFα (Shubayev et al., 2006; Chattopadhyay et al., 2007), from activation of the receptor for advanced glycation end products (RAGE) by axonal debris (Rong et al., 2004a, 2004b), and in response to LIF secreted by Schwann cells that have been stimulated by IL-6 (Sugiura et al., 2000; Galiano et al., 2001; Tofaris et al., 2002). Macrophages clearly respond to several signals, yet no one signal is sufficient to attract all macrophages.

Once macrophages have entered degenerating nerve, they require activation before they can target myelin for phagocytosis. IL-1β and TNFα have been found to stimulate phagocytosis in vitro, and MCP-1, MIP-1α, and IL-1β are required for effective myelin phagocytosis in vivo (Shamash et al., 2002; Perrin et al., 2005) (Figure 9-16). These factors may signal through upregulation of PLA_2; the resulting LPC can mark myelin for destruction much as the ubiquitins mark proteins, and may also activate the complement system to further enhance phagocytosis (Bruck, Friede, 1991; Hack et al., 1997; Dailey et al., 1998; Lauber et al., 2003; Rotshenker, 2003). Upregulation and display of specific macrophage receptors is also an important concomitant of myelin clearance. The receptors MAC-1, also known as complement receptor-3 (CR3), and scavenger receptor AI/II (SRAI/II) are displayed by activated macrophages, are necessary for phagocytosis, and are regulated in their efficiency by the level of intracellular cAMP (Reichert, Rotshenker, 2003; Makranz et al., 2004; Makranz et al., 2006). The galactose-specific lectin MAC-2 also contributes to phagocytosis. Unlike MAC-1 and SRAI/II, however, it is upregulated in response to the cytokine granulocyte macrophage-colony stimulating factor (GM-CSF), a product of activated fibroblasts (Saada et al., 1996). MAC-2 is also the

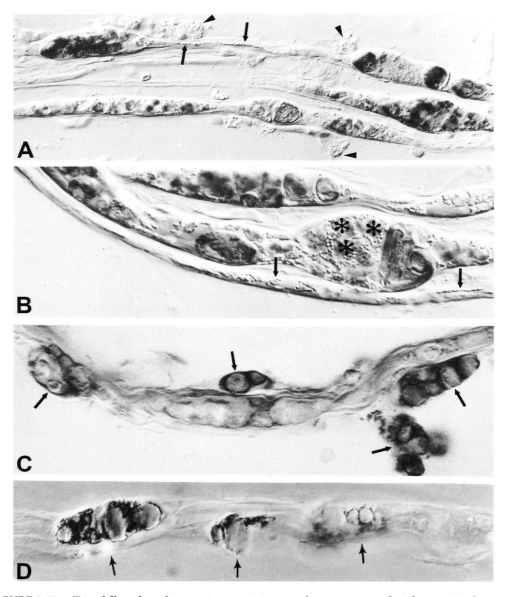

FIGURE 9-17   Teased fibers from degenerating rat sciatic nerve that was transected 14 days previously. A,B—osmium stain, Nomarsky optics; C,D—immunostaining for macrophage marker ED1. A. Schwann cell tubes contain large myelin ovoids (dark) and lipid droplets (arrows). Arrowheads identify cells that adhere to the outside of the Schwann cell tube. B. Asterisks mark cells within the Schwann cell tube, arrows identify lipid droplets. C. ED1-positive macrophages (arrows) adhere to the outside of the Schwann cell tube. D. Arrows point out foamy intratubal macrophages. From Griffin and Hoffman, 1993, with permission.

only one of the three to be expressed by Schwann cells, consistent with their ability to degrade myelin without the participation of macrophages (Stoll et al., 1989; Reichert et al., 1994; Fernandez-Valle et al., 1995).

Terminating Wallerian Degeneration

Although some macrophages undergo apoptosis within nerve, the majority migrate out across the basal lamina and enter the lymphatic circulation

(Kuhlmann et al., 2001). Recent experimental work provides a novel hypothesis to explain the transition from phagocytosis to diapedesis (Fry et al., 2007; David et al., 2008). The NGR has been mentioned previously in the context of interacting with the p75NTR to signal binding of the inhibitory myelin component MAG (Figure 9-3). The NGR is upregulated by macrophages 1 week after a crush injury, just as they are completing the process of phagocytosis, and is able to mediate repulsion of these macrophages by activating Rho (Figure 9-1). Contact with MAG in the newly formed myelin that ensheaths regenerating axons could thus repulse NGR-bearing macrophages, resulting in their departure from the nerve.

THE REGENERATING AXON

Regeneration Speed

The clinical significance of regeneration speed was recognized early in the practice of peripheral nerve surgery. Nerve repairs failed relatively often, and were frequently reexplored once deemed to be ineffective. Surgeons estimated regeneration speed to calculate the anticipated time-to-recovery of muscles a known distance from the repair site, and reoperated if these milestones were not met.

Early estimates of regeneration speed were based on clinical observation. The first measurements were made by Tinel, who recognized that tapping over the front of regenerating axons elicited paresthesias (Tinel, 1916). The progress of "Tinel's sign" down the course of a nerve could thus be used as a measure of regeneration speed. Estimates based on this technique ranged from 1–2 mm/day (Tinel, 1916) to 2–5 mm/day (Dustin, 1917). Early clinical estimates of regeneration speed were also derived by timing the reinnervation of muscles a known distance apart or by timing the progression of sensibility return along a longitudinally oriented strip of skin. By using the muscle reinnervation technique, the resulting estimates of regeneration speed after nerve suture were 1.6 +/- 0.2 mm per day for the radial nerve (Seddon et al., 1943), and 1.24 mm per day for a combined group of ulnar, median, and radial nerves (Marble et al., 1942). The progression of cutaneous reinnervation was found to occur at 1.3 mm/day for touch and 2.1 mm/day for pain (Trotter, Davies, 1913).

In an attempt to measure regeneration speed more precisely, Gutmann et al. (1942) identified the advancing front of regenerating axons by pinching rabbit sciatic nerve, working from the periphery toward the crush or repair site until a reflex was elicited. They found that regeneration proceeded at 3.5 mm/day after suture and 4.4 m/day after crush. This "pinch technique" is quite convenient, but can be used to measure the speed of only the most rapidly growing sensory axons. Subsequent application in the rat has yielded values of 3.5–4.3 mm/day after crush, 3.2 mm/day after transection and suture, and 1.5 mm/day after grafting (McQuarrie et al., 1977; Forman et al., 1979; Kanje et al., 1988; Holmquist et al., 1993).

In 1978 Forman and Berenberg introduced a technique that became the reference standard for determining the speed of axon regeneration (Forman, Berenberg, 1978a). Peripheral axons were radiolabeled by injecting tagged amino acids into the spinal cord. The front of axons regenerating after nerve crush could then be identified by quantifying the level of radioactivity in an ordered series of nerve segments (Figure 9-18). By localizing the front of advancing radiolabel at two distinct time periods, it was possible to calculate regeneration speed precisely without having to account for the delay between injury and the onset of regeneration. As these authors mapped the distribution of radiolabel at progressively longer time intervals after nerve crush, they found that axons became more dispersed as they moved distally. The sharp peak of radioactivity that represented the advancing axonal front at early time periods became progressively shorter, broader, and less well defined as it progressed distally (Figure 9-18). In effect, the leading edge of regeneration progressed more rapidly than the main body of the axon population. Most authors have chosen to measure the leading edge when calculating regeneration speed from this type of data, and have clocked motor axon regeneration at 3.0 to 3.8 mm/day (Forman, Berenberg, 1978a; Black, Lasek, 1979; Danielsen et al., 1986). When the effects of axonal dispersion are reduced by characterizing the regenerating front with a point on the leading edge of the curve midway between the baseline (fastest axons) and the peak itself (the largest volume of axoplasm) a speed of 3.27 +/- 0.9 mm/day is obtained (Brushart et al., 2002).

The crush/radiolabel technique was used to quantify the conditioning effect and to demonstrate the decline in regeneration speed that accompanies aging (McQuarrie, 1978; Black, Lasek, 1979; Pestronk et al., 1980). It proved more difficult,

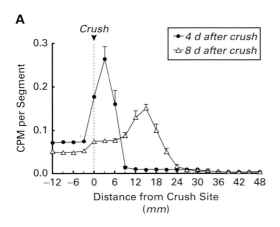
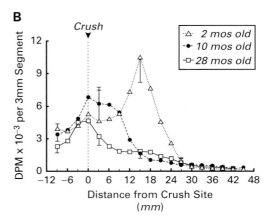

FIGURE 9-18   Use of radiolabel to measure the speed of axon regeneration. A. Sciatic nerve crush was followed in 3 or 7 days by injection of $[^{35}S]$methionine into the parent motoneuron pool. After an additional 24 hours, the sciatic nerves were harvested, cut into 3-mm-long segments, and counts of radioactivity were obtained from each segment. Twenty-four hours after injection the radiolabel has been transported distally and is concentrated at the growing axon tips. Counts per minute are plotted as a function of distance from the crush site. Each curve represents the mean of five nerves. In the interval from 4 to 8 days, the peak has broadened, indicating dispersion of axon tips as a result of different regeneration speeds. To compensate for the changing slope of the regenerating front, it is characterized by a point midway between the baseline (fastest axons) and the peak itself (the largest volume of axoplasm), resulting in a calculated regeneration speed of 3.27 +/- 0.9 mm/day (from Brushart et al., 2002). B. Similar technique used to examine the distribution of radiolabel within the peripheral nerves of rats ranging in age from 2 months to 28 months. Nerves were crushed 9 days before samples were harvested. A sharp peak is advancing rapidly in the 2-month-old rats, whereas the peaks in the older animals are still centered at or just distal to the crush site. Regeneration speed is shown to decrease markedly with advancing age. From Pestronk et al., 1980, with permission.

however, to apply this approach to nerve transection and repair. The small amount of radioactivity that was found in the distal stump at early time periods was dispersed and formed no clear peak (Forman, Berenberg, 1978a; Brushart, Hoffman, unpublished observations). Both of these deviations from the pattern seen after crush are consistent with staggered regeneration. To study regeneration after nerve repair more effectively, Fugleholm et al. (1994) implanted electrodes along the course of the cat sciatic nerve and took serial electrophysiologic measurements from each animal as regeneration proceeded. The cat sciatic nerve provided a longer pathway than any rodent model, and thus a longer time span over which to follow regeneration. Initial estimates of regeneration speed by using this complex technique (data presented in Figure 7-7) were 3–4 mm/day after crush and 2.5 mm/day after transection and suture. In subsequent experiments the model was used to compare the speed of sensory and motor axon regeneration. Although these had

been found to proceed at essentially equal speeds in early radiotracer experiments (Pestronk et al., 1980), indirect evidence had been presented for both faster motor (da Silva et al., 1985) and faster sensory (Suzuki et al., 1998; Madorsky et al., 1998) regeneration. Sequential data from the cat sciatic nerve confirmed the parity of both the regeneration and the maturation of the swiftest sensory and motor fibers (Moldovan et al., 2006).

The speed of axon regeneration has been studied with an evolving series of techniques that have yielded slightly varying estimates. In spite of these differences, each technique has shown regeneration after nerve transection and repair to be slower than after nerve crush. Rat and mouse experiments demonstrating this with the pinch test and radiolabeling are limited to the early days of regeneration, yet the relationship holds up over the longer distances and times measured in the cat sciatic nerve (Fugleholm et al., 1994). These observations confirm the importance of an early interaction between regenerating axons and some aspect of the repair environment—either the absence of basal lamina or the presence of wound products—that modifies the entire course of regeneration. A challenge for the future will be to determine the basis for the varying speeds of regeneration that are seen even after nerve crush, as exemplified by the increasing width of the peak of radiolabel as regeneration progresses (Figure 9-18) and the progressive dispersion of regenerating GFP-labeled axons (Figure 9-14). During development, axons that need to go farther grow faster (Davies, 1989); could these intrinsic differences persist into adulthood? Could mean regeneration speed be affected by axon modality? Similarly, it will be interesting to determine whether the slowing of regeneration over long distances such as the length of the sciatic nerve (Sunderland et al., 1993) is a property of the neuron or merely the consequence of progressive Schwann cell deterioration.

The Regenerating Bundle

The term "regenerating bundle" was introduced earlier in this chapter to describe the axons grouped within a single Schwann cell tube in the distal nerve stump (Figure 9-19). It is important to distinguish this structure from the "regenerating unit" described by Morris et al. in the proximal stump (Morris et al., 1972c). The regenerating unit as originally described is indeed a unit, as it contains only the daughter axons of a single proximal axon, all still contained within the original Schwann cell tube. The term "regenerating unit" was subsequently applied more broadly to characterize the axons regenerating within a single Schwann cell tube in the distal nerve stump (Hudson et al., 1972). A growing body of evidence implies, however, that Schwann cell tubes in the distal stump contain the progeny of two or more parent axons (Brushart, 1990; Witzel et al., 2005) (Figure 9-11). The term "regenerating bundle" describes the grouping of axons, but does not imply that they are derived from the same source. The distinction is functionally relevant: axons of the regenerating unit are derived from a single source but may enter multiple distal pathways, whereas axons of the regenerating bundle arise from multiple sources but are guided toward the same destination, where many will be unable to form functional connections.

Schwann cell tubes in the distal stump play a critical role at the advancing front of regeneration. They provide an optimal regeneration environment between the inner surface of the basal lamina and the Schwann cell membrane, and they provide physical constraint that directs regenerating axons within

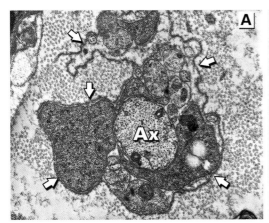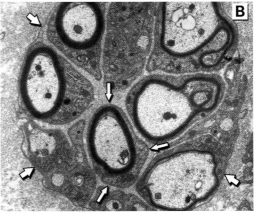

FIGURE 9-19   Electronmicrographs of regenerating axons. A. A collapsed basal lamina tube, seen in cross-section, is indicated by multiple arrows. It contains a single axon (Ax) and multiple Schwann cell process that constitute the Band of Bungner. Original magnification 20,000x. B. At a more advanced stage of regeneration a basal lamina tube similar to that on the left, marked by large arrows, is occupied by multiple axons in various stages of myelination. New basal lamina has been laid down by each of the Schwann cells (small arrows), so that the original Basal lamina is no longer in direct contact with either axons or Schwann cells. Original magnification 10,000x.

the confines of the tube itself (Haftek, Thomas, 1968; Meeker, Farel, 1993; Nguyen et al., 2002). As the progeny of myelinated axons that are confined within a given bundle mature and assume one-to-one relationships with Schwann cells, each is surrounded by newly synthesized basal lamina. The redundant outer basal lamina, which no longer has dedicated Schwann cells to sustain it, eventually fragments and ceases to function as a physical constraint. Whereas the landscape of the distal stump is dominated by regenerating bundles early on, no trace of them remains at later time periods (see Figure 8-5). The original Schwann cell tube must therefore vary in structure along its length, initially remaining intact in denervated segments and at the front of regenerating axons, then disintegrating more proximally as axons mature (Figure 9-20). Although there has been extensive investigation of the fate of chronically denervated Schwann cell tubes (see below), there appears to be little information regarding the shedding of the basal lamina chrysalis that initially surrounds regenerating axons. The interactions that may influence pruning of collaterals from the regenerating bundle are described in the context of regeneration specificity (Chapter 10).

Remyelination

The process of developmental myelination has been examined in great detail (reviewed in Melli, Hoke, 2007; Mirsky et al., 2008). Although much less is known about the remyelination of regenerating adult axons, several elements of the process have been defined. A key regulator of developmental myelination, the POU-domain transcription factor suppressed cAMP-inducible POU (SCIP/Oct-6) is upregulated by previously denervated adult Schwann cells when they are contacted by regenerating axons (Scherer et al., 1994). This process involves activation of the transcription factor NF-κB (Nickols et al., 2003), and may lead to either positive regulation of myelination through increased expression of the transcription factor Egr2/Krox-20 or, conversely, negative regulation by blocking expression of the myelin proteins P0 and MBP (discussed in Ryu et al., 2007). The predominance of the latter function is suggested by experiments in which Schwann cell production of SCIP/Oct-6 has been manipulated. Knockout animals fail to proceed beyond promyelination, and mice in which SCIP/Oct-6 is expressed constitutively display persistent hypomyelination

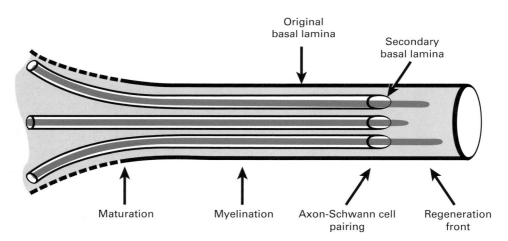

FIGURE 9-20   Schematic depiction of the changing relationship between Schwann cell tubes and regenerating axons. Axons are regenerating from left to right through the distal nerve stump. On the right, advancing axon tips proceed in direct contact with the inner surface of the original basal lamina, which signals to them through integrin receptors on their surface. Moving closer to the repair site (left), larger axons have formed 1:1 relationships with Schwann cells that have initiated myelination and generated new basal lamina. These newly synthesized basal lamina tubes separate each axon–Schwann cell unit from the others, but all are still grouped together within the original basal lamina tube. As these axons grow in size and are progressively myelinated, the original Schwann cell tube fragments and can no longer be recognized.

(Ghazvini et al., 2002; Ryu et al., 2007). For reasons that are not yet clear, transgenic modification of the SCIP/Oct-6 molecule so that only portions of it are functional results in both hypermyelination and accelerated axon regeneration after nerve crush, suggesting that the speed of axon regeneration may be enhanced genetically (Gondré et al., 1998).

A variety of environmental factors have also been found to influence remyelination. The integrin-linked kinase (ILK) promotes regenerative myelination in response to contact with the normal ECM through activation of the PI3K-Akt pathway, which has been shown to enhance myelination both in vitro and in vivo (Ogata et al., 2004; Pereira et al., 2009). After nerve injury, the ECM is modified by influx of fibrinogen, which is converted to fibrin, a potent inhibitor of remyelination (Akassoglou et al., 2000, 2002). Tissue plasminogen activator (tPA) produced by Schwann cells degrades fibrin and amelioriates this effect in vivo (Akassoglou et al., 2000). Growth factors may also play a significant role. During development, myelination is enhanced by BDNF acting through the p75NTR and is inhibited by NT-3 (Chan et al., 2001; Cosgaya et al., 2002). BDNF also activates the p75NTR to promote remyelination in adult rodents after both nerve crush and nerve grafting (Zhang et al., 2000; Song et al., 2006; Tomita et al., 2007b;). The process of remyelination may also be regulated by local administration of progesterone and thyroid hormone, although a role for these hormones at physiologic concentrations has not been established (Koenig et al., 1995; Voinesco et al., 1998; Panaite, Barakat-Walter, 2010).

Compartmentation and the Blood-Brain Barrier

In their pioneering electronmicroscopic study of early regenerative events in the proximal nerve stump, Morris and coworkers described the subdivision of fascicles into multiple small compartments, each surrounded by perineurium (Morris et al., 1972a). Similar architecture was also found near both the proximal and distal junctures of nerve autografts (Hudson et al., 1972) (Figure 9-21). Endoneurial fibroblasts contribute to the formation of these compartments, consistent with the fibroblastic origin of the developing perineurium (Nesbitt, Acland, 1980; Bunge et al., 1989; Popovic et al., 1994). Compartmentation was initially conceptualized as an attempt to restore the endoneurial environment through reconstruction of the perineurium (Morris et al., 1972a). The validity of this hypothesis was questioned by Nesbitt and Acland, who showed that perineurium regenerated from endoneurial fibroblasts without compartmentation if it was resected atraumatically (Nesbitt, Acland, 1980).

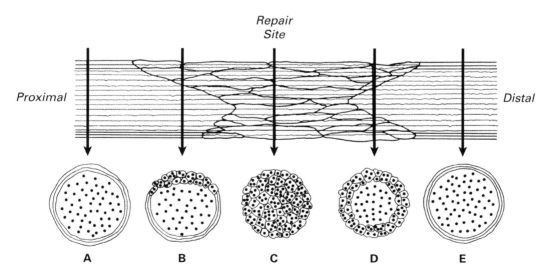

FIGURE 9-21   Compartmentation near a site of nerve repair. At the repair site (C) the entire nerve has been divided into multiple small perineurial compartments. Farther from the repair (B, D), only peripheral portions of the nerve are compartmented. Several millimeters proximal and distal to the repair (A, E) compartmentation is not observed. From Ahmed and Weller, 1979, with permission.

Taking into account the response to a variety of peripheral lesions, the degree of compartmentation appears to parallel the severity and duration of damage to both the perineurium and the nerve as a whole (Thomas, Bhagat, 1978; Nesbitt, Acland, 1980; Popovic et al., 1994).

The perineurium plays a critical role in maintaining the intraneural environment by serving as a peripheral extension of the blood-brain barrier (Shanthaveerappa, Bourne, 1962). A potential role for compartmentation in restoring this barrier seems unlikely, as disruption of the blood-brain barrier may persist for up to 6 months after nerve repair, long after compartments have formed and matured (Ahmed, Weller, 1979). Barrier function is abolished within 3 days of nerve injury in the entire distal stump and at least the distal 5 mm of the proximal stump (Omura et al., 2004). It is then restored in a gradual progression from proximal to distal, lagging behind the front of advancing axons (Bouldin et al., 1991; Omura et al., 2004). Drugs that cannot pass through the blood-brain barrier will thus have access to regenerating axons at the site of nerve repair for several weeks, and can presumably reach axons at the front of regeneration throughout their course. This attribute broadens the scope of potential therapies for nerve injury without subjecting the CNS to unwanted side effects.

THE REGENERATION ENVIRONMENT

In the first weeks after nerve repair the distal nerve stump provides regenerating axons with an evolving menu of soluble and contact interactions that influence the progress of regeneration (Figure 9-22). Denervated Schwann cells upregulate production

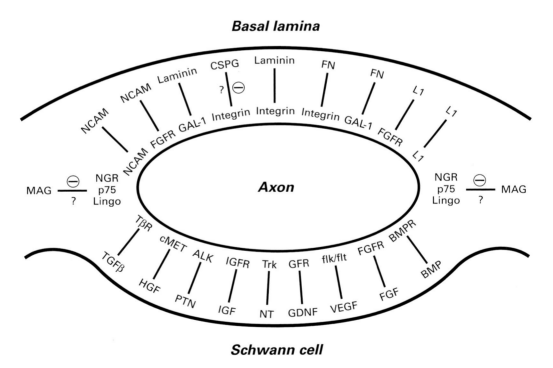

FIGURE 9-22   Possible molecular interactions between regenerating axons and their environment. Cross section of the periphery of a Schwann cell tube, showing a regenerating axon coursing between the inner surface of the basal lamina (above) and an adjacent Schwann cell (below). Abbreviations are those used in the text and listed at the beginning of the chapter; negative interactions are identified by (−). Growth factors produced by the Schwann cell may be displayed on the cell membrane or may diffuse from it. Interactions between the axon and basal lamina require direct contact. The inhibitory myelin protein MAG may be present in fragments of degenerating myelin or may be in soluble form.

of a variety of growth factors, several of which have been implicated in the support of regeneration. The structure and function of the neurotrophins and GDNF were described earlier in this chapter in the broad context of neuronal signaling; their specific roles in the PNS will be described here. Additional growth factors that may support regeneration include TGF-β, the BMPs, HGF, VEGF, PT, IGF-I and -2, and FGF. The myriad functions carried out by these factors in development and maintenance of the PNS are well beyond the scope of this chapter, so only the aspects of potential relevance to adult regeneration will be emphasized. As axons regenerate distally in the plane between Schwann cells and basal lamina, they will be exposed to the extracellular matrix molecules laminin, fibronectin, and tenascin-C. They will also encounter a variety of proteins and glycoproteins that act as recognition molecules, including Galectin-1, Netrin-1, the neuropilins, the neural cell adhesion molecule (NCAM), L1, and the potential regeneration inhibitors MAG and the CSPGs. The net effect of this complex environment must be positive, as axons pass through myelin debris containing MAG and confront newly synthesized CSPGs, yet proceed rapidly once they have entered the distal stump.

Neurotrophins

NERVE GROWTH FACTOR (NGF)

NGF structure and the process through which NGF signals from periphery to neuron were described in Part 2 of this chapter. Uninjured adult Schwann cells express very little NGF (Heumann et al., 1987a, 1987b). Soon after they are denervated by axotomy, however, they upregulate NGF production, a process that is stimulated by macrophage-derived interleukin-1 (Heumann et al., 1987a, 1987b; Lindholm et al., 1987). Recent studies in our laboratory localized this expression to dorsal root and cutaneous nerve, but found minimal upregulation by denervated muscle afferents, peripheral motor efferents, or ventral root (Brushart et al., 2006) (Figures 9-23, 9-24).

The NGF receptor TrkA is expressed by about 40% of rodent lumbar DRG neurons, with variability by both root level and animal model (Averill et al., 1995; Karchewski et al., 1999; Tucker, Mearow, 2008). Motoneurons do not express TrkA receptors. The p75NTR, normally expressed at very low levels by adult Schwann cells, is upregulated by denervation and may serve to display NGF to regenerating

axons (Taniuchi et al., 1988; Funakoshi et al., 1993). Motoneurons upregulate the p75NTR after peripheral axotomy, but not after the more severe injury of root avulsion, suggesting a correlation between p75NTR expression and the ability to regenerate (Ernfors et al., 1989; Yuan et al., 2006). On the basis of the expression patterns of NGF and the TrkA receptor, pathway-derived NGF could theoretically support the regeneration of dorsal root and peripheral cutaneous axons within their appropriate pathways.

Experiments performed on adult DRG neurons in vitro illustrate the effects of NGF on regeneration in a context that is potentially relevant to nerve repair. Although DRG neurons in both monolayer and explant form extend neurites spontaneously, NGF acts through both TrkA and p75NTR to enhance both neurite extension and branching beyond normal levels (Lindsay, 1988; Edstrom et al., 1996; Kimpinski et al., 1999). Neurons that express TrkA are able to extend neurites on a laminin substrate without the addition of growth factors, an effect that is integrin-dependent (Tucker et al., 2005, 2006). In this same NGF-sensitive population, addition of NGF to the culture enhanced neurite outgrowth only modestly (Tucker et al., 2005). This growth mode does not involve upregulation of GAP-43, and is thought to be responsible for branching or sprouting of NGF-sensitive neurons rather than for long-distance regeneration. Far more robust growth results from a previous conditioning lesion to the peripheral nerve with its attendant upregulation of GAP-43. Conditioning also empowers TrkA-expressing DRG neurons to turn on a laminin substrate in response to an NGF gradient, an activity they cannot perform without prior conditioning (Webber et al., 2008). NGF also produces secondary effects that could possibly influence regeneration. For instance, intrathecal administration of NGF increases the expression of both BDNF and TrkB by DRG neurons, potentially enhancing their regeneration state (Apfel et al., 1996; Michael et al., 1997) (Chapter 9, Part 1).

The effects of NGF on regeneration in vivo have been investigated in a variety of models. NGF clearly promotes local axon sprouting. Injection of NGF into skin stimulates sprouting of otherwise normal cutaneous innervation, whereas NGF antibodies block the sprouting response from normal axons into adjacent, denervated skin (Owen et al., 1989; Diamond et al., 1992a). Regeneration after nerve crush, in contrast, is neither enhanced by exogenous

Denervation Procedures

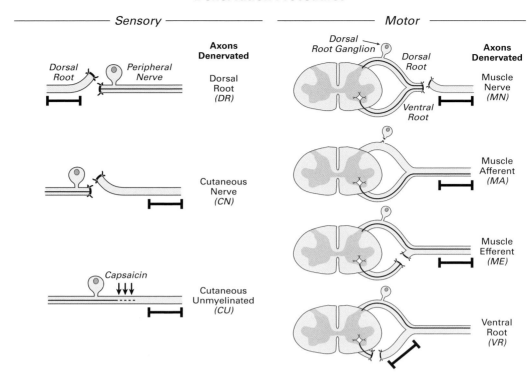

FIGURE 9-23   Procedures used to denervate specific Schwann cell populations for PCR evaluation. The cutaneous (CN) and muscle (MN) branches of the femoral nerve were denervated by proximal ligation and interruption of the femoral nerve trunk. L2, L3, and L4 laminectomies were performed to expose the distal roots and DRGs contributing to the femoral nerve. Dorsal root (DR) was denervated by interrupting it just proximal to the ganglia, muscle afferents in the femoral muscle branch (MA) by excising the exposed DRGs, and muscle efferents (ME) by interrupting the ventral root while preserving the dorsal root and DRG. Ventral root (VR) denervation required more proximal laminectomies to expose and interrupt the ventral roots as they exited the spinal cord. Cutaneous unmyelinated axons (CU) were denervated by direct application of capsaicin. From Brushart et al., 2006.

NGF (Gold, 1997) nor impeded by NGF function-blocking antibodies, although antibody treatment results in neuronal atrophy (Rich et al., 1984; Diamond et al., 1992b). When NGF is pumped onto the proximal stump of transected sciatic nerves, the normal post-axotomy increase in neuronal GAP-43 is diminished and the expression of p75NTR is increased rather than decreased, changes detrimental to regeneration (Mohiuddin et al., 1999). It is certainly possible that application of NGF in this context blunts the injury response that is triggered by the cessation of NGF transport (Raivich et al., 1991).

Addition of NGF to the nerve repair environment has produced variable results depending on the model and the mode of administration. Long-term delivery of NGF to the site of rat sciatic nerve repair or into a short intraneural gap increased distal axon numbers in the former case, but enhanced neither axon numbers nor function as measured by SFI in the latter (Santos et al., 1998; Young et al., 2001). Similarly, overexpression of NGF in the distal sciatic stump, resulting in an approximately fourfold increase in NGF protein levels over those in the proximal stump, did not increase the number of DRG neurons that reinnervated nerve 1 cm distal to the repair (Tannemaat et al., 2008). In the femoral nerve model, however, overexpression of NGF within the cutaneous branch enhanced its selective reinnervation by DRG neurons without increasing

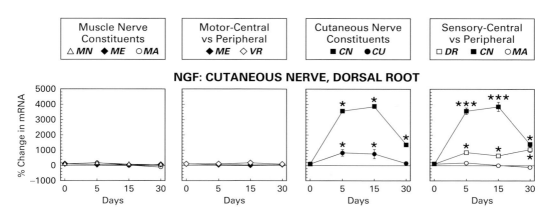

FIGURE 9-24 Expression of the gene encoding NGF by various components of the peripheral nervous system 5 days, 15 days, and 30 days after denervation. Overall patterns of expression are grouped within the four boxes as Muscle Nerve Constituents: muscle nerve (MN), muscle efferent (ME), muscle afferent (MA); Motor—Central vs. Peripheral: motor efferent (ME), ventral root (VR); Cutaneous Nerve Constituents: cutaneous nerve (CN), cutaneous unmyelinated (CU); and Sensory—Central vs. Peripheral: dorsal root (DR), cutaneous nerve (CN), muscle afferent (MA) (* $p < 0.005$ compared to baseline, ** $p < 0.005$ compared to one other value at the same time, *** $p < 0.005$ compared to both other values at the same time). From Brushart et al., 2006.

the total number of neurons that regenerated (Hu et al., 2010). Application of NGF to the site of nerve repair in fibrin glue, a less precise method of dosing, resulted in modest but significant increase in the number of motoneurons reinnervating the distal stump at 12 weeks but did not improve motor function (Jubran, Widenfalk, 2003).

In contrast to the minimal success in increasing the volume of peripheral regeneration with exogenous NGF, attempts to stimulate regeneration of dorsal root axons back into the spinal cord with NGF have been more successful (Oudega, Hagg, 1996; Ramer et al., 2000; Romero et al., 2001). Addition of NGF to enclosed neural gaps has also been fruitful; the numbers and caliber of axons in the tube and distal stump have been increased in several instances (Chen et al., 1989; Rich et al., 1989; Lee et al., 2003; Xu et al., 2003). NGF enhances the migration of Schwann cells into neural gaps bridged by tubes or fibronectin sheets (Derby et al., 1993; Whitworth et al., 1996), so it is difficult to ascertain whether NGF promotes regeneration across gaps through direct action on neurons or through indirect actions on Schwann cells. Inclusion of NGF in neural gaps has hastened the return of sensory function, but failed to increase the distance grown by fluorescent axons and did not improve

CMAP amplitude or SFI (Derby et al., 1993: Chen et al., 2006; Unezaki et al., 2009).

NGF SUMMARY

The failure of antibodies to NGF to hinder regeneration after nerve injury and the failure of increased NGF concentrations to promote it suggest that pathway-derived NGF is not essential for axon regeneration. Substantial evidence is consistent with a role for NGF in promoting regenerative collateral branching, however, a process that may increase axon numbers in the distal stump. It is possible that exposure of some collateral branches to high concentrations of NGF may stimulate the pruning of others that do not get this support, ultimately leading to selective collateral pruning and regeneration specificity. Stimulation of growth across neural gaps by NGF is consistent with its direct effects on Schwann cell migration, and promotion of dorsal root axons through CNS territory suggests the ability to enhance the regeneration state of DRG neurons as it relates to their central processes. Overall, upregulation of NGF by denervated Schwann cells in cutaneous nerve and dorsal root could support peripheral branching and enhance the regeneration state of dorsal root axons, but is unlikely to provide direct support for long-distance regeneration through peripheral nerve.

BRAIN-DERIVED NEUROTROPHIC FACTOR (BDNF)

Early studies failed to detect BDNF expression in uninjured peripheral nerve by Northern blot or RNAse protection analysis (Meyer et al., 1992; Funakoshi et al., 1993). RT-PCR, in contrast, revealed baseline BDNF expression that increased rapidly within 5 days of axotomy, reaching a peak at a 60-fold increase by 15 days, then returning to near baseline by 30 days (Hoke et al., 2006). Others have found this time course to be more prolonged (Michalski et al., 2008). In a recent evaluation of growth factor expression within functional subsets of axotomized peripheral nerve, we found that BDNF was expressed vigorously by denervated cutaneous nerve and dorsal root, moderately by muscle afferents, but was not expressed at all by ventral root or distal motor efferent axons (Brushart et al., 2006) (Figure 9-25).

Injured motoneurons upregulate the BDNF receptor TrkB over several days, with expression returning to normal within 3–4 weeks (Piehl et al., 1994; Kobayashi et al., 1996; Hammarberg et al., 2000a). TrkB is expressed by 33% of adult DRG neurons; 35% of these, in turn, also express BDNF, so that 10–20% of DRG neurons express both (Apfel et al., 1996; Karchewski et al., 1999). On the basis of the expression patterns of BDNF and the TrkB receptor, pathway-derived BDNF could theoretically support the functionally appropriate regeneration of a subset of DRG neurons within dorsal root and peripheral cutaneous nerve, as well as the inappropriate regeneration of motor axons within these pathways.

The effects of BDNF on axon regeneration in vivo have been subjected to intense scrutiny. Systemic treatment of mice with BDNF antibody after nerve crush reduced the length of the regenerate by 25% and the number of axons in the distal stump by 83%, indicating a critical requirement for endogenous BDNF in early regeneration (Zhang et al., 2000). Presumably, the BDNF antibodies exerted their effects at the site of nerve repair, where the blood-nerve barrier was disrupted, rather than at the neuronal cell body. Attempts to maximize regeneration after nerve repair with additional BDNF, however, have met with modest success at best. Sensory function was not enhanced by adding BDNF to a short (0.5-mm) gap repair of the cat lingual nerve (Yates et al., 2004). Slow release of BDNF from collagen matrices in the rat hastened the onset of facial nerve regeneration by three days without influencing ultimate function, and improved SFI from about -70 to -60, still a poor outcome (Utley et al., 1996; Kohmura et al., 1999). The importance of the BDNF dose was emphasized by Boyd and Gordon (2002), who found that low doses of BDNF (0.5–2 μg/day by osmotic pump) did not influence motoneuron regeneration, whereas higher doses (12–20 μg/day) inhibited regeneration by signaling through the p75NTR (Boyd, Gordon, 2002). Recently, an intermediate dose of 6 μg/day was found to increase the number of motoneurons that regenerated through a 20-mm rat tibial nerve graft (Hontanilla et al., 2007).

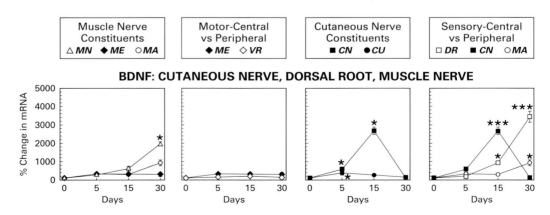

FIGURE 9-25   Expression of the gene encoding BDNF. Labeling as in Figure 9-24. From Brushart et al., 2006.

Further experimentation with other BMPs, especially BMP7, will be required to determine the contributions of this family of growth factors to nerve regeneration.

Hepatocyte Growth Factor (HGF)

HGF is a heterodimer comprising a 699-kDa α chain and a 34-kDa β chain (reviewed in Funakoshi, Nakamura, 2003). It is secreted as a single-chain pro-HGF that is modified by serine proteases. HGF acts through the receptor cMet, which consists of an α extracellular chain and a β intracellular tyrosine kinase chain. HGF signaling affects a wide variety of developmental and homeostatic functions; receptor specificity for particular pathways is mediated by association with cell-specific surface molecules including α6β4 integrin, Plexin B1, and CD44 (Bertotti, Comoglio, 2003).

Schwann cell expression of HGF was not detected by in situ hybridization (Hashimoto et al., 2001b). Using competitive RT-PCR, we found baseline expression of HGF and substantial upregulation by denervated cutaneous nerve and dorsal root, with modest upregulation by denervated muscle afferents (Hoke et al., 2006; Brushart et al., 2006) (Figure 9-27). Upregulation in cutaneous nerve was briskly reversed by contact with regenerating axons. HGF is expressed by 25% of DRG neurons, 80% of which co-express TrkA (Hashimoto et al., 2001a). The HGF receptor cMET has been localized to the dorsal horn, suggesting a role for HGF/cMET signaling in the regulation of sensory transmission. In the hypoglossal system, HGF is produced by the tongue, and cMET is gradually upregulated in hypoglossal motoneurons after axotomy (Okura et al., 1999).

Pumping HGF onto the proximal stump of the transected hypoglossal nerve reduces cMET expression and amelioriates the loss of ChAT (Okura et al., 1999). Similarly, HGF prevents motoneuron loss and normalizes ChAT expression after avulsion of facial or cervical nerves (Hayashi et al., 2006). In studies of regeneration after nerve crush or acellular nerve grafting, application of HGF improves the morphology and function of regenerated axons (Kato et al., 2005) but has little impact on limb function as measured with the SFI (Li et al., 2008).

Vascular Endothelial Growth Factor (Vegf)

VEGF is a 45-Da heparin binding glycoprotein (Rosenstein, Krum, 2004). Numerous splice variants have been described, $VEGF_{165}$ ($VEGF_{164}$ in rodents) being the most common in the nervous system (Ferrara, Alitalo, 1999). VEGF has four known receptors; the tyrosine kinases flt-1 (fms-like tyrosine kinase) and flk-1 (fetal liver tyrosine kinase), also known, respectively, as VEGF receptors 1 and 2, and the sema receptors neuropilin-1 and neuropilin-2 (reviewed in Meirer et al., 2001; Rosenstein, Krum, 2004). Additionally, heparin sulfate proteoglycans can promote VEGF signaling from the surface of adjacent cells (Jakobsson et al., 2006; Selleck, 2006).

Recent evidence suggests a tight linkage between the vascular and neural effects of VEGF. The semaphorins, axon guidance molecules, compete with VEGF for sites on the extracellular domain of neuropilin-1 (Yazawa et al., 1999), and the Slit proteins, also active in axon guidance, interfere with VEGF signaling (Jones et al., 2008). A dramatic example of the

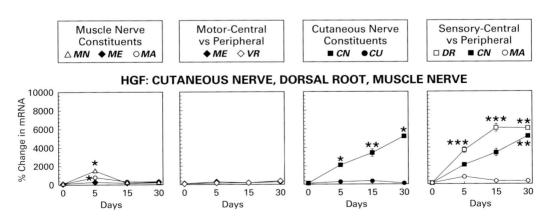

FIGURE 9-27   Expression of the gene encoding HGF. Labeling as in Figure 9-24. From Brushart et al., 2006.

SEMA-VEGF interaction has been found to regulate development of the facial nerve: VEGF164 directs migration of the neural somata, while SEMA3A guides the outgrowth of facial nerve axons (Schwarz et al., 2004).

VEGF and both neuropilin receptors are upregulated by denervated Schwann cells (Hoke et al., 2001; Scarlato et al., 2003). Absence of the VEGF response in old rats suggests that the decline in regenerative ability with age may be VEGF-related (Pola et al., 2004). Experiments in our laboratory demonstrated that upregulation of VEGF in response to Schwann cell denervation is dramatic in cutaneous nerve, where it is downregulated in response to reinnervation with cutaneous but not motor axons, significant but less pronounced in muscle nerve, and virtually absent in dorsal and ventral root under all conditions tested (Hoke et al., 2006; Brushart et al., 2006) (Figure 9-28).

In early postnatal life, all DRG neurons are immunoreactive for VEGF, but by P12 the adult proportion of 34% is achieved (Sondell, Kanje, 2001). Similarly, roughly one-half of neonatal DRG neurons express Flk-1, but by P12 this proportion is also reduced to the adult levels of 7%; some of these also express RT97, while others express CGRP (Sondell et al., 2000). Adult motoneurons display VEGF, Flk-1, and Flt-1 immunoreactivity (Islamov et al., 2004). VEGF and Flt-1, but not Flk-1, are upregulated by adult motoneurons in response to axotomy in vivo, leading to the speculation that VEGF may promote motoneuron regeneration through either paracrine or autocrine mechanisms (Islamov et al., 2004).

VEGF function has been explored in both sensory and motor systems. In cultures of adult DRG neurons the flk-1 receptor was found on neurons, axonal growth cones, and Schwann cells (Sondell et al., 1999a; Sondell et al., 2000). Exogenous VEGF promoted axonal outgrowth through interaction with the flk-1 receptor to activate the MAP kinase pathway, and enhanced both neuronal survival and Schwann cell proliferation. Experiments in two-compartment systems revealed VEGF effects on both axon and neuron, the latter mediated by retrograde transport. In the motor system of adult mammals, flk-1 receptors on regenerating axons and their growth cones can interact with VEGF produced locally by vascular sprouts to promote regeneration of motor axons (Bearden, Segal, 2004).

The effects of VEGF on end-to-end nerve repair have not been reported. Treatment of acellular nerve grafts with VEGF stimulates early ingrowth of vessels and Schwann cells, but not of axons (Sondell et al., 1999b). At later times, VEGF promotes axonal sprouting at the proximal end of an acellular graft, but does not enhance distal axon propagation (Rovak et al., 2004). Within a silicon tube containing Matrigel, progressive increase in axon numbers in response to increasing doses of VEGF closely parallels concomitant increases in vascularity (Hobson et al., 2000). VEGF is thus unlikely to have a substantial direct effect on axon regeneration after nerve repair, but can improve regeneration through unstructured spaces by stimulating vascular ingrowth.

Pleiotrophin (PTN)

PTN is an 18-Kd heparin-binding protein that was first isolated from bovine uterus and rat brain (Rauvala, 1989; Li et al., 1990). It is a member of the midkine family of cytokines, with which it shares

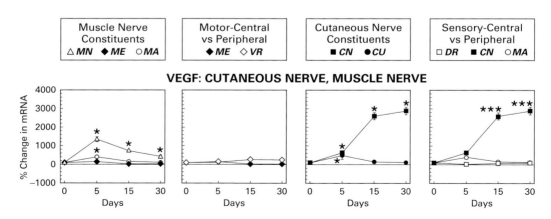

FIGURE 9-28   Expression of the gene encoding VEGF. Labeling as in Figure 9-24. From Brushart et al., 2006.

cysteine- and basic amino acid–rich residues that set it apart from other heparin-binding growth factors (Rauvala, 1989). Multiple PTN receptors have been described, although anaplastic lymphoma kinase (ALK) appears to be the most relevant in the PNS (Mi et al., 2007).

Seven days after transection of the rat sciatic nerve, pleiotrophin mRNA is upregulated in the distal nerve stump by 650% as determined by RT-PCR, but expression drops to subnormal levels by 3 months (Mi et al., 2007). PTN immunoreactivity is exhibited by Schwann cells 2 days after denervation, and then by macrophages after 1 week (Blondet et al., 2005). Both upregulation of PTN and resultant protein concentrations are highest in ventral root, intermediate in peripheral motor efferents, and minimal in cutaneous nerve (Hoke et al., 2006) (Figure 9-29). The ALK receptor is upregulated by motoneurons after peripheral nerve transection (Mi et al., 2007), but not after the more severe injury of ventral root avulsion (Chu et al., 2009); it is not upregulated by DRG neurons under either circumstance.

In spinal cord slice culture, pleiotrophin promoted vigorous motor axon outgrowth and provided tropic guidance for these axons (Mi et al., 2007). PTN expressed by HEK-293[PTN] cells promoted axons across a 15-mm rat sciatic nerve gap to reinnervate plantar muscles, whereas nonexpressing cells promoted significantly fewer axons, and these did not reinnervate muscle (Mi et al., 2007). Addition of pleitrophin to sensory nerve graft implanted in the spinal cord after ventral root avulsion stimulated motor axon outgrowth but not motoneuron survival (Chu et al., 2009). When high-dose pleiotrophin was applied to both the site of nerve crush and within muscle, however, muscle reinnervation was impeded (Blondet et al., 2006). This could result from the "candy store effect," the inability of axons to regenerate beyond a supraphysiologic concentration of growth factor described by Tannemaat and coworkers (2008). Overall, selective PTN expression in motor pathways and selective ALK expression by motoneurons suggest that PTN might contribute to the selective growth of motor axons within previously motor pathways.

Insulin-Like Growth Factors 1 and 2 (Igf-1, Igf-2)

IGF-1 and IGF-2 are single chain polypeptides with over 40% homology to human proinsulin (Russo et al., 2005; Cohen, 2006). IGF-1 binds to the IGF-1 receptor (IGF-1R), a cell-surface glycoprotein that responds by promoting intracellular tyrosine kinase activity and downstream signaling through MAPK and P13K pathways. Although IGF-2 also binds to this receptor, it interacts preferentially with the IGF-2 receptor, a single-chain polypeptide with no tyrosine kinase component that also serves as a receptor for LIF, TGFβ, and retinoic acid (Hawkes, Kar, 2003). Additionally, the IGF system includes a family of six IGF binding proteins that transport IGF in the bloodstream, increase its half-life, and modify IGF-receptor interactions (Russo et al., 2005).

The contributions of the IGFs to peripheral nerve regeneration have been investigated extensively. Increasing concentrations of IGF-I distal to a site of peripheral nerve injury were demonstrated by

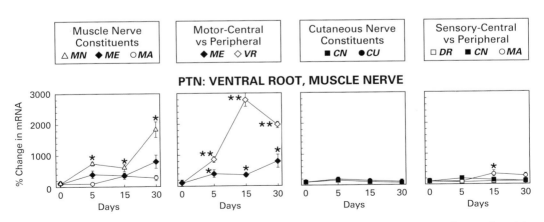

FIGURE 9-29   Expression of the gene encoding PTN. Labeling as in Figure 9-24. From Brushart et al., 2006.

immunohistochemistry (Hansson et al., 1986). Local upregulation of the genes for IGF-1 and IGF-2 was later confirmed by PCR; in the case of IGF-1, the predominant activity was found to shift from Schwann cells to macrophages 1 week after injury (Pu et al., 1995; Cheng et al., 1996). The expression patterns of IGF-1 and IGF-2, both temporally and topographically, suggest distinct functions for each factor. IGF-1 is upregulated rapidly and intensely in the distal stump by 4 days after crush of mixed nerve, then decreases with reinnervation (Pu et al., 1995). IGF-2 expression, in contrast, is characterized by a more gradual increase, beginning at 10 days and increasing to 20 days, and is greatest in distal portions of motor nerves. In the process of examining growth factor expression by subsets of denervated Schwann cells, we found that IGF-1 is expressed vigorously in cutaneous nerve, where it is downregulated by axonal ingrowth, but is expressed little by ventral root, dorsal root, distal muscle afferents, or distal muscle efferents (Hoke et al., 2006; Brushart et al., 2006) (Figure 9-30). IGF-2 is expressed predominantly by distal motor afferents and efferents, and to a lesser degree by cutaneous nerve after reinnervation by cutaneous but not by motor axons.

In the adult sensory system, IGF-1 and the IGF-1R are expressed predominately in small DRG neurons; after axotomy, neuronal IGF-1 levels decline, while expression of the IGF-1R is relatively unchanged (Russell et al., 1998; Delbono, 2003). In both dissociated and organotypic cultures, adult DRG neurons respond to IGF-1 with robust neurite outgrowth, an effect that is reduced by inhibitors of the MAPK and PI3K pathways (Fernyhough et al., 1993; Akahori, Horie, 1997; Kimpinski, Mearow, 2001). Local application of IGF-1 in vivo increases the distance covered by sensory axons regenerating into both otherwise unmodified and freeze-injured nerve in the first 3–4 days after it is crushed, whereas antibodies to IGF-1 decrease this distance (Kanje et al., 1989; Sjoberg, Kanje, 1989).

IGF-1 also promotes the survival and regeneration of adult motoneurons. The IGF-1R is expressed in the spinal cord, but has not been localized specifically to motoneurons (Lewis et al., 1993; Adem et al., 1994; Suliman et al., 1999). IGF-1 supports both the phenotype and the survival of mature motoneurons after a variety of physiologic insults (Pulford et al., 1999; Nakao et al., 2001), and has promoted motor axon regeneration in most studies

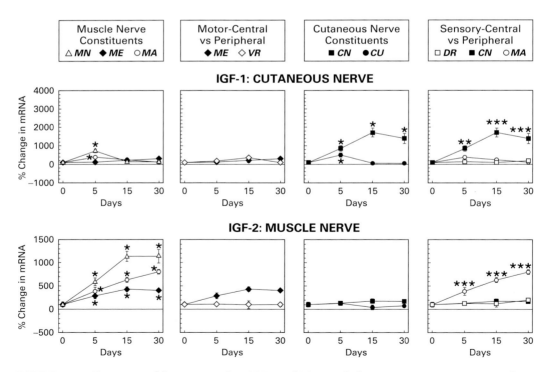

FIGURE 9-30   Expression of the gene encoding IGF-1 and IGF-2. Labeling as in Figure 9-24. From Brushart et al., 2006.

performed in vivo. When applied to sciatic nerve grafts, IGF-1 enhanced muscle weight, axon number, and g-ratio (Fansa et al., 2002). In the rat cross-facial nerve graft model, local infusion of IGF-1 hastened the return of blinking and improved both muscle and axon morphology (Thanos et al., 1999, 2001). Systemic infusion of IGF-1 hastened the return of motor function after mouse sciatic nerve crush (Contreras et al., 1995), but did not influence ultimate function after repair of the rat median nerve (Lutz et al., 1999).

The IGF-2 system in neurons has received less attention. IGF-2 receptors are present on both DRG and motoneurons in the adult (Hawkes, Kar, 2002). IGF binding protein-6 (IGFBP-6), which preferentially binds to IGF-2 and inhibits its actions, is also upregulated by injured motoneurons (Russo et al., 2005). Exogenous IGF-2 was found to increase the distance covered in the first 3–4 days after crush by regenerating sciatic motor axons as determined electrophysiologically (Near et al., 1992), and sciatic sensory axons as determined by the pinch test (Glazner et al., 1993), but had no effect on the regeneration of neurites from adult DRG explants (Akahori, Horie, 1997).

The IGFs play a complex role in neuromuscular homeostasis. Both IGF-1 and IGF-2 are synthesized by skeletal muscle (Sullivan et al., 2008). IGF-2 is expressed at high levels in fetal muscle, downregulated during synapse elimination, and upregulated by subsequent muscle denervation (Ishii, 1989). The levels of IGF-1 also increase significantly with denervation, but to a lesser degree (Glazner, Ishii, 1995). Both IGFs promote intramuscular sprouting of motor axons (Caroni, Grandes, 1990; Caroni et al., 1994), a repair response to partial denervation. Additionally, IGF-1 promotes muscle repair by inducing proliferation of interstitial cells (Caroni, Schneider, 1994), by inducing myogenesis (Florini et al., 1996), and by suppressing protein breakdown by the ubiquitin ligases atrogin-1 and MuRF-1 (Sacheck et al., 2004). Increasing IGF-1 expression within muscle enhances the speed and quality of muscle reinnervation (Shiotani et al., 1998; Rabinovsky et al., 2002). Serum IGF levels were not measured in these studies, so that the role of circulating IGF-I is unclear. These outcomes could also result from enhanced regeneration of the intramuscular portions of the nerve or from accelerated muscle reinnervation per se.

In addition to direct effects on axon regeneration and muscle reinnervation, the IGFs may also influence axon regeneration indirectly through their effects on Schwann cells and their interactions with other growth factors. In the culture environment, IGF-1 prevents the apoptotic death of Schwann cells and enhances their motility through the PI-3K/Akt pathway (Delaney et al., 1999; Syroid et al., 1999; Cheng et al., 2000). IGF-1 also upregulates expression of P_0 at the initiation of myelination, stimulates Schwann cell proliferation, and supports myelination over the long term (Stewart et al., 1996; Svenningsen, Kanje, 1996; Cheng et al., 1999). IGF expression is decreased in muscle by increasing levels of TNFα (Fernández-Celemín et al., 2002) but is increased by adding heparin or glycosaminoglycans (Gorio et al., 1998; Madaschi et al., 2003). In peripheral nerve, IGF-1 expression is diminished in the absence of LIF (De Pablo et al., 2000). Interactions may also include the IGF-1R, which is both upregulated in response to platelet-derived growth factor (PDGF) and is necessary for the function of the PDGF receptor PDGF-BB (DeAngelis et al., 1995; Carlberg, Larsson, 1996).

IGF-1,2 SUMMARY

IGF-1 clearly promotes the early stages of peripheral sensory axon regeneration. Focal upregulation of IGF-1 by Schwann cells in denervated cutaneous nerve is thus positioned to support functionally appropriate regeneration of cutaneous axons within these pathways. IGF-1 also enhances the overall process of motor axon regeneration/muscle reinnervation, although it is often difficult to determine which effect predominates, especially in experiments in which overexpression of IGF-1 by muscles is shown to hasten their reinnervation. At this point IGF-2 has been found to support early motor and sensory regeneration after crush in one experiment each. Prominent expression of IGF-2 by denervated Schwann cells in both afferent and efferent components of muscle nerve are consistent with a role in nerve/muscle interactions. The complexity of the IGF system will doubtless hamper definition of its precise role in nerve regeneration.

Fibroblast Growth Factors (FGFS)

FGFs are members of an extended family of more than 20 polypeptides that play diverse roles in development, homeostasis, and regeneration (Thisse, Thisse, 2005). Members of the FGF family bind with low affinity to heparin (Burgess, Maciag, 1989), and with high affinity to the fibroblast growth factor receptors (FGFR1-4). FGF-1 binds to all four FGFRs, while FGF-2 binds preferentially to isoforms 1c, 3c, and 4 Δ (Ornitz et al., 1996). Neurite outgrowth in response to L1, NCAM and N-cadherin is also dependent on the FGF receptor system (Williams et al., 1994). FGF signaling, which occurs largely through the Ras Map kinase pathway, can be modified additionally by the regulatory proteins Sprouty, XFLRT3, MKP3, and Sef (Thisse, Thisse, 2005). For example, Sef (similar expression to FGF genes) is a transmembrane protein that inhibits the mitogenic activity of FGF. Not normally present in peripheral nerve, it is upregulated focally at the site of nerve crush, where it may play a role in fine-tuning of FGF activity (Grothe et al., 2008). In addition to its role as a low-affinity receptor, heparin also plays a role in high affinity binding by bridging between FGF and FGFR (Ornitz, 2000). FGF signaling can thus be adapted to a variety of circumstances by varying the receptor isoforms present, by modulating the local concentration of heparin, and by differential upregulation of regulatory proteins.

Within uninjured peripheral nerve, low-level expression of FGF-2 and FGFR1-3 can be detected by RT-PCR (Grothe et al., 2001). After axotomy by crushing, FGF-2 and FGFR1-3 are upregulated by both Schwann cells and macrophages (Grothe et al., 1997, 2001). In recent RT-PCR studies, we found that expression in the distal stump was actually decreased 5 days after nerve transection and repair, a response that was slightly more prominent in sensory nerve than in ventral root (Brushart et al., 2006).

FGF-1 is expressed by adult DRG and motoneurons (Elde et al., 1991; Ji et al., 1995), and levels are altered minimally by axotomy (Piehl et al., 1993). Embryonic FGF-2 expression is shut off in most DRG neurons after birth, remaining in only 5% of small neurons (Ji et al., 1995). After axotomy, however, it is upregulated vigorously by 80% of all DRG neurons (Ji et al., 1995; Meisinger, Grothe, 1997). FGFR1 and FGFR-2 are normally expressed at high levels in the DRG, and this does not change after axotomy; FGFR-3 is upregulated strongly, and FGFR-4 expression is unchanged, remaining at low levels (Grothe et al., 2001, 2006). Motoneurons, like their DRG counterparts, shift from generalized expression of FGF-2 in the embryo to focal expression in subsets of adult motoneurons (reviewed by Grothe, Wewetzer, 1996), where FGF-2 immunoreactivity is confined to the nucleus and perinuclear

cytoplasm (Hassan et al., 1994). Following axotomy, FGF-2 immunoreactivity in motoneurons is reduced substantially (Grothe, Unsicker, 1992). FGF-2 is subject to retrograde transport within motor axons in the hypoglossal system (Grothe, Unsicker, 1992), but it does not appear to undergo retrograde transport within the sciatic nerve (Ferguson et al., 1990; discussed in Grothe, Wewetzer, 1996).

The availability of FGF-2 knockout mice has facilitated exploration of the contributions of FGF-2 to regeneration (Jungnickel et al., 2006, 2010). In comparison with controls, FGF-2 knockouts had increased numbers of axon sprouts just distal to a crush lesion after 1 week, and these were of increased size and were better-myelinated. By two weeks, however, relative axon numbers were no longer increased in the knockout animals, though increased axon size and myelin thickness persisted, and expression of the myelin protein P0 was elevated. Functional testing revealed a more rapid return of mechanosensory but not motor function in the knockout animals. The beneficial effects of FGF knockout were attributed to normal suppression of P0 expression by FGF-2, and thus increased P0 production in the knockout animals. This interpretation is consistent with the suppression of P0 by FGF-2 in vitro and reduced myelination by mice that overexpress FGF-2 (Morgan et al., 1994; Jungnickel et al., 2006).

The effects of exogenous fibroblast growth factors on peripheral nerve regeneration have varied according to the experimental setting. Both FGF-1 and FGF-2 increased the length of axon extension in the first 3–5 days after crush or freezing axotomy (Laird et al., 1995; Fujimoto et al., 1997). In the one study of end-to-end nerve repair, there was no improvement in sensory or motor function when FGF-1 containing fibrin glue was placed around the repair (Jubran, Widenfalk, 2003). Addition of FGF-1 or FGF-2 improved regeneration across enclosed neural gaps by a variety of criteria (Aebischer et al., 1989; Cordeiro et al., 1989; Walter et al., 1993; Coppola et al., 2001; Midha et al., 2003; Wang et al., 2003). Recently, experiments in which 15-mm sciatic nerve gaps were bridged with silicon tubes supplemented with Schwann cells expressing different FGF-2 isoforms revealed that the 18 KDa isoform inhibited myelination, whereas the 21/23 KDa isoform promoted early recovery of thermosensitivity and long-distance myelination (Haastert et al., 2006). Addition of similar Schwann cells to a

5-mm rat facial nerve gap, however, failed to improve functional recovery (Haastert et al., 2009).

FGF SUMMARY

The complex expression patterns of the FGFs and their receptors, their differential effects on regeneration and myelination, the modification of their actions by regulatory proteins and heparin, and the varying outcomes of regeneration experiments obfuscate the regenerative effects of these growth factors. It appears that the early positive effects of FGF-2 result from stimulation of Schwann cell proliferation, whereas in the longer term removal of FGF-2 speeds the return of sensory function by enhancing myelination through upregulation of the myelin protein P0.

Extracellular Matrix and Recognition Molecules

LAMININ

In the context of peripheral nerve regeneration, the glycoprotein laminin is the sine qua non of the extracellular matrix. The potent effect of laminin in promoting regeneration was first observed in cultures of central and peripheral neurons, including mouse DRG neurons and putative avian motoneurons (Manthorpe et al., 1983). Soon thereafter it was shown that laminin was produced by Schwann cells and was localized to their basal laminae, where it was found only on the inner, abaxonal surface (Cornbrooks et al., 1983; Tohyama, Ide, 1984). The strong preference of regenerating axons for this inner surface and the abolition of this preference by treatment with antibodies to laminin indicated a critical role for laminin in the promotion and guidance of peripheral regeneration (Ide et al., 1983; Wang et al., 1992a).

Laminin is a trimer composed of one alpha, one beta, and one gamma chain (Patton, 2000) (Chapter 1). The 5 alpha, 3 beta, and 3 gamma chain configurations that have been identified are known to associate in at least 15 distinct combinations. These were initially numbered in the chronological order of their discovery (Aumailley et al., 2005). Recently, a more descriptive nomenclature has been adopted in which laminins are denoted as the aggregate of their component chains, i.e., LM211 for alpha 2, beta1, gamma1, previously laminin 2, and LM411 for alpha 4, beta 1, gamma 1, previously laminin 8

(Aumailley et al., 2005). LM211 and LM411 are upregulated by Schwann cells soon after they are contacted by regenerating axons (Masaki et al., 2000; Wallquist et al., 2002). Mice lacking the gamma 1 chain, common to LM211 and LM411, cannot radially sort and myelinate axons, and respond to sciatic nerve crush with impaired regeneration (Chen, Strickland, 2003). Individual disruption of the alpha 2 chain (LM211; laminin 2) or the alpha 4 chain (LM411; laminin 8) reveals that the former promotes regeneration, whereas the latter directs radial sorting of Schwann cells and myelination (Uziyel et al., 2000; Wallquist et al., 2005).

Laminin within the basal lamina of the Schwann cell tube influences the behavior of regenerating axons directly by binding to integrins on the neuronal surface, and indirectly by binding to integrins displayed by Schwann cells. The 18 α and 8 β integrin subunits that have been identified are known to join in forming at least 24 different heterodimeric combinations (van der Flier, Sonnenberg, 2001). After axotomy both motoneurons and DRG neurons upregulate the components of the α6β1 and α7β1 integrins; DRG neurons may additionally upregulate the α3 chain to form the α3β1 integrin (Tomaselli et al., 1993; Hammarberg et al., 2000b; Wallquist et al., 2004). Schwann cells are known to display the α6β1 and α6β4 integrins (Dubovy et al., 2001; Van der Zee et al., 2008). Recent work has revealed that the α3β1 and α7β1 integrins are specific receptors for LM-111 (laminin 1) and LM-211 (laminin 2), and the α6β1 integrin is specific for LM411 (laminin 8) and LM511 (laminin 10) (Plantman et al., 2008). As will be shown below, the α7β1 receptor, which binds to LM-211 (laminin 2), has been shown to play a critical role in nerve regeneration. Furthermore, integrin and NGF signaling converge in their activation of the PI3K-Akt pathway to maximize regeneration (Tucker et al., 2008).

Integrin signaling has been shown to play a substantial role in the regeneration of adult mammalian peripheral nerve. In many instances this has been demonstrated by manipulating the α7 component of the receptor for LM-211 (laminin 2). In the motor system, the α7 gene is upregulated by motoneurons after injury; elimination of its function impedes facial nerve regeneration in vivo (Werner et al., 2000, Hammarberg et al., 2000b). In the sensory system, growth of DRG neurons from α7 knockout mice on laminin is reduced, and blocking α7 function with antibodies selectively inhibits the growth of large and medium-sized DRG neurons (Ekstrom et al., 2003; Gardiner et al., 2005). The relative importance of integrin signaling is emphasized by its role in influencing the growth state of neurons. DRG neurons upregulate α7β1 integrin after peripheral but not central axotomy, require α7β1 integrin for the conditioning effect both in vitro and in vivo, and can have their regenerative performance enhanced to equal that of young neurons by transgenic overexpression of integrin (Condic, 2001; Ekstrom et al., 2003; Wallquist et al., 2004).

Schwann cells interact with laminin to influence axon regeneration through both integrin-dependent and integrin-independent mechanisms. Knockout of the integrin β4 gene reduces the myelination of regenerating axons and impairs motor recovery (Van der Zee et al., 2008). The enzyme β-1,4-galactosyltransferase I (β-1,4-GalT-I) can also serve as a receptor for laminin (Thomas et al., 1990; Riopelle, Dow, 1991). A potential role for laminin/β-1,4-GalT-I binding in regeneration is supported by the observation that Schwann cells that overexpress β-1,4-GalT-I promote the growth of axons from cultured DRG neurons, whereas those transfected with an antisense plasmid inhibit outgrowth (Shen et al., 2003).

FIBRONECTIN (FN)

Fibronectins are large extracellular matrix glycoproteins (Schwarzbauer et al., 1983; Proctor, 1987). In uninjured peripheral nerve, fibronectin is localized to the endoneurium and outer surface of the Schwann cell basal lamina (Cornbrooks et al., 1983; Wang et al., 1992b). Its location and production by fibroblasts clearly differentiate it from laminin, a product of Schwann cells that is confined to the inner surface of the basal lamina (see above). Fibronectin gene expression is upregulated by nerve injury, but alternative splicing produces an embryonic rather than the adult form of the molecule (Lefcort et al., 1992; Vogelezang et al., 1999). Fibronectin within the extracellular matrix interacts with integrin receptors on Schwann cells and growing axons. The α5β1 integrin receptor has been localized to the filopodia of DRG growth cones in vitro; treatment with antibodies that block α5β1 reduces growth from DRG explants on fibronectin surfaces (Yanagida et al., 1999; Gardiner et al., 2007). Similarly, α4 integrins on adult mouse DRG neurons and the growing tips of crushed sciatic nerve axons contribute to enhanced growth on fibronectin (Vogelezang et al., 2001). Although fibronectin can

promote growth in some environments, its ability to do so is dwarfed by that of laminin. Growth promotion by fibronectin may be improved, however, by preconditioning DRG neurons in vivo, an effect that is mediated largely by the α5β1 integrin receptor (Gardiner et al., 2007).

Fibronectin has been used in a variety of constructs to enhance growth across neural gaps. When placed within a tube bridging a 5-mm rat sciatic nerve gap, exogenous fibronectin promoted Schwann cell migration; interference with fibronectin-integrin signaling, in contrast, inhibited bridge formation and axon ingrowth (Bailey et al., 1993; Liu et al., 2009). Across gaps of 1 cm, fibronectin mats promoted early axon regeneration, addition of fibronectin to an alginate hydrogel containing Schwann cells enhanced Schwann cell viability and early regeneration, and inclusion of fibrinogen within an unstructured gap improved both morphologic and electrophysiologic indices of regeneration (Whitworth et al., 1995; Mosahebi et al., 2003; Zhang et al., 2003). Current evidence thus suggests that fibronectin is required to form new neural structure, but functions primarily as a constituent of the endoneurium and only secondarily as a growth-promoting surface.

TENASCIN-C

Tenascin-C is a large extracellular matrix glycoprotein that serves as a recognition molecule during development of the nervous system (Faissner, 1997). It is confined to the perineurium and nodes of Ranvier in normal peripheral nerve, but is found throughout the endoneurium of the distal stump after axotomy (Martini et al., 1990). A potential role for tenascin-C in regeneration was indicated by experiments in the C57Bl/Wlds mouse, a model of delayed Wallerian degeneration (see "Wallerian Degeneration" above). Fruttiger and colleagues (1995) found that motor axons degenerate before sensory axons in this mouse. During regeneration, motor pathways also upregulate tenascin-C and are reinnervated more rapidly, thus linking tenascin-C expression with the support of regeneration. Experiments in tenascin-C knockout animals have focused on reinnervation of the neuromuscular junction, and have provided conflicting results. Reinnervation of the sternomastoid muscle after crush of its nerve was found to be normal by one group (Moscoso et al., 1998), yet others have demonstrated both abnormal development and regeneration of the neuromuscular junction in the same strain of mice (Cifuentes-Diaz et al., 1998, 2002). Experiments in the rat facial nerve have confirmed the prominent role of tenascin-C at the neuromuscular junction, in that tenascin-C knockouts regenerated normal numbers of motoneurons after facial nerve crush, yet still had poor vibrissal function (Guntinas-Lichius et al., 2005). Tenascin-C is thus likely to play a significant role in motor endplate reinnervation, but its contribution to axonal regeneration remains to be clarified.

GALECTIN-1

The galectins are a family of β-galactoside-binding lectins that are found throughout the peripheral nervous system. Galectin-1 (Gal1) is expressed by 57% of DRG neurons, the majority of which are of small diameter (McGraw et al., 2005). Peripheral axotomy stimulates expression within larger DRG neurons as well, so that over 80% of the total DRG population are Gal1-positive by 1 week after injury. Axotomy of the dorsal root, in contrast, does not enhance Gal1 expression by DRG neurons, suggesting a role for Gal1 in peripheral regeneration (McGraw et al., 2005). Gal1 is also present at low levels in uninjured motoneurons, where it is upregulated in response to axotomy (Hynes et al., 1990; McGraw et al., 2004). In peripheral nerve, Gal-1 is present in both axons and Schwann cells, but the evidence for upregulation after injury is largely circumstantial (Fukaya et al., 2003; Sango et al., 2004).

Two distinct roles have been proposed for Gal1 in peripheral nerve depending on its oxidation state. The reduced form is a homodimer of 14 kDa subunits that functions as a laminin- and fibronectin-binding lectin in vitro (Zhou, Cummings, 1990; Ozeki et al., 1995). The oxidized form (Gal1-Ox), in contrast, is a monomer that lacks lectin activity and appears to function as a cytokine (Gaudet et al., 2005). Exogenous Gal-1/Ox promotes sensory and motor axon regeneration after nerve crush/freeze, and into acellular autografts, allografts, and enclosed nerve gaps, activities that are blocked by antibodies to Gal-1 (Horie et al., 1999; Fukaya et al., 2003; McGraw et al., 2004). Gal-1/Ox also enhances Schwann cell migration (Fukaya et al., 2003). Horie and colleagues have proposed a model in which Gal-1 is secreted into the extracellular space by injured axons and Schwann cells, is oxidized, and stimulates macrophages to produce a growth-promoting factor that is ultimately responsible for the effects of Gal-1 on regeneration (Horie et al., 2004; Horie et al., 2005).

NETRIN-1

Netrin-1 is a diffusible protein of the laminin superfamily that plays several critical roles during development of the mammalian CNS (Tessier-Lavigne et al., 1988; Rajasekharan, Kennedy, 2009). Recently, the list has been expanded to include guidance of primary sensory axons as they enter the spinal cord (Watanabe et al., 2006; Masuda et al., 2008). Netrin-1 attracts axons by signaling through the deleted in colorectal cancer (DCC) receptors (Keino-Masu et al., 1996) and mediates axon repulsion through the receptor UNC5 (Hong et al., 1999). The expression of netrin-1 mRNA is upregulated by nerve transection, and increased concentrations of netrin-1 protein have been found in nerve that is undergoing reinnervation (Madison et al., 2000). The recent observations that adult DRG neurons express the UNC5 receptor and that netrin-1 inhibits outgrowth of neurites from DRG explant cultures (Park et al., 2007) suggest that netrin-1 may inhibit regeneration after nerve repair, a possibility that warrants further investigation.

NEUROPILINS

Neuropilins 1 (NP-1) and 2 (NP-2) are transmembrane receptors for members of the Semaphorin-3 (Sema-3) family of axon guidance molecules and the growth factor VEGF (Kolodkin et al., 1997; Meirer et al., 2001). The neuropilin/semaphorin system can mediate both attraction and repulsion, and participates in the guidance of both sensory and motor axons during development (Messersmith et al., 1995; Wright et al., 1995; Wolman et al., 2004; Huber et al., 2005). In adults, axotomy induces expression of NP-1 in large DRG neurons and NP-2 in motoneurons (Gavazzi et al., 2000; Lindholm et al., 2004). Sema-3 is upregulated by motoneurons after intraspinal axotomy, but is downregulated after peripheral axotomy (Pasterkamp et al., 1998; Lindholm et al., 2004). In the periphery, NP-1 and -2 are upregulated by denervated nerve (Ara et al., 2004). Sema 3A and Sema 3F are also upregulated, primarily in the epineurium and perineurium, suggesting that they could inhibit regenerating axons from entering these areas (Scarlato et al., 2003). The localization of NP-2 expression to Schwann cells and the observation of impaired regeneration in NP-2 knockout mice suggest that Schwann cell production of NP-2 may facilitate peripheral axon regeneration (Scarlato et al., 2003; Bannerman et al., 2008).

NCAM

The neural cell adhesion molecule (NCAM) is a member of the immunoglobulin superfamily that influences axon guidance and cell migration during development of the CNS (Maness, Schachner, 2007). NCAM is expressed widely in developing peripheral nerve, but in adults is only found in non-myelinating Schwann cells (Martini, 1994). NCAM itself is known to bind homophilically to activate the FGF receptor FGFR, and has been found to play a significant role in promoting axons across a 6-mm rat sciatic nerve gap (Remsen et al., 1990; Povlsen et al., 2003). More is known, however, about the specific role of two carbohydrate epitopes that attach to the NCAM backbone, polysialic acid (PSA) and HNK-1. PSA occupies a large volume, so increasing PSA concentrations on a cell will interfere progressively with membrane apposition and cell-to-cell interactions (Rutishauser et al., 1988). Reducing PSA synthesis decreases the number and size of myelinated axons that regenerate after nerve transection without altering myelination, whereas addition of a PSA glycomimetic to a 2-mm mouse femoral nerve gap promotes Schwann cell proliferation and enhances myelination and motor function (Jungnickel et al., 2009; Mehanna et al., 2009). PSA expression by subsets of motoneurons and HNK-1 expression by motor Schwann cells have been linked to PMR, and will be discussed in Chapter 10.

L1

L1, like NCAM, is a member of the immunoglobulin superfamily, and its expression in peripheral nerve mirrors that of NCAM (Martini, 1994). After nerve injury, expression increases in previously myelinating Schwann cells until they begin to form new myelin (Martini, Schachner, 1988). L1 is known to promote regeneration in the CNS (Maness, Schachner, 2007). It was thus unexpected that knockout of L1 would promote peripheral axon regeneration by enhancing Schwann cell proliferation (Guseva et al., 2009). L1 thus appears to be an inhibitor of regeneration that acts indirectly by restraining Schwann cell division.

MAG

The myelin-associated glycoprotein, MAG, is concentrated on the inner, adaxonal membrane of myelinating Schwann cells (Figure 1-2). The identification of MAG as a potent inhibitor of CNS regeneration stimulated interest in its mechanisms of action (McKerracher et al., 1994; Mukhopadhyay et al., 1994; Domeniconi, Filbin, 2005); current understanding of the pathway through which MAG signals to block regeneration is described in Part 1 of this chapter. A potential role for MAG in peripheral regeneration was suggested by experiments in which distal stump reinnervation in mice with delayed Wallerian degeneration (C57BL/Wlds) was enhanced when MAG was not present in the pathway (Schafer et al., 1996). Similarly, PNS myelin containing MAG was found to inhibit both the outgrowth and branching of adult DRG neurons in vitro (Shen et al., 1998). The effects of MAG on nerve repair in normal rats and mice appears to be context-dependent; application of MAG to the site of sciatic nerve repair in fibrin glue reduced axon branching and improved SFI, whereas long-term systemic application of MAG antibodies increased both the number of motoneurons regenerating and their ability to reinnervate the femoral muscle branch rather than the cutaneous branch (Mears et al., 2003; Tomita et al., 2007). It is possible that reduction of branching is beneficial when the potential targets are of a single modality, such as multiple muscles (sciatic nerve), whereas enhanced branching could be helpful when axons are sampling and choosing between fundamentally different environments, such as muscle and skin (femoral nerve).

CHONDROITIN SULFATE PROTEOGLYCANS (CSPGS)

CSPGs are components of the extracellular matrix that inhibit peripheral axon regeneration (reviewed in Muir, 2009). They consist of a protein core decorated with sulfated glycosaminoglycans, and are classified into three major categories based on the number and position of the sulfate groups: chondroitin 4-sulfate (CS-4 or CS-A), dermatin sulfate (DS or CS-B), and chondroitin 6-sulfate (CS-6 or CS-C) (Sugahara et al., 2003). CS-6 is confined to the endoneurium, whereas CS-4 is present in both endoneurium and epineurium in the rat, but only within the epineurium in humans (Tona et al., 1993; Muir, 2009). CSPGs bind to a wide range of ligands, including the extracellular matrix molecules collagen, hyaluronan, NCAM, and tenascin, and the growth factors FGF-2 and pleitrophin, and play diverse functions in the development of the nervous system (reviewed in Properzi, Fawcett, 2004).

In response to peripheral nerve injury, the concentration of CSPGs in the distal stump increases both in its normal location within the endoneurium and de novo within the basal lamina, where it is physically positioned to influence regenerating axons (Tona et al., 1993; Zuo et al., 1998; Morgenstern et al., 2003). The CSPGs signal through both integrin-dependent and integrin-independent pathways (Zhou et al., 2006). Recent experiments comparing the effects of deactivating CSPGs with those of elevating intracellular cAMP suggest that CSPG inhibition, similar to that posed by MAG (see above), can be overcome by enhancing the regeneration state of the neuron (Udina et al., 2009). In addition to their inhibitory effects, the focus of most recent research, CSPGs may also exert positive effects through mechanisms such as the facilitation of Schwann cell migration (Liu et al., 2006). The inhibitory effects of the CSPGs are mitigated by matrix metalloproteinases (MMPs), proteolytic enzymes that degrade a variety of extracellular matrix molecules. The observation that MMP upregulation in the distal stump coincides with axon regeneration suggests that MMPs render the pathway more permissive by removing proteoglycans (Platt et al., 2003; Pizzi, Crowe, 2007).

CSPGs can be deactivated by stripping their side chains from the protein core with the bacterial glycosaminoglycanase Chondroitinase ABC (ChABC), so named because of its action on CSPGs A, B, and C (Bertolotto et al., 1986). Injection of ChABC into the site of a rat sciatic nerve repair more than doubles the number of axons that reinnervate the distal stump after 4 days (Zuo et al., 2002). In the longer term, retrograde regeneration of axons into the extrafascicular compartment of the proximal sciatic stump is reduced significantly and hindpaw grip strength is enhanced by 8% over saline-treated controls (Graham et al., 2007). Enhanced distal stump reinnervation may, however, come at a price. In a recent series of mouse sciatic nerve repairs, inappropriate reinnervation of the peroneal nerve by tibial axons was increased by ChABC treatment by an as yet undetermined mechanism (English, 2005). This finding suggests that CSPGs normally constrain inappropriate reinnervation, a possibility that warrants further investigation.

Evolution of the Distal Pathway

THE FIRST MONTH OF DENERVATION

The capacity of the denervated distal stump to promote axon regeneration varies dramatically in the weeks and months after nerve repair. The permissiveness of nerve that has not undergone Wallerian degeneration is minimal (Langley, Anderson, 1904; Brown et al., 1992). In the early weeks after axotomy, however, the process of Wallerian degeneration transforms an initially inhibitory environment to one that promotes regeneration vigorously. This optimal environment is transitory, such that regeneration through rat nerve that has been denervated for 2–3 months is already reduced substantially.

Enhancement of nerve graft function by predegeneration was noted by Ramon y Cajal (1928), but was not confirmed by experiments carried out soon thereafter (Sanders, Young, 1942). As a result, this potentially important observation received little attention for more than 40 years. The effects of short periods of predegeneration have varied according to the rat model used. The delay in reinnervating sciatic nerve grafts was reduced from 2.31 days to 0.87 days, as determined by the pinch test, after only 3 days of graft predegeneration (Urabe et al., 1995). Extracts and exudates from sciatic nerve 7 days postdenervation provided both neurotrophic and neurotropic support for axons regenerating into enclosed neural gaps as assessed morphologically (Zhao, Kerns, 1994; Marcol et al., 2003). Predegeneration for 6 days enhanced reinnervation of sciatic nerve grafts (Hasan et al., 1996), yet facial nerves denervated for 1 week were not reinnervated as effectively as were freshly axotomized nerves (Guntinas-Lichius et al., 2000). The effects of denervation for 3–4 weeks have been more uniformly positive. Myelinated axon counts were increased in the facial-hypoglossal transfer model, the amplitude of the nerve action potential was increased at 4 but not at 8 weeks in the sciatic graft model, and both the volume and specificity of motoneuron regeneration were enhanced in the femoral nerve graft model (Figure 9-31) (Sorenson, Windebank, 1993; Brushart et al., 1998; Guntinas-Lichius et al., 2000).

Multiple factors may contribute to the enhancement of regeneration through grafts that have been predegenerated for 1–4 weeks. Schwann cell production of several growth factors is enhanced (Figures 9-24 to 9-30), the basal lamina is rendered more conducive to regeneration, and Schwann cell

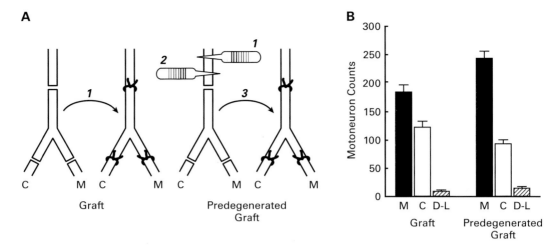

FIGURE 9-31 The effects of graft predegeneration on motoneuron regeneration in the rat femoral nerve model. M—motor; C—cutaneous; DL—double-labeled. A. In the graft group, the femoral nerve trunk was excised and immediately sewn in place on the opposite side of the animal. In the predegenerated graft group, grafts were predegenerated by proximal crushes 4 and 2 weeks before harvest, then transferred to the opposite side of the animal. B. After 8 weeks of regeneration, the mean number of motoneurons reinnervating the muscle branch, the cutaneous branch, or both branches (double-labeled) was determined by simultaneous retrograde double labeling. Both the volume and the specificity of regeneration were enhanced by 4 weeks of graft predegeneration. From Brushart et al., 1998.

motility is increased (Ochi et al., 1994; Danielsen et al., 1995; Tomita et al., 2009). Negative influences may also be reduced, as MAG can no longer be detected in the distal stump after 1 week (Schafer et al., 1996). It will be important to determine the relative contributions of these factors to optimization of the distal stump environment, as predegeneration results in the best environment for nerve regeneration yet identified.

CHRONIC DENERVATION

Delay between injury and nerve repair compromises patient outcomes (Chapter 5). The effects of chronic axotomy on the regenerative capacity of neurons was considered in Part 1 of this chapter. Chronic pathway denervation may also play a significant role, as Schwann cells may be denervated for extended periods of time before they are contacted by regenerating axons. After transection and repair of human nerve, the number of months that a Schwann cell will be denervated can be approximated by assuming that, after a 1 month delay at the repair site, regeneration proceeds at 1 inch per month. The denervation time in months will thus be equal to the distance between the injury and the

Schwann cell in inches, plus one month for delay at the repair site.

Several reports have documented the numbers of freshly axotomized axons and/or parent neurons that are able to regenerate through pathways that have been denervated for varying periods. In a rat sciatic graft model, myelinated axon counts distal to a 2-cm graft were not affected by up to 3 months of graft denervation, but decreased modestly after 6 months of denervation and were reduced by 62% after denervation was prolonged for 12 months (Gulati, 1996). When the peroneal nerve was denervated and then reinnervated with freshly cut tibial axons, the reduction in distal myelinated axon counts from those seen after immediate suture was approximately 30% after 12 weeks of peroneal denervation and 80% when the peroneal nerve had been denervated for 24 weeks (Sulaiman, Gordon, 2000). In the same set of experiments, the number of motoneurons that reinnervated the peroneal nerve was reduced by approximately 75% in the 12-week group; regeneration was negligible in the 24-week group. In a similar model, the number of motor units reinnervated after 6 months of pathway denervation was only 10% of that found after immediate suture (Fu, Gordon, 1995a). In the rat model, the ability of peripheral nerve to support regeneration diminishes rapidly after only 3 months of denervation. No equivalent estimates are currently available for human nerve.

Denervation of peripheral nerve for more than 3–4 weeks is accompanied by progressive morphologic, ultrastructural, and physiologic changes that may contribute to the observed regeneration deficits. Peripheral nerve atrophy was first quantified by Sunderland and Bradley (1950a, 1950b), who noted that intrafascicular area was reduced by 50% after only 50 days of denervation, by 60–70% from 50 to 250 days, and by 70–80% thereafter. Shrinkage of Schwann cell tubes by 80–90% in the first 3 months, as determined by light microscopy, was cited as a major contributor. The ultrastructural changes that underlie neural atrophy were clarified by subsequent electronmicroscopic studies of rat and rabbit nerve. Schwann cell basal lamina tubes collapse inward as axon and myelin debris are cleared, and begin to fragment between 4 and 8 weeks (Thomas, 1964; Giannini, Dyck, 1990). Laminin remains immunoreactive for up to a year, but its tubular configuration is lost by 20 weeks, and by 1 year only fine longitudinal threads remain (Salonen et al., 1987). Schwann cells are markedly atrophied by 20 weeks, after which they begin to die off (Weinberg, Spencer, 1978; Roytta, Salonen, 1988; Bradley et al., 1998). As the Schwann cell tube and its contents contract, new collagen is laid down outside the basal lamina (Thomas, 1964). After 1 year of denervation, remnants of the Schwann cell tube form the axis for cylindrical "collagen domains" that are encircled by fibroblasts and perineurium-like cells (Roytta, Salonen, 1988; Vuorinen et al., 1995; Bradley et al., 1998). Many of these changes have also been identified in biopsies of chronically denervated human nerve, with the exception that fragmentation of the basal lamina is not prominent in human tissue (Terenghi et al., 1998).

The process of Schwann cell atrophy is accompanied by a series of physiologic changes in the rat sciatic nerve. The initial burst of growth factor expression gradually subsides, many Schwann cell markers are downregulated, axon/Schwann cell signaling is impaired, and the nerve environment becomes hypoperfused. GDNF expression by chronically denervated nerve was found by in situ hybridization to persist at relatively high levels for 5 months (Hammarberg et al., 1996), but more recent PCR and ELISA studies have found that both upregulation of the GDNF gene and GDNF protein levels return to baseline after 5–6 months of denervation, and, most importantly, do not increase in response to freshly axotomized axons (Hoke et al., 2002; Michalski et al., 2008). Expression of markers consistent with the denervated Schwann cell phenotype, p75NTR and S100, is undetectable by 6 months even though Schwann cells can still be found within the nerve (You et al., 1997). The failure of chronically denervated Schwann cells to respond to axon ingrowth may be due to a breakdown in signaling between the two, as suggested by parallel decreases in expression of the c-erbB neuregulin receptors, Schwann cell proliferation, and distal stump reinnervation after progressively long periods of denervation (Li et al., 1997). For as yet unexplained reasons, the erbB receptors on rat facial nerve Schwann cells are reexpressed in response to axon contact after even prolonged denervation (Rueger et al., 2008). Additionally, blood flow within chronically denervated nerve is reduced, though this has not been correlated with local PO^2 (Hoke et al., 2001). A process of physiologic deterioration thus accompanies Schwann cell atrophy and has been implicated in poor support of axon regeneration by chronically denervated nerve.

CONCLUSIONS

The regenerative response of an injured neuron has come to be viewed as the summation of positive and negative external influences in the context of the neuron's intrinsic "regeneration state." The results of clinical and experimental nerve repair presented earlier suggest that age is the single most important determinant of intrinsic regeneration state, whereas integrity of the basal lamina is the most important external influence. Regeneration is dramatically more effective in children than in adults (Chapter 5), and after nerve crush, which preserves basal lamina integrity, than after nerve transection (Chapter 7). This chapter has presented several correlates of age and basal lamina status that could mediate the regenerative response.

For many years aging has been known to slow the speed of axonal transport, and thus the speed of regeneration (Black, Lasek, 1979; Pestronk et al., 1980). Subsequently, a number of processes have been shown to deteriorate or slow with aging, such as Wallerian degeneration, axonal sprouting, and the production of growth factors by Schwann cells (reviewed in Verdu et al., 2000; Kovacic et al., 2009). Mechanisms underlying the beneficial effects of young age, in contrast, have only emerged within the last decade. A seminal observation was the finding that levels of endogenous cAMP are higher in neurons from young animals, in which axonal growth is promoted by MAG and myelin, and decrease substantially as the neurons mature and switch to being inhibited by these substrates (Cai et al., 2001). Similarly, the intrinsic activity of Arginase I, a rate-limiting enzyme in the regeneration-enhancing polyamine pathway, is high in the DRGs of young animals, decreasing with age in parallel with the cAMP concentration (Cai et al., 2002). Recently, it has been shown that increasing neuronal cAMP through systemic administration of rolipram, an inhibitor of PDE-4 (Figure 9-1), promotes motoneurons across the site of nerve repair and into the distal nerve stump (Udina et al., 2009). Neuronal age has also been found to influence neurite guidance, in that embryonic DRG neurites turn briskly in a gradient of NGF without the need for interaction with laminin, whereas adult DRG neurites require both a preconditioning lesion and a laminin substrate to do so (Gunderson, Barrett, 1979; Webber et al., 2008). Additionally, young age has been correlated with increased expression of the integrin receptors through which growing neurites interact with laminin displayed by the basal lamina (Condic, 2001; Lemons et al., 2005).

Regeneration after axotomy proceeds more rapidly when the basal lamina remains intact than when it is disrupted (Forman, Berenberg, 1978b; Forman et al., 1979; Fugleholm et al., 1994). This remains true even when Schwann cells within the pathway have been killed to eliminate their production of growth-promoting substances (Sketelj et al., 1989; Fugleholm et al., 1994). Axons that cross the basal lamina gap separating proximal and distal nerve stumps will regain a spatial relationship with Schwann cells and basal lamina in the distal stump identical to that maintained consistently by their crushed counterparts, but will not regenerate as quickly. The critical interaction that reduces the relative regeneration speed after nerve repair, in analogy to the conditioning effect, has been termed "de-conditioning." Where there is a gap in the basal lamina, signaling from laminin to axonal $\alpha7\beta1$ integrins will be disrupted. Specific contributions of this signaling to nerve regeneration were detailed in Part 3 of this chapter.

Disruption of the basal lamina could potentially inhibit regeneration through a variety of mechanisms (Figure 9-32). Slit2, a protein that is a potent stimulus to axon collateral sprouting, is upregulated by Schwann cells after nerve transection but not after nerve crush (Wang et al., 1999; Tanno et al., 2005). As discussed in Part 2 of this chapter, excess collateral sprouting may be detrimental to regeneration. Similarly, Netrin-1, a guidance molecule that may promote or defeat regeneration depending on the receptor it activates, is upregulated by denervated Schwann cells after nerve transection but not after nerve crush (Madison et al., 2000). Recent work has shown that adult DRG neurons upregulate the receptor Unc5h, which is associated with the repulsive actions of netrin-1, but not deleted in colorectal cancer (DCC), the receptor that mediates axon attraction (Park et al., 2007). As a result, growth from adult DRG explants is inhibited strongly by Netrin-1.

Disruption of the basal lamina may also impede regeneration by modifying the neuronal response to the CSPGs and MAG, inhibitory molecules that are normally present in the regeneration environment. Destruction of CSPGs with chondroitinase ABC was found to enhance regeneration when the basal lamina was disrupted by nerve transection, but not after nerve crush when it remained intact (Zuo et al., 2002). This observation is consistent with experiments demonstrating that CSPGs inhibit regeneration by interfering with integrin signaling, and that this inhibition can be overcome by increased integrin expression (Condic, 2001). Similarly, inhibition of regeneration by MAG in vitro can be overcome by contact with laminin (David et al., 1995). In PC12 cells, integrin signaling downregulates expression of the p75NTR, a component of the MAG receptor, suggesting a mechanism for the laminin effect (Rankin et al., 2008). As long as axons are traveling along a laminin-containing surface they are relatively resistant to MAG inhibition, but at a site of basal lamina discontinuity this "rescue" would be lacking. Nerve transection in vivo presents both a gap in the basal lamina and soluble MAG in the interstump gap (Torigoe, Lundborg, 1998), so that inhibition through this mechanism is likely.

In addition to its role in overcoming the negative effects of pathway inhibitors, laminin-induced integrin signaling is important because of its positive contributions to neuronal regeneration state. DRG neurons upregulate the $\alpha7\beta1$ integrin after peripheral but not central axotomy, require the $\alpha7\beta1$ integrin for the conditioning effect both in vitro and in vivo, and can have their regenerative performance enhanced to equal that of young neurons by

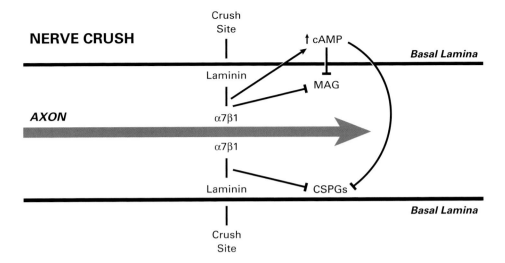

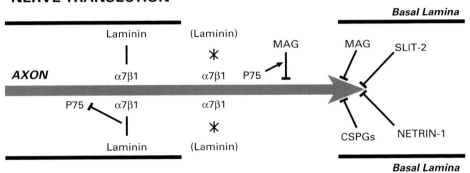

FIGURE 9-32   Molecular events that may enhance regeneration after nerve crush and impede it after nerve transection. Maintenance of the basal lamina after nerve crush ensures ongoing activation of the α7β1 integrin, which serves to enhance the intrinsic growth state of the neuron directly, and indirectly by increasing cAMP levels. As a result, the regenerating axon can overcome the inhibition posed by MAG and CSPGs in the distal stump. Nerve transection, in contrast, interrupts the basal lamina. The effects of MAG and the CSPGs can no longer be blunted through integrin signaling, and upregulation of the p75 component of the MAG receptor is no longer suppressed by contact with laminin. Additionally, Slit-2 and Netrin-1 are upregulated after nerve transection but not after nerve crush, and could pose an additional impediment to regeneration.

transgenic integrin overexpression (Condic, 2001; Ekstrom et al., 2003; Wallquist et al., 2004). Additionally, integrin and NGF signaling converge in their activation of the PI3K-Akt pathway to maximize regeneration (Tucker et al., 2008).

This discussion has attempted to fulfill a goal laid out in Chapter 5: to explore the biological underpinnings of important clinical findings. Age and basal lamina integrity were shown to be the two most important determinants of clinical outcome

after routine nerve repair. Both variables have been analyzed from the perspective of neural regeneration state, and a preliminary hypothesis relating each to regeneration success has been formulated. Simply stated, axons that maintain continuous contact with laminin achieve a relatively high regeneration state that empowers them to overcome inhibitors within the pathway. Axons that must cross a gap, and are therefore initially devoid of integrin signaling from laminin, have a lower regeneration state and are more susceptible to inhibitory interactions, which are more numerous and of potentially greater magnitude when the basal lamina has been breached. As this chapter has indicated, many additional interactions shape the outcome of regeneration and may assume primary importance in special circumstances such as prolonged delay in nerve repair.

REFERENCES

Abe N, Cavalli V (2008) Nerve injury signaling. Curr Opin Neurobiol 18: 276–283.

Abernethy DA, Thomas PK, Rud A, King RHM (1994) Mutual attraction between emigrant cells from transected denervated nerve. J Anat 184: 239–249.

Adams DH, Lloyd AR (1997) Chemokines: leucocyte recruitment and activation cytokines. Lancet 349: 490–495.

Adem A, Ekblom J, Gillberg PG, Jossan SS, Hoog A, Winblad B, Aquilonius SM, Wang LH, Sara V (1994) Insulin-like growth factor-1 receptors in human spinal cord: changes in amyotrophic lateral sclerosis. J Neural Transm Gen Sect 97: 73–84.

Aebischer P, Salessiotis AN, Winn SR (1989) Basic fibroblast growth factor released from synthetic guidance channels facilitates peripheral nerve regeneration across long nerve gaps. J Neurosci Res 23: 282–289.

Agthong S, Kaewsema A, Tanomsridejchai N, Chentanez V (2006) Activation of MAPK ERK in peripheral nerve after injury. BMC Neurosci 7: 45.

Aguayo AJ, Epps J, Charron L, Bray G (1976) Multipotentiality of Schwann cells in cross-anastomosed and grafted myelinated and unmyelinated nerves: quantitative microscopy and radioautography. Brain Res 104: 1–20.

Ahmed AM, Weller RO (1979) The blood-nerve barrier and reconstitution of the perineurium following nerve grafting. Neuropathol Appl Neurobiol 5: 469–483.

Airaksinen MS, Saarma M (2002) The GDNF family: signalling, biological functions and therapeutic value. Nat Rev Neurosci 3: 383–394.

Akahori Y, Horie H (1997) IGF-I enhances neurite regeneration but is not required for its survival in adult DRG explant. Neuroreport 8: 2265–2269.

Akassoglou K, Kombrinck KW, Degen JL, Strickland S (2000) Tissue plasminogen activator-mediated fibrinolysis protects against axonal degeneration and demyelination after sciatic nerve injury. J Cell Biol 149: 1157–1166.

Akassoglou K, Yu WM, Akpinar P, Strickland S (2002) Fibrin inhibits peripheral nerve remyelination by regulating Schwann cell differentiation. Neuron 33: 861–875.

Al-Majed AA, Neumann CM, Brushart TM, Gordon T (2000) Brief electrical stimulation promotes the speed and accuracy of motor axonal regeneration. J Neurosci 20: 2602–2608.

Al-Majed AA, Tam SL, Gordon T (2004) Electrical stimulation accelerates and enhances expression of regeneration-associated genes in regenerating rat femoral motoneurons. Cell Mol Neurobiol 24: 379–402.

Anderson PN, Mitchell J, Mayor D, Stauber VV (1983) An ultrastructural study of the early stages of axonal regeneration through rat nerve grafts. Neuropathol Appl Neurobiol 9: 455–466.

Anderson PN, Nadim W, Turmaine M (1991) Schwann cell migration through freeze-killed peripheral nerve grafts without accompanying axons. Acta Neuropath (Berl) 82: 193–199.

Apfel SC, Wright DE, Wiideman AM, Dormia C, Snider WD, Kessler JA (1996) Nerve growth factor regulates the expression of brain-derived neurotrophic factor mRNA in the peripheral nervous system. Mol Cell Neurosci 7: 134–142.

Ara J, Bannerman P, Hahn A, Ramirez S, Pleasure D (2004) Modulation of sciatic nerve expression of class 3 semaphorins by nerve injury. Neurochem Res 29: 1153–1159.

Araki K, Shiotani A, Watabe K, Saito K, Moro K, Ogawa K (2006) Adenoviral GDNF gene transfer enhances neurofunctional recovery after recurrent laryngeal nerve injury. Gene Therapy 13: 296–303.

Arevalo JC, Wu SH (2006) Neurotrophin signaling: many exciting surprises! Cell Mol Life Sci 63: 1523–1537.

Arevalo JC, Waite J, Rajagopal R, Beyna M, Chen ZY, Lee FS, Chao MV (2006) Cell survival through Trk neurotrophin receptors is differentially regulated by ubiquitination. Neuron 50: 549–559.

Atanasoski S, Notterpek L, Lee HY, Castagner F, Young P, Ehrengruber MU, Meijer D, Sommer L, Stavnezer E, Colmenares C, Suter U (2004) The protooncogene Ski Schwann cell proliferation controls and myelination. Neuron 43: 499–511.

Atanasoski S, Scherer SS, Sirkowski E, Leone D, Garratt AN, Birchmeier C, Suter U (2006) ErbB2 signaling in Schwann cells is mostly dispensable for maintenance of myelinated peripheral nerves and proliferation of adult Schwann cells after injury. J Neurosci 26: 2124–2131.

Atkins S, Smith KG, Loescher AR, Boissonade FM, O'Kane S, Ferguson MW, Robinson PP (2006) Scarring impedes regeneration at sites of peripheral nerve repair. Neuroreport 17: 1245–1249.

Atkins S, Smith KG, Loescher AR, Boissonade FM, Ferguson MW, Robinson PP (2006) The effect of antibodies to TGF-beta1 and TGF-beta2 at a site of sciatic nerve repair. J Peripher Nerv Syst 11: 286–293.

Atkins S, Loescher AR, Boissonade FM, Smith KG, Occleston N, O'Kane S, Ferguson MW, Robinson PP (2007) Interleukin-10 reduces scarring and enhances regeneration at a site of sciatic nerve repair. J Peripher Nerv Syst 12: 269–276.

Atwal JK, Pinkston-Gosse J, Syken J, Stawicki S, Wu Y, Shatz C, Tessier-Lavigne M (2008) PirB is a functional receptor for myelin inhibitors of axonal regeneration. Science 322: 967–970.

Augsburger A, Schuchardt A, Hoskins S, Dodd J, Butler S (1999) BMPs as mediators of roof plate repulsion of commissural neurons. Neuron 24: 127–141.

Aumailley M, Bruckner-Tuderman L, Carter WG, Deutzmann R, Edgar D, Ekblom P, Engel J, Engvall E, Hohenester E, Jones JCR, Kleinman HK, Marinkovich MP, Martin GR, Mayer U, Meneguzzi G, Miner JH, Miyazaki K, Patarroyo M, Paulsson M, Quaranta V, Sanes JR, Sasaki T, Sekiguchi K, Sorokin LM (2005) A simplified laminin nomenclature. Matrix Biol 24: 326–332.

Averill S, McMahon SB, Clary DO, Reichardt LF, Priestley JV (1995) Immunocytochemical localization of TrkA receptors in chemically identified subgroups of adult rat sensory neurons. Eur J Neurosci 7: 1484–1494.

Averill S, Michael GJ, Shortland PJ, Leavesley RC, King VR, Bradbury EJ, McMahon SB, Priestley JV (2004) NGF and GDNF ameliorate the increase in ATF3 expression which occurs in dorsal root ganglion cells in response to peripheral nerve injury Eur.J.Neurosci. 19: 1437–1445.

Axelrad TW, Einhorn TA (2009) Bone morphogenetic proteins in orthopaedic surgery. Cytokine Growth Factor Rev 20: 481–488.

Bailey SB, Eichler ME, Villadiego A, Rich KM (1993) The influence of fibronectin and laminin during Schwann cell migration and peripheral nerve regeneration through silicon chambers. J Neurocytol 22: 176–184.

Bajrovic F, Bresjanac M, Sketelj J (1994) Long-term effects of deprivation of cell support in the distal stump on peripheral nerve regeneration. J Neurosci Res 39: 23–30.

Ballin RH, Thomas PK (1969) Changes at the nodes of Ranvier during Wallerian degeneration: an electron microscope study. Acta Neuropathol 14: 237–249.

Bannerman P, Ara J, Hahn A, Hong L, McCauley E, Friesen K, Pleasure D (2008) Peripheral nerve regeneration is delayed in neuropilin 2-deficient mice. J Neurosci Res 86: 3163–3169.

Barde YA, Edgar D, Thoenen H (1982) Purification of a new neurotrophic factor from mammalian brain. Embo J 1: 549–553.

Barker PA (2009) Whither proBDNF? Nat Neurosci 12: 105–106.

Barnett MW, Fisher CE, Perona-Wright G, Davies JA (2002) Signalling by glial cell line-derived neurotrophic factor (GDNF) requires heparan sulphate glycosaminoglycan. J Cell Sci 115: 4495–4503.

Barras FM, Kuntzer T, Zurn AD, Pasche P (2009) Local delivery of glial cell line-derived neurotrophic factor improves facial nerve regeneration after late repair. Laryngoscope 119: 846–855.

Bearden SE, Segal SS (2004) Microvessels promote motor nerve survival and regeneration through local VEGF release following ectopic reattachment. Microcirculation 11: 633–644.

Bendszus M, Stoll G (2003) Caught in the act: in vivo mapping of macrophage infiltration in nerve injury by magnetic resonance imaging. J Neurosci 23: 10892–10896.

Bennett DLH, Boucher TJ, Armanini MP, Poulsen KT, Michael GJ, Priestley JV, Phillips HS, McMahon SB, Shelton DL (2000) The glial cell line-derived neurotrophic factor family receptor components are differentially regulated within sensory neurons after nerve injury. J Neurosci 20: 427–437.

Berkemeier LR, Winslow JW, Kaplan DR, Nikolics K, Goeddel DV, Rosenthal A (1991) Neurotrophin-5: a novel neurotrophic factor that activates Trk and TrkB. Neuron 7: 857–866.

Bertolotto A, Palmucci L, Gagliano A, Mongini T, Tarone G (1986) Immunohistochemical localization of chondroitin sulfate in normal and pathological human muscle. J Neurol Sci 73: 233–244.

Bertotti A, Comoglio PM (2003) Tyrosine kinase signal specificity: lessons from the HGF receptor. Trends Biochem Sci 28: 527–533.

Besset V, Scott RP, Ibanez CF (2000) Signaling complexes and protein-protein interactions involved in the activation of the Ras and phosphatidylinositol 3-kinase pathways by the c-Ret receptor tyrosine kinase. J Biol Chem 275: 39159–39166.

Beuche W, Friede RL (1984) The role of non-resident cells in Wallerian degeneration. J Neurocytol 13: 767–796.

Beuche W, Friede RL (1986) Myelin phagocytosis in Wallerian degeneration of peripheral nerves depends on silica-sensitive, bg/bg-negative and Fc-positive monocytes. Brain Res 378: 97–106.

Bhakar AL, Roux PP, Lachance C, Kryl D, Zeindler C, Barker PA (1999) The p75 neurotrophin receptor (p75NTR) alters tumor necrosis factor-mediated NF-kappaB activity under physiological conditions, but direct p75NTR-mediated NF-kappaB activation requires cell stress. J Biol Chem 274: 21443–21449.

Bibel M, Hoppe E, Barde YA (1999) Biochemical and functional interactions between the neurotrophin receptors Trk and p75NTR. Embo J 18: 616–622.

Black MM, Lasek RJ (1979) Slowing of the rate of axonal regeneration during growth and maturation. Exp Neurol 63: 108–119.

Blesch A, Tuszynski MH (2001) GDNF gene delivery to injured adult CNS motor neurons promotes axonal growth, expression of the trophic neuropeptide CGRP, and cellular protection. J Comp Neurol 436: 399–410.

Blits B, Carlstedt TP, Ruitenberg MJ, De Winter F, Hermens WTJMC, Dijkhuizen PA, Claasens JWC, Eggers R, Van der Sluis R, Tenenbaum L, Boer GJ, Verhaagen J (2004) Rescue and sprouting of motoneurons following ventral root avulsion and reimplantation combined with intraspinal adeno-associated viral vector-mediated expression of glial cell line-derived neurotrophic factor or brain-derived neurotrophic factor. Exp Neurol 189: 303–316.

Blizzard CA, Haas MA, Vickers JC, Dickson TC (2007) Cellular dynamics underlying regeneration of damaged axons differs from initial axon development. Eur J Neurosci 26: 1100–1108.

Bloch J, Fine EG, Bouche N, Zurn AD, Aebischer P (2001) Nerve growth factor- and neurotrophin-3-releasing guidance channels promote regeneration of the transected rat dorsal root. Exp Neurol 172: 425–432.

Blondet B, Carpentier G, Lafdil F, Courty J (2005) Pleiotrophin cellular localization in nerve regeneration after peripheral nerve injury. J Histochem Cytochem 53: 971–977.

Blondet B, Carpentier G, Ferry A, Courty J (2006) Exogenous pleiotrophin applied to lesioned nerve impairs muscle reinnervation. Neurochem Res 31: 907–913.

Boivin A, Pineau I, Barrette B, Filali M, Vallieres N, Rivest S, Lacroix S (2007) Toll-like receptor signaling is critical for Wallerian degeneration and functional recovery after peripheral nerve injury. J Neurosci 27: 12565–12576.

Bosse F, Hasenpusch-Theil K, Kury P, Muller HW (2006) Gene expression profiling reveals that peripheral nerve regeneration is a consequence of both novel injury-dependent and reactivated developmental processes. J Neurochem 96: 1441–1457.

Bouldin T, Earnhardt AB, Goines N (1991) Restoration of blood-nerve barrier in neuropathy is associated with axonal regeneration and remyelination. J Neuropathology 50: 719–728.

Boyd JG, Gordon T (2001) The neurotrophin receptors, TrkB and p75, differentially regulate motor axonal regeneration. J Neurobiol 49: 314–325.

Boyd JG, Gordon T (2002) A dose-dependent facilitation and inhibition of peripheral nerve regeneration by brain-derived neurotrophic factor. Eur J Neurosci 15: 613–626.

Boyd JG, Gordon T (2003a) Neurotrophic factors and their receptors in axonal regeneration and functional recovery after peripheral nerve injury. Mol Neurobiol 27: 277–323.

Boyd JG, Gordon T (2003b) Glial cell line-derived neurotrophic factor and brain-derived neurotrophic factor sustain the axonal regeneration of chronically axotomized motoneurons in vivo. Exp Neurol 183: 610–619.

Bradley JL, Abernethy DA, King RHM, Muddle JR, Thomas PK (1998) Neural architecture in transected rabbit sciatic nerve after prolonged nonreinnervation. J Anat 192: 529–538.

Broude E, McAtee M, Kelley MS, Bregman BS (1997) c-Jun expression in adult rat dorsal root ganglion neurons: differential response after central or peripheral axotomy. Exp Neurol 148: 367–377.

Brown DL, Bennett TM, Dowsing BJ, Hayes A, Abate M, Morrison WA (2002) Immediate and delayed nerve repair: Improved muscle mass and function with leukemia inhibitory factor. J Hand Surg [Am] 27A: 1048–1055.

Brown MC, Lunn ER, Perry VH (1992) Consequences of slow Wallerian degeneration for regenerating motor and sensory axons. J Neurobiol 23: 521–536.

Bruck W, Friede RL (1991) The role of complement in myelin phagocytosis during PNS Wallerian degeneration. J Neurol Sci 103: 182–187.

Brunet A, Datta SR, Greenberg ME (2001) Transcription-dependent and -independent control of neuronal survival by the PI3K-Akt signaling pathway. Curr Opin Neurobiol 11: 297–305.

Brunet I, Weinl C, Piper M, Trembleau A, Volovitch M, Harris W, Prochiantz A, Holt C (2005) The transcription factor Engrailed-2 guides retinal axons. Nature 438: 94–98.

Brushart TM (1990) Preferential motor reinnervation: a sequential double-labeling study. Restor Neuro Nsci 1: 281–287.

Brushart, TM. (1998) Nerve repair and grafting. In: *Green's Operative Hand Surgery*, pp. 1381–1403, New York: Churchill Livingston.

Brushart TM, Gerber J, Kessens P, Chen YG, Royal R (1998) Contributions of pathway and neuron to preferential motor reinnervation. J Neurosci 18: 8674–8681.

Brushart TM, Hoffman PN, Royall RM, Murinson BB, Witzel C, Gordon T (2002) Electrical stimulation promotes motoneuron regeneration without increasing its speed or conditioning the neuron. J Neurosci 22: 6631–6638.

Brushart TM, Jari R, Verge V, Rohde C, Gordon T (2005) Electrical stimulation restores the specificity of sensory axon regeneration. Exp Neurol 194: 221–229.

Brushart, T.M., R. Redett, H. Hameed, C. Zhou, and A. Hoke (2006) *Differential Growth Factor Expression in Subsets of Schwann Cells*. Program No. 787.3. 2006 Neuroscience meeting planner. Atlanta, GA: Society for Neuroscience, online.

Buck CR, Seburn KL, Cope TC (2000) Neurotrophin expression by spinal motoneurons in adult and developing rats. J Comp Neurol 416: 309–318.

Buck K, Zheng JQ (2002) Growth cone turning induced by direct local modification of microtubule dynamics. J Neurosci 22: 9358–9367.

Bucko CD, Joynt RL, Grabb WC (1981) Peripheral nerve regeneration in primates during D-penicillamine-induced lathyrism. Plast Reconstr Surg 67: 23–30.

Bunge MB, Wood PM, Tynan LB, Bates ML, Sanes JR (1989) Perineurium originates from fibroblasts: demonstration in vitro with a retroviral marker. Science 243: 229–231.

Bungner Ov (1891) Ueber die degeneratuins-und regenerationsvorgange am nerven nach verletzungen. Beitr Pathol Anat 10: 312–393.

Burazin TCD, Gundlach AL (1998) Up-regulation of GDNFR-alpha and c-ret mRNA in facial motor neurons following facial nerve injury in the rat. Mol Brain Res 55: 331–336.

Burgess WH, Maciag T (1989) The heparin-binding (fibroblast) growth factor family of proteins. Annu Rev Biochem 58: 575–606.

Burnette DT, Ji L, Schaefer AW, Medeiros NA, Danuser G, Forscher P (2008) Myosin II activity facilitates microtubule bundling in the neuronal growth cone neck. Dev Cell 15: 163–169.

Cafferty WB, Gardiner NJ, Gavazzi I, Powell J, McMahon SB, Heath JK, Munson J, Cohen J, Thompson SW (2001) Leukemia inhibitory factor determines the growth status of injured adult sensory neurons. J Neurosci 21: 7161–7170.

Cafferty WBJ, Gardiner NJ, Das P, Qiu J, McMahon SB, Thompson SWN (2004) Conditioning injury-induced spinal axon regeneration fails in interleukin-6 knock-out mice. J Neurosci 24: 4432–4443.

Cai CM, Qiu J, Cao ZX, McAtee M, Bregman BS, Filbin MT (2001) Neuronal cyclic AMP controls the developmental loss in ability of axons to regenerate. J Neurosci 21: 4731–4739.

Cai D, Deng K, Mellado W, Lee J, Ratan RR, Filbin MT (2002) Arginase I and polyamines act downstream from cyclic AMP in overcoming inhibition of axonal growth MAG and myelin in vitro. Neuron 35: 711–719.

Campbell JB, Bassett CA, Husby J, Thulin CA, Feringa ER (1961) Microfilter sheaths in peripheral nerve surgery: a laboratory report and preliminary clinical study. J Trauma 1: 139–158.

Campenot RB (1977) Local control of neurite development by nerve growth factor. Proc Natl Acad Sci U S A 74: 4516–4519.

Campenot RB (1982a) Development of sympathetic neurons in compartmentalized cultures. I. Local control of neurite growth by nerve growth factor Dev Biol 93: 1–12.

Campenot RB (1982b) Development of sympathetic neurons in compartmentalized cultures. II. Local control of neurite survival by nerve growth factor Dev Biol 93: 13–21.

Cao ZX, Gao Y, Bryson JB, Hou JW, Chaudhry N, Siddiq M, Martinez J, Spencer T, Carmel J, Hart RB, Filbin MT (2006) The cytokine interleukin-6 is sufficient but not necessary to mimic the peripheral conditioning lesion effect on axonal growth. J Neurosci 26: 5565–5573.

Carlberg M, Larsson O (1996) Stimulatory effect of PDGF on HMG-CoA reductase activity and N-linked glycosylation contributes to increased expression of IGF-1 receptors in human fibroblasts. Exp Cell Res 223: 142–148.

Carnevale KA, Cathcart MK (2001) Calcium-independent phospholipase A(2) is required for human monocyte chemotaxis to monocyte chemoattractant protein 1. J Immunol 167: 3414–3421.

Caroni P, Grandes P (1990) Nerve sprouting in innervated adult skeletal muscle induced by exposure to elevated levels of insulin-like growth factors. J Cell Biol 110: 1307–1317.

Caroni P, Schneider C (1994) Signaling by insulin-like growth factors in paralyzed skeletal muscle: rapid induction of IGF1 expression in muscle fibers and prevention of interstitial cell proliferation by IGF-BP5 and IGF-BP4. J Neurosci 14: 3378–3388.

Caroni P, Schneider C, Kiefer MC, Zapf J (1994) Role of muscle insulin-like growth factors in nerve sprouting: suppression of terminal sprouting in paralyzed muscle by IGF-binding protein 4. J Cell Biol 125: 893–902.

Carter BD, Kaltschmidt C, Kaltschmidt B, Offenhauser N, Bohm-Matthaei R, Baeuerle PA, Barde YA (1996) Selective activation of NF-kappa B by nerve growth factor through the neurotrophin receptor p75. Science 272: 542–545.

Carter DA, Lisney SJ (1991) Changes in myelinated and unmyelinated axon numbers in the proximal parts of rat sural nerves after two types of injury. Restor Neurol Neurosci 3: 65–73.

Casademunt E, Carter BD, Benzel I, Frade JM, Dechant G, Barde YA (1999) The zinc finger protein NRIF interacts with the neurotrophin receptor p75(NTR) and participates in programmed cell death. Embo J 18: 6050–6061.

Cavalli V, Kujala P, Klumperman J, Goldstein LS (2005) Sunday Driver links axonal transport to damage signaling. J Cell Biol 168: 775–787.

Chan JR, Cosgaya JM, Wu YJ, Shooter EM (2001) Neurotrophins are key mediators of the myelination program in the peripheral nervous system. Proc Natl Acad Sci U S A 98: 14661–14668.

Chattopadhyay S, Myers RR, Janes J, Shubayev V (2007) Cytokine regulation of MMP-9 in peripheral glia: implications for pathological processes and pain in injured nerve. Brain Behav Immun 21: 561–568.

Chen MH, Chen PR, Chen MH, Hsieh ST, Lin FH (2006) Gelatin-tricalcium phosphate membranes immobilized with NGF, BDNF, or IGF-1 for peripheral nerve repair: an in vitro and in vivo study. J Biomed Mater Res A 79: 846–857.

Chen YS, Wang-Bennett L, Coker N (1989) Facial nerve regeneration in the silicon chamber: the influence of nerve growth factor. Exp Neurol 103: 52–60.

Chen YY, McDonald D, Cheng C, Magnowski B, Durand J, Zochodne DW (2005) Axon and Schwann cell partnership during nerve regrowth. J Neuropathol Exp Neurol 64: 613–622.

Chen ZL, Strickland S (2003) Laminin gamma1 is critical for Schwann cell differentiation, axon myelination, and regeneration in the peripheral nerve. J Cell Biol 163: 889–899.

Chen ZL, Yu WM, Strickland S (2007) Peripheral regeneration. Annu Rev Neurosci 30: 209–233.

Cheng HL, Russell JW, Feldman EL (1999) IGF-I promotes peripheral nervous system myelination. Ann NY Acad Sci 883: 124–130.

Cheng HL, Randolph A, Yee D, Delafontaine P, Tennekoon G, Feldman EL (1996) Characterization of insulin-like growth factor-I and its receptor and binding proteins in transected nerves and cultured Schwann cells. J Neurochem 66: 525–536.

Cheng HL, Steinway M, Delaney CL, Franke TF, Feldman EL (2000) IGF-I promotes Schwann cell motility and survival via activation of Akt. Mol Cell Endocrinol 170: 211–215.

Chierzi S, Ratto GM, Verma P, Fawcett JW (2005) The ability of axons to regenerate their growth cones depends on axonal type and age, and is regulated by calcium, cAMP and ERK. Eur J Neurosci 21: 2051–2062.

Chilton JK (2006) Molecular mechanisms of axon guidance. Dev Biol 292: 13–24.

Chong M, Reynolds M, Irwin N, Coggeshall R, Emson P, Benowitz L, Woolf C (1994) GAP-43 expression in primary sensory neurons following central axotomy. J Neurosci 14: 4375–4384.

Chu GK, Tator CH (2001) Calcium influx is necessary for optimal regrowth of transected neurites of rat sympathetic ganglion neurons in vitro. Neuroscience 102: 945–957.

Chu TH, Li SY, Guo A, Wong WM, Yuan Q, Wu W (2009) Implantation of neurotrophic factor-treated sensory nerve graft enhances survival and axonal regeneration of motoneurons after spinal root avulsion. J Neuropathol Exp Neurol 68: 94–101.

Cifuentes-Diaz C, Velasco E, Meunier FA, Goudou D, Belkadi L, Faille L, Murawsky M, Angaut-Petit D, Molgo J, Schachner M, Saga Y, Aizawa S, Rieger F (1998) The peripheral nerve and the neuromuscular junction are affected in the tenascin-C-deficient mouse. Cell Mol Biol (Noisy-le-grand) 44: 357–379.

Cifuentes-Diaz C, Faille L, Goudou D, Schachner M, Rieger F, Angaut-Petit D (2002) Abnormal reinnervation of skeletal muscle in a tenascin-C-deficient mouse. J Neurosci Res 67: 93–99.

Cohen P (2006) Overview of the IGF-I system. Horm Res 65 (Suppl 1): 3–8.

Condic ML (2001) Adult neuronal regeneration induced by transgenic integrin expression. J Neurosci 21: 4782–4788.

Contreras PC, Steffler C, Yu EY, Callison K, Stong D, Vaught JL (1995) Systemic administration of rhIGF-I enhanced regeneration after sciatic nerve crush in mice. J Pharmacol Exp Ther 274: 1443–1449.

Coppola V, Kucera J, Palko ME, Martinez-De Velasco J, Lyons WE, Fritzsch B, Tessarollo L (2001) Dissection of NT3 functions in vivo by gene replacement strategy. Development 128: 4315–4327.

Cordeiro PG, Seckel BR, Lipton S, D'Amore P, Wagner J, Madison R (1989) Acidic fibroblast growth factor enhances peripheral nerve regeneration *in vivo*. Plast Reconstr Surg 83: 1013–1019.

Cornbrooks CJ, Carey DJ, McDonald JA, Timpl R, Bunge RP (1983) In vivo and in vitro observations on laminin production by Schwann cells. Proc Natl Acad Sci U S A 80: 3850–3854.

Cosgaya JM, Chan JR, Shooter EM (2002) The neurotrophin receptor p75NTR as a positive modulator of myelination. Science 298: 1245–1248.

Cottin P, Vidalenc PL, Ducastaing A (1981) Ca2+-dependent association between a Ca2+-activated neutral proteinase (CaANP) and its specific inhibitor. FEBS Lett 136: 221–224.

Court FA, Hendriks WT, Macgillavry HD, Alvarez J, van Minnen J (2008) Schwann cell to axon transfer of ribosomes: toward a novel understanding of the role of glia in the nervous system. J Neurosci 28: 11024–11029.

Cui Q (2006) Actions of neurotrophic factors and their signaling pathways in neuronal survival and axonal regeneration. Mol Neurobiol 33: 155–179.

Curtis R, Adryan KM, Stark JL, Park JS, Compton DL, Weskamp G, Huber LJ, Chao MV, Jaenisch R, Lee KF, et al. (1995) Differential role of the low affinity neurotrophin receptor (p75) in retrograde axonal transport of the neurotrophins. Neuron 14: 1201–1211.

da Silva CF, Madison R, Dikkes P, Chiu TH, Sidman RL (1985) An in vivo model to quantify motor and sensory peripheral nerve regeneration using bioresorbable nerve guide tubes. Brain Res 342: 307–315.

D'Antonio M, Droggiti A, Feltri ML, Roes J, Wrabetz L, Mirsky R, Jessen KR (2006) TGFbeta type II receptor signaling controls Schwann cell death and proliferation in developing nerves. J Neurosci 26: 8417–8427.

Dahlin L (1992) Stimulation of regeneration of the sciatic nerve by experimentally induced inflammation in rats. Scand J Plast Reconstr Hand Surg 26: 121–125.

Dahlin L, Kanje M (1992) Conditioning effect induced by chronic nerve compression. Scand J Plast Reconstr Hand Surg 26: 37–41.

Dahlin L, Necking L, Lundstrom R, Lundborg G (1992) Vibration exposure and conditioning lesion effect in nerves: an experimental study in rats. J Hand Surg 17A: 858–861.

Dailey AT, Avellino AM, Benthem L, Silver J, Kliot M (1998) Complement depletion reduces macrophage infiltration and activation during Wallerian degeneration and axonal regeneration. J Neurosci 18: 6713–6722.

Danielsen N, Lundborg G, Frizell M (1986) Nerve repair and axonal transport: outgrowth delay and regeneration rate after transection and repair of rabbit hypoglossal nerve. Brain Res 376: 125–132.

Danielsen N, Kerns JM, Holmquist B, Zhao Q, Lundborg G, Kanje M (1994) Pre-degenerated nerve grafts enhance regeneration by shortening the initial delay period. Brain Res 666: 250–254.

Danielsen N, Kerns JM, Holmquist B, Zhao Q, Lundborg G, Kanje M (1995) Predegeneration enhances regeneration into acellular nerve grafts. Brain Res 681: 105–108.

David S, Braun PE, Jackson DL, Kottis V, McKerracher L (1995) Laminin overrides the inhibitory effects of peripheral nervous system and central nervous system myelin-derived inhibitors of neurite growth. J Neurosci Res 42: 594–602.

David S, Fry EJ, Lopez-Vales R (2008) Novel roles for Nogo receptor in inflammation and disease. Trends Neurosci 31: 221–226.

Davies AM (1989) Intrinsic differences in the growth rate of early nerve fibres related to target distance. Nature 337: 553–555.

Davies AM, Lee KF, Jaenisch R (1993) p75-deficient trigeminal sensory neurons have an altered response to NGF but not to other neurotrophins. Neuron 11: 565–574.

Davison SP, McCaffrey TV, Porter MN, Manders E (1999) Improved nerve regeneration with neutralization of transforming growth factor-beta1. Laryngoscope 109: 631–635.

De S, Trigueros MA, Kalyvas A, David S (2003) Phospholipase A2 plays an important role in myelin breakdown and phagocytosis during Wallerian degeneration. Mol Cell Neurosci 24: 753–765.

DeAngelis T, Ferber A, Baserga R (1995) Insulin-like growth factor I receptor is required for the mitogenic and transforming activities of the platelet-derived growth factor receptor. J Cell Physiol 164: 214–221.

De Pablo F, Banner LR, Patterson PH (2000) IGF-I expression is decreased in LIF-deficient mice after peripheral nerve injury. Neuroreport 11: 1365–1368.

Delaney CL, Cheng HL, Feldman EL (1999) Insulin-like growth factor-I prevents caspase-mediated apoptosis in Schwann cells. J Neurobiol 41: 540–548.

Delbono O (2003) Neural control of aging skeletal muscle. Aging Cell 2: 21–29.

Deng K, He H, Qiu J, Lorber B, Bryson JB, Filbin MT (2009) Increased synthesis of spermidine as a result of upregulation of arginase I promotes axonal regeneration in culture and in vivo. J Neurosci 29: 9545–9552.

Dent EW, Gertler FB (2003) Cytoskeletal dynamics and transport in growth cone motility and axon guidance. Neuron 40: 209–227.

Derby A, Engleman VW, Frierdich GE, Neises G, Rapp SR, Roufa DG (1993) Nerve growth factor facilitates regeneration across nerve gaps: morphological and behavioral studies in rat sciatic nerve. Exp Neurol 119: 176–191.

Dergham P, Ellezam B, Essagian C, Avedissian H, Lubell WD, McKerracher L (2002) Rho signaling pathway targeted to promote spinal cord repair. J Neurosci 22: 6570–6577.

Diamond J, Holmes M, Coughlin M (1992a) Endogenous NGF and nerve impulses regulate the collateral sprouting of sensory axons in the skin of the adult rat. J Neurosci 12: 1454–1466.

Diamond J, Foerster A, Holmes M, Coughlin M (1992b) Sensory nerves in adult rats regenerate and restore sensory function to the skin independently of endogenous NGF. J Neurosci 12: 1467–1476.

Dohm S, Streppel M, Guntinas-Lichius O, Pesheva P, Probstmeier R, Walther M, Neiss W, Stennert E, Angelov DN (2000) Local application of extracellular matrix proteins fails to reduce the number of axonal branches after varying reconstructive surgery on rat facial nerve. Restor Neuro Nsci 16: 117–126.

Domeniconi M, Filbin MT (2005) Overcoming inhibitors in myelin to promote axonal regeneration. J Neurol Sci 233: 43–47.

Dowsing BJ, Hayes A, Bennett TM, Morrison WA, Messina A (2000) Effects of LIF dose and laminin plus fibronectin on axotomized sciatic nerves. Muscle & Nerve 23: 1356–1364.

Dubový and Svízenská (1994) Denervated skeletal muscle stimulates migration of Schwann cells from the distal stump of transected peripheral nerve: an in vivo study. Glia 12: 99–107.

Dubový P, Svízenská I, Klusáková I, Zítková A, Haninec P (2001) Laminin molecules in freeze-treated nerve segments are associated with migrating Schwann cells that display the corresponding α6β1 integrin receptor. Glia 33: 36–44.

Ducker TB, Ludwig GK, Hayes GJ (1969) The metabolic background for peripheral nerve surgery. J Neurosurg 30: 270–280.

Dustin, A.P. (1917) Le service de neurologie a l'ambulance ocean. Paris: Masson et Cie.

Eberhardt KA, Irintichev A, Al-Majed AA, Simova O, Brushart TM, Gordon T, Schachner M (2006) BDNF/TrkB signaling regulates HNK-1 carbohydrate expression in regenerating motor nerves and promotes functional recovery after peripheral nerve repair. Exp Neurol 198: 500–510.

Edstrom A, Ekstrom PA (2003) Role of phosphatidylinositol 3-kinase in neuronal survival and axonal outgrowth of adult mouse dorsal root ganglia explants. J Neurosci Res 74: 726–735.

Edstrom A, Ekstrom PA, Tonge D (1996) Axonal outgrowth and neuronal apoptosis in cultured adult mouse dorsal root ganglion preparations: effects of neurotrophins, of inhibition of neurotrophin actions and of prior axotomy. Neuroscience 75: 1165–1174.

Eggers R, Hendriks WT, Tannemaat MR, van Heerikhuize JJ, Pool CW, Carlstedt TP, Zaldumbide A, Hoeben RC, Boer GJ, Verhaagen J (2008) Neuroregenerative effects of lentiviral vector-mediated GDNF expression in reimplanted ventral roots. Mol Cell Neurosci 39: 105–117.

Ehlers MD (2004) Deconstructing the axon: Wallerian degeneration and the ubiquitin-proteasome system. Trends Neurosci 27: 3–6.

Eickholt BJ, Ahmed AI, Davies M, Papakonstanti EA, Pearce W, Starkey ML, Bilancio A, Need AC, Smith AJ, Hall SM, Hamers FP, Giese KP, Bradbury EJ, Vanhaesebroeck B (2007) Control of axonal growth and regeneration of sensory neurons by the p110delta PI3-kinase. PLoS ONE 2 e869.

Ekstrom PA, Mayer U, Panjwani A, Pountney D, Pizzey J, Tonge DA (2003) Involvement of alpha7beta1 integrin in the conditioning-lesion effect on sensory axon regeneration. Mol Cell Neurosci 22: 383–395.

Elde R, Cao YH, Cintra A, Brelje TC, Pelto-Huikko M, Junttila T, Fuxe K, Pettersson RF, Hokfelt T (1991) Prominent expression of acidic fibroblast growth factor in motor and sensory neurons. Neuron 7: 349–364.

English AW (2005) Enhancing axon regeneration in peripheral nerves also increases functionally inappropriate reinnervation of targets. J Comp Neurol 490: 427–441.

English AW, Meador W, Carrasco DI (2005) Neurotrophin-4/5 is required for the early growth of regenerating axons in peripheral nerves. Eur J Neurosci 21: 2624–2634.

English AW, Schwartz G, Meador W, Sabatier MJ, Mulligan A (2007) Electrical stimulation promotes peripheral axon regeneration by enhanced neuronal neurotrophin signaling. Dev Neurobiol 67: 158–172.

Ensslen-Craig SE, Brady-Kalnay SM (2004) Receptor protein tyrosine phosphatases regulate neural development and axon guidance. Dev Biol 275: 12–22.

Ernfors P, Henschen A, Olson L, Persson H (1989) Expression of nerve growth factor receptor mRNA is developmentally regulated and increased after axotomy in rat spinal cord motoneurons. Neuron 2: 1605–1613.

Esper RM, Loeb JA (2004) Rapid axoglial signaling mediated by neuregulin and neurotrophic factors. J Neurosci 24: 6218–6227.

Esposito D, Patel P, Stephens RM, Perez P, Chao MV, Kaplan DR, Hempstead BL (2001) The cytoplasmic and transmembrane domains of the p75 and Trk A receptors regulate high affinity binding to nerve growth factor. J Biol Chem 276: 32687–32695.

Evans DH, Murray JG (1956) A study of regeneration in a motor nerve with a unimodal fiber diameter distribution. Anat Rec 126: 311–329.

Faissner A (1997) The tenascin gene family in axon growth and guidance. Cell Tissue Res 290: 331–341.

Fan YJ, Wu LL, Li HY, Wang YJ, Zhou XF (2008) Differential effects of pro-BDNF on sensory neurons after sciatic nerve transection in neonatal rats. Eur J Neurosci 27: 2380–2390.

Fansa H, Schneider W, Wolf G, Keilhoff G (2002) Influence of insulin-like growth factor-I (IGF-I) on nerve autografts and tissue-engineered nerve grafts. Muscle & Nerve 26: 87–93.

Farrar NR, Spencer GE (2008) Pursuing a "turning point" in growth cone research. Dev Biol 318: 102–111.

Fawcett JW, Mathews G, Housden E, Goedert M, Matus A (1994) Regenerating sciatic nerve axons contain the adult rather than the embryonic pattern of microtubule associated proteins. Neuroscience 61: 789–804.

Ferguson IA, Schweitzer JB, Johnson EM, Jr. (1990) Basic fibroblast growth factor: receptor-mediated internalization, metabolism, and anterograde axonal transport in retinal ganglion cells. J Neurosci 10: 2176–2189.

Fernández-Celemín L, Pasko N, Blomart V, Thissen JP (2002) Inhibition of muscle insulin-like growth factor I expression by tumor necrosis factor-α. Am J Physiol Endocrinol Metab 283: E1279–E1290.

Fernandez-Valle C, Bunge RP, Bunge MB (1995) Schwann cells degrade myelin and proliferate in the absence of macrophages: evidence from in vitro studies of Wallerian degeneration. J Neurocytol 24: 667–679.

Fernyhough P, Willars GB, Lindsay RM, Tomlinson DR (1993) Insulin and insulin-like growth factor I enhance regeneration in cultured adult rat sensory neurones. Brain Res 607: 117–124.

Ferrara N, Alitalo K (1999) Clinical applications of angiogenic growth factors and their inhibitors. Nat Med 5: 1359–1364.

Finn JT, Weil M, Archer F, Siman R, Srinivasan A, Raff MC (2000) Evidence that Wallerian degeneration and localized axon degeneration induced by local neurotrophin deprivation do not involve caspases. J Neurosci 20: 1333–1341.

Florini JR, Ewton DZ, Coolican SA (1996) Growth hormone and the insulin-like growth factor system in myogenesis. Endocr Rev 17: 481–517.

Flumerfelt BA, Lewis PR (1975) Cholinesterase activity in the hypoglossal nucleus of the rat and the changes produced by axotomy: a light and electron microscopic study. J Anat 119: 309–331.

Forman DS, Berenberg RA (1978) Regeneration of motor axons in the rat sciatic nerve studied by labeling with axonally transported radioactive proteins. Brain Res 156: 213–225.

Forman DS, Wood DK, DeSilva S (1979) Rate of regeneration of sensory axons in transected rat sciatic nerve repaired with epineurial sutures. J Neurol Sci 44: 55–59.

Friede RL, Bischhausen R (1980) The fine structure of stumps of transected nerve fibers in subserial sections. J Neurol Sci 44: 181–203.

Frizell M, Sjostrand J (1974) Transport of proteins, glycoproteins and cholinergic enzymes in regenerating hypoglossal neurons. J Neurochem 22: 845–850.

Fruttiger M, Schachner M, Martini R (1995) Tenascin-C expression during Wallerian degeneration in C57BL/Wlds mice: possible implications for axonal regeneration. J Neurocytol 24: 1–14.

Fry EJ, Ho C, David S (2007) A role for Nogo receptor in macrophage clearance from injured peripheral nerve. Neuron 53: 649–662.

Fu SY, Gordon T (1995a) Contributing factors to poor functional recovery after delayed nerve repair: prolonged denervation. J Neurosci 15: 3886–3895.

Fu SY, Gordon T (1995b) Contributing factors to poor functional recovery after delayed nerve repair: prolonged axotomy. J Neurosci 15: 3876–3885.

Fu SY, Gordon T (1997) The cellular and molecular basis of peripheral nerve regeneration. Mol Neurobiol 14: 67–116.

Fugleholm K, Schmalbruch H, Krarup C (1994) Early peripheral nerve regeneration after crushing, sectioning, and freeze studied by implanted electrodes in the cat. J Neurosci 14: 2659–2673.

Fujimoto E, Mizoguchi A, Hanada K, Yajima M, Ide C (1997) Basic fibroblast growth factor promotes extension of regenerating axons of peripheral nerve: in vivo experiments using a Schwann cell basal lamina tube model. J Neurocytol 26: 511–528.

Fukaya K, Hasegawa M, Mashitani T, Kadoya T, Horie H, Hayashi Y, Fujisawa H, Tachibana O, Kida S, Yamashita J (2003) Oxidized galectin-1 stimulates the migration of Schwann cells from both proximal and distal stumps of transected nerves and promotes axonal regeneration after peripheral nerve injury. J Neuropathol Exp Neurol 62: 162–172.

Fukuda T, Kiuchi K, Takahashi M (2002) Novel mechanism of regulation of Rac activity and lamellipodia formation by RET tyrosine kinase. J Biol Chem 277: 19114–19121.

Funakoshi H, Nakamura T (2003) Hepatocyte growth factor: from diagnosis to clinical applications. Clin Chim Acta 327: 1–23.

Funakoshi H, Frisen J, Barbany G, Timmusk T, Zachrisson O, Verge V, Persson H (1993) Differential expression of mRNAs for neurotrophins and their receptors after axotomy of the sciatic nerve. J Cell Biol 123: 455–465.

Funakoshi H, Risling M, Carlstedt T, Lendahl U, Timmusk T, Metsis M, Yamamoto Y, Ibamez CF (1998) Targeted expression of a multifunctional chimeric neurotrophin in the lesioned sciatic nerve accelerates regeneration of sensory and motor axons. PNAS 95: 5269–5274.

Fundin BT, Mikaels A, Westphal H, Ernfors P (1999) A rapid and dynamic regulation of GDNF-family ligands and receptors correlate with the developmental dependency of cutaneous sensory innervation. Development 126: 2597–2610.

Furey MJ, Midha R, Xu QG, Belkas J, Gordon T (2007) Prolonged target deprivation reduces the capacity of injured motoneurons to regenerate. Neurosurgery 60: 723–732; discussion 732–733.

Galiano M, Liu ZQ, Kalla R, Bohatschek M, Koppius A, Gschwendtner A, Xu SL, Werner A, Kloss CUA, Jones LL, Bluethmann H, Raivich G (2001) Interleukin-6 (IL-6) and cellular response to facial nerve injury: effects on lymphocyte recruitment, early microglial activation and axonal outgrowth in IL6-deficient mice. Eur J Neurosci 14: 327–341.

Gao Y, Nikulina E, Mellado W, Filbin MT (2003) Neurotrophins elevate cAMP to reach a threshold required to overcome inhibition by MAG through extracellular signal-regulated kinase-dependent inhibition of phosphodiesterase. J Neurosci 23: 11770–11777.

Gao Y, Deng KW, Hou JW, Bryson JB, Barco A, Nikulina E, Spencer T, Mellado W, Kandel ER, Filbin MT (2004) Activated CREB is sufficient to overcome inhibitors in myelin and promote spinal axon regeneration in vivo. Neuron 44: 609–621.

Garcia-Mata R, Burridge K (2007) Catching a GEF by its tail. Trends Cell Biol 17: 36–43.

Gardiner NJ, Fernyhough P, Tomlinson DR, Mayer U, von der Mark H, Streuli CH (2005) Alpha7 integrin mediates neurite outgrowth of distinct populations of adult sensory neurons. Mol Cell Neurosci 28: 229–240.

Gardiner NJ, Moffatt S, Fernyhough P, Humphries MJ, Streuli CH, Tomlinson DR (2007) Preconditioning injury-induced neurite outgrowth of adult rat sensory neurons on fibronectin is mediated by mobilisation of axonal alpha5 integrin. Mol Cell Neurosci 35: 249–260.

Gaudet AD, Steeves JD, Tetzlaff W, Ramer MS (2005) Expression and functions of galectin-1 in sensory and motoneurons. Curr Drug Targets 6: 419–425.

Gavazzi I, Kumar RD, McMahon SB, Cohen J (1999) Growth responses of different subpopulations of adult sensory neurons to neurotrophic factors in vitro. Eur J Neurosci 11: 3405–3414.

Gavazzi I, Stonehouse J, Sandvig A, Reza JN, Appiah-Kubi LS, Keynes R, Cohen J (2000) Peripheral, but not central, axotomy induces neuropilin-1 mRNA expression in adult large diameter primary sensory neurons. J Comp Neurol 423: 492–499.

Gentry JJ, Rutkoski NJ, Burke TL, Carter BD (2004) A functional interaction between the p75 neurotrophin receptor interacting factors, TRAF6 and NRIF. J Biol Chem 279: 16646–16656.

Geremia NM, Gordon T, Brushart TM, Al-Majed A, Verge V (2007) Electrical stimulation promotes sensory neuron regeneration and growth-associated gene expression. Exp Neurol 205: 347–359.

Geremia NM, Pettersson LM, Hasmatali JC, Hryciw T, Danielsen N, Schreyer DJ, Verge VM (2010) Endogenous BDNF regulates induction of intrinsic neuronal growth programs in injured sensory neurons. Exp Neurol 223: 128–142.

George EB, Glass JD, Griffin JW (1995) Axotomy-induced axonal degeneration is mediated by calcium influx through ion-specific channels. J Neurosci 15: 6445–6452.

Ghazvini M, Mandemakers W, Jaegle M, Piirsoo M, Driegen S, Koutsourakis M, Smit X, Grosveld F,

Meijer D (2002) A cell type-specific allele of the POU gene Oct-6 reveals Schwann cell autonomous function in nerve development and regeneration. Embo J 21: 4612–4620.

Gilad VH, Tetzlaff WG, Rabey JM, Gilad GM (1996) Accelerated recovery following polyamines and aminoguanidine treatment after facial nerve injury in rats. Brain Res 724: 141–144.

Giannini C, Dyck P (1990) The fate of Schwann cell basement membranes in permanently transected nerves. J Neuropath 49: 550–563.

Gilliatt RW, Hjorth RJ (1972) Nerve conduction during Wallerian degeneration in the baboon. J Neurol Nsurg Psych 35: 335–341.

Ginty DD, Segal RA (2002) Retrograde neurotrophin signaling: Trk-ing along the axon. Curr Opin Neurobiol 12: 268–274.

Girolami EI, Bouhy D, Haber M, Johnson H, David S (2009) Differential expression and potential role of SOCS1 and SOCS3 in Wallerian degeneration in injured peripheral nerve. Exp Neurol 223: 173–182.

Glass JD, Brushart TM, George EB, Griffin JW (1993) Prolonged survival of transected nerve fibres in C57BL/Ola mice is an intrinsic characteristic of the axon. J Neurocytol 22: 311–321.

Glass JD, Schryer BL, Griffin JW (1994) Calcium-mediated degeneration of the axonal cytoskeleton in the Ola mouse. J Neurochem 62: 2472–2475.

Glass JD, Culver DG, Levey AI, Nash NR (2002) Very early activation of m-calpain in peripheral nerve during Wallerian degeneration. J Neurol Sci 196: 9–20.

Glazner GW, Lupien S, Miller JA, Ishii DN (1993) Insulin-like growth factor II increases the rate of sciatic nerve regeneration in rats. Neuroscience 54: 791–797.

Glazner GW, Ishii DN (1995) Insulinlike growth factor gene expression in rat muscle during reinnervation. Muscle & Nerve 18: 1433–1442.

Glickman MH, Ciechanover A (2002) The ubiquitin-proteasome proteolytic pathway: destruction for the sake of construction. Physiol Rev 82: 373–428.

Gold BG (1997) Axonal regeneration of sensory nerves is delayed by continuous intrathecal infusion of nerve growth factor. Neuroscience 76: 1153–1158.

Gomez TM, Zheng JQ (2006) The molecular basis for calcium-dependent axon pathfinding. Nat Rev Neurosci 7: 115–125.

Gondré M, Burrola P, Weinstein DE (1998) Accelerated nerve regeneration mediated by Schwann cells expressing a mutant form of the POU protein SCIP. J Cell Biol 141: 493–501.

Goold RG, Gordon-Weeks PR (2005) The MAP kinase pathway is upstream of the activation of GSK3beta that enables it to phosphorylate MAP1B and contributes to the stimulation of axon growth. Mol Cell Neurosci 28: 524–534.

Gordon T (2009) The role of neurotrophic factors in nerve regeneration. Neurosurg Focus 26: E3.

Gordon-Weeks PR (2004) Microtubules and growth cone function. J Neurobiol 58: 70–83.

Gorio A, Vergani L, De Tollis A, Di Giulio AM, Torsello A, Cattaneo L, Muller EE (1998) Muscle reinnervation following neonatal nerve crush, interactive effects of glycosaminoglycans and insulin-like growth factor-I. Neuroscience 82: 1029–1037.

Govek EE, Newey SE, Van Aelst L (2005) The role of the Rho GTPases in neuronal development. Genes Dev 19: 1–49.

Graham JB, Neubauer D, Xue QS, Muir D (2007) Chondroitinase applied to peripheral nerve repair averts retrograde axonal regeneration. Exp Neurol 203: 185–195.

Gregson NA, Hall SM (1973) A quantitative analysis of the effects of the intraneural injection of lysophosphatidyl choline. J Cell Sci 13: 257–277.

Griffin, J.W. and P.N. Hoffman (1993) Degeneration and regeneration in the peripheral nervous system. In: *Peripheral Neuropathy*, P.J. Dyck and P.K. Thomas, eds., pp. 361–376, Philadelphia: Saunders.

Griffin JW, Price DL, Engel WK, Drachman DB (1977) The pathogenesis of reactive axonal swellings: role of axonal transport. J Neuropathol Exp Neurol 36: 214–227.

Griffin JW, George R, Lobato C, Tyor WR, Yan LC, Glass JD (1992) Macrophage responses and myelin clearance during Wallerian degeneration: relevance to immune-mediated demyelination. J Neuroimmunol 40: 153–165.

Griffin, J.W., E.B. George, S. Hsieh, and Glass D.J. (1995) Axonal degeneration and disorders of the axonal cytoskeleton. In: *The Axon*, S.G. Waxman, J.D. Kocsis and P.K. Stys, eds., pp. 375–390, New York: Oxford University Press.

Grothe C, Unsicker K (1992) Basic fibroblast growth factor in the hypoglossal system: specific retrograde transport, trophic, and lesion-related responses. J Neurosci 32: 317–328.

Grothe C, Wewetzer K (1996) Fibroblast growth factor and its implications for developing and regenerating neurons. Int J Dev Biol 40: 403–410.

Grothe C, Meisinger C, Hertenstein A, Kurz H, Wewetzer K (1997) Expression of fibroblast growth factor-2 and fibroblast growth factor receptor 1 messenger RNAs in spinal ganglia and sciatic nerve: regulation after peripheral nerve lesion. Neuroscience 76: 123–135.

Grothe C, Meisinger C, Claus P (2001) In vivo expression and localization of the fibroblast growth factor system in the intact and lesioned rat peripheral nerve and spinal ganglia. J Comp Neurol 434: 342–357.

Grothe C, Haastert K, Jungnickel J (2006) Physiological function and putative therapeutic impact of the FGF-2 system in peripheral nerve regeneration: lessons from in vivo studies in mice and rats. Brain Res Rev 51: 293–299.

Grothe C, Claus P, Haastert K, Lutwak E, Ron D (2008) Expression and regulation of Sef, a novel signaling inhibitor of receptor tyrosine kinases-mediated signaling in the nervous system. Acta Histochem 110: 155–162.

Gu X, Thomas PK, King RHM (1995) Chemotropism in nerve regeneration studied in tissue culture. J Anat 186: 153–163.

Guertin AD, Zhang DP, Mak KS, Alberta JA, Kim HA (2005) Microanatomy of axon/glial signaling during Wallerian degeneration. J Neurosci 25: 3478–3487.

Guha U, Gomes WA, Samanta J, Gupta M, Rice FL, Kessler JA (2004) Target-derived BMP signaling limits sensory neuron number and the extent of peripheral innervation in vivo. Development 131: 1175–1186.

Gulati AK (1996) Peripheral nerve regeneration through short- and long-term degenerated nerve transplants. Brain Res 742: 265–270.

Gunderson RW, Barrett JN (1979) Neuronal chemotaxis: chick dorsal root axons turn toward high concentrations of nerve growth factor. Science 206: 1079–1080.

Guntinas-Lichius O, Effenberger K, Angelov DN, Klein J, Streppel M, Stennert E, Neiss WF (2000) Delayed rat facial nerve repair leads to accelerated and enhanced muscle reinnervation with reduced collateral axonal sprouting during a definite denervation period using a cross-anastomosis paradigm. Exp Neurol 162: 98–111.

Guntinas-Lichius O, Angelov DN, Morellini F, Lenzen M, Skouras E, Schachner M, Irintchev A (2005) Opposite impacts of tenascin-C and tenascin-R deficiency in mice on the functional outcome of facial nerve repair. Eur J Neurosci 22: 2171–2179.

Guseva D, Angelov DN, Irintchev A, Schachner M (2009) Ablation of adhesion molecule L1 in mice favours Schwann cell proliferation and functional recovery after peripheral nerve injury. Brain 132: 2180–2195.

Guth L (1956) Regeneration in the mammalian peripheral nervous system. Physiol Rev 36: 441–478.

Gutmann E, Sanders FK (1943) Recovery of fiber numbers and diameters in the regeneration of peripheral nerves. J Physiol 101: 489–518.

Gutmann E, Young JZ (1944) The re-innervation of muscle after various periods of atrophy. J Anat 78: 15–43.

Gutmann E, Guttman L, Medawar PB, Young JZ (1942) The rate of regeneration of nerve. J Exp Biol 19: 14–44.

Haase G, Dessaud E, Garcäs A, De Bovis B, Birling MC, Filippi P, Schmalbruch H, Arber S, DeLapeyriäre O (2002) GDNF acts through PEA3 to regulate cell body positioning and muscle innervation of specific motor neuron pools. Neuron 35: 893–905.

Haastert K, Lipokatic E, Fischer M, Timmer M, Grothe C (2006) Differentially promoted peripheral nerve regeneration by grafted Schwann cells over-expressing different FGF-2 isoforms. Neurobiol Dis 21: 138–153.

Haastert K, Grosheva M, Angelova SK, Guntinas-Lichius O, Skouras E, Michael J, Grothe C, Dunlop SA, Angelov DN (2009) Schwann cells overexpressing FGF-2 alone or combined with manual stimulation do not promote functional recovery after facial nerve injury. J Biomed Biotechnol 2009: 408794.

Hack CE, Wolbink GJ, Schalkwijk C, Speijer H, Hermens WT, van den Bosch H (1997) A role for secretory phospholipase A2 and C-reactive protein in the removal of injured cells. Immunol Today 18: 111–115.

Haftek J, Thomas PK (1968) Electron-microscope observations on the effects of localized crush injuries on the connective tissue of peripheral nerve. J Anat 103: 233–243.

Haggiag S, Zhang P, Slutzky G, Kumar A, Chebath J, Revel M (2001) Stimulation of myelin gene expression in vitro and of sciatic nerve remyelination by interleukin-6 receptor-interleukin-6 chimera. J Neurosci Res 64: 564–574.

Hall SM (1986) The effect of inhibiting Schwann cell mitosis on the reinnervation of acellular autografts in the peripheral nervous system of the mouse. Neuropathol Appl Neurobiol 12: 401–414.

Hall SM, Gregson NA (1971) The in vivo and ultrastructural effects of injection of lysophosphatidyl choline into myelinated peripheral nerve fibres of the adult mouse. J Cell Sci 9: 769–789.

Hall SM (2001) Nerve repair: a neurobiologist's view. J Hand Surg [Br Eur] 26: 129–136.

Hallbook F, Ibanez CF, Persson H (1991) Evolutionary studies of the nerve growth factor family reveal a novel member abundantly expressed in Xenopus ovary. Neuron 6: 845–858.

Hammarberg H, Piehl F, Cullheim S, Fjell J, Hokfelt T, Fried K (1996) GDNF mRNA in Schwann cells and DRG satellite cells after chronic sciatic nerve injury. Neuroreport 7: 857–860.

Hammarberg H, Risling M, Hokfelt T, Cullheim S, Piehl F (1998) Expression of insulin-like growth factors and corresponding binding proteins (IGFBP 1-6) in rat spinal cord and peripheral nerve after axonal injuries. J Comp Neurol 400: 57–72.

Hammarberg H, Piehl F, Risling M, Cullheim S (2000a) Differential regulation of trophic factor receptor mRNAs in spinal motoneurons after sciatic nerve transection and ventral root avulsion in the rat. J Comp Neurol 426: 587–601.

Hammarberg H, Wallquist W, Piehl F, Risling M, Cullheim S (2000b) Regulation of laminin-associated integrin subunit mRNAs in rat spinal motoneurons during postnatal development and after axonal injury. J Comp Neurol 428: 294–304.

Han PJ, Shukla S, Subramanian PS, Hoffman PN (2004) Cyclic AMP elevates tubulin expression without increasing intrinsic axon growth capacity. Exp Neurol 189: 293–302.

Hanna-Mitchell AT, O'Leary D, Mobarak MS, Ramer MS, McMahon SB, Priestley JV, Kozlova EN, Aldskogius H, Dockery P, Fraher JP (2008) The impact of neurotrophin-3 on the dorsal root transitional zone following injury. Spinal Cord 46: 804–810.

Hannila SS, Filbin MT (2008) The role of cyclic AMP signaling in promoting axonal regeneration after spinal cord injury. Exp Neurol 209: 321–332.

Hansson HA, Dahlin LB, Danielsen N, Fryklund L, Nachemson AK, Polleryd P, Rozell B, Skottner A, Stemme S, Lundborg G (1986) Evidence indicating trophic importance of IGF-I in regenerating peripheral nerves. Acta Physiol Scand 126: 609–614.

Hanz S, Perlson E, Willis D, Zheng JQ, Massarwa R, Huerta JJ, Koltzenburg M, Kohler M, van-Minnen J, Twiss JL, Fainzilber M (2003) Axoplasmic importins enable retrograde injury signaling in lesioned nerve. Neuron 40: 1095–1104.

Hanz S, Fainzilber M (2006) Retrograde signaling in injured nerve: the axon reaction revisited. J Neurochem 99: 13–19.

Hasan NA, Neumann MM, De Souky MA, So KF, Bedi KS (1996) The influence of predegenerated nerve grafts on axonal regeneration from prelesioned peripheral nerves. J Anat 189: 293–302.

Hassan S, Kerkhoff H, Troost D, Veldman H, Jennekens F (1994) Basic fibroblast growth factor immunoreactivity in the peripheral motor system of the rat. Acta Neuropathol.(Berl.) 87: 405–410.

Hashimoto N, Yamanaka H, Fukuoka T, Obata K, Mashimo T, Noguchi K (2001a) Expression of hepatocyte growth factor in primary sensory neurons of adult rats. Brain Res Mol Brain Res 97: 83–88.

Hashimoto N, Yamanaka H, Fukuoka T, Dai Y, Obata K, Mashimo T, Noguchi K (2001b) Expression of HGF and cMet in the peripheral nervous system of adult rats following sciatic nerve injury. Neuroreport 12: 1403–1407.

Hawkes C, Kar S (2002) Insulin-like growth factor-II/mannose-6-phosphate receptor in the spinal cord and dorsal root ganglia of the adult rat. Eur J Neurosci 15: 33–39.

Hawkes C, Kar S (2003) Insulin-like growth factor-II/mannose-6-phosphate receptor: widespread distribution in neurons of the central nervous system including those expressing cholinergic phenotype. J Comp Neurol 458: 113–127.

Hayashi H, Ichihara M, Iwashita T, Murakami H, Shimono Y, Kawai K, Kurokawa K, Murakumo Y, Imai T, Funahashi H, Nakao A, Takahashi M (2000) Characterization of intracellular signals via tyrosine 1062 in RET activated by glial cell line-derived neurotrophic factor. Oncogene 19: 4469–4475.

Hayashi Y, Kawazoe Y, Sakamoto T, Ojima M, Wang W, Takazawa T, Miyazawa D, Ohya W, Funakoshi H, Nakamura T, Watabe K (2006) Adenoviral gene transfer of hepatocyte growth factor prevents death of injured adult motoneurons after peripheral nerve avulsion. Brain Res 1111: 187–195.

Heasman SJ, Ridley AJ (2008) Mammalian Rho GTPases: new insights into their functions from in vivo studies. Nat Rev Mol Cell Biol 9: 690–701.

Heidemann SR, Lamoureux P, Buxbaum RE (1990) Growth cone behavior and production of traction force. J Cell Biol 111: 1949–1957.

Heinrich PC, Behrmann I, Haan S, Hermanns HM, Muller-Newen G, Schaper F (2003) Principles of interleukin (IL)-6-type cytokine signalling and its regulation. Biochem J 374: 1–20.

Heldin CH, Miyazono K, ten Dijke P (1997) TGF-beta signalling from cell membrane to nucleus through SMAD proteins. Nature 390: 465–471.

Hempstead BL (2006) Dissecting the diverse actions of pro- and mature neurotrophins. Curr Alzheimer Res 3: 19–24.

Herdegen T, Claret FX, Kallunki T, Martin-Villalba A, Winter C, Hunter T, Karin M (1998) Lasting N-terminal phosphorylation of c-Jun and activation of c-Jun N-terminal kinases after neuronal injury. J Neurosci 18: 5124–5135.

Heumann R, Korsching S, Bandtlow C, Thoenen H (1987a) Changes of nerve growth factor synthesis in nonneuronal cells in response to sciatic nerve transection. J Cell Biol 104: 1623–1631.

Heumann R, Lindholm D, Bandtlow C, Meyer M, Radeke MJ, Misko TP, Shooter E, Thoenen H (1987b) Differential regulation of mRNA encoding nerve growth factor and its receptor in rat sciatic nerve during development, degeneration, and regeneration: role of macrophages. PNAS 84: 8735–8739.

Hirata A, Masaki T, Motoyoshi K, Kamakura K (2002) Intrathecal administration of nerve growth factor delays GAP 43 expression and early phase regeneration of adult rat peripheral nerve. Brain Res 944: 146–156.

Hirota H, Kiyama H, Kishimoto T, Taga T (1996) Accelerated nerve regeneration in mice by upregulated expression of interleukin (IL) 6 and IL-6 receptor after trauma. J Exp Med 183: 2627–2634.

Hobson MI, Green CJ, Terenghi G (2000) VEGF enhances intraneural angiogenesis and improves nerve regeneration after axotomy. J Anat 197: 591–605.

Hodge LK, Klassen MP, Han BX, Yiu G, Hurrell J, Howell A, Rousseau G, Lemaigre F, Tessier-Lavigne M, Wang F (2007) Retrograde BMP signaling regulates trigeminal sensory neuron identities and the formation of precise face maps. Neuron 55: 572–586.

Hoffman PN, Lasek RJ (1980) Axonal transport of the cytoskeleton in regenerating motor neurons: constancy and change. Brain Res 202: 317–333.

Hohn A, Leibrock J, Bailey K, Barde YA (1990) Identification and characterization of a novel member of the nerve growth factor/brain-derived neurotrophic factor family. Nature 344: 339–341.

Hoke A, Cheng C, Zochodne W (2000) Expression of glial cell line-derived neurotrophic factor family of growth factors in peripheral nerve injury in rats. Neuroreport 11: 1651–1654.

Hoke A, Sun HS, Gordon T, Zochodne DW (2001) Do denervated peripheral nerve trunks become ischemic? The impact of chronic denervation on vasa nervorum. Exp Neurol 172: 398–406.

Hoke A, Gordon T, Zochodne DW, Sulaiman OAR (2002) A decline in glial cell-line-derived neurotrophic factor expression is associated with impaired regeneration after long-term Schwann cell denervation. Exp Neurol 173: 77–85.

Hoke A, Ho T, Crawford TO, LeBel C, Hilt D, Griffin JW (2003) Glial cell line-derived neurotrophic factor alters axon Schwann cell units and promotes myelination in unmyelinated nerve fibers. J Neurosci 23: 561–567.

Hoke A, Redett R, Hameed H, Jari R, Li JB, Griffin JW, Brushart TM (2006) Schwann cells express motor and sensory phenotypes that regulate axon regeneration. J Neurosci 26: 9646–9655.

Holmes FE, Mahoney SA, Wynick D (2005) Use of genetically engineered transgenic mice to investigate the role of galanin in the peripheral nervous system after injury. Neuropeptides 39: 191–199.

Holmes W, Young JZ (1942) Nerve regeneration after immediate and delayed suture. J Anat 77: 63–106.

Holmquist B, Kanje M, Kerns J, Danielsen N (1993) A mathematical model for regeneration rate and initial delay following surgical repair of peripheral nerves. J Neurosci Methods 48: 27–33.

Hong K, Hinck L, Nishiyama M, Poo MM, Tessier-Lavigne M, Stein E (1999) A ligand-gated association between cytoplasmic domains of UNC5 and DCC family receptors converts netrin-induced growth cone attraction to repulsion. Cell 97: 927–941.

Hong K, Nishiyama M (2009) From guidance signals to movement: signaling molecules governing growth cone turning. Neuroscientist 16: 65–78.

Hontanilla B, Auba C, Gorria O (2007) Nerve regeneration through nerve autografts after local administration of brain-derived neurotrophic factor with osmotic pumps. Neurosurgery 61: 1268–1274; discussion 1274–1265.

Horch KW, Lisney SJW (1981) On the number and nature of regenerating myelinated axons after lesions of cutaneous nerves in the cat. J Physiol 313: 275–286.

Horie H, Inagaki Y, Sohma Y, Nozawa R, Okawa K, Hasegawa M, Muramatsu N, Kawano H, Horie M, Koyama H, Sakai I, Takeshita K, Kowada Y, Takano M, Kadoya T (1999) Galectin-1 regulates initial axonal growth in peripheral nerves after axotomy. J Neurosci 19: 9964–9974.

Horie H, Kadoya T, Hikawa N, Sango K, Inoue H, Takeshita K, Asawa R, Hiroi T, Sato M, Yoshioka T, Ishikawa Y (2004) Oxidized galectin-1 stimulates macrophages to promote axonal regeneration in peripheral nerves after axotomy. J Neurosci 24: 1873–1880.

Horie H, Kadoya T, Sango K, Hasegawa M (2005) Oxidized galectin-1 is an essential factor for peripheral nerve regeneration. Curr Drug Targets 6: 385–394.

Hu X, Cai J, Yang J, Smith GM (2010) Sensory axon targeting is increased by NGF gene therapy within the lesioned adult femoral nerve. Exp Neurol 223(1): 153–165.

Huber AB, Kania A, Tran TS, Gu CH, Garcia ND, Lieberam I, Johnson D, Jessell TM, Ginty DD, Kolodkin AL (2005) Distinct roles for secreted semaphorin signaling in spinal motor axon guidance. Neuron 48: 949–964.

Hudson AR, Morris J, Weddell G, Drury A (1972) Peripheral nerve autografts. J Surg Res 12: 267–274.

Huse M, Muir TW, Xu L, Chen YG, Kuriyan J, Massague J (2001) The TGF beta receptor activation process: an inhibitor- to substrate-binding switch. Mol Cell 8: 671–682.

Hynes MA, Gitt M, Barondes SH, Jessell TM, Buck LB (1990) Selective expression of an endogenous lactose-binding lectin gene in subsets of central and peripheral neurons. J Neurosci 10: 1004–1013.

Ide C, Tohyama K, Yokota R, Nitatori T, Onodepa H (1983) Schwann cell basal lamina and nerve regeneration. Brain Res 288: 61–65.

Inserra MM, Yao M, Murray R, Terris DJ (2000) Peripheral nerve regeneration in interleukin 6-deficient mice. Arch Otolaryngol Head Neck Surg 126: 1112–1116.

Irintchev A, Simova O, Eberhardt KA, Morellini F, Schachner M (2005) Impacts of lesion severity and tyrosine kinase receptor B deficiency on functional outcome of femoral nerve injury assessed by a novel single-frame motion analysis in mice. Eur J Neurosci 22: 802–808.

Ishii DN (1989) Relationship of insulin-like growth factor ii gene expression in muscle to synaptogenesis. PNAS 86: 2898–2902.

Islamov RR, Chintalgattu V, Pak ES, Katwa LC, Murashov AK (2004) Induction of VEGF and its Flt-1 receptor after sciatic nerve crush injury. Neuroreport 15: 2117–2121.

Jacob JM, McQuarrie IG (1993) Acceleration of axonal outgrowth in rat sciatic nerve at one week after axotomy. J Neurobiol 24: 356–367.

Jacob JM, Croes SA (1998) Acceleration of axonal outgrowth in motor axons from mature and old F344 rats after a conditioning lesion. Exp Neurol 152: 231–237.

Jaffe AB, Hall A (2005) Rho GTPases: biochemistry and biology. Annu Rev Cell Dev Biol 21: 247–269.

Jakobsson L, Kreuger J, Holmborn K, Lundin L, Eriksson I, Kjellen L, Claesson-Welsh L (2006) Heparan sulfate in trans potentiates VEGFR-mediated angiogenesis. Dev Cell 10: 625–634.

Jankowski MP, Cornuet PK, McIlwrath S, Koerber HR, Albers KM (2006) SRY-box containing gene 11 (Sox11) transcription factor is required for neuron survival and neurite growth. Neuroscience 143: 501–514.

Jankowski MP, McIlwrath SL, Jing X, Cornuet PK, Salerno KM, Koerber HR, Albers KM (2009) Sox11 transcription factor modulates peripheral nerve regeneration in adult mice. Brain Res 1256: 43–54.

Jenq CB, Coggeshall RE (1984) Regeneration of axons in tributary nerves. Brain Res 310: 107–121.

Jessen KR, Mirsky R (2005) The origin and development of glial cells in peripheral nerves. Nat Rev Neurosci 6: 671–682.

Ji RR, Zhang Q, Zhang X, Piehl F, Reilly T, Pettersson RF, Hökfelt T (1995) Prominent expression of bFGF in dorsal root ganglia after axotomy. Eur J Neurosci 7: 2458–2468.

Johnson H, Hökfelt T, Ulfhake B (1996) Decreased expression of TrkB and TrkC mRNAs in spinal motoneurons of aged rats. Eur J Neurosci 8: 494–499.

Jones CA, London NR, Chen H, Park KW, Sauvaget D, Stockton RA, Wythe JD, Suh W, Larrieu-Lahargue F, Mukouyama YS, Lindblom P, Seth P, Frias A, Nishiya N, Ginsberg MH, Gerhardt H, Zhang K, Li DY (2008) Robo4 stabilizes the vascular network by inhibiting pathologic angiogenesis and endothelial hyperpermeability. Nat Med 14: 448–453.

Jones DM, Tucker BA, Rahimtula M, Mearow KM (2003) The synergistic effects of NGF and IGF-1 on neurite growth in adult sensory neurons: convergence on the PI 3-kinase signaling pathway. J Neurochem 86: 1116–1128.

Jones SL, Selzer ME, Gallo G (2006) Developmental regulation of sensory axon regeneration in the absence of growth cones. J Neurobiol 66: 1630–1645.

Jongen JL, Jaarsma D, Hossaini M, Natarajan D, Haasdijk ED, Holstege JC (2007) Distribution of RET immunoreactivity in the rodent spinal cord and changes after nerve injury. J Comp Neurol 500: 1136–1153.

Jubran M, Widenfalk J (2003) Repair of peripheral nerve transections with fibrin sealant containing neurotrophic factors. Exp Neurol 181: 204–212.

Jungnickel J, Haase K, Konitzer J, Timmer M, Grothe C (2006) Faster nerve regeneration after sciatic nerve injury in mice over-expressing basic fibroblast growth factor. J Neurobiol 66: 940–948.

Jungnickel J, Bramer C, Bronzlik P, Lipokatic-Takacs E, Weinhold B, Gerardy-Schahn R, Grothe C (2009) Level and localization of polysialic acid is critical for early peripheral nerve regeneration. Mol Cell Neurosci 40: 374–381.

Jungnickel J, Haastert K, Grzybek M, Thau N, Lipokatic-Takacs E, Ratzka A, Nolle A, Claus P, Grothe C (2010) Mice lacking basic fibroblast growth factor showed faster sensory recovery. Exp Neurol 223: 166–172.

Kang Q, Sun MH, Cheng H, Peng Y, Montag AG, Deyrup AT, Jiang W, Luu HH, Luo J, Szatkowski JP, Vanichakarn P, Park JY, Li Y, Haydon RC, He TC (2004) Characterization of the distinct orthotopic bone-forming activity of 14 BMPs using recombinant adenovirus-mediated gene delivery. Gene Ther 11: 1312–1320.

Kanje M, Lundborg G, Edstrom A (1988) A new method for studies of the effects of locally applied drugs on peripheral nerve regeneration in vivo. Brain Res 439: 116–121.

Kanje M, Skottner A, Sjoberg J, Lundborg G (1989) Insulin-like growth factor I (IGF-I) Stimulates regeneration of the rat sciatic nerve. Brain Res 486: 396–398.

Karanth S, Yang G, Yeh J, Richardson PM (2006) Nature of signals that initiate the immune response during Wallerian degeneration of peripheral nerves. Exp Neurol 202: 161–166.

Karchewski LA, Kim FA, Johnston J, McKnight RM, Verge VMK (1999) Anatomical evidence supporting the potential for modulation by multiple neurotrophins in the majority of adult lumbar sensory neurons. J Comp Neurol 413: 327–341.

Karchewski LA, Gratto KA, Wetmore C, Verge VMK (2002) Dynamic patterns of BDNF expression in injured sensory neurons: differential modulation by NGF and NT-3. Eur J Neurosci 16: 1449–1462.

Kato N, Nemoto K, Nakanishi K, Morishita R, Kaneda Y, Uenoyama M, Ikeda T, Fujikawa K (2005) Nonviral HVJ (hemagglutinating virus of Japan) liposome-mediated retrograde gene transfer of human hepatocyte growth factor into rat nervous system promotes functional and histological recovery of the crushed nerve. Neurosci Res 52: 299–310.

Kauffmann-Zeh A, Rodriguez-Viciana P, Ulrich E, Gilbert C, Coffer P, Downward J, Evan G (1997) Suppression of c-Myc-induced apoptosis by Ras signalling through PI(3)K and PKB. Nature 385: 544–548.

Keino-Masu K, Masu M, Hinck L, Leonardo ED, Chan SS, Culotti JG, Tessier-Lavigne M (1996) Deleted in colorectal cancer (DCC) encodes a netrin receptor. Cell 87: 175–185.

Kelleher MO, Myles LM, Al-Abri RK, Glasby MA (2006) The use of ciliary neurotrophic factor to promote recovery after peripheral nerve injury by delivering it at the site of the cell body. Acta Neurochir 148: 55–61.

Kenney AM, Kocsis JD (1998) Peripheral axotomy induces long-term c-Jun amino-terminal kinase-1 activation and activator protein-1 binding activity by c-Jun and junD in adult rat dorsal root ganglia in vivo. J Neurosci 18: 1318–1328.

Kerekes N, Landry M, Hokfelt T (1999) Leukemia inhibitory factor regulates galanin/galanin message-associated peptide expression in cultured mouse dorsal root ganglia; with a note on in situ hybridization methodology. Neuroscience 89: 1123–1134.

Kerns JM, Danielsen N, Holmquist B, Kanje M, Lundborg G (1993) The influence of predegeneration on regeneration through peripheral nerve grafts in the rat. Exp Neurol 122: 28–36.

Kerschensteiner M, Schwab ME, Lichtman JW, Misgeld T (2005) In vivo imaging of axonal degeneration and regeneration in the injured spinal cord. Nat Med 11: 572–577.

Kilvington B (1912) An investigation on the regeneration of nerves, with regard to the surgical treatment of certain paralyses. Brit Med J I: 177–179.

Kim HA, Pomeroy SL, Whoriskey W, Pawlitzky I, Benowitz LI, Sicinski P, Stiles CD, Roberts TM (2000) A developmentally regulated switch directs regenerative growth of Schwann cells through cyclin D1. Neuron 26: 405–416.

Kimpinski K, Mearow K (2001) Neurite growth promotion by nerve growth factor and insulin-like growth factor-1 in cultured adult sensory neurons: role of phosphoinositide 3-kinase and mitogen activated protein kinase. J Neurosci Res 63: 486–499.

Kimpinski K, Campenot RB, Mearow K (1997) Effects of the neurotrophins nerve growth factor, neurotrophin-3, and brain-derived neurotrophic factor (BDNF) on neurite growth from adult sensory neurons in compartmented cultures. J Neurobiol 33: 395–410.

Kimpinski K, Jelinski S, Mearow K (1999) The anti-p75 antibody, MC192, and brain-derived neurotrophic factor inhibit nerve growth factor-dependent neurite growth from adult sensory neurons. Neuroscience 93: 253–263.

Kingham PJ, Hughes A, Mitchard L, Burt R, Murison P, Jones A, Terenghi G, Birchall MA (2007) Effect of neurotrophin-3 on reinnervation of the larynx using the phrenic nerve transfer technique. Eur J Neurosci 25: 331–340.

Kirsch M, Terheggen U, Hofmann HD (2003) Ciliary neurotrophic factor is an early lesion-induced retrograde signal for axotomized facial motoneurons. Mol Cell Neurosci 24: 130–138.

Kishino A, Ishige Y, Tatsuno T, Nakayama C, Noguchi H (1997) BDNF prevents and reverses adult rat motor neuron degeneration and induces axonal outgrowth. Exp Neurol 144: 273–286.

Klimaschewski L, Nindl W, Feurle J, Kavakebi P, Kostron H (2004) Basic fibroblast growth factor isoforms promote axonal elongation and branching of adult sensory neurons in vitro. Neuroscience 126: 347–353.

Kline DG, Hudson AR, Lassmann H (1981) Experimental study of fascicular nerve repair with and without epineurial closure. J Neurosurg 54: 513–520.

Kobayashi NR, Bedard AM, Hincke MT, Tetzlaff W (1996) Increased expression of BDNF and TrkB mRNA in rat facial motoneurons after axotomy. Eur J Neurosci 8: 1018–1029.

Koenig E, Martin R, Titmus M, Sotelo-Silveira JR (2000) Cryptic peripheral ribosomal domains distributed intermittently along mammalian myelinated axons. J Neurosci 20: 8390–8400.

Koenig HL, Schumacher M, Ferzaz B, Thi AN, Ressouches A, Guennoun R, Jung-Testas I, Robel P, Akwa Y, Baulieu EE (1995) Progesterone synthesis and myelin formation by Schwann cells. Science 268: 1500–1503.

Koh CG (2006) Rho GTPases and their regulators in neuronal functions and development. Neurosignals 15: 228–237.

Kohmura E, Yuguchi T, Yoshimine T, Fujinaka T, Koseki N, Sano A, Kishino A, Nakayama C, Sakaki T, Nonaka M, Takemoto O, Hayakawa T (1999) BDNF atelocollagen mini-pellet accelerates facial nerve regeneration. Brain Res 849: 235–238.

Kolodkin AL, Levengood DV, Rowe EG, Tai YT, Giger RJ, Ginty DD (1997) Neuropilin is a semaphorin III receptor. Cell 90: 753–762.

Korsching S (1993) The neurotrophic factor concept: a reexamination. J Neurosci 13: 2739–2748.

Kotulska K, Larysz-Brysz M, Marcol W, Malinowska I, Matuszek I, Grajkowska W, Lewin-Kowalik J (2006) TrkB deficiency increases survival and regeneration of spinal motoneurons after axotomy in mice. Folia Neuropathol 44: 251–256.

Kovacic U, Sketelj J, Bajrovic FF (2009) Chapter 26: age-related differences in the reinnervation after peripheral nerve injury. Int Rev Neurobiol 87: 465–482.

Kramer ER, Knott L, Su F, Dessaud E, Krull CE, Helmbacher F, Klein R (2006) Cooperation between GDNF/Ret and ephrinA/EphA4 signals for motor-axon pathway selection in the limb. Neuron 50: 35–47.

Krekoski CA, Neubauer D, Zuo J, Muir D (2001) Axonal regeneration into acellular nerve grafts is enhanced by degradation of chondroitin sulfate proteoglycan. J Neurosci 21: 6206–6213.

Krieglstein K, Henheik P, Farkas L, Jaszai J, Galter D, Krohn K, Unsicker K (1998) Glial cell line-derived neurotrophic factor requires transforming growth factor-β for exerting its full neurotrophic potential on peripheral and CNS neurons. J Neurosci 18: 9822–9834.

Kuhlmann T, Bitsch A, Stadelmann C, Siebert H, Bruck W (2001) Macrophages are eliminated from the injured peripheral nerve via local apoptosis and circulation to regional lymph nodes and the spleen. J Neurosci 21: 3401–3408.

Kurokawa K, Nakamura T, Aoki K, Matsuda M (2005) Mechanism and role of localized activation of Rho-family GTPases in growth factor-stimulated fibroblasts and neuronal cells. Biochem Soc Trans 33: 631–634.

Kuruvilla R, Ye H, Ginty DD (2000) Spatially and functionally distinct roles of the PI3-K effector pathway during NGF signaling in sympathetic neurons. Neuron 27: 499–512.

Laird JMA, Mason GS, Thomas KA, Hargreaves RJ, Hill RG (1995) Acidic fibroblast growth factor stimulates motor and sensory axon regeneration after sciatic nerve crush in the rat. Neuroscience 65: 209–216.

Lang EM, Asan E, Plesnila N, Hofmann GO, Sendtner M (2005) Motoneuron survival after C7 nerve root avulsion and replantation in the adult rabbit: effects of local ciliary neurotrophic factor and brain-derived neurotrophic factor application. Plast Reconstr Surg 115: 2042–2050.

Lang EM, Schlegel N, Reiners K, Hofmann GO, Sendtner M, Asan E (2008) Single-dose application of CNTF and BDNF improves remyelination of regenerating nerve fibers after C7 ventral root avulsion and replantation. J Neurotrauma 25: 384–400.

Langley JN, Anderson HK (1904) The union of different kinds of nerve fibers. J Physiol 31: 365–391.

Lauber K, Bohn E, Krober SM, Xiao YJ, Blumenthal SG, Lindemann RK, Marini P, Wiedig C, Zobywalski A,

Baksh S, Xu Y, Autenrieth IB, Schulze-Osthoff K, Belka C, Stuhler G, Wesselborg S (2003) Apoptotic cells induce migration of phagocytes via caspase-3-mediated release of a lipid attraction signal. Cell 113: 717–730.

Leah JD, Herdegen T, Bravo R (1991) Selective expression of Jun proteins following axotomy and axonal transport block in peripheral nerves in the rat: evidence for a role in the regeneration process. Brain Res 566: 198–207.

LeBlanc AC, Poduslo JF (1990) Axonal modulation of myelin gene expression in the peripheral nerve. J Neurosci Res 26: 317–326.

Leclere P, Ekstrom P, Edstrom A, Priestley J, Averill S, Tonge DA (1998) Effects of glial cell line-derived neurotrophic factor on axonal growth and apoptosis in adult mammalian sensory neurons in vitro. Neuroscience 82: 545–558.

Lee AC, Yu VM, Lowe JB, III, Brenner MJ, Hunter DA, Mackinnon SE, Sakiyama-Elbert SE (2003) Controlled release of nerve growth factor enhances sciatic nerve regeneration. Exp Neurol 184: 295–303.

Lee AC, Suter DM (2008) Quantitative analysis of microtubule dynamics during adhesion-mediated growth cone guidance. Dev Neurobiol 68: 1363–1377.

Lee H, Jo EK, Choi SY, Oh SB, Park K, Kim JS, Lee SJ (2006) Necrotic neuronal cells induce inflammatory Schwann cell activation via TLR2 and TLR3: implication in Wallerian degeneration. Biochem Biophys Res Commun 350: 742–747.

Lee R, Kermani P, Teng KK, Hempstead BL (2001) Regulation of cell survival by secreted proneurotrophins. Science 294: 1945–1948.

Lefcort F, Venstrom K, McDonald JA, Reichardt LF (1992) Regulation of expression of fibronectin and its receptor, alpha 5 beta 1, during development and regeneration of peripheral nerve. Development 116: 767–782.

Leibrock J, Lottspeich F, Hohn A, Hofer M, Hengerer B, Masiakowski P, Thoenen H, Barde YA (1989) Molecular cloning and expression of brain-derived neurotrophic factor. Nature 341: 149–152.

Lemons ML, Barua S, Abanto ML, Halfter W, Condic ML (2005) Adaptation of sensory neurons to hyalectin and decorin proteoglycans. J Neurosci 25: 4964–4973.

Letourneau PC (1983) Differences in the organization of actin in the growth cones compared with the neurites of cultured neurons from chick embryos. J Cell Biol 97: 963–973.

Levi-Montalcini R, Hamburger V (1951) Selective growth stimulating effects of mouse sarcoma on the sensory and sympathetic nervous system of the chick embryo. J Exp Zool 116: 321–361.

Levi-Montalcini R, Booker B (1960) Destruction of the sympathetic ganglia in mammals by an antiserum to a nerve-growth protein. Proc Natl Acad Sci U S A 46: 384–391.

Levi-Montalcini R (1987) The nerve growth factor 35 years later. Science 237: 1154–1162.

Levy D, Hoke A, Zochodne DW (1999) Local expression of inducible nitric oxide synthase in an animal model of neuropathic pain. Neurosci Lett 260: 207–209.

Levy D, Kubes P, Zochodne DW (2001) Delayed peripheral nerve degeneration, regeneration, and pain in mice lacking inducible nitric oxide synthase. J Neuropathol Exp Neurol 60: 411–421.

Lewis ME, Neff NT, Contreras PC, Stong DB, Oppenheim RW, Grebow PE, Vaught JL (1993) Insulin-like growth factor-I: potential for treatment of motor neuronal disorders. Exp Neurol 124: 73–88.

Li H, Terenghi G, Hall SM (1997) Effects of delayed re-innervation on the expression of c-erbB receptors by chronically denervated rat Schwann cells in vivo. Glia 20: 333–347.

Li XQ, Gonias SL, Campana WM (2005) Schwann cells express erythropoietin receptor and represent a major target for Epo in peripheral nerve injury. Glia 51: 254–265.

Li YS, Milner PG, Chauhan K, Watson MA, Hoffman RM, Kodner CM, Millibrandt CM, Duel TF (1990) Cloning and expression of a developmentally regulated protein that induces mitogenic and neurite outgrowth activity. Science 250: 1690–1694.

Li Z, Peng J, Wang G, Yang Q, Yu H, Guo Q, Wang A, Zhao B, Lu S (2008) Effects of local release of hepatocyte growth factor on peripheral nerve regeneration in acellular nerve grafts. Exp Neurol 214: 47–54.

Lieberman AR (1971) The axon reaction: a review of the principal features of perikaryal responses to axon injury. Int Rev Neurobiol 14: 49–124.

Lin AC, Holt CE (2008) Function and regulation of local axonal translation. Curr Opin Neurobiol 18: 60–68.

Lindholm D, Heumann R, Meyer M, Thoenen H (1987) Interleukin-1 regulates synthesis of nerve growth factor in non-neuronal cells of rat sciatic nerve. Nature 330: 658–659.

Lindholm T, Skold MK, Suneson A, Carlstedt T, Cullheim S, Risling M (2004) Semaphorin and neuropilin expression in motoneurons after intraspinal motoneuron axotomy. Neuroreport 15: 649–654.

Lindsay RM (1988) Nerve growth factors (NGF, BDNF) enhance axonal regeneration but are not required for survival of adult sensory neurons. J Neurosci 8: 2394–2405.

Lindwall C, Dahlin L, Lundborg G, Kanje M (2004) Inhibition of c-Jun phosphorylation reduces axonal outgrowth of adult rat nodose ganglia and dorsal root ganglia sensory neurons. Mol Cell Neurosci 27: 267–279.

Liu J, Chau CH, Liu HY, Jang BR, Li XG, Chan YS, Shum DKY (2006) Upregulation of chondroitin 6-sulphotransferase-1 facilitates Schwann cell migration during axonal growth. J Cell Sci 119: 933–942.

Liu RY, Snider WD (2001) Different signaling pathways mediate regenerative versus developmental sensory axon growth. J Neurosci 21:RC164.

Liu WQ, Martinez JA, Durand J, Wildering W, Zochodne DW (2009) RGD-mediated adhesive interactions are important for peripheral axon outgrowth in vivo. Neurobiol Dis 34: 11–22.

Longo FM, Manthorpe M, Skaper SD, Lundborg G, Varon S (1983a) Neuronotrophic activities accumulate in vivo within silicone nerve regeneration chambers. Brain Res 261: 109–117.

Longo FM, Skaper SD, Manthorpe M, Williams LR, Lundborg G, Varon S (1983b) Temporal changes in neuronotrophic activities accumulating in vivo within nerve regeneration chambers. Exp Neurol 81: 756–769.

Lonze BE, Ginty DD (2002) Function and regulation of CREB family transcription factors in the nervous system. Neuron 35: 605–623.

Lowery LA, Van Vactor D (2009) The trip of the tip: understanding the growth cone machinery. Nat Rev Mol Cell Biol 10: 332–343.

Lu VB, Biggs JE, Stebbing MJ, Balasubramanyan S, Todd KG, Lai AY, Colmers WF, Dawbarn D, Ballanyi K, Smith PA (2009) Brain-derived neurotrophic factor drives the changes in excitatory synaptic transmission in the rat superficial dorsal horn that follow sciatic nerve injury. J Physiol 587: 1013–1032.

Lubinska L (1977) Early course of Wallerian degeneration in myelinated fibers of the rat phrenic nerve. Brain Res 130: 47–63.

Lundborg G, Hansson HH (1979) Regeneration of peripheral nerve through a preformed tissue space: preliminary observations on the reorganization of regenerating nerve fibers and perineurium Brain Res 178: 573–576.

Lundborg G, Dahlin L, Danielsen N, Hansson H, Larsson K (1981) Reorganization and orientation of regenerating nerve fibers, perineurium, and epineurium in preformed mesothelial tubes: an experimental study on the sciatic nerve of rats. J Neurosci Res 6: 265–281.

Lunn ER, Perry VH, Brown MC, Rosen H, Gordon S (1989) Absence of Wallerian degeneration does not hinder regeneration in peripheral nerve. Eur J Neurosci 1: 27–33.

Luo XG, Rush RA, Zhou XF (2001) Ultrastructural localization of brain-derived neurotrophic factor in rat primary sensory neurons. Neurosci Res 39: 377–384.

Lutz BS, Wei FC, Ma SF, Chuang DC (1999) Effects of insulin-like growth factor-1 in motor nerve regeneration after nerve transection and repair vs. nerve crushing injury in the rat. Acta Neurochir (Wien) 141: 1101–1106.

Lutz M, Knaus P (2002) Integration of the TGF-β pathway into the cellular signalling network. Cell Signal 14: 977–988.

Mack TGA, Reiner M, Beirowski B, Mi WQ, Emanuelli M, Wagner D, Thomson D, Gillingwater T, Court F, Conforti L, Fernando FS, Tarlton A, Andressen C, Addicks K, Magni G, Ribchester RR, Perry VH, Coleman MP (2001) Wallerian degeneration of injured axons and synapses is delayed by a Ube4b/Nmnat chimeric gene. Nat Neurosci 4: 1199–1206.

Mackinnon S, Dellon L, O'Brien J (1991) Changes in nerve fiber numbers distal to a nerve repair in the rat sciatic nerve model. Muscle & Nerve 14: 1116–1122.

Madaschi L, Di Giulio AM, Gorio A (2003) Muscle reinnervation and IGF-I synthesis are affected by exposure to heparin: an effect partially antagonized by anti-growth hormone-releasing hormone. Neurochem Res 28: 163–168.

Madison RD, Zomorodi A, Robinson GA (2000) Netrin-1 and peripheral nerve regeneration in the adult rat. Exp Neurol 161: 563–570.

Madorsky SJ, Swett JE, Crumley RL (1998) Motor versus sensory neuron regeneration through collagen tubules. Plast Reconstr Surg 102: 430–436; discussion 437–438.

Makranz C, Cohen G, Baron A, Levidor L, Kodama T, Reichert F, Rotshenker S (2004) Phosphatidylinositol 3-kinase, phosphoinositide-specific phospholipase-Cgamma and protein kinase-C signal myelin phagocytosis mediated by complement receptor-3 alone and combined with scavenger receptor-AI/II in macrophages. Neurobiol Dis 15: 279–286.

Makranz C, Cohen G, Reichert F, Kodama T, Rotshenker S (2006) cAMP cascade (PKA, Epac, adenylyl cyclase, Gi, and phosphodiesterases) regulates myelin phagocytosis mediated by complement receptor-3 and scavenger receptor-AI/II in microglia and macrophages. Glia 53: 441–448.

Mandolesi G, Madeddu F, Bozzi Y, Maffei L, Ratto GM (2004) Acute physiological response of mammalian central neurons to axotomy: ionic regulation and electrical activity. Faseb J 18: 1934–1936.

Maness PF, Schachner M (2007) Neural recognition molecules of the immunoglobulin superfamily: signaling transducers of axon guidance and neuronal migration. Nat Neurosci 10: 19–26.

Manthorpe M, Engvall E, Ruoslahti E, Longo FM, Davis GE, Varon S (1983) Laminin promotes neuritic regeneration from cultured peripheral and central neurons. J Cell Biol 97: 1882–1890.

Marble HC, Hamlin E, Watkins AL (1942) Regeneration in the ulnar, median and radial nerves. Am J Surg 55: 274–294.

Marcol W, Kotulska K, Swiech-Sabuda E, Larysz-Brysz M, Golka B, Górka D, Lewin-Kowalik J (2003) Regeneration of sciatic nerves of adult rats induced by extracts from distal stumps of pre-degenerated peripheral nerves. J Neurosci Res 72: 417–424.

Marte BM, Downward J (1997) PKB/Akt: connecting phosphoinositide 3-kinase to cell survival and beyond. Trends Biochem Sci 22: 355–358.

Martini R, Schachner M (1988) Immunoelectron microscopic localization of neural cell adhesion molecules (L1, N-CAM, and myelin-associated glycoprotein) in regenerating adult mouse sciatic nerve. J Cell Biol 106: 1735–1746.

Martini R, Schachner M, Faissner A (1990) Enhanced expression of the extracellular matrix molecule J1/tenascin in the regenerating adult mouse sciatic nerve. J Neurocytol 19: 601–616.

Martini R (1994) Expression and functional roles of neural cell surface molecules and extracellular matrix components during development and regeneration of peripheral nerves. J Neurocytol 23: 1–28.

Martini R, Fischer S, Lopez-Vales R, David S (2008) Interactions between Schwann cells and macrophages in injury and inherited demyelinating disease. Glia 56: 1566–1577.

Masaki T, Matsumura K, Saito F, Sunada Y, Shimizu T, Yorifuji H, Motoyoshi K, Kamakura K (2000) Expression of dystroglycan and laminin-2 in peripheral nerve under axonal degeneration and regeneration. Acta Neuropathol (Berl) 99: 289–295.

Mason CA, Wang LC (1997) Growth cone form is behavior-specific and, consequently, position-specific along the retinal axon pathway. J Neuroscience 17: 1086–1100.

Masuda T, Watanabe K, Sakuma C, Ikenaka K, Ono K, Yaginuma H (2008) Netrin-1 acts as a repulsive guidance cue for sensory axonal projections toward the spinal cord. J Neurosci 28: 10380–10385.

McDonald D, Cheng C, Chen Y, Zochodne D (2006) Early events of peripheral nerve regeneration. Neuron Glia Biol 2: 139–147.

McDonald DS, Cheng C, Martinez JA, Zochodne DW (2007) Regenerative arrest of inflamed peripheral nerves: role of nitric oxide. Neuroreport 18: 1635–1640.

McGraw J, McPhail LT, Oschipok LW, Horie H, Poirier F, Steeves JD, Ramer MS, Tetzlaff W (2004) Galectin-1 in regenerating motoneurons. Eur J Neurosci 20: 2872–2880.

McGraw J, Gaudet AD, Oschipok LW, Kadoya T, Horie H, Steeves JD, Tetzlaff W, Ramer MS (2005) Regulation of neuronal and glial galectin-1 expression by peripheral and central axotomy of rat primary afferent neurons. Exp Neurol 195: 103–114.

McKay Hart A, Wiberg M, Terenghi G (2003) Exogenous leukaemia inhibitory factor enhances nerve regeneration after late secondary repair using a bioartificial nerve conduit. Br J Plast Surg 56: 444–450.

McKerracher L, David S, Jackson DL, Kottis V, Dunn RJ, Braun PE (1994) Identification of myelin-associated glycoprotein as a major myelin-derived inhibitor of neurite growth. Neuron 13: 805–811.

McKerracher L, Chamoux M, Arregui CO (1996) Role of laminin and integrin interactions in growth cone guidance. Mol Neurobiol 12: 95–116.

McQuarrie IG, Grafstein B (1973) Axon outgrowth enhanced by a previous nerve injury. Arch Neurol 29: 53–55.

McQuarrie I, Grafstein B, Gershon M (1977) Axonal regeneration in the rat sciatic nerve: effect of a conditioning lesion and of dbcAMP. Brain Res 132: 442–453.

McQuarrie IG (1978) The effect of a conditioning lesion on the regeneration of motor axons. Brain Res 152: 597–602.

McQuarrie IG (1979) Accelerated axonal sprouting after nerve transection. Brain Res 167: 185–188.

McQuarrie IG (1985) Effect of a conditioning lesion on axonal sprout formation at nodes of Ranvier. J Comp Neurol 231: 239–230.

McQuarrie I, Jacob J (1991) Conditioning nerve crush accelerates cytoskeletal protein transport in sprouts that form after a subsequent crush. J Comp Neurol 305: 139–147.

Mears S, Schachner M, Brushart TM (2003) Antibodies to myelin-associated glycoprotein accelerate preferential motor reinnervation. JPNS 8: 91–99.

Medeiros NA, Burnette DT, Forscher P (2006) Myosin II functions in actin-bundle turnover in neuronal growth cones. Nat Cell Biol 8: 215–226.

Meeker ML, Farel PB (1993) Coincidence of Schwann cell-derived basal lamina development and loss of regenerative specificity of spinal motoneurons. J Comp Neurol 329: 257–268.

Mehanna A, Mishra B, Kurschat N, Schulze C, Bian S, Loers G, Irintchev A, Schachner M (2009) Polysialic acid glycomimetics promote myelination and functional recovery after peripheral nerve injury in mice. Brain 132: 1449–1462.

Mehta NR, Lopez PH, Vyas AA, Schnaar RL (2007) Gangliosides and Nogo receptors independently mediate myelin-associated glycoprotein inhibition of neurite outgrowth in different nerve cells. J Biol Chem 282: 27875–27886.

Meirer R, Gurunluoglu R, Siemionow M (2001) Neurogenic perspective on vascular endothelial growth factor: review of the literature. J Reconstr Microsurg 17: 625–630.

Meisinger C, Grothe C (1997) Differential regulation of FGF-2 and FGF receptor 1 mRNAs and FGF-2 isoforms in spinal ganglia and sciatic nerve after peripheral nerve lesion. J Neurochem 68: 1150–1158.

Melli G, Hoke A (2007) Canadian Association of Neurosciences review: regulation of myelination by trophic factors and neuron-glial signaling. Can J Neurol Sci 34: 288–295.

Menager C, Arimura N, Fukata Y, Kaibuchi K (2004) PIP3 is involved in neuronal polarization and axon formation. J Neurochem 89: 109–118.

Merianda TT, Lin AC, Lam JS, Vuppalanchi D, Willis DE, Karin N, Holt CE, Twiss JL (2009) A functional equivalent of endoplasmic reticulum and Golgi in axons for secretion of locally synthesized proteins. Mol Cell Neurosci 40: 128–142.

Messersmith EK, Leonardo ED, Shatz CJ, Tessier-Lavigne M, Goodman CS, Kolodkin AL (1995) Semaphorin III can function as a selective chemorepellent to pattern sensory projections in the spinal cord. Neuron 14: 949–959.

Meyer M, Matsuoka I, Wetmore C, Olson L, Thoenen H (1992) Enhanced synthesis of brain-derived neurotrophic factor in the lesioned peripheral nerve: different mechanisms are responsible for the regulation of BDNF and NGF mRNA. J Cell Biol 119: 45–54.

Mi R, Chen W, Hoke A (2007) Pleitrophin is a neurotrophic factor for spinal motor neurons. PNAS 104: 4664–4669.

Miao T, Wu D, Zhang Y, Bo X, Subang MC, Wang P, Richardson PM (2006) Suppressor of cytokine signaling-3 suppresses the ability of activated signal transducer and activator of transcription-3 to stimulate neurite growth in rat primary sensory neurons. J Neurosci 26: 9512–9519.

Michael GJ, Averill S, Nitkunan A, Rattray M, Bennett DL, Yan Q, Priestley JV (1997) Nerve growth factor treatment increases brain-derived neurotrophic factor selectively in TrkA-expressing dorsal root ganglion cells and in their central terminations within the spinal cord. J.Neurosci. 17: 8476–8490.

Michael GJ, Averill S, Shortland PJ, Yan Q, Priestley JV (1999) Axotomy results in major changes in BDNF expression by dorsal root ganglion cells: BDNF expression in large TrkB and TrkC cells, in pericellular baskets, and in projections to deep dorsal horn and dorsal column nuclei. Eur J Neurosci 11: 3539–3551.

Michalski B, Bain JR, Fahnestock M (2008) Long-term changes in neurotrophic factor expression in distal nerve stump following denervation and reinnervation with motor or sensory nerve. J Neurochem 105: 1244–1252.

Midha R, Munro CA, Dalton PD, Tator CH, Shoichet MS (2003) Growth factor enhancement of peripheral nerve regeneration through a novel synthetic hydrogel tube. J Neurosurg 99: 555–565.

Miledi R, Slater CR (1970) On the degeneration of rat neuromuscular junctions after nerve section. J Physiol (Lond) 207: 507–528.

Miller KE, Samuels DC (1997) The axon as a metabolic compartment: protein degradation, transport, and maximum length of an axon. J Theor Biol 186: 373–379.

Mills CD, Allchorne AJ, Griffin RS, Woolf CJ, Costigan M (2007) GDNF selectively promotes regeneration of injury-primed sensory neurons in the lesioned spinal cord. Mol Cell Neurosci 36: 185–194.

Mirsky R, Woodhoo A, Parkinson DB, Arthur-Farraj P, Bhaskaran A, Jessen KR (2008) Novel signals controlling embryonic Schwann cell development, myelination and dedifferentiation. J Peripher Nerv Syst 13: 122–135.

Mitchison T, Kirschner M (1988) Cytoskeletal dynamics and nerve growth. Neuron 1: 761–772.

Mograbi B, Bocciardi R, Bourget I, Busca R, Rochet N, Farahi-Far D, Juhel T, Rossi B (2001)

Glial cell line-derived neurotrophic factor-stimulated phosphatidylinositol 3-kinase and Akt activities exert opposing effects on the ERK pathway: importance for the rescue of neuroecodermic cells. J Biol Chem 276: 45307–45319.

Mohiuddin L, Delcroix JD, Fernyhough P, Tomlinson DR (1999) Focally administered nerve growth factor suppresses molecular regenerative responses of axotomized peripheral afferents in rats. Neuroscience 91: 265–271.

Moises T, Dreier A, Flohr S, Esser M, Brauers E, Reiss K, Merken D, Weis J, Kruttgen A (2007) Tracking TrkA's trafficking: NGF receptor trafficking controls NGF receptor signaling. Mol Neurobiol 35: 151–159.

Moldovan M, Sorensen J, Krarup C (2006) Comparison of the fastest regenerating motor and sensory myelinated axons in the same peripheral nerve. Brain 129: 2471–2483.

Monaco S, Gehrmann J, Raivich G, Kreutzberg GW (1992) MHC-positive, ramified macrophages in the normal and injured rat peripheral nervous system. J Neurocytol 21: 623–634.

Morgan L, Jessen KR, Mirsky R (1994) Negative regulation of the P0 gene in Schwann cells: suppression of P0 mRNA and protein induction in cultured Schwann cells by FGF2 and TGF beta 1, TGF beta 2 and TGF beta 3. Development 120: 1399–1409.

Morgenstern DA, Asher RA, Naidu M, Carlstedt T, Levine JM, Fawcett JW (2003) Expression and glycanation of the NG2 proteoglycan in developing, adult, and damaged peripheral nerve. Mol Cell Neurosci 24: 787–802.

Morris JH, Hudson AR, Weddell G (1972a) A study of degeneration and regeneration in the divided rat sciatic nerve based on electron microscopy. IV. Changes in fascicular microtopography, perineurium and endoneurial fibroblasts. Z Zellforsch Mikrosk Anat 124: 165–203.

Morris JH, Hudson AR, Weddell G (1972b) A study of degeneration and regeneration in the divided rat sciatic nerve based on electron microscopy. III. Changes in the axons of the proximal stump. Z Zellforsch Mikrosk Anat 124: 131–164.

Morris JH, Hudson AR, Weddell G (1972c) A study of degeneration and regeneration in the divided rat sciatic nerve based on electron microscopy. II. The development of the "regenerating unit." Z Zellforsch Mikrosk Anat 124: 103–130.

Morris JH, Hudson AR, Weddell G (1972d) A study of degeneration and regeneration in the divided rat sciatic nerve based on electron microscopy. I. The traumatic degeneration of myelin in the proximal stump of the divided nerve. Z Zellforsch Mikrosk Anat 124: 76–102.

Mosahebi A, Wiberg M, Terenghi G (2003) Addition of fibronectin to alginate matrix improves peripheral nerve regeneration in tissue-engineered conduits. Tissue Eng 9: 209–218.

Moscoso LM, Cremer H, Sanes JR (1998) Organization and reorganization of neuromuscular junctions in mice lacking neural cell adhesion molecule, tenascin-C, or fibroblast growth factor-5. J Neurosci 18: 1465–1477.

Mueller M, Leonhard C, Wacker K, Ringelstein EB, Okabe M, Hickey WF, Kiefer R (2003) Macrophage response to peripheral nerve injury: the quantitative contribution of resident and hematogenous macrophages. Lab Invest 83: 175–185.

Muir D (2010) The potentiation of peripheral nerve sheaths in regeneration and repair. Exp Neurol 223: 102–111.

Mukhopadhyay G, Doherty P, Walsh FS, Crocker PR, Filbin MT (1994) A novel role for myelin-associated glycoprotein as an inhibitor of axonal regeneration. Neuron 13: 757–767.

Murphy PG, Borthwick LA, Altares M, Gauldie J, Kaplan D, Richardson PM (2000) Reciprocal actions of interleukin-6 and brain-derived neurotrophic factor on rat and mouse primary sensory neurons. Eur J Neurosci 12: 1891–1899.

Nachemson AK, Lundborg G, Myrhage R, Rank F (1985) Nerve regeneration and pharmacological suppression of the scar reaction at the suture site. An experimental study on the effect of estrogen-progesterone, methylprednisolone-acetate and cis-hydroxyproline in rat sciatic nerve. Scand J Plast Reconstr Surg 19: 255–260.

Nakao Y, Otani H, Yamamura T, Hattori R, Osako M, Imamura H (2001) Insulin-like growth factor 1 prevents neuronal cell death and paraplegia in the rabbit model of spinal cord ischemia. J Thorac Cardiovasc Surg 122: 136–143.

Namikawa K, Honma M, Abe K, Takeda M, Mansur K, Obata T, Miwa A, Okado H, Kiyama H (2000) Akt/protein kinase B prevents injury-induced motoneuron death and accelerates axonal regeneration. J Neurosci 20: 2875–2886.

Naveilhan P, ElShamy VM, Emfors P (1997) Differential regulation of mRNAs for GDNF and its receptors Ret and GDNFRα after sciatic nerve lesion in the mouse. Eur J Neurosci 9: 1450–1460.

Near SL, Whalen LR, Miller JA, Ishii DN (1992) Insulin-like growth factor II stimulates motor nerve regeneration. Proc Natl Acad Sci U S A 89: 11716–11720.

Neet KE, Campenot RB (2001) Receptor binding, internalization, and retrograde transport of neurotrophic factors. Cell Mol Life Sci 58: 1021–1035.

Nesbitt JA, Acland RD (1980) Histopathological changes following removal of the perineurium. J Neurosurg 53: 233–238.

Neumann S, Woolf CJ (1999) Regeneration of dorsal column fibers into and beyond the lesion site following adult spinal cord injury. Neuron 23: 83–91.

Neumann S, Bradke F, Tessier-Lavigne M, Basbaum AI (2002) Regeneration of sensory axons within the injured spinal cord induced by intraganglionic cAMP elevation. Neuron 34: 885–893.

Newman JP, Verity AN, Hawatmeh S, Fee WE, Jr., Terris DJ (1996) Ciliary neurotrophic factor enhances peripheral nerve regeneration. Arch Otolaryngol Head Neck Surg 122: 399–403.

Nguyen QT, Sanes JR, Lichtman JW (2002) Pre-existing pathways promote precise projection patterns. Nat Neurosci 5: 861–867.

Nickols JC, Valentine W, Kanwal S, Carter BD (2003) Activation of the transcription factor NF-kappaB in Schwann cells is required for peripheral myelin formation. Nat Neurosci 6: 161–167.

Nielsen J, Gotfryd K, Li S, Kulahin N, Soroka V, Rasmussen KK, Bock E, Berezin V (2009) Role of glial cell line-derived neurotrophic factor (GDNF)-neural cell adhesion molecule (NCAM) interactions in induction of neurite outgrowth and identification of a binding site for NCAM in the heel region of GDNF. J Neurosci 29: 11360–11376.

Nilsson A, Moller K, Dahlin L, Lundborg G, Kanje M (2005) Early changes in gene expression in the dorsal root ganglia after transection of the sciatic nerve: effects of amphiregulin and PAI-1 on regeneration. Brain Res Mol Brain Res 136: 65–74.

Nissl F (1894) Uber eine neue untersuchungsmethode des centralorgans speziell zur fesstellung der lokalisation der nervenzellen. Zentralbl Nervenheilkd Psychiatr 17: 337–344.

Novikov L, Novikova L, Kellerth JO (1997) Brain-derived neurotrophic factor promotes axonal regeneration and long-term survival of adult rat spinal motoneurons in vivo. Neuroscience 79: 765–774.

Nykjaer A, Lee R, Teng KK, Jansen P, Madsen P, Nielsen MS, Jacobsen C, Kliemannel M, Schwarz E, Willnow TE, Hempstead BL, Petersen CM (2004) Sortilin is essential for proNGF-induced neuronal cell death. Nature 427: 843–848.

Oaklander AL, Miller MS, Spencer PS (1987) Rapid anterograde spread of premitotic activity along degenerating cat sciatic nerve. J Neurochem 48: 111–114.

O'Brien JJ, Nathanson NM (2007) Retrograde activation of STAT3 by leukemia inhibitory factor in sympathetic neurons. J Neurochem 103: 288–302.

Ochi M, Wakasa M, Ikuta Y, Kwong WH (1994) Nerve regeneration in predegenerated basal lamina graft: The effect of duration of predegeneration on axonal extension. Exp Neurol 128: 216–225.

Ochs S (1975) Waller's concept of the trophic dependence of the nerve fiber on the cell body in the light of early neuron theory. Clio Med 10: 253–265.

Ogata T, Iijima S, Hoshikawa S, Miura T, Yamamoto S, Oda H, Nakamura K, Tanaka S (2004) Opposing extracellular signal-regulated kinase and Akt pathways control Schwann cell myelination. J Neurosci 24: 6724–6732.

Ogata T, Yamamoto S, Nakamura K, Tanaka S (2006) Signaling axis in Schwann cell proliferation and differentiation. Mol Neurobiol 33: 51–61.

Ohta K, Inokuchi T, Gen E, Chang JW (2001) Ultrastructural study of anterograde transport of glial cell line-derived neurotrophic factor from dorsal root ganglion neurons of rats towards the nerve terminal. Cells Tissues Organs 169: 410–421.

Okura Y, Arimoto H, Tanuma N, Matsumoto K, Nakamura T, Yamashima T, Miyazawa T, Matsumoto Y (1999) Analysis of neurotrophic effects of hepatocyte growth factor in the adult hypoglossal nerve axotomy model. Eur J Neurosci 11: 4139–4144.

Okuyama N, Kiryu-Seo S, Kiyama H (2007) Altered expression of Smad family members in injured motor neurons of rat. Brain Res 1132: 36–41.

Omura K, Ohbayashi M, Sano M, Omura T, Hasegawa T, Nagano A (2004) The recovery of blood-nerve barrier in crush nerve injury: a quantitative analysis utilizing immunohistochemistry. Brain Res 1001: 13–21.

Omura T, Omura K, Sano M, Sawada T, Hasegawa T, Nagano A (2005a) Spatiotemporal quantification of recruit and resident macrophages after crush nerve injury utilizing immunohistochemistry. Brain Res 1057: 29–36.

Omura T, Sano M, Omura K, Hasegawa T, Doi M, Sawada T, Nagano A (2005b) Different expressions of BDNF, NT3, and NT4 in muscle and nerve after various types of peripheral nerve injuries. J Peripher Nerv Syst 10: 293–300.

Oppenheim RW (1996a) Neurotrophic survival molecules for motoneurons: an embarrassment of riches. Neuron 17: 195–197.

Oppenheim RW (1996b) The concept of uptake and retrograde transport of neurotrophic molecules during development: history and present status. Neurochem Res 21: 769–777.

Ornitz DM (2000) FGFs, heparan sulfate and FGFRs: complex interactions essential for development. Bioessays 22: 108–112.

Ornitz DM, Xu J, Colvin JS, McEwen DG, MacArthur CA, Coulier F, Gao G, Goldfarb M (1996) Receptor specificity of the fibroblast growth factor family. J Biol Chem 271: 15292–15297.

Oudega M, Hagg T (1996) Nerve growth factor promotes regeneration of sensory axons into adult rat spinal cord. Exp Neurol 140: 218–229.

Ousman SS, David S (2001) MIP-1alpha, MCP-1, GM-CSF, and TNF-alpha control the immune cell response that mediates rapid phagocytosis of myelin from the adult mouse spinal cord. J Neurosci 21: 4649–4656.

Owen DJ, Logan A, Robinson PP (1989) A role for nerve growth factor in collateral reinnervation from sensory nerves in the guinea pig. Brain Res 476: 248–255.

Ozeki Y, Matsui T, Yamamoto Y, Funahashi M, Hamako J, Titani K (1995) Tissue fibronectin is an endogenous ligand for galectin-1. Glycobiology 5: 255–261.

Ozturk G, Tonge DA (2001) Effects of leukemia inhibitory factor on galanin expression and on axonal growth in adult dorsal root ganglion neurons in vitro. Exp Neurol 169: 376–385.

Panaite PA, Barakat-Walter I (2010) Thyroid hormone enhances transected axonal regeneration and muscle reinnervation following rat sciatic nerve injury. J Neurosci Res 88: 1751–1763.

Paratcha G, Ledda F, Ibanez CF (2003) The neural cell adhesion molecule NCAM is an alternative signaling receptor for GDNF family ligands. Cell 113: 867–879.

Park JI, Seo IA, Lee HK, Park HT, Shin SW, Park YM, Ahn KJ (2007) Netrin inhibits regenerative axon growth of adult dorsal root ganglion neurons in vitro. J Korean Med Sci 22: 641–645.

Park KK, Liu K, Hu Y, Smith PD, Wang C, Cai B, Xu B, Connolly L, Kramvis I, Sahin M, He Z (2008) Promoting axon regeneration in the adult CNS by modulation of the PTEN/mTOR pathway. Science 322: 963–966.

Park KK, Liu K, Hu Y, Kanter JL, He Z (2010) PTEN/mTOR and axon regeneration. Exp Neurol 223: 45–50.

Parkinson DB, Bhaskaran A, Arthur-Farraj P, Noon LA, Woodhoo A, Lloyd AC, Feltri ML, Wrabetz L, Behrens A, Mirsky R, Jessen KR (2008) c-Jun is a negative regulator of myelination. J Cell Biol 181: 625–637.

Pasterkamp RJ, Giger RJ, Verhaagen J (1998) Regulation of semaphorin III collapsin-1 gene expression during peripheral nerve regeneration. Exp Neurol 153: 313–327.

Patton BL (2000) Laminins of the neuromuscular system. Microsc Res Tech 51: 247–261.

Pearson AG, Gray CW, Pearson JF, Greenwood JM, During MJ, Dragunow M (2003) ATF3 enhances c-Jun-mediated neurite sprouting. Brain Res Mol Brain Res 120: 38–45.

Pellegrino RG, Politis MJ, Ritchie JM, Spencer PS (1986) Events in degenerating cat peripheral nerve: induction of Schwann cell S phase and its relation to nerve fibre degeneration. J Neurocytol 15: 17–28.

Pereira DB, Chao MV (2007) The tyrosine kinase Fyn determines the localization of TrkB receptors in lipid rafts. J Neurosci 27: 4859–4869.

Pereira JA, Benninger Y, Baumann R, Goncalves AF, Ozcelik M, Thurnherr T, Tricaud N, Meijer D, Fassler R, Suter U, Relvas JB (2009) Integrin-linked kinase is required for radial sorting of axons and Schwann cell remyelination in the peripheral nervous system. J Cell Biol 185: 147–161.

Perlson E, Hanz S, Ben-Yaakov K, Segal-Ruder Y, Seger R, Fainzilber M (2005) Vimentin-dependent spatial translocation of an activated MAP kinase in injured nerve. Neuron 45: 715–726.

Perlson E, Michaelevski I, Kowalsman N, Ben-Yaakov K, Shaked M, Seger R, Eisenstein M, Fainzilber M (2006) Vimentin binding to phosphorylated Erk sterically hinders enzymatic dephosphorylation of the kinase. J Mol Biol 364: 938–944.

Perrin FE, Lacroix S, Avilés-Trigueros M, David S (2005) Involvement of monocyte chemoattractant protein-1, macrophage inflammatory protein-1α and interleukin-1β in Wallerian degeneration. Brain 128: 854–866.

Pertz OC, Wang Y, Yang F, Wang W, Gay LJ, Gristenko MA, Clauss TR, Anderson DJ, Liu T, Auberry KJ, Camp DG, 2nd, Smith RD, Klemke RL (2008) Spatial mapping of the neurite and soma proteomes reveals a functional Cdc42/Rac regulatory network. Proc Natl Acad Sci U S A 105: 1931–1936.

Pestronk A, Drachman DB, Griffin JW (1980) Effects of aging on nerve sprouting and regeneration. Exp Neurol 70: 65–82.

Peterziel H, Unsicker K, Krieglstein K (2002) TGF-β induces GDNF responsiveness in neurons by recruitment of GFR-α1 to the plasma membrane. J Cell Biol 159: 157–167.

Piehl F, Arvidsson U, Johnson H, Cullheim S, Dagerlind A, Ulfhake B, Cao Y, Elde R, Pettersson RF, Terenius L, Hokfelt T (1993) GAP-43, aFGF, CCK and alpha- and beta-CGRP in rat spinal motoneurons subjected to axotomy and/or dorsal root severance. Eur J Neurosci 5: 1321–1333.

Piehl F, Frisen J, Risling M, Hokfelt T, Cullheim S (1994) Increased TrkB mRNA expression by axotomised motoneurons. Neuroreport 5: 697–700.

Pizzi MA, Crowe MJ (2007) Matrix metalloproteinases and proteoglycans in axonal regeneration. Exp Neurol 204: 496–511.

Plantman S, Patarroyo M, Fried K, Domogatskaya A, Tryggvason K, Hammarberg H, Cullheim S (2008) Integrin-laminin interactions controlling neurite outgrowth from adult DRG neurons in vitro. Mol Cell Neurosci 39: 50–62.

Platt CI, Krekoski CA, Ward RV, Edwards DR, Gavrilovic J (2003) Extracellular matrix and matrix metalloproteinases in sciatic nerve. J Neurosci Res 74: 417–429.

Pleasure D, Bora FW, Jr., Lane J, Prockop D (1974) Regeneration after nerve transection: effect of inhibition of collagen synthesis. Exp Neurol 45: 72–78.

Pola R, Aprahamian TR, Bosch-Marcé M, Curry C, Gaetani E, Flex A, Smith RC, Isner JM, Losordo DW (2004) Age-dependent VEGF expression and intraneural neovascularization during regeneration of peripheral nerves. Neurobiol Aging 25: 1361–1368.

Popovic M, Bresjanac M, Sketelj J (1994) Regenerating axons enhance differentiation of perineurial-like cells involved in minifascicle formation in the injured peripheral nerve. J Neuropath Exp Neurol 53: 590–597.

Poteryaev D, Titievsky A, Sun YF, Thomas-Crusells J, Lindahl M, Billaud M, Arumäe U, Saarma M (1999a) GDNF triggers a novel Ret-independent Src kinase family-coupled signaling via a GPI-linked GDNF receptor α1. FEBS Lett 463: 63–66.

Poteryaev D, Titievsky A, Sun YF, Thomas-Crusells J, Lindahl M, Billaud M, Arumäe U, Saarma M (1999b) GDNF triggers a novel ret-independent Src kinase family-coupled signaling via a GPI-linked GDNF receptor α1. FEBS Lett 463: 63–66.

Povlsen GK, Ditlevsen DK, Berezin V, Bock E (2003) Intracellular signaling by the neural cell adhesion molecule. Neurochem Res 28: 127–141.

Price DL, Porter KR (1972) The response of ventral horn neurons to axonal transection. J Cell Biol 53: 24–37.

Proctor RA (1987) Fibronectin: a brief overview of its structure, function, and physiology. Rev Infect Dis 9 (Suppl 4): S317–321.

Properzi F, Fawcett JW (2004) Proteoglycans and brain repair. News Physiol Sci 19: 33–38.

Pu SF, Zhuang HX, Ishii DN (1995) Differential spatio-temporal expression of the insulin-like growth factor genes in regenerating sciatic nerve. Brain Res Mol Brain Res 34: 18–28.

Pulford BE, Whalen LR, Ishii DN (1999) Peripherally administered insulin-like growth factor-I preserves hindlimb reflex and spinal cord noradrenergic circuitry following a central nervous system lesion in rats. Exp Neurol 159: 114–123.

Qiu J, Cai CM, Dai HN, McAtee M, Hoffman PN, Bregman BS, Filbin MT (2002) Spinal axon regeneration induced by elevation of cyclic AMP. Neuron 34: 895–903.

Qiu J, Cafferty WBJ, McMahon SB, Thompson SWN (2005) Conditioning injury-induced spinal axon regeneration requires signal transducer and activator of transcription 3 activation. J Neurosci 25: 1645–1653.

Qui J, Cai D, Filbin M (2002) A role for cAMP on regeneration during development and after injury. Prog Brain Res 137: 381–387.

Rabinovsky ED, Smith GM, Browder DP, Shine HD, McManaman JL (1992) Peripheral nerve injury down-regulates CNTF expression in adult rat sciatic nerves. J Neurosci Res 31: 188–192.

Rabinovsky ED, Gelir E, Gelir S, Lui H, Kattash M, DeMayo FJ, Shenaq SM, Schwartz RJ (2002) Targeted expression of IGF-1 transgene to skeletal muscle accelerates muscle and motor neuron regeneration. FASEB J 16: NIL556–NIL579.

Radeke MJ, Misko TP, Hsu C, Herzenberg LA, Shooter EM (1987) Gene transfer and molecular cloning of the rat nerve growth factor receptor. Nature 325: 593–597.

Raff MC, Hornby-Smith A, Brockes JP (1978) Cyclic AMP as a mitogenic signal for cultured rat Schwann cells. Nature 273: 672–673.

Raftopoulou M, Hall A (2004) Cell migration: Rho GTPases lead the way. Dev Biol 265: 23–32.

Raivich G, Hellweg R, Kreutzberg G (1991) NGF receptor-mediated decrease in axonal uptake and retrograde transport of endogenous NGF following sciatic nerve injury and during regeneration. Neuron 7: 151–164.

Raivich G, Bohatschek M, Da Costa C, Iwata O, Galiano M, Hristova M, Nateri AS, Makwana M, Riera-Sans L, Wolfer DP, Lipp HP, Aguzzi A,

Wagner EF, Behrens A (2004) The AP-1 transcription factor c-jun is required for efficient axonal regeneration. Neuron 43: 57–67.

Rajasekharan S, Kennedy TE (2009) The netrin protein family. Genome Biol 10: 239.

Ramer MS, Priestley JV, McMahon SB (2000) Functional regeneration of sensory axons into the adult spinal cord. Nature 403: 312–316.

Ramer MS, Bishop T, Dockery P, Mobarak MS, O'Leary D, Fraher JP, Priestley JV, McMahon SB (2002) Neurotrophin-3-mediated regeneration and recovery of proprioception following dorsal rhizotomy. Mol Cell Neurosci 19: 239–249.

Ramon y Cajal, S. (1928) *Degeneration and Regeneration of the Nervous System*. London: Oxford University Press.

Rankin SL, Guy CS, Mearow KM (2008) Neurite outgrowth is enhanced by laminin-mediated down-regulation of the low affinity neurotrophin receptor, p75NTR. J Neurochem 107: 799–813.

Rauvala H (1989) An 18-Kd heparin-binding protein of developing brain that is distinct from fibroblast growth factors. EMBO J 8: 2933–2941.

Redett R, Jari R, Crawford T, Chen YG, Rohde C, Brushart T (2005) Peripheral pathways regulate motoneuron collateral dynamics. J Neurosci 25: 9406–9412.

Reichardt LF (2006) Neurotrophin-regulated signalling pathways. Philos Trans R Soc Lond B Biol Sci 361: 1545–1564.

Reichert F, Rotshenker S (2003) Complement-receptor-3 and scavenger-receptor-AI/II mediated myelin phagocytosis in microglia and macrophages. Neurobiol Dis 12: 65–72.

Reichert F, Saada A, Rotshenker S (1994) Peripheral nerve injury induces Schwann cells to express two macrophage phenotypes: phagocytosis and the galactose-specific lectin MAC-2. J Neurosci 14: 3231–3245.

Reid AJ, Welin D, Wiberg M, Terenghi G, Novikov LN (2010) Peripherin and ATF3 genes are differentially regulated in regenerating and non-regenerating primary sensory neurons. Brain Res 1310: 1–7.

Remsen LG, Strain GM, Newman MJ, Satterlee N, Daniloff JK (1990) Antibodies to the neural cell adhesion molecule disrupt functional recovery in injured nerves. Exp Neurol 110: 268–273.

Rich KM, Yip HK, Osborne PA, Schmidt RE, Johnson EM, Jr. (1984) Role of nerve growth factor in the adult dorsal root ganglia neuron and its response to injury. J Comp Neurol 230: 110–118.

Rich KM, Alexander T, Pryor J, Hollowell J (1989) Nerve growth factor enhances regeneration through silicon chambers. Exp Neurol 105: 162–170.

Richardson PM, Issa VM (1984) Peripheral injury enhances central regeneration of primary sensory neurones. Nature 309: 791–793.

Ridley AJ, Davies JB, Stroobant P, Land H (1989) Transforming growth factors B-1 and B-2 are mitogens for rat Schwann cells. J Cell Biol 109: 3419–3424.

Riederer BM (2007) Microtubule-associated protein 1B, a growth-associated and phosphorylated scaffold protein. Brain Res Bull 71: 541–558.

Rind HB, Von Bartheld CS (2002) Anterograde axonal transport of internalized GDNF in sensory and motor neurons. Neuroreport 13: 659–664.

Riopelle RJ, Dow KE (1991) Neurite formation on laminin: effects of a galactosyltransferase on primary sensory neurons. Brain Res 541: 265–272.

Robinson PP, Yates JM, Smith KG (2004) An electrophysiological study into the effect of neurotrophin-3 on functional recovery after lingual nerve repair. Arch Oral Biol 49: 763–775.

Robles E, Gomez TM (2006) Focal adhesion kinase signaling at sites of integrin-mediated adhesion controls axon pathfinding. Nat Neurosci 9: 1274–1283.

Romero MI, Rangappa N, Garry MG, Smith GM (2001) Functional regeneration of chronically injured sensory afferents into adult spinal cord after neurotrophin gene therapy. J Neurosci 21: 8408–8416.

Rong LL, Trojaborg W, Qu W, Kostov K, Du Yan S, Gooch C, Szabolcs M, Hays AP, Schmidt AM (2004a) Antagonism of RAGE suppresses peripheral nerve regeneration. FASEB J 18: 1812–1817.

Rong LL, Yan SF, Wendt T, Hans D, Pachydaki S, Bucciarelli LG, Adebayo A, Qu W, Lu Y, Kostov K, Lalla E, Yan SD, Gooch C, Szabolcs M, Trojaborg W, Hays AP, Schmidt AM (2004b) RAGE modulates peripheral nerve regeneration via recruitment of both inflammatory and axonal outgrowth pathways. FASEB J 18: 1818–1825.

Rosenstein JM, Krum JM (2004) New roles for VEGF in nervous tissue: beyond blood vessels. Exp Neurol 187: 246–253.

Rotshenker S (2003) Microglia and macrophage activation and the regulation of complement-receptor-3 (CR3/MAC-1)-mediated myelin phagocytosis in injury and disease. J Mol Neurosci 21(1): 65–72.

Rovak JM, Mungara AK, Aydin MA, Cederna PS (2004) Effects of vascular endothelial growth factor on nerve regeneration in acellular nerve grafts. J Reconstr Microsurg 20: 53–58.

Roytta M, Salonen V (1988) Long-term endoneurial changes after nerve transection. Acta Neuropathol 76: 35–45.

Rueger MA, Aras S, Guntinas-Lichius O, Neiss WF (2008) Re-activation of atrophic motor Schwann cells after hypoglossal-facial nerve anastomosis. Neurosci Lett 434: 253–259.

Runeberg-Roos P, Saarma M (2007) Neurotrophic factor receptor RET: structure, cell biology, and inherited diseases. Ann Med 39: 572–580.

Russell FD, Koishi K, Jiang Y, McLennan IS (2000) Anterograde axonal transport of glial cell line-derived neurotrophic factor and its receptors in rat hypoglossal nerve. Neuroscience 97: 575–580.

Russell JW, Windebank AJ, Schenone A, Feldman EL (1998) Insulin-like growth factor-I prevents apoptosis in neurons after nerve growth factor withdrawal. J Neurobiol 36: 455–467.

Russo VC, Gluckman PD, Feldman EL, Werther GA (2005) The insulin-like growth factor system and its pleiotropic functions in brain. Endocr Rev 26: 916–943.

Rutishauser U, Acheson A, Hall AK, Mann DM, Sunshine J (1988) The neural cell adhesion molecule (NCAM) as a regulator of cell-cell interactions. Science 240: 53–57.

Rydevik M, Bergstrom F, Mitts C, Danielsen N (2002) Locally-applied collagenase and regeneration of transsected and repaired rat sciatic nerves. Scand J Plast Reconstr Surg Hand Surg 36: 193–196.

Ryu EJ, Wang JY, Le N, Baloh RH, Gustin JA, Schmidt RE, Milbrandt J (2007) Misexpression of Pou3f1 results in peripheral nerve hypomyelination and axonal loss. J Neurosci 27: 11552–11559.

Saada A, Reichert F, Rotshenker S (1996) Granulocyte macrophage colony stimulating factor produced in lesioned peripheral nerves induces the up-regulation of cell surface expression of MAC-2 by macrophages and Schwann cells. J Cell Biol 133: 159–167.

Sacheck JM, Ohtsuka A, McLary SC, Goldberg AL (2004) IGF-I stimulates muscle growth by suppressing protein breakdown and expression of atrophy-related ubiquitin ligases, atrogin-1 and MuRF1. Am J Physiol Endocrinol Metab 287: E591–E601.

Sahenk Z, Seharaseyon J, Mendell JR (1994) CNTF potentiates peripheral nerve regeneration. Brain Res 655: 246–250.

Sahenk Z, Oblinger J, Edwards C (2008) Neurotrophin-3 deficient Schwann cells impair nerve regeneration. Exp Neurol 212: 552–556.

Saika T, Senba E, Noguchi K, Sato M, Kubo T, Matsunaga T, Tohyama M (1991) Changes in expression of peptides in rat facial motoneurons after facial nerve crushing and resection. Brain Res Mol Brain Res 11: 187–196.

Saito H, Dahlin LB (2008) Expression of ATF3 and axonal outgrowth are impaired after delayed nerve repair. BMC Neurosci 9: 88.

Sakamoto T, Kawazoe Y, Shen JS, Takeda Y, Arakawa Y, Ogawa J, Oyanagi K, Ohashi T, Watanabe K, Inoue K, Eto Y, Watabe K (2003) Adenoviral gene transfer of GDNF, BDNF and TGF-β2, but not CNTF, cardiotrophin-1 or IGF1, protects injured adult motoneurons after facial nerve avulsion. J Neurosci Res 72: 54–64.

Salehi AH, Roux PP, Kubu CJ, Zeindler C, Bhakar A, Tannis LL, Verdi JM, Barker PA (2000) NRAGE, a novel MAGE protein, interacts with the p75 neurotrophin receptor and facilitates nerve growth factor-dependent apoptosis. Neuron 27: 279–288.

Salonen V, Peltonen J, Roytta M, Virtanen I (1987) Laminin in traumatized peripheral nerve: basement membrane changes during degeneration and regeneration. J Neurocytol 16: 713–720.

Sanders FK, Young JZ (1942) The degeneration and re-innervation of grafted nerves. J Anat 76: 143–170.

Sango K, Tokashiki A, Ajiki K, Horie M, Kawano H, Watabe K, Horie H, Kadoya T (2004) Synthesis, localization and externalization of galectin-1 in mature dorsal root ganglion neurons and Schwann cells. Eur J Neurosci 19: 55–64.

Santos X, Rodrigo J, Hontanilla B, Bilbao G (1998) Evaluation of peripheral nerve regeneration by nerve growth factor locally administered with a novel system. J Neurosci Methods 85: 119–127.

Sarmiere PD, Bamburg JR (2004) Regulation of the neuronal actin cytoskeleton by ADF/cofilin. J Neurobiol 58: 103–117.

Scarisbrick IA, Isackson PJ, Windebank AJ (1999) Differential expression of brain-derived neurotrophic factor, neurotrophin-3, and neurotrophin-4/5 in the adult rat spinal cord: regulation by the glutamate receptor agonist kainic acid. J Neurosci 19: 7757–7769.

Scarlato M, Ara J, Bannerman P, Scherer S, Pleasure D (2003) Induction of neuropilins-1 and-2 and their ligands, Sema3A, Sema3F, and VEGF, during Wallerian degeneration in the peripheral nervous system. Exp Neurol 183: 489–498.

Schaefer AW, Schoonderwoert VT, Ji L, Mederios N, Danuser G, Forscher P (2008) Coordination of actin filament and microtubule dynamics during neurite outgrowth. Dev Cell 15: 146–162.

Schafer M, Fruttiger M, Montag D, Schachner M, Martini R (1996) Disruption of the gene for the myelin-associated glycoprotein improves axonal regrowth along myelin in C57BL/Wld mice. Neuron 16: 1107–1113.

Scherer SS, Kamholz J, Jakowlew SB (1993) Axons modulate the expression of transforming growth factor-betas in Schwann cells. Glia 8: 265–276.

Scherer SS, Wang D, Kuhn R, Lemke G, Wrabetz L, Kamholz J (1994) Axons regulate Schwann cell expression of the POU transcription factor SCIP. J Neurosci 14: 1930–1942.

Schlaepfer WW, Micko S (1979) Calcium-dependent alterations of neurofilament proteins of rat peripheral nerve. J Neurochem 32: 211–219.

Schwaiger FW, Hager G, Schmitt AB, Horvat A, Hager G, Streif R, Spitzer C, Gamal S, Breuer S, Brook GA, Nacimiento W, Kreutzberg GW (2000) Peripheral but not central axotomy induces changes in Janus kinases (JAK) and signal transducers and activators of transcription (STAT). Eur J Neurosci 12: 1165–1176.

Schwarz Q, Gu C, Fujisawa H, Sabelko K, Gertsenstein M, Nagy A, Taniguchi M, Kolodkin AL, Ginty DD, Shima DT, Ruhrberg C (2004) Vascular endothelial growth factor controls neuronal migration and cooperates with Sema3A to pattern distinct compartments of the facial nerve. Genes Dev 18: 2822–2834.

Schwarzbauer JE, Tamkun JW, Lemischka IR, Hynes RO (1983) Three different fibronectin mRNAs arise by alternative splicing within the coding region. Cell 35: 421–431.

Seddon HJ, Medawar PB, Smith H (1943) Rate of regeneration of peripheral nerves in man. J Physiol 102: 191–215.

Seijffers R, Allchorne AJ, Woolf CJ (2006) The transcription factor ATF-3 promotes neurite outgrowth. Mol Cell Neurosci 32: 143–154.

Seijffers R, Mills CD, Woolf CJ (2007) ATF3 increases the intrinsic growth state of DRG neurons to enhance peripheral nerve regeneration. J Neurosci 27: 7911–7920.

Selleck SB (2006) Signaling from across the way: transactivation of VEGF receptors by HSPGs. Mol Cell 22: 431–432.

Sendtner M, Stockli KA, Thoenen H (1992) Synthesis and localization of ciliary neurotrophic factor in the sciatic nerve of the adult rat after lesion and during regeneration. J Cell Biol 118: 139–148.

Seniuk N, Altares M, Dunn R, Richardson PM (1992) Decreased synthesis of ciliary neurotrophic factor in degenerating peripheral nerves. Brain Res 572: 300–302.

Shadiack AM, Sun Y, Zigmond RE (2001) Nerve growth factor antiserum induces axotomy-like changes in neuropeptide expression in intact sympathetic and sensory neurons. J Neurosci 21: 363–371.

Shah M, Foreman DM, Ferguson MW (1992) Control of scarring in adult wounds by neutralising antibody to transforming growth factor beta. Lancet 339: 213–214.

Shamash S, Reichert F, Rotshenker S (2002) The cytokine network of Wallerian degeneration: tumor necrosis factor-α, interleukin-1α, and interleukin-1β. J Neurosci 22: 3052–3060.

Shanthaveerappa TR, Bourne GH (1962) The "perineurial epithelium," a metabolically active, continuous, protoplasmic cell barrier surrounding peripheral nerve fasciculi. J Anat 96: 527–520.

Shao Y, Akmentin W, Toledo-Aral JJ, Rosenbaum J, Valdez G, Cabot JB, Hilbush BS, Halegoua S (2002) Pincher, a pinocytic chaperone for nerve growth factor/TrkA signaling endosomes. J Cell Biol 157: 679–691.

Shawe GDH (1955) On the number of branches formed by regenerating nerve-fibers. Brit J Surg 42: 474–488.

Shen A, Yan J, Ding F, Gu X, Zhu D, Gu J (2003) Overexpression of beta-1,4-galactosyltransferase I in rat Schwann cells promotes the growth of co-cultured dorsal root ganglia. Neurosci Lett 342: 159–162.

Shen YJ, DeBellard ME, Salzer JL, Roder J, Filbin MT (1998) Myelin-associated glycoprotein in myelin and expressed by Schwann cells inhibits axonal regeneration and branching. Mol Cell Neurosci 12: 79–91.

Sherren, J. (1908) *Injuries of Nerves and Their Treatment*. London: James Nisbit.

Shi Y, Massague J (2003) Mechanisms of TGF-beta signaling from cell membrane to the nucleus. Cell 113: 685–700.

Shiotani A, O'Malley BW, Jr., Coleman ME, Alila HW, Flint PW (1998) Reinnervation of motor endplates and increased muscle fiber size after human insulin-like growth factor I gene transfer into the paralyzed larynx. Hum Gene Ther 9: 2039–2047.

Shubayev VI, Angert M, Dolkas J, Campana WM, Palenscar K, Myers RR (2006) TNFα-induced MMP-9 promotes macrophage recruitment into injured peripheral nerve. Mol Cell Neurosci 31: 407–415.

Siegel SG, Patton B, English AW (2000) Ciliary neurotrophic factor is required for motoneuron sprouting. Exp Neurol 166: 205–212.

Sisken BF, Kanje M, Lundborg G, Herbst E, Kurtz W (1989) Stimulation of rat sciatic nerve regeneration with pulsed electromagnetic fields. Brain Res 485: 309–316.

Sivasankaran R, Pei J, Wang KC, Zhang YP, Shields CB, Xu XM, He Z (2004) PKC mediates inhibitory effects of myelin and chondroitin sulfate proteoglycans on axonal regeneration. Nat Neurosci 7: 261–268.

Sjoberg J, Kanje M (1989) Insulin-like growth factor (IGF-I) as a stimulator of regeneration in the freeze-injured rat sciatic nerve. Brain Res 485: 102–108.

Skaper SD (2008) The biology of neurotrophins, signalling pathways, and functional peptide mimetics of neurotrophins and their receptors. CNS Neurol Disord Drug Targets 7: 46–62.

Skene J, Willard M (1981) Axonally transported proteins associated with axon growth in rabbit central and peripheral nervous systems. J Cell Biol 89: 96–103.

Skene J, Jacobson RD, Snipes GJ, McGuire CB, Norden JJ, Freeman JA (1986) A protein induced during nerve growth (GAP-43) is a major component of growth-cone membranes. Science 233: 783–786.

Sketelj J, Bresjanac M, Popovic M (1989) Rapid growth of regenerating axons across the segments of sciatic nerve devoid of Schwann cells. J Neurosci Res 24: 153–162.

Sondell M, Lundborg G, Kanje M (1999a) Vascular endothelial growth factor has neurotrophic activity and stimulates axonal outgrowth, enhancing cell survival and Schwann cell proliferation in the peripheral nervous system. J Neurosci 19: 5731–5740.

Sondell M, Lundborg G, Kanje M (1999b) Vascular endothelial growth factor stimulates Schwann cell invasion and neovascularization of acellular nerve grafts. Brain Res 846: 219–228.

Sondell M, Sundler F, Kanje M (2000) Vascular endothelial growth factor is a neurotrophic factor which stimulates axonal outgrowth through the flk-1 receptor. Eur J Neurosci 12: 4243–4254.

Sondell M, Kanje M (2001) Postnatal expression of VEGF and its receptor flk-1 in peripheral ganglia. Neuroreport 12: 105–108.

Song HJ, Ming GL, Poo MM (1997) cAMP-induced switching in turning direction of nerve growth cones. Nature 388: 275–279.

Song HJ, Ming GL, He ZG, Lehmann M, McKerracher L, Tessier-Lavigne M, Poo MM (1998) Conversion of neuronal growth cone responses from repulsion to attraction by cyclic nucleotides. Science 281: 1515–1518.

Song XY, Zhou FHH, Zhong JH, Wu LLY, Zhou XF (2006) Knockout of p75NTR impairs re-myelination of injured sciatic nerve in mice. J Neurochem 96: 833–842.

Sorenson E, Windebank A (1993) Relative importance of basement membrane and soluble growth factors in delayed and immediate regeneration of rat sciatic nerve. J Neuropathology 52: 216–222.

Sorensen J, Fugleholm K, Moldovan M, Schmalbruch H, Krarup G (2001) Axonal elongation through long acellular nerve segments depends on recruitment of phagocytic cells from the near-nerve environment: electrophysiological and morphological studies in the cat. Brain Res 903: 185–197.

Staniszewska I, Sariyer IK, Lecht S, Brown MC, Walsh EM, Tuszynski GP, Safak M, Lazarovici P, Marcinkiewicz C (2008) Integrin alpha9 beta1 is a receptor for nerve growth factor and other neurotrophins. J Cell Sci 121: 504–513.

Stark B, Carlstedt T, Risling M (2001) Distribution of TGF-beta, the TGF-beta type I receptor and the R-II receptor in peripheral nerves and mechanoreceptors: observations on changes after traumatic injury. Brain Res 913: 47–56.

Stephens RM, Loeb DM, Copeland TD, Pawson T, Greene LA, Kaplan DR (1994) Trk receptors use redundant signal transduction pathways involving SHC and PLC-gamma 1 to mediate NGF responses. Neuron 12: 691–705.

Sterne GD, Brown RA, Green CJ, Terenghi G (1997a) Neurotrophin-3 delivered locally via fibronectin mats enhances peripheral nerve regeneration. Eur J Neurosci 9: 1388–1396.

Sterne GD, Coulton GR, Brown RA, Green CJ, Terenghi G (1997b) Neurotrophin-3-enhanced nerve regeneration selectively improves recovery of muscle fibers expressing myosin heavy chains 2b. J Cell Biol 139: 709–715.

Stewart HJS, Bradke F, Tabernero A, Morrell D, Jessen KR, Mirsky R (1996) Regulation of rat Schwann cell Po expression and DNA synthesis by insulin-like growth factors in vitro. Eur J Neurosci 8: 553–564.

Stoll G, Mueller HW (1999) Nerve injury, axonal degeneration and neural regeneration: Basic insights. Brain Pathol 9: 313–325.

Stoll G, Griffin JW, Li CY, Trapp B (1989) Wallerian degeneration in the peripheral nervous system: participation of both Schwann cells and macrophages in myelin degradation. J Neurocytol 18: 671–683.

Stoll G, Jander S, Myers RR (2002) Degeneration and regeneration of the peripheral nervous system: from Augustus Waller's observations to neuroinflammation. J Peripher Nerv Syst 7: 13–27.

Streppel M, Azzolin N, Dohm S, Guntinas-Lichius O, Haas C, Grothe C, Wevers A, Neiss WF, Angelov DN (2002) Focal application of neutralizing antibodies to soluble neurotrophic factors reduces collateral axonal branching after peripheral nerve lesion. Eur J Neurosci 15: 1327–1342.

Subang MC, Richardson PM (2001) Influence of injury and cytokines on synthesis of monocyte chemoattractant protein-1 mRNA in peripheral nervous tissue. Eur J Neurosci 13: 521–528.

Sugahara K, Mikami T, Uyama T, Mizuguchi S, Nomura K, Kitagawa H (2003) Recent advances in the structural biology of chondroitin sulfate and dermatan sulfate. Curr Opin Struct Biol 13: 612–620.

Sugiura S, Lahav R, Han J, Kou SY, Banner LR, de Pablo F, Patterson PH (2000) Leukaemia inhibitory factor is required for normal inflammatory responses to injury in the peripheral and central nervous systems in vivo and is chemotactic for macrophages in vitro. Eur J Neurosci 12: 457–466.

Sulaiman OAR, Gordon T (2000) Effects of short- and long-term Schwann cell denervation on peripheral nerve regeneration, myelination, and size. Glia 32: 234–246.

Sulaiman OA, Gordon T (2002) Transforming growth factor-beta and forskolin attenuate the adverse effects of long-term Schwann cell denervation on peripheral nerve regeneration in vivo. Glia 37: 206–218.

Suliman IA, Lindgren JU, Gillberg PG, Elhassan AM, Monneron C, Adem A (1999) Alteration of spinal cord IGF-I receptors and skeletal muscle IGF-I after hind-limb immobilization in the rat. Neuroreport 10: 1195–1199.

Sullivan KA, Kim B, Feldman EL (2008) Insulin-like growth factors in the peripheral nervous system. Endocrinology 149: 5963–5971.

Sun Y, Zigmond RE (1996) Leukaemia inhibitory factor induced in the sciatic nerve after axotomy is involved in the induction of galanin in sensory neurons. Eur J Neurosci 8: 2213–2220.

Sunderland S, Bradley KC (1950a) Denervation atrophy of the distal stump of a severed nerve. J Comp Neurol 93: 401–409.

Sunderland S, Bradley KC (1950b) Endoneurial tube shrinkage in the distal segment of a severed nerve. J Comp Neurol 93: 411–420.

Sunderland S, McArthur RA, Nam DA (1993) Repair of a transected sciatic nerve. A study of nerve regeneration and functional recovery: report of a case. J Bone Joint Surg Am 75: 911–914.

Sung YJ, Chiu DT, Ambron RT (2006) Activation and retrograde transport of protein kinase G in rat nociceptive neurons after nerve injury and inflammation. Neuroscience 141: 697–709.

Suter DM, Forscher P (2000) Substrate-cytoskeletal coupling as a mechanism for the regulation of growth cone motility and guidance. J Neurobiol 44: 97–113.

Suzuki G, Ochi M, Shu N, Uchio Y, Matsuura Y (1998) Sensory neurons regenerate more dominantly than motoneurons during the initial stage of the regenerating process after peripheral axotomy. Neuroreport 9: 3487–3492.

Suzuki S, Numakawa T, Shimazu K, Koshimizu H, Hara T, Hatanaka H, Mei L, Lu B, Kojima M (2004) BDNF-induced recruitment of TrkB receptor into neuronal lipid rafts: roles in synaptic modulation. J Cell Biol 167: 1205–1215.

Svenningsen AF, Kanje M (1996) Insulin and the insulin-like growth factors I and II are mitogenic to cultured rat sciatic nerve segments and stimulate [3H]thymidine incorporation through their respective receptors. Glia 18: 68–72.

Svenningsen AF, Kanje M (1998) Regulation of Schwann cell proliferation in cultured segments of the adult rat sciatic nerve. J Neurosci Res 52: 530–537.

Symons NA, Danielsen N, Harvey AR (2001) Migration of cells into and out of peripheral nerve isografts in the peripheral and central nervous systems of the adult mouse. Eur J Neurosci 14: 522–532.

Syroid DE, Zorick TS, Arbet-Engels C, Kilpatrick TJ, Eckhart W, Lemke G (1999) A role for insulin-like growth factor-I in the regulation of Schwann cell survival. J Neurosci 19: 2059–2068.

Tanabe K, Bonilla I, Winkles JA, Strittmatter SM (2003) Fibroblast growth factor-inducible-14 is induced in axotomized neurons and promotes neurite outgrowth. J Neurosci 23: 9675–9686.

Tanaka E, Ho T, Kirschner MW (1995) The role of microtubule dynamics in growth cone motility and axonal growth. J Cell Biol 128: 139–155.

Taniuchi M, Clark H, Schweitzer J, Johnson E (1988) Expression of nerve growth factor receptors by Schwann cells of axotomized peripheral nerves: ultrastructural location, suppression by axonal contact, and binding properties. J Neurosci 8: 664–681.

Tannemaat MR, Eggers R, Hendriks WT, de Ruiter GC, van Heerikhuize JJ, Pool CW, Malessy MJ, Boer GJ, Verhaagen J (2008) Differential effects of lentiviral vector-mediated overexpression of nerve growth factor and glial cell line-derived neurotrophic factor on regenerating sensory and motor axons in the transected peripheral nerve. Eur J Neurosci 28: 1467–1479.

Tanno T, Fujiwara A, Takenaka S, Kuwamura M, Tsuyama S (2005) Expression of a chemorepellent factor, Slit2, in peripheral nerve regeneration. Biosci Biotechnol Biochem 69: 2431–2434.

Tansey MG, Baloh RH, Milbrandt J, Johnson EM, Jr. (2000) GFRalpha-mediated localization of RET to lipid rafts is required for effective downstream signaling, differentiation, and neuronal survival. Neuron 25: 611–623.

Tcherkezian J, Lamarche-Vane N (2007) Current knowledge of the large RhoGAP family of proteins. Biol Cell 99: 67–86.

Terenghi G, Calder JS, Birch R, Hall SM (1998) A morphological study of Schwann cells and axonal regeneration in chronically transected human peripheral nerves. J Hand Surg [Br Eur] 23B: 583–587.

Tessier-Lavigne M, Placzek M, Lumsden AG, Dodd J, Jessell TM (1988) Chemotropic guidance of developing axons in the mammalian central nervous system. Nature 336: 775–778.

Tetzlaff W, Bisby MA, Kreutzberg GW (1988) Changes in cytoskeletal proteins in the rat facial nucleus following axotomy. J Neurosci 8: 3181–3189.

Tham S, Dowsing B, Finkelstein D, Donato R, Cheema SS, Bartlett PF, Morrison WA (1997) Leukemia inhibitory factor enhances the regeneration of transected rat sciatic nerve and the function of reinnervated muscle. J Neurosci Res 47: 208–215.

Thanos PK, Okajima S, Tiangco DA, Terzis JK (1999) Insulin-like growth factor-I promotes nerve regeneration through a nerve graft in an experimental model of facial paralysis. Restor Neurol Neurosci 15: 57–71.

Thanos PK, Tiangco DA, Terzis JK (2001) Enhanced reinnervation of the paralyzed orbicularis oculi muscle after insulin-like growth factor-I (IGF-I) delivery to a nerve graft. J Reconstr Microsurg 17: 357–362.

Thisse B, Thisse C (2005) Functions and regulations of fibroblast growth factor signaling during embryonic development. Dev Biol 287: 390–402.

Thoenen H, Barde YA (1980) Physiology of nerve growth factor. Physiol Rev 60: 1284–1335.

Thomas PK (1964) Changes in the endoneurial sheaths of peripheral myelinated nerve fibers during Wallerian degeneration. J Anat 98: 175–182.

Thomas PK, Bhagat S (1978) The effect of extraction of the intrafascicular contents of peripheral nerve trunks on perineurial structure. Acta Neuropathol 43: 135–141.

Thomas RW, Davenport HA (1949) Axon branching in nerve regeneration and its trophic effect on muscle. Q Bull Northw Univ Med Sch 23: 170–176.

Thomas SM, DeMarco M, D'Arcangelo G, Halegoua S, Brugge JS (1992) Ras is essential for nerve growth factor- and phorbol ester-induced tyrosine phosphorylation of MAP kinases. Cell 68: 1031–1040.

Thomas WA, Schaefer AW, Treadway RM, Jr. (1990) Galactosyl transferase-dependence of neurite outgrowth on substratum-bound laminin. Development 110: 1101–1114.

Tinel, J. (1916) Les blessures des nerfs. Paris: Masson et Cie.

Toews AD, Barrett C, Morell P (1998) Monocyte chemoattractant protein 1 is responsible for macrophage recruitment following injury to sciatic nerve. J Neurosci Res 53: 260–267.

Tofaris GK, Patterson PH, Jessen KR, Mirsky R (2002) Denervated Schwann cells attract macrophages by secretion of leukemia inhibitory factor (LIF) and monocyte chemoattractant protein-1 in a process regulated by interleukin-6 and LIF. J Neurosci 22: 6696–6703.

Tohyama K, Ide C (1984) The localization of laminin and fibronectin of the Schwann cell basal lamina. Arch Hist Jap 47: 519–532.

Tomaselli KJ, Doherty P, Emmett CJ, Damsky CH, Walsh FS, Reichardt LF (1993) Expression of beta 1 integrins in sensory neurons of the dorsal root ganglion and their functions in neurite outgrowth on two laminin isoforms. J Neurosci 13: 4880–4888.

Tomita K, Kubo T, Matsuda K, Yano K, Tohyama M, Hosokawa K (2007a) Myelin-associated glycoprotein reduces axonal branching and enhances functional recovery after sciatic nerve transection in rats. Glia 55: 1498–1507.

Tomita K, Kubo T, Matsuda K, Fujiwara T, Yano K, Winograd JM, Tohyama M, Hosokawa K (2007b) The neurotrophin receptor p75NTR in Schwann cells is implicated in remyelination and motor recovery after peripheral nerve injury. Glia 55: 1199–1208.

Tomita K, Hata Y, Kubo T, Fujiwara T, Yano K, Hosokawa K (2009) Effects of the in vivo predegenerated nerve graft on early Schwann cell migration: quantitative analysis using S100-GFP mice. Neurosci Lett 461: 36–40.

Tona A, Perides G, Rahemtulla F, Dahl D (1993) Extracellular matrix in regenerating rat sciatic nerve: a comparative study on the localization of laminin, hyaluronic acid, and chondroitin sulfate proteoglycans, including versican. J Histochem Cytochem 41: 593–599.

Torigoe K, Tanaka HF, Takahashi A, Awaya A, Hashimoto K (1996) Basic behavior of migratory Schwann cells in peripheral nerve regeneration. Exp Neurol 137: 301–308.

Torigoe K, Lundborg G (1998) Selective inhibition of early axonal regeneration by myelin-associated glycoprotein. Exp Neurol 150: 254–262.

Toth C, Martinez JA, Liu WQ, Diggle J, Guo GF, Ramji N, Mi R, Hoke A, Zochodne DW (2008) Local erythropoietin signaling enhances regeneration in peripheral axons. Neuroscience 154: 767–783.

Toth CC, Willis D, Twiss JL, Walsh S, Martinez JA, Liu WQ, Midha R, Zochodne DW (2009) Locally synthesized calcitonin gene-related Peptide has a critical role in peripheral nerve regeneration. J Neuropathol Exp Neurol 68: 326–337.

Trapp BD, Hauer P, Lemke G (1988) Axonal regulation of myelin protein mRNA levels in actively myelinating Schwann cells. J Neurosci 8: 3515–3521.

Trotter W, Davies WM (1913) Peculiarities of sensibility in cutaneous areas supplied by regenerating nerves. Zellforsch Fur Psychol U Neurol 20: 102–150.

Trupp M, Ryden M, Jornvall H, Funakoshi H, Timmusk T, Arenas E, Ibanez C (1995) Peripheral expression and biological activities of GDNF, a new neurotrophic factor for avian and mammalian peripheral neurons. J Cell Biol 130: 137–148.

Trupp M, Scott R, Whittemore SR, Ibanez CF (1999) Ret-dependent and -independent mechanisms of glial cell line-derived neurotrophic factor signaling in neuronal cells. J Biol Chem 274: 20885–20894.

Tsui-Pierchala B, Milbrandt J, Johnson EM, Jr. (2002) NGF utilizes c-Ret via a novel GFL-independent, inter-RTK signaling mechanism to maintain the trophic status of mature sympathetic neurons. Neuron 33: 261–273.

Tsujii M, Akeda K, Iino T, Uchida A (2009) Are BMPs involved in normal nerve and following transection? A pilot study. Clin Orthop Relat Res 467: 3183–3189.

Tsujino H, Kondo E, Fukuoka T, Dai Y, Tokunaga A, Miki K, Yonenobu K, Ochi T, Noguchi K (2000) Activating transcription factor 3 (ATF3) induction by axotomy in sensory and motoneurons: a novel neuronal marker of nerve injury. Mol Cell Neurosci 15: 170–182.

Tucker BA, Rahimtula M, Mearow KM (2005) Integrin activation and neurotrophin signaling cooperate to enhance neurite outgrowth in sensory neurons. J Comp Neurol 486: 267–280.

Tucker BA, Rahimtula M, Mearow KM (2006) Laminin and growth factor receptor activation stimulates differential growth responses in subpopulations of adult DRG neurons. Eur J Neurosci 24: 676–690.

Tucker BA, Mearow KM (2008) Peripheral sensory axon growth: from receptor binding to cellular signaling. Can J Neurol Sci 35: 551–566.

Tucker BA, Rahimtula M, Mearow KM (2008) Src and FAK are key early signalling intermediates required for neurite growth in NGF-responsive adult DRG neurons. Cell Signal 20: 241–257.

Uchida M, Enomoto A, Fukuda T, Kurokawa K, Maeda K, Kodama Y, Asai N, Hasegawa T, Shimono Y, Jijiwa M, Ichihara M, Murakumo Y, Takahashi M (2006) Dok-4 regulates GDNF-dependent neurite outgrowth through downstream activation of Rap1 and mitogen-activated protein kinase. J Cell Sci 119: 3067–3077.

Udina E, Ladak A, Furey M, Brushart T, Tyreman N, Gordon T (2010) Rolipram-induced elevation of cAMP or chondroitinase ABC breakdown of inhibitory proteoglycans in the extracellular matrix promotes peripheral nerve regeneration. Exp Neurol 223: 143–152.

Unezaki S, Yoshii S, Mabuchi T, Saito A, Ito S (2009) Effects of neurotrophic factors on nerve regeneration monitored by in vivo imaging in thy1-YFP transgenic mice. J Neurosci Methods 178: 308–315.

Urabe T, Zhao Q, Lundborg G, Danielsen N (1995) Effects of delayed nerve repair on regeneration of rat sciatic nerve. Restor Neurol Neurosci 9: 1–5.

Utley DS, Lewin SL, Cheng ET, Verity AN, Sierra D, Terris DJ (1996) Brain-derived neurotrophic factor and collagen tubulization enhance functional recovery after peripheral nerve transection and repair. Arch Otolaryngol Head Neck Surg 122: 407–413.

Uziyel Y, Hall S, Cohen J (2000) Influence of laminin-2 on Schwann cell-axon interactions. Glia 32: 109–121.

van der Flier A, Sonnenberg A (2001) Function and interactions of integrins. Cell Tissue Res 305: 285–298.

van der Veen RC, Roberts LJ (1999) Contrasting roles for nitric oxide and peroxynitrite in the peroxidation of myelin lipids. J Neuroimmunol 95: 1–7.

Van der Zee CE, Kreft M, Beckers G, Kuipers A, Sonnenberg A (2008) Conditional deletion of the Itgb4 integrin gene in Schwann cells leads to delayed peripheral nerve regeneration. J Neurosci 28: 11292–11303.

Verdu E, Ceballos D, Vilches JJ, Navarro X (2000) Influence of aging on peripheral nerve function and regeneration. J Peripher Nerv Syst 5: 191–208.

Verge VM, Richardson PM, Benoit R, Riopelle RJ (1989) Histochemical characterization of sensory neurons with high-affinity receptors for nerve growth factor. J Neurocytol 18: 583–591.

Verge VM, Richardson PM, Wiesenfeld-Hallin Z, Hokfelt T (1995) Differential influence of nerve growth factor on neuropeptide expression in vivo: a novel role in peptide suppression in adult sensory neurons. J Neurosci 15: 2081–2096.

Verma P, Chierzi S, Codd AM, Campbell DS, Meyer RL, Holt CE, Fawcett JW (2005) Axonal protein synthesis and degradation are necessary for efficient growth cone regeneration. J Neurosci 25: 331–342.

Vogelaar CF, Gervasi NM, Gumy LF, Story DJ, Raha-Chowdhury R, Leung KM, Holt CE, Fawcett JW (2009) Axonal mRNAs: characterisation and role in the growth and regeneration of dorsal root ganglion axons and growth cones. Mol Cell Neurosci 42: 102–115.

Vogelezang MG, Scherer SS, Fawcett JW, ffrench-Constant C (1999) Regulation of fibronectin alternative splicing during peripheral nerve repair. J Neurosci Res 56: 323–333.

Vogelezang MG, Liu ZQ, Relvas JB, Raivich G, Scherer SS, ffrench-Constant C (2001) α4 Integrin is expressed during peripheral nerve regeneration and enhances neurite outgrowth. J Neurosci 21: 6732–6744.

Voinesco F, Glauser L, Kraftsik R, Barakat-Walter I (1998) Local administration of thyroid hormones in silicone chamber increases regeneration of rat transected sciatic nerve. Exp Neurol 150: 69–81.

Volosin M, Trotter C, Cragnolini A, Kenchappa RS, Light M, Hempstead BL, Carter BD, Friedman WJ (2008) Induction of proneurotrophins and activation of p75NTR-mediated apoptosis via neurotrophin receptor-interacting factor in hippocampal neurons after seizures. J Neurosci 28: 9870–9879.

Vuorinen V, Siironen J, Röyttä M (1995) Axonal regeneration into chronically denervated distal stump. 1. Electron microscope studies. Acta Neuropathol (Berl) 89: 209–218.

Vuppalanchi D, Willis DE, Twiss JL (2009) Regulation of mRNA transport and translation in axons. Results Probl Cell Differ 48: 193–224.

Vyas A, Li Z, Aspalter M, Feiner J, Hoke A, Zhou C, O'Daly A, Abdullah M, Rohde C, Brushart TM (2010) An in vitro model of adult mammalian nerve repair. Exp Neurol 223: 112–118.

Waller A (1850) Experiments on the section of the glossopharyngeal and hypoglossal nerves of the frog, and observations of the alterations produced thereby in the structure of their primitive fibers. Phil Trans Roy Soc Lond 140: 423–429.

Wallquist W, Patarroyo M, Thams S, Carlstedt T, Stark B, Cullheim S, Hammarberg H (2002) Laminin chains in rat and human peripheral nerve: Distribution and regulation during development and after axonal injury. J.Comp.Neurol. 454: 284–293.

Wallquist W, Zelano J, Plantman S, Kaufman SJ, Cullheim S, Hammarberg H (2004) Dorsal root ganglion neurons up-regulate the expression of laminin-associated integrins after peripheral but not central axotomy. J Comp Neurol 480: 162–169.

Wallquist W, Plantman S, Thams S, Thyboll J, Kortesmaa J, Lännergren J, Domogatskaya A, Ogren SO, Risling M, Hammarberg H, Tryggvason K, Cullheim S (2005) Impeded interaction between Schwann cells and axons in the absence of laminin α4. J Neurosci 25: 3692–3700.

Walter MA, Kurouglu R, Caulfield JB, Vasconez LO, Thompson JA (1993) Enhanced peripheral nerve regeneration by acidic fibroblast growth factor. Lymphokine Cytokine Res 12: 135–141.

Wang GY, Hirai KI, Shimada H (1992a) The role of laminin, a component of Schwann cell basal lamina, in rat sciatic nerve regeneration within antiserum-treated nerve grafts. Brain Res 570: 116–125.

Wang GY, Hirai KI, Shimada H, Taji S, Zhong SZ (1992b) Behavior of axons, Schwann cells and perineurial cells in nerve regeneration within transplanted nerve grafts: effects of anti-laminin and anti-fibronectin antisera. Brain Res 583: 216–226.

Wang KC, Kim JA, Sivasankaran R, Segal R, He ZG (2002) p75 interacts with the Nogo receptor as a co-receptor for Nogo, MAG and OMgp. Nature 420: 74–78.

Wang KH, Brose K, Arnott D, Kidd T, Goodman CS, Henzel W, Tessier-Lavigne M (1999) Biochemical purification of a mammalian slit protein as a positive regulator of sensory axon elongation and branching. Cell 96: 771–784.

Wang L, Lee HK, Seo IA, Shin YK, Lee KY, Park HT (2009) Cell type-specific STAT3 activation by gp130-related cytokines in the peripheral nerves. Neuroreport 20: 663–668.

Wang PY, Koishi K, McLennan IS (2007) BMP6 is axonally transported by motoneurons and supports their survival in vitro. Mol Cell Neurosci 34: 653–661.

Wang SG, Cai Q, Hou JW, Bei JZ, Zhang T, Yang J, Wan YQ (2003) Acceleration effect of basic fibroblast growth factor on the regeneration of peripheral nerve through a 15-mm gap. J Biomed Mater Res 66A:522–531.

Wang YL, Wang DZ, Nie X, Lei DL, Liu YP, Zhang YJ, Suwa F, Tamada Y, Fang YR, Jin Y (2007) The role of bone morphogenetic protein-2 in vivo in regeneration of peripheral nerves. Br J Oral Maxillofac Surg 45(3): 197–202.

Watanabe K, Tamamaki N, Furuta T, Ackerman SL, Ikenaka K, Ono K (2006) Dorsally derived netrin 1 provides an inhibitory cue and elaborates the "waiting period" for primary sensory axons in the developing spinal cord. Development 133: 1379–1387.

Watson DF, Hoffman PN, Fittro KP, Griffin JW (1989) Neurofilament and tubulin transport slows along the course of mature motor axons. Brain Res 477: 225–232.

Watson FL, Heerssen HM, Moheban DB, Lin MZ, Sauvageot CM, Bhattacharyya A, Pomeroy SL, Segal RA (1999) Rapid nuclear responses to target-derived neurotrophins require retrograde transport of ligand-receptor complex. J Neurosci 19: 7889–7900.

Webber CA, Xu Y, Vanneste KJ, Martinez JA, Verge VM, Zochodne DW (2008) Guiding adult mammalian sensory axons during regeneration. J Neuropathol Exp Neurol 67: 212–222.

Weinberg HJ, Spencer PS (1978) The fate of Schwann cells isolated from axonal contact. J Neurocytol 7: 555–569.

Wen ZX, Zheng JQ (2006) Directional guidance of nerve growth cones. Curr Opin Neurobiol 16: 52–58.

Werner A, Willem M, Jones LL, Kreutzberg GW, Mayer U, Raivich G (2000) Impaired axonal regeneration in α7 integrin-deficient mice. J Neurosci 20: 1822–1830.

Whitworth IH, Brown RA, Dore C, Green CJ, Terenghi G (1995) Orientated mats of fibronectin as a conduit material for use in peripheral nerve repair. J Hand Surg [Br Eur] 20B: 429–436.

Whitworth IH, Brown RA, Dore CJ, Anand P, Green CJ, Terenghi G (1996) Nerve growth factor enhances nerve regeneration through fibronectin grafts. J Hand Surg [Br Eur] 21B: 514–522.

Widerberg A, Lundborg G, Dahlin LB (2001) Nerve regeneration enhancement by tourniquet. J Hand Surg [Br Eur] 26: 347–351.

Wiesenfeld-Hallin Z, Bartfai T, Hokfelt T (1992) Galanin in sensory neurons in the spinal cord. Front Neuroendocrinol 13: 319–343.

Wiklund P, Ekstrom PA, Edstrom A (2002) Mitogen-activated protein kinase inhibition reveals differences in signalling pathways activated by neurotrophin-3 and other growth-stimulating conditions of adult mouse dorsal root ganglia neurons. J Neurosci Res 67: 62–68.

Williams EJ, Furness J, Walsh FS, Doherty P (1994) Activation of the FGF receptor underlies neurite outgrowth stimulated by L1, N-CAM, and N-cadherin. Neuron 13: 583–594.

Williams KL, Rahimtula M, Mearow KM (2005) Hsp27 and axonal growth in adult sensory neurons in vitro. BMC Neurosci 6: 24.

Williams KL, Rahimtula M, Mearow KM (2006) Heat shock protein 27 is involved in neurite extension and branching of dorsal root ganglion neurons in vitro. J Neurosci Res 84: 716–723.

Willis DE, van Niekerk EA, Sasaki Y, Mesngon M, Merianda TT, Williams GG, Kendall M, Smith DS, Bassell GJ, Twiss JL (2007) Extracellular stimuli specifically regulate localized levels of individual neuronal mRNAs. J Cell Biol 178: 965–980.

Wilson-Gerwing TD, Johnston JM, Verge VM (2009) p75 neurotrophin receptor is implicated in the ability of neurotrophin-3 to negatively modulate activated ERK1/2 signaling in TrkA-expressing adult sensory neurons. J Comp Neurol 516: 49–58.

Witzel C, Rohde C, Brushart TM (2005) Pathway sampling by regenerating peripheral axons. J Comp Neurol 485: 183–190.

Wolman MA, Liu Y, Tawarayama H, Shoji W, Halloran MC (2004) Repulsion and attraction of axons by Semaphorin3D are mediated by different neuropilins in vivo. J Neurosci 24: 8428–8435.

Wong ST, Henley JR, Kanning KC, Huang KH, Bothwell M, Poo M (2002) A p75NTR and Nogo receptor complex mediates repulsive signaling by myelin-associated glycoprotein. Nat Neurosci 5: 1302–1308.

Woodhoo A, Alonso MB, Droggiti A, Turmaine M, D'Antonio M, Parkinson DB, Wilton DK, Al-Shawi R, Simons P, Shen J, Guillemot F, Radtke F, Meijer D, Feltri ML, Wrabetz L, Mirsky R, Jessen KR (2009) Notch controls embryonic Schwann cell differentiation, postnatal myelination and adult plasticity. Nat Neurosci 12: 839–847.

Woolf CJ, Salter MW (2000) Neuronal plasticity: increasing the gain in pain. Science 288: 1765–1769.

Wrana JL, Attisano L, Carcamo J, Zentella A, Doody J, Laiho M, Wang XF, Massague J (1992) TGF beta signals through a heteromeric protein kinase receptor complex. Cell 71: 1003–1014.

Wright DE, White FA, Gerfen RW, Silos-Santiago I, Snider WD (1995) The guidance molecule semaphorin III is expressed in regions of spinal cord and periphery avoided by growing sensory axons. J Comp Neurol 361: 321–333.

Wright MC, Son YJ (2007) Ciliary neurotrophic factor is not required for terminal sprouting and compensatory reinnervation of neuromuscular synapses: re-evaluation of CNTF null mice. Exp Neurol 205: 437–448.

Wu D, Zhang Y, Bo X, Huang W, Xiao F, Zhang X, Miao T, Magoulas C, Subang MC, Richardson PM (2007) Actions of neuropoietic cytokines and cyclic AMP in regenerative conditioning of rat primary sensory neurons. Exp Neurol 204: 66–76.

Wu KY, Hengst U, Cox LJ, Macosko EZ, Jeromin A, Urquhart ER, Jaffrey SR (2005) Local translation of RhoA regulates growth cone collapse. Nature 436: 1020–1024.

Wu WT, Li LX, Yick LW, Chai H, Xie YY, Yang Y, Prevette DM, Oppenheim RW (2003) GDNF and BDNF alter the expression of neuronal NOS, c-Jun, and p75 and prevent motoneuron death following spinal root avulsion in adult rats. J Neurotrauma 20: 603–612.

Xu QG, Forden J, Walsh SK, Gordon T, Midha R (2009) Motoneuron survival after chronic and sequential peripheral nerve injuries in the rat. J Neurosurg 112: 890–899.

Xu XY, Yee WC, Hwang PYK, Yu H, Wan ACA, Gao SJ, Boon KL, Mao HQ, Leong KW, Wang S (2003) Peripheral nerve regeneration with sustained release of poly(phosphoester) microencapsulated nerve growth factor within nerve guide conduits. Biomaterials 24: 2405–2412.

Yamada Y, Shimizu K, Nitta A, Soumiya H, Fukumitsu H, Furukawa S (2004) Axonal regrowth downregulates the synthesis of glial cell line-derived neurotrophic factor in the lesioned rat sciatic nerve. Neurosci Lett 364: 11–15.

Yamashita T, Tucker KL, Barde YA (1999) Neurotrophin binding to the p75 receptor modulates Rho activity and axonal outgrowth. Neuron 24: 585–593.

Yamashita T, Higuchi H, Tohyama M (2002) The p75 receptor transduces the signal from myelin-associated glycoprotein to Rho. J Cell Biol 157: 565–570.

Yamashita T, Tohyama M (2003) The p75 receptor acts as a displacement factor that releases Rho from Rho-GDI. Nat Neurosci 6: 461–467.

Yamashita T, Fujitani M, Yamagishi S, Hata K, Mimura F (2005) Multiple signals regulate axon regeneration through the Nogo receptor complex. Mol Neurobiol 32: 105–111.

Yan Q, Matheson C, Lopez O (1995) In vivo neurotrophic effects of GDNF on neonatal and adult facial motoneurons. Nature 373: 341–344.

Yanagida H, Tanaka J, Maruo S (1999) Immunocytochemical localization of a cell adhesion molecule, integrin alpha5beta1, in nerve growth cones. J Orthop Sci 4: 353–360.

Yang DP, Zhang DP, Mak KS, Bonder DE, Pomeroy SL, Kim HA (2008) Schwann cell proliferation during Wallerian degeneration is not necessary for regeneration and remyelination of the peripheral nerves: axon-dependent removal of newly generated Schwann cells by apoptosis. Mol Cell Neurosci 38: 80–88.

Yang LX, Nelson PG (2004) Glia cell line-derived neurotrophic factor regulates the distribution of acetylcholine receptors in mouse primary skeletal muscle cells. Neuroscience 128: 497–509.

Yao M, Moir MS, Wang MZ, To MP, Terris DJ (1999) Peripheral nerve regeneration in CNTF knockout mice. Laryngoscope 109: 1263–1268.

Yates JM, Smith KG, Robinson PP (2004) The effect of brain-derived neurotrophic factor on sensory and autonomic function after lingual nerve repair. Exp Neurol 190: 495–505.

Yazawa S, Ikeda A, Kaji R, Terada K, Nagamine T, Toma K, Kubori T, Kimura J, Shibasaki H (1999) Abnormal cortical processing of voluntary muscle relaxation in patients with focal hand dystonia studied by movement-related potentials. Brain 122: 1357–1366.

Yeiser EC, Rutkoski NJ, Naito A, Inoue J, Carter BD (2004) Neurotrophin signaling through the p75 receptor is deficient in traf6-/- mice. J Neurosci 24: 10521–10529.

Yin Q, Kemp GJ, Yu LG, Wagstaff SC, Frostick SP (2001) Neurotrophin-4 delivered by fibrin glue promotes peripheral nerve regeneration. Muscle & Nerve 24: 345–351.

Yoo S, van Niekerk EA, Merianda TT, Twiss JL (2009) Dynamics of axonal mRNA transport and implications for peripheral nerve regeneration. Exp Neurol 223: 19–27.

You SJ, Petrov T, Chung PH, Gordon T (1997) The expression of the low affinity nerve growth factor receptor in long-term denervated Schwann cells. Glia 20: 87–100.

Young C, Miller E, Nicklous DM, Hoffman JR (2001) Nerve growth factor and neurotrophin-3 affect functional recovery following peripheral nerve injury differently. Restor Neurol Neurosci 18: 167–175.

Young JZ (1949) Factors influencing the regeneration of nerves. Advances in Surgery 11: 165–220.

Yu T, Scully S, Yu YB, Fox GM, Jing SQ, Zhou RP (1998) Expression of GDNF family receptor components during development: implications in the mechanisms of interaction. J Neurosci 18: 4684–4696.

Yuan J, Lipinski M, Degterev A (2003) Diversity in the mechanisms of neuronal cell death. Neuron 40: 401–413.

Yuan QJ, Hu B, So KF, Wu WT (2006) Age-related reexpression of p75 in axotomized motoneurons. Neuroreport 17: 711–715.

Yuen EC, Howe CL, Li YW, Holtzman DM, Mobley WC (1996) Nerve growth factor and the neurotrophic factor hypothesis. Brain Dev 18: 362–368.

Zhai Q, Wang J, Kim A, Liu Q, Watts R, Hoopfer E, Mitchison T, Luo L, He Z (2003) Involvement of the ubiquitin-proteasome system in the early stages of Wallerian degeneration. Neuron 39: 217–225.

Zhang J, Oswald TM, Lineaweaver WC, Chen Z, Zhang G, Chen Z, Zhang F (2003) Enhancement of rat sciatic nerve regeneration by fibronectin and laminin through a silicone chamber. J Reconstr Microsurg 19: 467–472.

Zhang JY, Luo XG, Xian CJ, Liu ZH, Zhou XF (2000) Endogenous BDNF is required for myelination and regeneration of injured sciatic nerve in rodents. Eur J Neurosci 12: 4171–4180.

Zhang Y, Dijkhuizen PA, Anderson PN, Lieberman AR, Verhaagen J (1998) NT-3 delivered by an adenoviral vector induces injured dorsal root axons to regenerate into the spinal cord of adult rats. J Neurosci Res 54: 554–562.

Zhao Q, Kerns JM (1994) Effects of predegeneration on nerve regeneration through silicone Y-chambers. Brain Res 633: 97–104.

Zheng JQ, Felder M, Connor JA, Poo M (1994) Turning of nerve growth cones induced by neurotransmitters. Nature 368: 140–144.

Zheng JQ, Kelly TK, Chang BS, Ryazantsev S, Rajasekaran AK, Martin KC, Twiss JL (2001) A functional role for intra-axonal protein synthesis during axonal regeneration from adult sensory neurons. J Neurosci 21: 9291–9303.

Zhong J, Dietzel ID, Wahle P, Kopf M, Heumann R (1999) Sensory impairments and delayed regeneration of sensory axons in interleukin-6-deficient mice. J Neurosci 19: 4305–4313.

Zhou FQ, Zhou J, Dedhar S, Wu YH, Snider WD (2004) NGF-induced axon growth is mediated by localized inactivation of GSK-3beta and functions of the microtubule plus end binding protein APC. Neuron 42: 897–912.

Zhou FQ, Snider WD (2006) Intracellular control of developmental and regenerative axon growth. Philos Trans R Soc Lond B Biol Sci 361: 1575–1592.

Zhou FQ, Walzer M, Wu YH, Zhou J, Dedhar S, Snider WD (2006) Neurotrophins support regenerative axon assembly over CSPGs by an ECM-integrin-independent mechanism. J Cell Sci 119: 2787–2796.

Zhou Q, Cummings RD (1990) The S-type lectin from calf heart tissue binds selectively to the carbohydrate chains of laminin. Arch Biochem Biophys 281: 27–35.

Zhou XF, Rush RA (1996) Endogenous brain-derived neurotrophic factor is anterogradely transported in primary sensory neurons. Neuroscience 74: 945–951.

Zicha D, Dobbie IM, Holt MR, Monypenny J, Soong DY, Gray C, Dunn GA (2003) Rapid actin transport during cell protrusion. Science 300: 142–145.

Zimmerman UJ, Schlaepfer WW (1982) Characterization of a brain calcium-activated protease that degrades neurofilament proteins. Biochemistry 21: 3977–3982.

Zochodne DW, Cheng C (2000) Neurotrophins and other growth factors in the regenerative milieu of proximal nerve stump tips. J Anat 196: 279–283.

Zochodne DW, Cheng C, Miampamba M, Hargreaves K, Sharkey KA (2001) Peptide accumulations in proximal endbulbs of transected axons. Brain Res 902: 40–50.

Zou H, Ho C, Wong K, Tessier-Lavigne M (2009) Axotomy-induced Smad1 activation promotes axonal growth in adult sensory neurons. J Neurosci 29: 7116–7123.

Zuo J, Hernandez YJ, Muir D (1998) Chondroitin sulfate proteoglycan with neurite-inhibiting activity is up-regulated following peripheral nerve injury. J Neurobiol 34: 41–54.

Zuo J, Neubauer D, Graham J, Krekoski CA, Ferguson TA, Muir D (2002) Regeneration of axons after nerve transection repair is enhanced by degradation of chondroitin sulfate proteoglycan. Exp Neurol 176: 221–228.

Zou T, Ling CC, Xiao Y, Tao XM, Ma D, Chen ZL, Strickland S, Song HY (2006) Exogenous tissue plasminogen activator enhances peripheral nerve regeneration and functional recovery after injury in mice. J Neuropathol Exp Neurol 65: 78–86.

Zweifel LS, Kuruvilla R, Ginty DD (2005) Functions and mechanisms of retrograde neurotrophin signalling. Nat Rev Neurosci 6: 615–625.

10

SPECIFICITY IN NERVE REGENERATION

THE POTENTIAL exists for regeneration specificity at several levels within the peripheral nervous system: tissue, nerve trunk, sensory/motor, topographic, and end organ. Specificity may be generated by mechanical alignment of nerve stumps, contact recognition, neurotropism, or neurotrophism. Tissue specificity directs the growth of large numbers of axons as a group; neurotropism is likely to be the underlying mechanism. The existence of specificity at the nerve trunk level is debated, with electrophysiologic experiments in favor and axon counts against. Sensory/motor specificity results in preferential motor reinnervation (PMR), the tendency for motor axons regenerating in mixed nerve to reinnervate motor pathways and/or muscle. PMR is likely to result from initially random reinnervation of muscle and cutaneous nerve by motoneuron collaterals, followed by selective pruning of incorrect collaterals from cutaneous nerve and continued support of those in muscle nerve. PMR is more prominent in young animals and when motor axons are permitted to reinnervate muscle. PMR in response to muscle nerve alone, without muscle contact, has been demonstrated reproducibly in young rats; in adults, pathway specificity has been confirmed in some model systems but not in others. Within the motor system, topographic specificity can be enhanced by mechanical alignment of nerve stumps, but is not an inherent property of regeneration except during the experimental reinnervation of segmental muscles. Fast and slow muscles are usually reinnervated on a random basis in adults, although more specific reinnervation may occur in juveniles. There is no evidence for topographic specificity in cutaneous reinnervation. The majority of sensory end organ reinnervation appears to be random, although evidence of selective reinnervation of tendon organs by Ib afferents has been presented. There is currently insufficient experimental or clinical evidence to suggest that inherent topographic or end organ specificity has a positive influence on the outcome of nerve repair in humans.

INTRODUCTION

This chapter reviews the evidence for and against pathway and target specificity during peripheral axon regeneration. The types of specificity that would be required to restore normal function can be organized in a theoretical framework, progressing from gross through progressively finer distinctions (Brushart, 1988, 1991) (Figure 10-1). Specificity at the tissue level is characterized by the preferential growth of axons into nerve as opposed to other tissues, such as tendon, muscle, or bone. The next level at which pathfinding decisions could be made is at the nerve trunk, for instance a choice between the tibial and peroneal branches of the sciatic nerve. Within mixed nerve, sensory/motor specificity would be needed to separate afferent and efferent fibers, and thus determine the makeup of individual sensory and motor tributaries. Finally, within both sensory and motor systems, axons need to exhibit topographic and end organ specificity. Topographic specificity requires that axons return to the individual muscle or patch of skin that they innervated before they were injured. End organ specificity involves reinnervation of the correct type of sensory receptor within the sensory system, and the correct fiber type in the motor system. The distinction between topographic and end organ specificity cannot be absolute, as end organs may be limited in their distribution to a specific topographic area.

Several mechanisms have been described that could theoretically influence the specificity of peripheral axon regeneration (Figure 10-2). The mechanical control of specificity, physically aligning axons in the proximal and distal nerve stumps to maximize the chances of appropriate reinnervation,

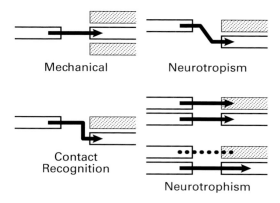

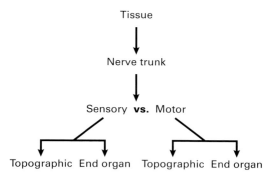

FIGURE 10-1 Organizational levels within the peripheral nervous system at which regeneration specificity could theoretically occur.

FIGURE 10-2 Potential mechanisms of specificity generation. Mechanical alignment of proximal and distal nerve stumps increases the chances that regenerating axons will enter functionally appropriate Schwann cell tubes in the distal stump. Contact recognition requires that an axon randomly sample multiple Schwann cell tubes, then enter one with an appropriate molecular signature. Neurotropism involves directed growth of an axon up a concentration gradient to reinnervate the Schwann cell tube producing the tropic substance. Neurotrophism provides support for axons or axon collaterals in appropriate pathways, and leads to the pruning of axons or collaterals in inappropriate pathways that do not receive that support.

is the self-assigned task of the surgeon. Fortunately, as this approach has had only limited success, there are other physiologic mechanisms that might be harnessed to influence regeneration specificity. These mechanisms can function only if the growth cone has access to multiple distal Schwann cell tubes (Figure 9-12). Contact recognition would require a growth cone to explore the cut edge of the distal stump, to recognize an appropriate molecular signature on Schwann cells or basal lamina, and to enter and course distally within the labeled Schwann cell tube. Whereas the exploration leading to contact recognition is presumably random, neurotropism requires growth that is directed precisely. Growth cones might detect a gradient of a diffusable factor, regenerate up that gradient, and reinnervate the Schwann cell tube from which the factor emanated. Both contact recognition and neurotropism would result in the immediate reinnervation of correct Schwann cell tubes. Neurotrophism, in contrast, is a more gradual process. Axons could enter distal Schwann cell tubes on a random basis. Those entering a correct pathway, or reinnervating an appropriate end organ, would receive trophic (nutritive) support in the form of growth factors. These axons would increase in size and become well myelinated, while those in pathways that failed to produce the required growth factor would be resorbed. Neurotrophism could be potentiated by the formation of multiple sprouts from each regenerating axon; if one sprout received the correct trophic support, it would survive at the expense of its siblings. This mechanism of sampling multiple pathways, then choosing one, would require the expenditure of far more energy and material than the others, but could increase the probability that a regenerating axon would eventually reinnervate an appropriate Schwann cell tube.

TISSUE SPECIFICITY

The possibility that regenerating axons could identify and grow toward nervous rather than other tissue—tissue specificity—was first explored in the context of debate over the existence of neurotropism. The earliest experiments to shed light on tissue specificity were performed by Forssman, who demonstrated that regenerating rat sciatic axons grew toward pieces of brain, but away from pieces of liver (Forssman, 1898). He attributed this selective attraction to elaboration of a neurotropic substance by degenerating myelin. Substantial experimental evidence of the selective reinnervation of nerve was also provided by Ramon y Cajal in his seminal work *Degeneration and Regeneration of the Nervous System* (Ramon y Cajal, 1928).

The theory of neurotropism was subsequently attacked by Weiss and Taylor (1944), who used a rat aortic graft in the shape of an inverted "Y" in an attempt to give regenerating rat sciatic axons equal access to nerve and tendon (Figure 10-3). In the two specimens with this construct that were examined, neural growth was equal to both tissues. These and similar experiments led Weiss and Taylor to conclude that regenerating axons could not be guided by neurotropic influences, a view that remained unchallenged until Goran Lundborg revived the debate 40 years later. To avoid the potentially confounding effects of vascular endothelium and inflammatory reaction to an allograft that may have influenced the Weiss and Taylor experiments, Lundborg substituted an inert silicon "Y" chamber for the aortic allograft and found clear evidence for preferential growth of axons toward nerve (Figure 10-3) (Lundborg et al., 1986). These results

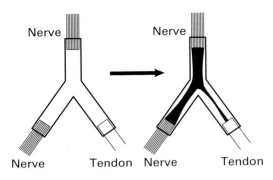

FIGURE 10-3   Experiments designed to elicit evidence of regeneration specificity at the tissue level. A silicon chamber in the form of an inverted "Y" ensures that axons entering the chamber will have equal access to nerve and a second tissue, in this case tendon, in the distal legs of the "Y." Once regeneration has occurred, as shown on the right, all or the majority of axons will have grown back to nerve as opposed to the other tissue.

were confirmed in a similar silicon chamber model (Mackinnon et al., 1986). It was subsequently found that tissue specificity was evident even when Weiss and Taylor's experiments were replicated precisely, casting further doubt on the original findings (Ochi et al., 1992). More recent work on tissue specificity has shown that NGF is not the factor responsible for the neurotropic guidance of axons from one nerve to another (Doubleday, Robinson 1995), and that Schwann cells may have a significant role in the guidance process (Abernethy et al. 1992).

NERVE TRUNK SPECIFICITY

In 1946 Paul Weiss returned to the rat aortic "Y" graft model to determine if muscle was reinnervated preferentially by its own nerve (Weiss, Hoag, 1946). In this case the Y was upright, with both tibial and peroneal fascicles providing axons proximally, but only the denervated stump of the tibial nerve as a target distally. After 4 months of regeneration, neither fascicle was found to have a competitive advantage over the other in reinnervating the distal tibial stump.

In the modern era, the inverted silicon "Y" chamber has been used by several investigators to explore the potential for regeneration specificity at the nerve trunk level (Figure 10-4). Ideally, the model provides either tibial or peroneal nerve axons in the inflow portal with equal access to both distal stumps

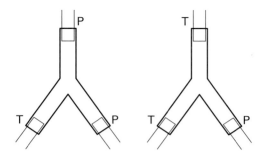

FIGURE 10-4   The same type of inverted "Y" tube used to demonstrate tissue specificity has been used in attempts to elicit specificity at the level of the nerve trunk. Axons regenerating from the rat tibial or peroneal sciatic fascicle are given equal access to the tibial and peroneal fascicles distally. The results of these experiments have varied widely as discussed in the text.

in the outflow portals. The initial experiments performed by Politis (1985) produced overwhelming evidence in favor of nerve trunk specificity, with no axons whatsoever in the inappropriate distal stump in 6/7 cases with regenerating peroneal axons and in 6/7 with regenerating tibial axons. Zhao et al. (1992a) evaluated similar experiments electrophysiologically and found that the force exerted by the tibialis anterior muscle was significantly greater when it had been reinnervated by the native peroneal nerve, whereas the gastrocnemius was strongest when reinnervated by its native tibial nerve. In separate experiments evaluated only by the size of the cables projecting to the distal tibial and peroneal stumps, they found that specificity was evident only when axons were permitted to reinnervate muscle, suggesting that the pathway itself contributed little to specificity at the nerve trunk level (Zhao et al., 1992c). In sharp disagreement with these findings, those who evaluated outcome on the basis of axon counts found no evidence of specificity (Abernethy et al., 1992; Iwabuchi et al., 1999). Clearly, no authors subsequent to Politis have found all-or-none specificity at the level of the nerve trunk. Although the results of electrophysiologic testing and axon counts seem incongruous, they are not necessarily inconsistent. The former measured only motor function, and thus the regeneration specificity of motor axons within the nerve trunk. Given that motor axons are in the minority in both tibial and peroneal nerves, and that branching is not accounted for by axon counts, specificity of motor axon regeneration

could well exist in these experiments, but remain concealed within the far larger afferent fiber population.

The possibility of nerve trunk specificity can also be investigated by varying the orientation of proximal and distal tibial and peroneal fascicles within an enclosed gap. Initial experiments in which the fascicles were unconstrained led to the conclusion that reinnervation of the tibial fascicle was specific, but reinnervation of the peroneal fascicle was not (Evans et al., 1991). Examination of the construct, however, revealed that the larger tibial fascicles overlap within the tube irrespective of their orientation, whereas the proximal and distal ends of the smaller peroneal fascicles are far removed from one another when fascicular orientation is reversed (Figure 10-5). If the fascicles are aligned around a neutral midplane, the volume of regeneration is determined by fascicular size rather than by fascicular identity, providing no evidence for specificity at the fascicular level (Brushart et al., 1995).

It is not yet possible to state firmly that nerve trunk specificity does or does not exist. In practical terms, however, the inaccuracy of regeneration across an enclosed gap (Chapter 8) indicates that whatever specificity there may be, it is not robust enough to shape the outcome of routine gap repair.

SENSORY-MOTOR SPECIFICITY

Preferential Motor Reinnervation

Preferential motor reinnervation (PMR) is the tendency for motor axons regenerating in mixed nerve to reinnervate motor pathways and/or muscle. PMR was first demonstrated in the rat femoral nerve model by single labeling with horseradish peroxidase (HRP) (Brushart, 1988) (Figure 7-12). Even with the relative inefficiency of this technique, it was possible to show that PMR shaped regeneration in both juvenile and adult animals, that it was not defeated by misalignment of proximal and distal nerve stumps, and that it was not affected by imposing a short gap at the repair. These experiments were performed in the femoral nerve for several reasons described in more detail in Brushart (1988): (1) The femoral nerve bifurcates into terminal cutaneous and muscle branches that are evenly matched in terms of axon number and size, so they will present targets that are as morphologically equivalent as is biologically possible, (2) All motor axons are normally in the muscle branch, so any motoneurons reinnervating the cutaneous branch have made a

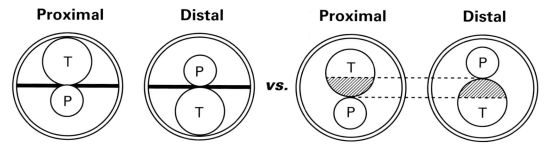

Proximal **Distal** **Proximal** **Distal**

vs.

FIGURE 10-5   The importance of model design when attempting to elicit regeneration specificity. The transected rat tibial and peroneal fascicles are inserted into the opposite ends of a silicon tube, leaving a gap of 5–10 mm that will be bridged by regenerating neural structure. The figures represent the alignment of the fascicles on cross section at either end of the tube. In the construct on the left, the distal fascicles have been rotated 180°. The tibial fascicle is much larger than the peroneal, so if the fascicles are not constrained a portion of the proximal tibial fascicle will be directly aligned with the tibial fascicle distally, facilitating some degree of regeneration specificity through mechanical alignment. The ends of the smaller peroneal fascicle, in contrast, are separated widely on either side of the tube. There is no overlap of proximal and distal peroneal fascicles, and thus no chance for specificity based on alignment alone. The results of these experiments were interpreted as showing fascicular specificity for the tibial fascicle, but not for the peroneal (Evans et al., 1991), an outcome that could have been determined by mechanical factors alone. In the construct on the right, the fascicles are oriented on either side of a neutral midplane to eliminate fascicular overlap and thus minimize the contribution of mechanical alignment to regeneration specificity. Altering the model in this way, it was shown that the destination of regenerating axons was controlled by the relative size of the distal stumps and not by any type of fascicular specificity. From Brushart et al., 1995.

pathfinding error, and can be quantified easily, and (3) At the site of nerve repair, proximally in the femoral trunk (Figure 7-11), sensory and motor axons intermingle within the nerve. As a result, motor axons that regenerate across the repair will have access to Schwann cell tubes leading both correctly to muscle and incorrectly to skin. The observation that purposeful misalignment of the nerve repair does not modify the outcome is consistent with a lack of functional topography within the nerve at this level. As a general rule, if purposeful misalignment of an experimental nerve repair modifies the outcome of regeneration, there is functional localization of axons within the nerve, and the nature of the repair itself becomes a variable in the experiment.

The effectiveness of the femoral nerve model was enhanced substantially by the introduction of simultaneous double labeling with HRP/Fluoro-Gold; the destination of all motoneurons regenerating in each nerve could be accounted for, and motoneurons that had projected collaterals into both cutaneous and muscle pathways could be identified (Brushart, 1990a). Two weeks after repair, equal numbers of motoneurons were labeled with

only HRP or Fluoro-Gold, and thus projected correctly to the muscle branch or incorrectly to the cutaneous branch (Figure 10-6). Additionally, nearly 100 motoneurons were double-labeled, or contained both tracers (Figure 6-3). These were neurons that had projected collaterals into both cutaneous and muscle branches. At later time periods, the progressive decrease in double labeling was coincident with a steady increase in the number of correct projections, suggesting the pruning hypothesis: *regenerating motor axons generate multiple collateral sprouts, which reinnervate previously sensory or motor Schwann cell tubes on a random basis. Over time, specific projections are generated by pruning collaterals from cutaneous pathways while maintaining those in muscle pathways. A motoneuron that initially samples both pathways is thus converted to one projecting correctly to muscle. Motoneurons limited to cutaneous pathways have no means of correcting their error, and their number remains relatively constant.*

The potential role of pruning in the generation of PMR might not have been detected had these experiments been performed in adult rats. In older animals PMR is still observed, but fewer motoneurons are double labeled, and there is no significant decline

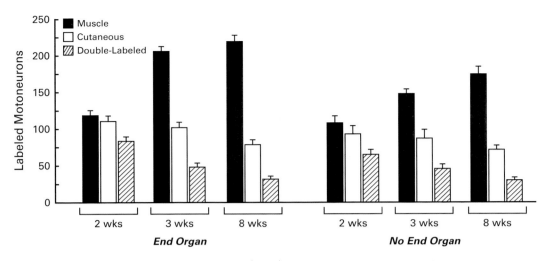

FIGURE 10-6   Preferential motor reinnervation (PMR). Motoneuron counts resulting from simultaneous double-labeling of the femoral cutaneous and muscle branches 2, 3, and 8 weeks after nerve repair. Surgeries were performed in 3-week-old female SD rats with the distal pathway intact (Left) or blocked off to prevent end-organ contact (Right). Each triad of vertical bars represents the mean count from 20 nerves. With the end organ present, initial regeneration is random, with equal numbers of motoneurons projecting correctly to muscle and incorrectly to skin at 2 weeks. By three weeks, however, the number of correct projections increases dramatically while the number of incorrect projections to skin is little changed. There is a further slight increase in the number of correct projections by 8 weeks. The number of double-labeled neurons, those with projections to both branches, decreases significantly at each time period. Axon collaterals are thus pruned from the cutaneous branch, increasing the number of correct projections at the expense of double-labeled neurons. This process is similar, although less pronounced, when end-organ contact is denied (Right). Regenerating motor axons are thus able to identify and respond to muscle nerve without the need to contact muscle.

in double labeling between 3 weeks and 3 months (Brushart et al., 1998). The pruning hypothesis is difficult to verify with currently available techniques. Dual projections only become evident when both collaterals have regenerated far down femoral cutaneous and muscle branches to the site of tracer application. Pruning that takes place in the femoral trunk or tributaries proximal to the labeling sites will escape detection, as will a collateral that extends as far as the labeling site but is pruned back between labeling intervals. It is possible, for instance, that pruning requires contact with a specific length of pathway; in an older, larger animal this length could be reached before collaterals reinnervate the distal tributaries. Simultaneous double labeling of different groups of animals at different times provides, in effect, snapshots of a very dynamic process that have been taken from a single perspective.

Subsequent experiments explored the biological underpinnings of PMR (Figures 10-6 and 10-7). In young animals, PMR was found to occur in response to the peripheral nerve pathway without the need for end organ contact. Juvenile motor axons are thus able to detect and respond to modality-specific cues in muscle nerve. Conditioning the neuron by crushing the sensory and motor branches 4 and 2 weeks before repair did not alter the outcome of regeneration, suggesting that PMR is not dependent on the growth state of the neuron (Brushart et al., 1998). Removing the femoral nerve as a graft and shifting it from one side of the animal to the other diminished the magnitude of PMR. This deterioration in specificity could be abrogated entirely, however, by predegenerating the graft to remove inhibitory components and upregulate growth factor expression. When grafts were exchanged among juvenile (1-month-old) and aged (10-month-old) rats, the age of the neuron emerged as the dominant factor, with young rats expressing substantial PMR in both young and old grafts (Le et al., 2001). Pathway was nonetheless important, as old animals could generate PMR through young grafts, but not through old grafts.

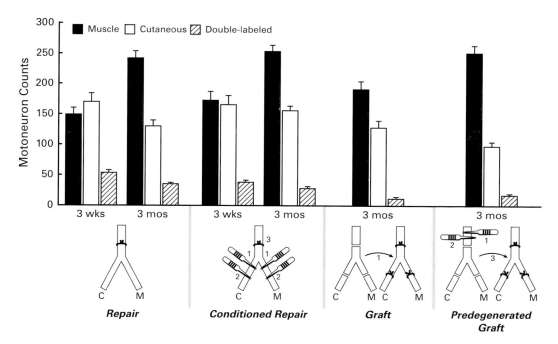

FIGURE 10-7   Motoneuron counts obtained by double labeling the muscle and cutaneous branches of the adult rat femoral nerve after various manipulations. After routine repair of the femoral trunk, motor axon regeneration is random at 3 weeks, but significant PMR has developed by 3 months. Conditioning the motoneurons by crushing the distal femoral branches before the repair does not enhance PMR. PMR is present but reduced when the opposite femoral nerve is used as a graft. Predegeneration of this graft, however, restores the number of regenerating motoneurons and the magnitude of PMR to normal levels.

The phenomenon of PMR has been confirmed in other laboratories by using retrograde tracing techniques in the rat (Madison et al. 1996; Al-Majed et al., 2000; Franz et al., 2005) and electrophysiologic techniques in the primate (Madison et al., 1999). Studies evaluated only with axon counts, in contrast, were interpreted as showing preferential growth of motor axons into sensory nerve (e.g., Maki 1991; Maki et al., 1996), a finding consistent with increased sprouting of motor axons in sensory pathways (Redett et al., 2005) (Figure 7-2).

Potential Mechanisms of Preferential Motor Reinnervation

Agreement as to the reproducibility of PMR was followed by a robust debate concerning the relative roles of the peripheral nerve pathway, the muscle end organ, and the parent motoneuron in its generation. A direct role for pathway involvement was demonstrated early on by the finding that PMR could be generated in young animals even when axons were prevented from contacting sensory or motor end organs (Brushart, 1993) (Figure 10-6). That motor axons can detect and respond to motor pathways in this age group was confirmed by experiments that reversed the orientation of the femoral sensory and motor branches (Brushart, 1993). Under these circumstances, significantly fewer motoneurons reinnervated muscle through the inappropriate cutaneous nerve than had done so previously through the appropriate muscle nerve. These experiments were repeated recently in adult Lewis rats, using fresh and predegenerated grafts of the entire femoral nerve trunk and its tributaries (Abdullah et al., 2010) (Figure 10-8). When freshly harvested grafts were used, PMR was not observed, and purposeful mismatch of pathway and end organ did not modify outcome. When grafts were predegenerated, in contrast, PMR was dramatic when grafts were oriented correctly, but was abolished by graft reversal, demonstrating a significant role for pathway identity in adult animals. Evidence for a motoneuron response to pathway identity was also

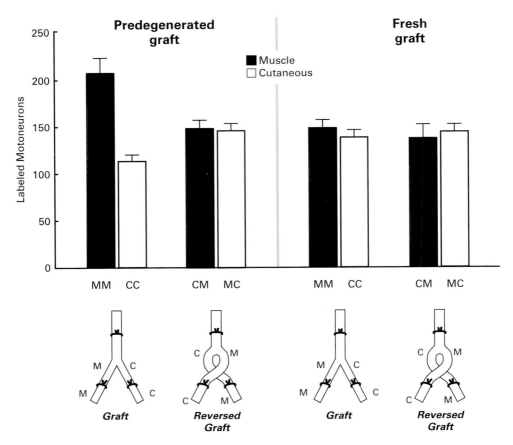

FIGURE 10-8 Adult motor axons recognize and respond to adult muscle pathways. Fresh and predegenerated grafts of the entire femoral nerve trunk and its tributaries were transferred to previously uninjured Lewis rats. Grafts were sewn in place in correct alignment, with the muscle branch leading to muscle and the cutaneous branch leading to skin, or with the alignment reversed, with the cutaneous branch leading to muscle and the muscle branch leading to skin. When freshly harvested grafts were used, PMR was not observed, and purposeful mismatch of pathway and end organ did not modify outcome. When grafts were predegenerated, in contrast, PMR was dramatic when grafts were oriented correctly, but was abolished by graft reversal. Pathway identity can thus play a substantial role in generating PMR in adult animals, but only after predegeneration has removed inhibitory debris and upregulated growth factors. (Abdullah et al., 2010).

provided by experiments that compared the number of collateral sprouts generated by each motoneuron in blocked cutaneous and muscle nerve (Redett et al., 2005) (Figure 7-2).

The potential for specific pathway identity has been explored more generally in the context of searching for grafts that facilitate muscle reinnervation. Although these investigations have focused on the ability of nerve to support motor axon regeneration, rather than on PMR per se, several have provided evidence of sensory/motor differences that could provide selective trophic support of motor axons in motor pathways. In the femoral nerve

model, reinnervation of femoral cutaneous or muscle nerve grafts by femoral motor branch axons (both sensory and motor) was similar at 2 weeks (Ghalib et al., 2001), whereas ventral root was twice as effective as cutaneous nerve in supporting motor axon regeneration as assayed by retrograde labeling at 3 weeks (Hoke et al., 2006). In the tibial nerve, 5-mm-long grafts of motor nerve were reinnervated by more axons at 3 weeks than were grafts of cutaneous nerve, irrespective of the number of cables used or the presence or absence of functioning Schwann cells, implicating a role for the basal lamina itself in promoting specificity

(Nichols et al., 2004; Moradzadeh et al., 2008). One additional study that was evaluated with retrograde labeling after one month revealed that motor neuron regeneration after root avulsion and nerve graft insertion within the anterior horn was superior if the graft was harvested from ventral root, as opposed to cutaneous nerve (Chu et al., 2008). It is difficult to assess motor axon regeneration with axon counts, as muscle nerve, and especially a nerve trunk such as the tibial, contains many afferent axons that cannot be differentiated from motor axons after 3–4 weeks of regeneration. Additionally, there is the issue of pathway-dependent sprouting discussed above. The retrograde labeling studies, both of which demonstrate improved motor axon regeneration in motor pathways, provide the most concrete evidence for modality-specific support of motor axon regeneration.

PMR is also linked to pathway identity by the preferential expression of the HNK-1 carbohydrate epitope in muscle nerve. An acidic glycan (3-sulfoglucuronyl β1-3-galactoside), HNK-1 binds to several of the neural recognition molecules described in Chapter 1 including NCAM, MAG, laminin, and P0 (reviewed in Kleene, Schachner, 2004). HNK-1 is expressed by Schwann cells in ventral root but not by those in dorsal root, and preferentially supports the growth of motor neurites in culture (Martini et al., 1992). In grafting experiments performed on the mouse femoral nerve, HNK-1 was expressed by Schwann cells in muscle nerve when they were reinnervated by motor, but not by sensory axons; expression by Schwann cells in cutaneous nerve was minimal under all circumstances (Martini et al., 1994). Subsequently, mice heterozygous for TrkB or BDNF were found to have less prominent HNK-1 expression, a reduction in PMR, and delayed functional recovery after femoral nerve repair (Eberhardt et al., 2006). In spite of these positive findings, other experimental evidence has failed to link HNK-1 expression with PMR. In the C57BL/6 mouse, the strain used in the initial experiments on HNK-1 expression (Martini et al., 1994), PMR is not evident after suture repair of the femoral nerve (Mears et al., 2003; Robinson, Madison, 2003; Simova et al., 2006). It is thus possible to have robust differences in HNK-1 expression between cutaneous and muscle nerve, but still no PMR. Similarly, administration of antibodies to HNK-1 resulted in substantial PMR when there was none in untreated animals, the opposite of what one would expect if HNK-1 played a critical role in generating PMR (Mears et al., 2003). Lastly, a peptide mimetic of HNK-1 was not found to enhance PMR over treatment with a scrambled control peptide (Simova et al., 2006). The role of HNK-1 in the generation of PMR thus awaits clarification.

The relative contributions of pathway and muscle to PMR have also been studied in a series of experiments in which the length of the femoral cutaneous and muscle branches was manipulated by transection and capping with a silicon tube (Robinson, Madison, 2004; Uschold et al., 2007). The authors concluded that the accuracy of motoneuron regeneration depended on the relative balance of trophic influences provided by pathways and end organs (Figure 10-9), and confirmed both the decline in

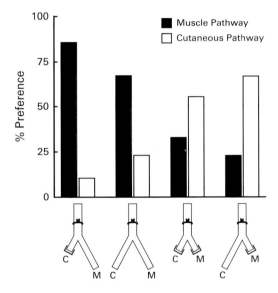

FIGURE 10-9 Motoneuron pathway preference after femoral nerve repair. The diagrams indicate a progression from the greatest preference for the muscle pathway when the cutaneous pathway is blocked, on the left, to the greatest preference for the cutaneous pathway when the muscle pathway is blocked, on the right. Intermediate values are obtained when neither pathway is interrupted, demonstrating PMR, and when both are blocked, favoring the cutaneous pathway. These experiments are interpreted to mean that relative pathway length, not identity, determines specificity. An alternative interpretation is that the block-off serves as a powerful stop signal that reroutes axons into the other, unblocked branch. Modified from Uschold et al., 2007.

PMR with aging and the paramount importance of the end organ as a trophic influence. Additionally, however, they rejected the concept of specific pathway identity, advancing in its place the hypothesis that the "relative level of trophic support" would determine how a regenerating motor axon responded to its environment. Another, equally valid interpretation of these experiments is that blocking a pathway not only denies access to a potentially positive influence, but adds a strikingly negative one, a stop signal that could have a far greater relative effect than the more subtle differences experienced by two axon collaterals as they regenerate, without hindrance, in cutaneous and muscle nerve. The closer this stop signal is to the nerve repair, the greater its effect, so that the preferential reinnervation of the opposite pathway could be seen as a negative response to the block-off, rather than as the result of comparing the magnitude of two positive effects.

The "relative level of support" hypothesis was pursued further in mice by increasing the relative size of the cutaneous nerve (Robinson, Madison, 2009) and by reducing the Schwann cell population in the distal pathways (Madison et al., 2009). After femoral nerve repair in transgenic mice that have a substantial increase in the size of the cutaneous nerve, most motoneurons reinnervate the cutaneous branch at early time periods, with the number of correct and incorrect projections equalizing by 8 weeks. This is interpreted as an initial active preference for the cutaneous nerve based on the volume of trophic support from the increased number of Schwann cells, followed by equalization as contact with muscle exerts its dominant influence. An alternative interpretation is that the initial "preference" for the cutaneous nerve is merely the consequence of mechanical factors. Before introduction of the femoral nerve as a model of regeneration specificity, the size and number of myelinated axons in the femoral cutaneous and muscle branches were evaluated in juvenile and adult rats to ensure their relative parity as targets for regenerating axons (Brushart, 1988). When the relative size of the cutaneous branch is increased, its axons make a bigger physical target on the cut surface of the distal nerve stump; one would expect random axon behavior to result in more motor axons entering the cutaneous nerve than would normally be the case. Motoneurons that have collaterals in both branches will correct this error when one collateral innervates muscle, as was seen by 8 weeks. Conversely, when the

number of Schwann cells was reduced in the distal nerve stumps, PMR proceeded normally in the intact femoral system, with normal numbers of motoneurons regenerating (Madison et al., 2009). Given that Schwann cells were not completely eliminated from the distal stumps, and that nothing is known about their phenotype, it is difficult to reach firm conclusions on the basis of this model.

The contribution of the motoneuron to specificity generation has been investigated in recent studies of the relationship between polysialic acid (PSA) expression and PMR (Franz et al., 2005, 2008). These authors found that PMR is absent in mice that express neither NCAM nor polysialic acid (PSA), and is abolished in wild type mice if PSA is removed enzymatically. The tendency for motoneurons to generate PMR was found to correlate with their ability to upregulate PSA after injury. Conversely, the number of motoneuron collateral sprouts and the ability to withdraw incorrect projections to cutaneous nerve were attenuated in mice lacking PSA. These elegant studies have emphasized the importance of giving equal consideration to all components of the regenerating system when attempting to understand its behavior.

A Mouse Is Not a Rat

PMR was first described in the rat (Brushart, 1988). A critical characteristic of the model was repair of the femoral nerve proximally, where cutaneous and motor axons intermingle, to avoid generating specificity by physically aligning concentrations of motor axons in proximal and distal nerve stumps. The validity of this strategy was demonstrated by the observation that purposeful misalignment of the nerve repair did not influence PMR. In the mouse, however, motor axons appear to be more localized within the femoral nerve than they are in the rat (Franz et al., 2005). The mouse also differs from the rat in the physical properties of its peripheral nerve; it is much harder to perform a suture repair in the mouse without significant mushrooming of the nerve stumps. Clearly, the conditions of nerve repair must be taken into account when interpreting the results of mouse PMR experiments.

In the mouse, suture repair at the proximal level used in the rat does not result in PMR (Mears et al., 2003; Robinson, Madison, 2003). The inability of PMR to overcome the relative axonal disorganization imposed by suture repair in the mouse thus differs from the robust response to intentional misalignment in the rat. Fibrin glue repair, a potentially less traumatic procedure, does result in PMR when performed at this level (Robinson, Madison, 2003). As discussed previously, when the nature of the repair determines regeneration specificity, mechanical factors are usually implicated. If suture repair is performed distally, where intraneural localization differs from that proximally, PMR results in spite of imprecise alignment of the nerve stumps (Franz et al., 2005). Differing outcomes of suture at two levels in the setting of known changes in intraneural organization again suggest that mechanical factors are at play.

The Present and Future of PMR

There is general agreement that PMR shapes the outcome of nerve repair, and that its influence diminishes with age. There is also agreement that contact with muscle is the most powerful stimulus to pruning of misdirected axon collaterals, and that PMR may be influenced additionally by the nerve pathway in young rats. The function of the pathway in older rats is still debated. In considering the evidence, experiments that vary minimally from those used routinely to demonstrate PMR should be given more weight than those requiring the introduction of manipulations that have been characterized incompletely. Pathway effects have been elicited by mismatching distal femoral muscle and cutaneous branches, altering only the axon population that reinnervates each distal pathway. Models used to deny pathway identity involve shortening nerve by adding a unilateral stop signal or killing an undefined population of Schwann cells, both maneuvers that introduce new variables with unknown consequences.

The ability of axons regenerating in adult animals to respond to pathway identity suggests significant therapeutic potential. Clinically, motor axons must often regenerate over distances of a foot or more, and will thus travel for months before they have the opportunity to establish muscle contact, the strongest impetus for collateral pruning. During this process growth factor production in the pathway decreases as Schwann cells are denervated for progressively longer periods (Chapter 9). Interventions that sustain Schwann cell activity might thus hasten the pruning of inappropriate motor axon collaterals and focus neuronal activity on the growth of the remaining correct projections.

MOTOR-TOPOGRAPHIC SPECIFICITY

The disordered function that follows regeneration of the human facial nerve (Kimura et al., 1975; Chapter 5), ulnar nerve (Thomas et al., 1987), and neonatal brachial plexus (Roth, 1983) are all consistent with a failure of topographic specificity in motor axon regeneration. Significant deterioration in the topographic specificity of motor reinnervation has been documented experimentally after repair of the adult rat sciatic (Bernstein, Guth, 1961; Brushart, Mesulam, 1980; Zhao et al., 1992b; Lago, Navarro, 2006), facial (Aldskogius, Thomander, 1986; Choi, Raisman, 2002), and intercostal nerves (Hardman, Brown, 1987), and after repair of the cat hypoglossal nerve (Mizuno et al., 1980) and lumbar roots (Ungar-Sargon, Goldberger, 1987). The reinnervation of segmental muscles, in contrast, provides evidence for topographic specificity at the root level. Adult muscles maintain rostrocaudal markers (Suzue et al., 1990; Donoghue et al., 1992), and can be reinnervated selectively by sympathetic and motor axons from appropriate segmental levels (Wigston, Sanes, 1982, 1985; Hardman, Brown, 1987; Laskowski, Sanes, 1988). This selectivity results from synaptic competition, with neuromuscular topography expressed as a gradient in nerve terminal size, and requires that the nerve lesion be close to muscle (Laskowski et al., 1998; Potluri et al., 2006). As human nerve lesions are usually far removed from their muscle targets, segmental specificity probably has little role in determining the response to nerve injuries in humans.

MOTOR–END ORGAN SPECIFICITY

In adult mammals, there is substantial evidence that fast and slow motor units are not reinnervated selectively by fast and slow motoneurons (Miledi, Stefani, 1969; Gillespie et al., 1986; Ostberg et al., 1986; Foehring et al., 1987), although evidence has also been presented in favor of some degree of specificity (Ip, Vrbova, 1983; Wang et al., 2002). Selectivity is demonstrated more readily in neonatal and juvenile animals (Hoh, 1975; Soileau et al., 1987), suggesting the presence of a developmental cue that is lost, or that axons become insensitive to as animals mature. Regeneration of gamma motoneurons is less robust that that of alpha and beta motoneurons, with significant reduction in both the speed of regeneration and in the number of motoneurons that reinnervate muscle spindles (Thulin, 1960; Takano, 1976; Brushart,

Mesulam, 1980; Wolf, English, 2000). Although regenerating gamma motor axons may return to appropriate locations within the spindle (DeSantis, Norman, 1993), muscle spindle function does not return to normal (Gregory et al., 1982; Banks et al., 1985).

SENSORY-TOPOGRAPHIC SPECIFICITY

False sensory localization is a frequent consequence of human median nerve injury and repair (Hawkins, 1948) (Figure 5-11), suggesting a lack of topographic specificity in the regeneration of afferent axons. This lack of specificity has been confirmed experimentally. After transection and repair of the cat femoral nerve, only 53% of type I fibers returned to the correct fascicle in the distal stump (Horch, 1979). In the rat, a recent sequential double labeling study of the specificity of cutaneous reinnervation found that the third digit was reinnervated correctly by L5 neurons 44–72% of the time, and by L4 neurons only 14–44% of the time (Puigdellívol-Sánchez et al., 2005). Lack of regeneration specificity is also indicated by a decrease or lack of somatotopic organization of the central projections of afferent fibers (Arvidsson, Johansson, 1988). The dorsal horn projection of afferents in the tibialis anterior muscle expands to include that of the peroneal-innervated skin after transection and repair of the peroneal nerve (Brushart et al., 1981) (Figure 10-10); when the entire sciatic nerve is repaired, it expands even further. In the femoral nerve, the percentage of muscle afferents that return to muscle rather than skin has been measured as 40% and 49% by using two different techniques of sequential double labeling (Madison et al., 1996; Brushart et al., 2004), again providing little evidence for topographic specificity.

SENSORY–END ORGAN SPECIFICITY

Conclusions regarding specific reinnervation of sensory end organs vary according to the model used. Cutaneous receptors are usually reinnervated by axons with conduction velocities and dorsal column projections similar to their native innervation after regeneration of the transected cat sural nerve (Burgess, Horch, 1973). This is not surprising, in that the sural nerve supplies a limited receptor population, making appropriate reinnervation fairly likely. In larger mixed nerve, where more types of receptor are represented, reinnervation is much

less specific. The most elegant studies to evaluate the specificity of receptor reinnervation combined electrophysiological characterization of individual receptors with neuroanatomical tracing to define their central projections (Koerber et al., 1989, 1994). Fifty-one percent of regenerated fibers reinnervated inappropriate receptors; mismatches included reinnervation of muscle receptors by cutaneous afferents and vice versa, reinnervation of low threshold cutaneous receptors by nociceptive afferents, and reinnervation of slowly adapting receptors by fibers that previously served rapidly adapting receptors. Given the variety of axons regenerating and the diversity of possible targets, however, the observation that one-half of the axons reached functionally appropriate end organs suggests that some specificity must be possible. In more focal studies of muscle reinnervation, muscle spindles were reinnervated randomly by appropriate Ia and inappropriate Ib afferents, while most tendon organs were reinnervated appropriately by Ib afferents (Munson et al., 1988; Collins et al., 1986).

POTENTIAL MECHANISMS OF SPECIFICITY GENERATION

Contact Recognition

Contact interactions are critical to the overall process of nerve regeneration, yet there are no proven examples in which an axon is able to recognize and selectively reinnervate a Schwann cell tube based on the activity of recognition molecules. There are, however, examples of adhesion molecules supporting the regeneration of a subset of neurons. A prime example is the HNK-1 carbohydrate discussed above. It is normally expressed in motor but only minimally in sensory pathways, and is upregulated selectively only when motor axons reenter previously motor Schwann cell tubes (Martini et al., 1994). In the sensory system, the α7 integrin, a receptor for laminin, is upregulated after sciatic nerve crush in medium-large diameter NF200+ neurons and in medium diameter CGRP+ neurons, but not in smaller neurons (Gardiner et al., 2005). The outgrowth of these neurons in vitro in response to NGF and NT-3 is reduced in the absence of α7 integrin signaling, yet their response to GDNF is unchanged. It is likely that more examples of specific interactions between defined axon populations and particular substrates will be discovered, increasing

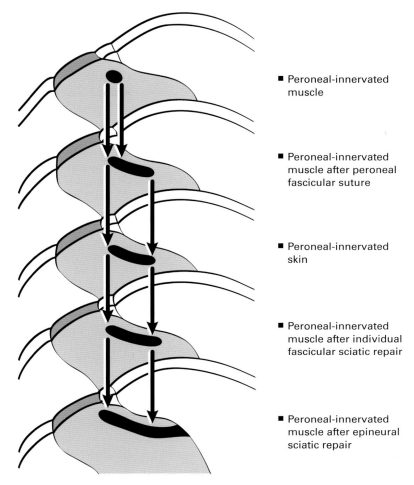

■ Peroneal-innervated
  muscle

■ Peroneal-innervated
  muscle after peroneal
  fascicular suture

■ Peroneal-innervated
  skin

■ Peroneal-innervated
  muscle after individual
  fascicular sciatic repair

■ Peroneal-innervated
  muscle after epineural
  sciatic repair

FIGURE 10-10   Dorsal horn projections of muscle innervated by the rat peroneal nerve. The central processes of primary sensory neurons project topographically to the dorsal horn of the spinal cord. The normal projection from peroneal-innervated muscle is quite narrow. This projection is much wider after epineurial repair of the sciatic nerve, reflecting reinnervation of peroneal muscle by axons from the tibial and sural fascicles. Individual fascicular sciatic suture narrows this projection significantly by providing mechanical control of topographic specificity at the fascicular level. This projection, however, is still much wider than that of normal peroneal-innervated muscle. This widening persists even if only the peroneal fascicle itself is transected and repaired. The widened projection overlaps with that of peroneal-innervated skin, demonstrating lack of control of topographic specificity within the fascicle itself.

the potential for purposeful manipulation of axon behavior.

Neurotropism

Ramon y Cajal believed that neurotropism could guide regeneration both at the tissue and end organ levels:

> We believe ... that the action exerted by the peripheral stump—the cells of Schwann,

etc.—on the growth of the young fibers is not individual and specific, that is, from tube to tube, but is general and collective, similarly directing the new axons towards the periphery ... Once the axons are near the terminal structures, no matter what their position in the distal segment, the terminal clubs are influenced by another neurotropic influence which now has an individual and specific character ... Among the specific orienting substances, those which appear especially necessary are those elaborated by the spindles of Kuhne and the musculotendinous structures of Golgi, and those also which are produced by the various categories of sensory organs of the skin and mucous membranes. (Ramon y Cajal, 1928, p278).

The potential for neurotropic guidance of regenerating axons was subsequently dismissed by Weiss and Taylor (1944) and not revisited for nearly 40 years.

Interest in neurotropism, or chemotaxis, was revived by the classic experiment in which Gunderson and Barrett redirected the growth of chick DRG neurites by moving a point source of NGF across their path (Gunderson, Barrett, 1979). In the same year, Lundborg's early work on regeneration through enclosed neural gaps raised the possibility that axons might be guided to the distal nerve stump by neurotropic influences (Lundborg, Hansson, 1979; Lundborg et al., 1982). The action of neurotropism could not be proven by Lundborg's experiments, however, as the construct was evaluated after the completion of regeneration. Neurotropism can only be implicated when axons are seen growing toward a target, but have not yet reached it. Once the target is contacted, it may exert a neurotrophic influence, supporting only those axons that reach it at the expense of others that do not. In this way, initially random behavior could be converted to a projection that is focused on the target. This criterion was met by the contemporaneous experiments of Politis, which demonstrated preferential growth toward a normal versus a metabolically compromised distal stump, even when a 0.2-μm millipore filter obstructed the pathway (Politis et al., 1982). The direction of axon growth was thus controlled by a diffusible substance that required living cells for its elaboration.

The majority of subsequent experiments on peripheral neurotropism in vivo were performed in the frog. Kuffler found that regenerating motor axons can be guided by diffusible substances emanating either from muscle or segments of nerve, and provided ample evidence of directional growth before target contact was made (Kuffler, 1986, 1989). He went on to show that medium conditioned by peripheral nerve could direct the regeneration of both motoneurons and DRG neurons in culture, and motor axons in the previous assay in vivo (Pérez et al., 1997; Hill et al., 1999; Zheng,

Kuffler, 2000). The specific factors responsible for this behavior have yet to be characterized.

The potential for neurotropism in peripheral nerve regeneration has also been suggested by experiments in a variety of in vitro preparations. Critical roles for the neurotrophins in guiding developing sensory and motor axons into the limb bud were confirmed by implanting ectopic neurotrophin sources in the embryo or treating embryos with function-blocking antibodies (Tucker et al., 2001). Cultured DRG neurons grow toward degenerating but not toward fresh segments of peripheral nerve (Gu et al., 1995), and selectively reinnervate appropriate target regions when co-cultured with slices of fetal spinal cord (Crain, Peterson, 1982). Repetition of the Gunderson and Barrett experiments with adult tissue has been particularly instructive. The initial demonstration of growth cone turning in response to a point source of NGF involved embryonic chick DRG neurons. When TrkA-expressing adult DRG neurons are challenged in the same way, however, they must be both preconditioned and growing on laminin before they respond to an NGF gradient (Webber et al., 2008). The discrepancy between the findings with embryonic and adult neurons is an example of the risk incurred when generalizing from in vitro experiments on fetal neurons to the behavior of adult tissue. In a more inclusive model, motoneurons regenerating from organotypic slice culture of postnatal spinal cord are directed over substantial distances to a point source of the growth factor pleiotrophin (Mi et al., 2007).

The manipulation of peripheral regeneration with gradients of growth factors and/or adhesion molecules is a potentially attainable goal. Recent research in this area has shifted from soluble to bound gradients, as these are much easier to control once established (Kapur, Shoichet, 2004; Rosoff et al., 2004; Yu et al., 2008; Mai et al., 2009). The ability to separate and redirect modality-specific axon populations would greatly enhance the potential for functional restoration after nerve injury.

Mechanical Alignment

The clinical experience documented in Chapter 5 is consistent with a role for mechanical alignment in influencing the outcome of nerve repair. Introduction of microsurgical techniques resulted in substantial improvement in outcomes, and there is preliminary evidence that techniques of fascicular matching have the potential to take this a step further.

Although some of these changes may have resulted from reduction of operative trauma and from the use of finer and therefore less reactive suture material, the organizational component probably dominates.

When mechanical alignment is essentially perfect, as it is after crush or freezing injury of peripheral nerve, recovery is often complete. Most axons remain within their initial Schwann cell tubes, and are directed back to their original end organs (Brown, Hopkins, 1981; Brown, Hardman, 1987; Nguyen et al., 2002; Valero-Cabré et al., 2004). The functional consequences of this precision are exemplified by uniform restoration of normal or nearly normal sciatic functional index (SFI) (Chapter 7, Table 7-1).

Restoration of function after nerve transection and repair rarely if ever equals the recovery after nerve crush. This divide is so pronounced that continuity of the basal lamina rivals age as a determinant of outcome. A potential exception is injury of a proper muscle nerve in which all motor axons are destined to innervate the same muscle, and the consequences of axonal disorganization at the suture line are minimal (Rafuse, Gordon, 1996). After transection injury of multifascicular nerve that subserves many distal functions, the accuracy of regeneration is influenced by the alignment of the nerve stumps. This was demonstrated initially by using HRP to compare the organization of motoneuron pools serving the peroneal muscles after various forms of sciatic nerve repair (Figures 7-10, 8-7). Reinnervation was 89% correct after individual fascicular suture, 74% correct after epineurial suture, and only 47% correct after regeneration across an intubated gap (Brushart et al., 1983; Brushart, 1990b). In similar studies, the accuracy of sensory axon regeneration was evaluated using the tracer HRP-WGA to label the dorsal horn projections of the peroneal muscles in normal animals, and after epineurial and individual fascicular sciatic nerve repair (Brushart et al., 1981) (Figure 10-10). Although quantification was not attempted, individual fascicular suture was clearly more effective than epineurial suture at limiting expansion of the peroneal dorsal horn projection into tibial nerve territory.

The importance of mechanical alignment is demonstrated most convincingly by experiments with the "nerve reconnection" technique described by de Medinaceli (de Medinaceli et al., 1983a, 1983b; de Medinaceli, Freed, 1983; de Medinaceli, Church, 1984). The nerve to be reconnected is first anchored to background material with slack between the anchor points so that it is completely tension-free in the repair zone. It is then gradually cooled to slightly below freezing in solutions that limit metabolic damage and calcium influx, and is transected with a vibrating blade. The nerve ends, still frozen and thus unchanged in their contour, are realigned and allowed to thaw in perfect alignment with one another. The dramatic improvements in SFI resulting from use of this technique were confirmed by two independent groups (Terzis, Smith, 1987; Zellem et al., 1989), and were associated with significant improvements in the specificity of muscle reinnervation by motoneurons that had served it previously (Wikholm et al., 1988). The primacy of mechanical alignment over the physiologic protection offered by the technique is indicated by the poor results when the stumps are misaligned before thawing (Amara et al., 2000), and by the failure to obtain good results when reconnecting nerves that were transected with scissors before initiation of the reconnection procedure (de Medinaceli, Seaber, 1989). Unfortunately, these findings also indicate that reconnection is unlikely to be helpful in the clinical setting. A series of 10 patients with maximum follow-up of 5 months was reported over a decade ago, yet no further follow-up is available (de Medinaceli, Merle, 1991).

Neurotrophism and Pruning

Detailed analysis of growth factor expression patterns in the various functional divisions of the peripheral nervous system was presented in Chapter 9. Clearly, a motor axon collateral regenerating in the femoral muscle branch will have access to a substantially different combination of growth factors than will another collateral from the same neuron that regenerates down the cutaneous branch. This differential trophic support could then result in differential growth of the two collaterals (Hoke et al., 2006). Under these conditions, it is possible that "sibling neurite bias" will contribute to collateral pruning (Smalheiser, Crain, 1984). The "sibling neurite" model states that a finite pool of structural precursors is available within the neuron (Devor, Schneider, 1975). Growing neurites that consume structural components at higher rates would deplete the pool available to their less vigorous "siblings." A neurite growing successfully down the femoral muscle branch, attaining larger size because of positive interaction with the pathway (Goldberg,

Schacher, 1987), would deplete the resources available to its sibling in the cutaneous branch, ultimately leading to resorption of the incorrect sensory projection. In this way a projection can be removed from a neutral environment, such as the cutaneous pathway, without the need for negative interaction. Similarly, when all collaterals of a motoneuron are trapped in this neutral environment, "sibling neurite bias" provides no mechanism for eliminating them all and starting over; this prediction is confirmed by the stability of motoneurons that project only to the femoral cutaneous branch (Brushart, 1993).

The molecular basis for pruning axon collaterals regenerating within peripheral nerve is little understood. Once one of the collaterals has made contact with muscle, however, mechanisms that control synaptic competition could potentially initiate pruning. The refinement of neuromuscular connections during development was one of the first examples of collateral pruning to be studied. In the neonatal limb, muscle cells are innervated by several axons (Redfern, 1970). Terminal axon collaterals are then pruned to "fine tune" the motor unit (Brown, Booth, 1983). Recent work has demonstrated that pruning favors the more active of two competing synapses (Buffelli et al., 2003; Hua et al., 2005), and that under some circumstances BDNF secreted in an activity-dependent fashion by winning collaterals binds to the p75NTR on adjacent collaterals, resulting in their demise (Singh et al., 2008). To the extent that regenerating axons explore distal environments with multiple collateral sprouts, the ability to manipulate collateral pruning could play a significant role in improving regeneration specificity.

CONCLUSIONS

Few areas of regeneration research spark the level of controversy engendered by specificity experiments. From the early refutation of Ramon y Cajal and Forssman by Paul Weiss to the current debate over the role of the pathway in the generation of PMR, investigators have presented arguments for and against many of the potential types of regeneration specificity. In most instances where controversy has arisen, differing interpretations of outcome have been derived from different experimental models. Ideally, a model should unleash the potential for regenerating axons to demonstrate the specificity in question without introducing extraneous,

uncontrolled variables. It is thus of paramount importance that specificity models be characterized as fully as possible to appreciate the variables that influence experimental outcome. They must also use the best tools available to answer the experimental question. For instance, unless an all-or-none answer is desired, axon counts are rarely an accurate indicator of regeneration specificity. Axon counts alone cannot differentiate one modality from another, and cannot account for differential generation of collateral sprouts at the repair site. In most instances, an electrophysiologic or neuroanatomical measure of neuron behavior provides more meaningful information.

Should any of these experiments change surgical behavior? In recent years, the pressure of dwindling reinbursements and the availability of tubular prostheses have resulted in less, rather than more, attention being paid to the actual process of nerve repair. Nonetheless, the possibility remains that a technique of correctly matching fascicles, and restricting axons to the intended fascicle, could result in incremental improvements in outcome. Clearly, the opposite approach of providing axons with more room to maneuver within a tube has not resulted in discernable change (Chapter 8), confirming the relative paucity of intrinsic regeneration specificity within the human sensory and motor systems. To be accepted, however, a technique of fascicular matching would need to provide measurably superior outcomes in order to justify the commitment of increased operating time.

Although improving mechanical alignment has the potential to enhance outcomes somewhat, substantial changes will require biological manipulations at the level of the individual axon and Schwann cell tube. A first step in this direction will be identification of neuronal receptors and Schwann cell–derived recognition or growth factors that are not distributed evenly throughout the PNS. If receptor-ligand pairs are found in which either or both are distributed in a modality- or location-specific fashion, it might be possible to generate specificity by enhancing their expression. If no such pairs exist, it may be necessary to induce expression of a receptor or ligand in a limited distribution so that a specific interaction can occur. At the opposite extreme, recent research suggests that the use of artificially generated gradients of growth factors and/or recognition molecules to guide the regeneration of specific axon populations is a realistic possibility.

REFERENCES

Abdullah MA, O'Daly A, Vyas AA, Brushart TM (2010) Adult motor axons preferentially reinnervate adult motor pathways. Orthopaedic Research Society Annual Meeting, New Orleans, Louisiana: poster 1615.

Abernethy DA, Rud A, Thomas PK (1992) Neurotropic influence of the distal stump of transected peripheral nerve on axonal regeneration: absence of topographic specificity in adult nerve. J Anat 180 (Pt 3): 395–400.

Al-Majed AA, Neumann CM, Brushart TM, Gordon T (2000) Brief electrical stimulation promotes the speed and accuracy of motor axonal regeneration. J Neurosci 20: 2602–2608.

Aldskogius H, Thomander L (1986) Selective reinnervation of somatotopically appropriate muscles after facial nerve transection and regeneration in the neonatal rat. Brain Res 375: 126–134.

Amara B, de Medinaceli L, merle M (2000) Functional assessment of misdirected axon growth after nerve repair in the rat. J Reconstr Microsurg 16: 563–567.

Arvidsson J, Johansson K (1988) Changes in the central projection pattern of vibrissae innervating primary sensory neurons after peripheral nerve injury in the rat. Neurosci Lett 84: 120–124.

Banks RW, Barker D, Brown HG (1985) Sensory reinnervation of muscles following nerve section and suture in cats. J Hand Surg 10B: 340–344.

Bernstein JJ, Guth L (1961) Nonselectivity in establishment of neuromuscular connections following nerve regeneration in the rat. Exp Neurol 4: 262–275.

Brown MC, Hopkins WG (1981) Role of degenerating axon pathways in regeneration of mouse soleus motor axons. J Physiol 318: 365–373.

Brown MC, Booth CM (1983) Postnatal development of the adult pattern of motor axon distribution in rat muscle. Nature 304: 741–742.

Brown MC, Hardman V (1987) A reassessment of the accuracy of reinnervation by motoneurons following crushing or freezing of the sciatic or lumbar spinal nerves of rats. Brain 110: 695–705.

Brushart TM, Mesulam MM (1980) Alteration in connections between muscle and anterior horn motoneurons after peripheral nerve repair. Science 208: 603–605.

Brushart TM, Henry EW, Mesulam MM (1981) Reorganization of muscle afferent projections accompanies peripheral nerve regeneration. Neuroscience 6: 2053–2061.

Brushart TM, Tarlov EC, Mesulam MM (1983) Specificity of muscle reinnervation after epineurial and individual fascicular suture of the rat sciatic nerve. J Hand Surg 8: 248–253.

Brushart TM (1988) Preferential reinnervation of motor nerves by regenerating motor axons. J Neurosci 8: 1026–1031.

Brushart TM (1990a) Preferential motor reinnervation: a sequential double-labeling study. Res Neurol Neurosci 1: 281–287.

Brushart TM (1990b) Topographic specificity of peripheral axon regeneration across enclosed gaps. Soc Neurosc Abstr 16: 806–800.

Brushart TM (1991) The mechanical and humoral control of specificity in nerve repair. In: *Operative Nerve Repair and Reconstruction*, pp. 215–230, Philadelphia: Lippincott.

Brushart TM (1993) Motor axons preferentially reinnervate motor pathways. J Neurosci 13: 2730–2738.

Brushart TM, Mathur V, Sood R, Koschorke GM (1995) Dispersion of regenerating axons across enclosed neural gaps. J Hand Surg [Am] 20A: 557–564.

Brushart TM, Gerber J, Kessens P, Chen YG, Royall RM (1998) Contributions of pathway and neuron to preferential motor reinnervation. J Neurosci 18: 8674–8681.

Brushart TM, Jari R, Verge V, Rohde C, Gordon T (2004) Electrical stimulation restores the specificity of sensory axon regeneration. Exp Neurol 194: 221–229.

Buffelli M, Burgess RW, Feng G, Lobe CG, Lichtman JW, Sanes JR (2003) Genetic evidence that relative synaptic efficacy biases the outcome of synaptic competition. Nature 424: 430–434.

Burgess PR, Horch KW (1973) Specific regeneration of cutaneous fibers in the cat. J Neurophysiol 36: 101–114.

Choi D, Raisman G (2002) Somatotopic organization of the facial nucleus is disrupted after lesioning and regeneration of the facial nerve: the histological representation of synkinesis. Neurosurgery 50: 355–362.

Chu TH, Du Y, Wu W (2008) Motor nerve graft is better than sensory nerve graft for survival and regeneration of motoneurons after spinal root avulsion in adult rats. Exp Neurol 212: 562–565.

Collins WF, Mendell LM, Munson JB (1986) On the specificity of sensory reinnervation of cat skeletal muscle. J Physiol 375: 587–609.

Crain SM, Peterson ER (1982) Selective innervation of target regions within fetal mouse spinal cord and medulla explants by isolated dorsal root ganglia in organotypic co-cultures. Dev Brain Res 2: 341–362.

de Medinaceli L, Freed WJ (1983) Peripheral nerve reconnection: immediate histologic consequences of distributed mechanical support. Exp Neurol 81: 459–468.

de Medinaceli L, Church AC (1984) Peripheral nerve reconnection: inhibition of early degenerative processes through the use of a novel fluid medium. Exp Neurol 84: 396–408.

de Medinaceli L, Merle M (1991) Applying "Cell Surgery" to Nerve Repair: A Preliminary Report on the First Ten Human Cases. J Hand Surg 16B:499–504.

de Medinaceli L, Wyatt RJ, Freed WJ (1983a) Peripheral nerve reconnection: Mechanical, thermal, and ionic conditions that promote the return of function. Exp Neurol 81: 469–487.

de Medinaceli L, Freed W, Wyatt R (1983b) Peripheral nerve reconnection: Improvement of long-term functional effects under simulated clinical conditions in the rat. Exp Neurol 81: 488–496.

de Medinaceli L, Seaber AV (1989) Experimental nerve reconnection: importance of initial repair. Microsurgery 10: 56–70.

DeSantis M, Norman WP (1993) Location and completeness of reinnervation by two types of neurons at a single target: the feline muscle spindle. J Comp Neurol 336: 66–76.

Devor, M. and G. Schneider (1975) Neuroanatomical plasticity: the principle of conservation of total axonal arborization. In: *Aspects of Neural Plasticity* (INSERM Colloquia, Vol. 43), F. Vital-Durand and M. Jeannerod, eds., pp 191–200, Paris: INSERM.

Donoghue MJ, Morris-Valero R, Johnson YR, Merlie JP, Sanes JR (1992) Mammalian muscle cells bear a cell-autonomous, heritable memory of their rostrocaudal position. Cell 69: 67–77.

Doubleday B, Robinson PP (1995) The effect of NGF depletion on the neurotropic influence exerted by the distal stump following nerve transection. J Anat 186: 593–605.

Eberhardt KA, Irintichev A, Al-Majed AA, Simova O, Brushart TM, Gordon T, Schachner M (2006) BDNF/TrkB signaling regulates HNK-1 carbohydrate expression in regenerating motor nerves and promotes functional recovery after peripheral nerve repair. Exp Neurol 198: 500–510.

Evans P, Bain J, Mackinnon S, Makino A, Hunter D (1991) Selective reinnervation: a comparison of recovery following microsuture and conduit nerve repair. Brain Res 559: 315–321.

Foehring RC, Sypert GW, Munson JB (1987) Motor-unit properties following cross-reinnervation of cat lateral gastrocnemius and soleus muscles with medial gastrocnemius nerve. II. Influence of muscle on motoneurons. J Neurophysiol 57: 1227–1245.

Forssman J (1898) Ueber die Ursachen, welche die Wachstumsrichtung der peripheren Nervenfasern bei der Regeneration bestimmen. Beitrz Pathol Anat 24: 56–100.

Franz CK, Rutishauser U, Rafuse VF (2005) Polysialylated neural cell adhesion molecule is necessary for selective targeting of regenerating motor neurons. J Neurosci 25: 2081–2091.

Franz CK, Rutishauser U, Rafuse VF (2008) Intrinsic neuronal properties control selective targeting of regenerating motoneurons. Brain 131(Pt 6): 1492–1505.

Gardiner NJ, Fernyhough P, Tomlinson DR, Mayer U, von der Mark H, Streuli CH (2005) Alpha7 integrin mediates neurite outgrowth of distinct populations of adult sensory neurons. Mol Cell Neurosci 28: 229–240.

Ghalib N, Houstava L, Haninec P, Dubovy P (2001) Morphometric analysis of early regeneration of motor axons through motor and cutaneous nerve grafts. Ann Anat 183: 363–368.

Gillespie MJ, Gordon T, Murphy PR (1986) Reinnervation of the lateral gastrocnemius and soleus muscles in the rat by their common nerve. J Physiol 372: 485–500.

Goldberg DJ, Schacher S (1987) Differential growth of the branches of a regenerating bifurcate axon is associated with differential axonal transport of organelles. Dev Biol 124: 35–40.

Gregory JE, Luff AR, Proske U (1982) Muscle receptors in the cross-reinnervated soleus muscle of the cat. J Physiol 331: 367–383.

Gu X, Thomas PK, King RHM (1995) Chemotropism in nerve regeneration studied in tissue culture. J Anat 186: 153–163.

Gunderson RW, Barrett JN (1979) Neuronal chemotaxis: chick dorsal root axons turn toward high concentrations of nerve growth factor. Science 206: 1079–1080.

Hardman VJ, Brown MC (1987) Accuracy of reinnervation of rat intercostal muscles by their own segmental nerves. J Neurosci 7: 1031–1036.

Hawkins GL (1948) Faulty sensory localization in nerve regeneration. J Neurosurg 5: 11–18.

Hill ES, Latalladi G, Kuffler DP (1999) Dissociated adult Rana pipiens motoneuron growth cones turn up concentration gradients of denervated peripheral nerve-released factors. Neurosci Lett 277: 87–90.

Hoh JFY (1975) Selective and non-selective reinnervation of fast-twitch and slow-twitch rat skeletal muscle. J Physiol 251: 791–801.

Hoke A, Redett R, Hameed H, Jari R, Li JB, Griffin JW, Brushart TM (2006) Schwann cells express motor and sensory phenotypes that regulate axon regeneration. J Neurosci 26: 9646–9655.

Horch K (1979) Guidance of regrowing sensory axons after cutaneous nerve lesions in the cat. J Neurophysiol 42: 1437–1449.

Hua JY, Smear MC, Baier H, Smith SJ (2005) Regulation of axon growth in vivo by activity-based competition. Nature 434: 1022–1026.

Ip MC, Vrbova G (1983) Reinnervation of the soleus muscle by its own or by an alien nerve. Neuroscience 10: 1463–1469.

Iwabuchi Y, Maki Y, Yoshizu T, Narisawa H (1999) Lack of topographical specificity in peripheral nerve regeneration in rats. Scand J Plast Reconstr Surg Hand Surg 33: 181–185.

Kapur TA, Shoichet MS (2004) Immobilized concentration gradients of nerve growth factor guide neurite outgrowth. J Biomed Mater Res A 68: 235–243.

Kimura J, Rodnitzky RL, Okawara SH (1975) Electrophysiologic analysis of aberrant regeneration after facial nerve paralysis. Neurology 25: 989–993.

Kleene R, Schachner M (2004) Glycans and neural cell interactions. Nat Rev Neurosci 5: 195–208.

Koerber HR, Mirnics K, Brown P, Mendell L (1994) Central sprouting and functional plasticity of regenerated primary afferents. J Neurosci 14: 3655–3671.

Koerber HR, Seymour AW, Mendell LM (1989) Mismatches between peripheral receptor type and central projections after peripheral nerve regeneration. Neurosci Lett 99: 67–72.

Kuffler DP (1986) Isolated satellite cells of a peripheral nerve direct the growth of regenerating frog axons. J Comp Neurol 249: 57–64.

Kuffler DP (1989) Regeneration of muscle axons in the frog is directed by diffusible factors from denervated muscle and nerve tubes. J Comp Neurol 281: 416–425.

Lago N, Navarro X (2006) Correlation between target reinnervation and distribution of motor axons in the injured rat sciatic nerve. J Neurotrauma 23: 227–240.

Laskowski MB, Sanes JR (1988) Topographically selective reinnervation of adult mammalian skeletal muscles. J Neurosci 8: 3094–3099.

Laskowski MB, Colman H, Nelson C, Lichtman JW (1998) Synaptic competition during the reformation of a neuromuscular map. J Neurosci 18: 7328–7335.

Le TB, Aszmann O, Chen YG, Royall RM, Brushart TM (2001) Effects of pathway and neuronal aging on the specificity of motor axon regeneration. Exp Neurol 167: 126–132.

Lundborg G, Hansson HH (1979) Regeneration of peripheral nerve through a preformed tissue space: preliminary observations on the reorganization of regenerating nerve fibers and perineurium. Brain Res 178: 573–576.

Lundborg, G., L.B. Dahlin, N. Danielsen, A. Johannesson and H.A. Hansson (1982) Regenerating nerve fibers in preformed mesothelial chambers: influence of the distal segment of a transected nerve on growth an direction. In: Clinical Applications of Biomaterials, T. Albrektsson, P.-I. Branemark and A.J.C. Lee, eds., pp. 323–329. Chichester, UK: Wiley.

Lundborg GL, Dahlin N, Danielsen N, Nachemson AK (1986) Tissue specificity in nerve regeneration. Scand J Plast Reconstr Surg 20: 279–283.

Mackinnon SE, Dellon AL, Lundborg G, Hudson AR, Hunter DA (1986) A study of neurotrophism in a primate model. J Hand Surg 11A:888–894.

Madison RD, Archibald SJ, Brushart TM (1996) Reinnervation accuracy of the rat femoral nerve by motor and sensory neurons. J Neurosci 16: 5698–5703.

Madison RD, Archibald SJ, Lacin R, Krarup C (1999) Factors contributing to preferential motor reinnervation in the primate peripheral nervous system. J Neurosci 19: 11007–11016.

Madison RD, Sofroniew MV, Robinson GA (2009) Schwann cell influence on motor neuron regeneration accuracy. Neuroscience 163: 213–221.

Mai J, Fok L, Gao H, Zhang X, Poo MM (2009) Axon initiation and growth cone turning on bound protein gradients. J Neurosci 29: 7450–7458.

Maki Y (1991) Experimental study of selective motor and sensory nerve regeneration (Part 2). J Jpn Soc Surg Hand 7: 975–978.

Maki Y, Yoshizu T, Tajima T, Narisawa H (1996) The selectivity of regenerating motor and sensory axons. J Reconstr Microsurg 12: 547–551.

Martini R, Xin Y, Schmitz B, Schachner M (1992) The L2/HNK-1 carbohydrate epitope is involved in the preferential outgrowth of motor neurons on ventral roots and motor nerves. Eur J Neurosci 4: 628–639.

Martini R, Schachner M, Brushart TM (1994) The L2/HNK-1 carbohydrate is preferentially expressed by previously motor axon-associated

Schwann cells in reinnervated peripheral nerves. J Neurosci 14: 7180–7191.

Mears S, Schachner M, Brushart TM (2003) Antibodies to myelin-associated glycoprotein accelerate preferential motor reinnervation. JPNS 8: 91–99.

Mi R, Chen W, Hoke A (2007) Pleiotrophin is a neurotrophic factor for spinal motor neurons. PNAS 104: 4664–4669.

Miledi R, Stefani E (1969) Non-selective re-innervation of slow and fast muscle fibers in the rat. Nature 222: 569–571.

Mizuno N, Uemura-Sumi M, Matsuda K, Takeuchi Y, Kume M, Matsushima R (1980) Non-selective distribution of hypoglossal nerve fibers after section and resuture: a horseradish peroxidase study in the cat. Neurosci Lett 19: 33–37.

Moradzadeh A, Borschel GH, Luciano JP, Whitlock EL, Hayashi A, Hunter DA, Mackinnon SE (2008) The impact of motor and sensory nerve architecture on nerve regeneration. Exp Neurol 212: 370–376.

Munson, J.B., W.F. Collins and L.M. Mendell (1988) Reinnervation of muscle spindles by groups Ia and Ib fibers is consistent with specificity in the reinnervation process. In: The Current Status of Peripheral Nerve Regeneration, T. Gordon, R.B. Stein and PA Smith, eds., pp. 259–268, New York: Liss.

Nguyen QT, Sanes JR, Lichtman JW (2002) Pre-existing pathways promote precise projection patterns. Nat Neurosci 5: 861–867.

Nichols CM, Brenner MJ, Fox IK, Tung TH, Hunter DA, Rickman SR, Mackinnon SE (2004) Effect of motor versus sensory nerve grafts on peripheral nerve regeneration. Exp Neurol 190: 347–355.

Ochi M, Ikuta Y, Miyamoto Y, Takeno S (1992) Experimental evidence of selective axonal regeneration in allogenic and isogenic Y-chambers. Exp Neurol 115: 260–265.

Ostberg AJ, Vrbova G, O'Brien RA (1986) Reinnervation of fast and slow mammalian muscles by a superfluous number of motor axons. Neuroscience 18: 205–213.

Pérez NL, Sosa MA, Kuffler DP (1997) Growth cones turn up concentration gradients of diffusible peripheral target-derived factors. Exp Neurol 145: 196–202.

Politis MJ, Ederle K, Spencer PS (1982) Tropism in nerve regeneration in vivo: attraction of regenerating axons by diffusable factors derived from cells in distal nerve stumps of transected peripheral nerves. Brain Res 253: 1–12.

Politis MJ (1985) Specificity in mammalian peripheral nerve regeneration at the level of the nerve trunk. Brain Res 328: 271–276.

Potluri S, Lampa SJ, Norton AS, Laskowski MB (2006) Morphometric analysis of neuromuscular topography in the serratus anterior muscle. Muscle & Nerve 33: 398–408.

Puigdellívol-Sánchez A, Prats-Galino A, Molander C (2005) On regenerative and collateral sprouting to hind limb digits after sciatic nerve injury in the rat. Res Neurol Neurosci 23: 97–107.

Rafuse VF, Gordon T (1996) Self-reinnervated cat medial gastrocnemius muscles 0.1. Comparisons of the capacity for regenerating nerves to form enlarged motor units after extensive peripheral nerve injuries. J Neurophysiol 75: 268–281.

Ramon y Cajal, S. (1928) *Degeneration and Regeneration of the Nervous System*. London: Oxford University Press.

Redett R, Jari R, Crawford T, Chen YG, Rohde C, Brushart TM (2005) Peripheral pathways regulate motoneuron collateral dynamics. J Neurosci 25: 9406–9412.

Redfern PA (1970) Neuromuscular transmission in newborn rats. J Physiol (Lond) 209: 701–709.

Robinson GA, Madison RD (2003) Preferential motor reinnervation in the mouse: comparison of femoral nerve repair using a fibrin sealant or suture. Muscle & Nerve 28: 227–231.

Robinson GA, Madison RD (2004) Motor neurons can preferentially reinnervate cutaneous pathways. Exp Neurol 190: 407–413.

Robinson GA, Madison RD (2009) Influence of terminal nerve branch size on motor neuron regeneration accuracy. Exp Neurol 215: 228–235.

Rosoff WJ, Urbach JS, Esrick MA, McAllister RG, Richards LJ, Goodhill GJ (2004) A new chemotaxis assay shows the extreme sensitivity of axons to molecular gradients. Nat Neurosci 7: 678–682.

Roth G (1983) Reinnervation in obstetrical brachial plexus paralysis. J Neurol Sci 58: 103–115.

Simova O, Irintchev A, Mehanna A, Liu J, Dihne M, Bachle D, Sewald N, Loers G, Schachner M (2006) Carbohydrate mimics promote functional recovery after peripheral nerve repair. Ann Neurol 60: 430–437.

Singh KK, Park KJ, Hong EJ, Kramer BM, Greenberg ME, Kaplan DR, Miller FD (2008) Developmental axon pruning mediated by BDNF-p75NTR-dependent axon degeneration. Nat Neurosci 11: 649–658.

Smalheiser NR, Crain SM (1984) The possible role of "sibling neurite bias" in the coordination of neurite extension, branching, and survival. J Neurobiol 15: 517–529.

Soileau LC, Silberstein L, Blau HM, Thompson WJ (1987) Reinnervation of muscle fiber types in the newborn rat soleus. J Neurosci 7: 4176–4194.

Suzue T, Kaprielian Z, Patterson P (1990) A monoclonal antibody that defines rostrocaudal gradients in the mammalian nervous system. Neuron 5: 421–431.

Takano K (1976) Absence of gamma-spindle loop in the reinnervated hind leg muscles of the cat: "alpha muscle." Exp Brain Res 26: 343–354.

Terzis JK, Smith K (1987) Repair of severed peripheral nerves: comparison of the "deMedinaceli" and standard microsuture methods. Exp Neurol 96: 672–680.

Thomas CK, Stein RB, Gordon T, Lee RG, Elleker MG (1987) Patterns of reinnervation and motor unit recruitment in human hand muscles after complete ulnar and median nerve section and resuture. J Neurol Neurosurg Psychiatry 50: 259–268.

Thulin CA (1960) Electrophysiological studies of peripheral nerve regeneration with special reference to the small diameter (gamma) fibers. Exp Neurol 2: 598–612.

Tucker KL, Meyer M, Barde YA (2001) Neurotrophins are required for nerve growth during development. Nat Neurosci 4: 29–37.

Ungar-Sargon J, Goldberger ME (1987) Maintenance of specificity by sprouting and regenerating peripheral nerves. II. Variability after lesions. Brain Res 407: 124–136.

Uschold T, Robinson GA, Madison RD (2007) Motor neuron regeneration accuracy: balancing trophic influences between pathways and end-organs. Exp Neurol 205: 250–256.

Valero-Cabré A, Tsironis K, Skouras E, Navarro X, Neiss W (2004) Peripheral and spinal motor reorganization after nerve injury and repair. J Neurotrauma 21: 95–108.

Wang LC, Copray S, Brouwer N, Meek MF, Kernell D (2002) Regional distribution of slow-twitch muscle fibers after reinnervation in adult rat hindlimb muscles. Muscle & Nerve 25: 805–815.

Webber CA, Xu Y, Vanneste KJ, Martinez JA, Verge VM, Zochodne DW (2008) Guiding adult mammalian sensory axons during regeneration. J Neuropathol Exp Neurol 67: 212–222.

Weiss P, Taylor AC (1944) Further experimental evidence against neurotropism in nerve regeneration. J Exp Zool 95: 233–257.

Weiss P, Hoag A (1946) Competitive reinnervation of rat muscles by their own and foreign nerves. J Neurophysiol 9: 413–418.

Wigston DJ, Sanes JR (1982) Selective reinnervation of adult mammalian muscle by axons from different segmental levels. Nature 299: 464–467.

Wigston DJ, Sanes JR (1985) Selective reinnervation of intercostal muscles transplanted from different segmental levels to a common site. J Neurosci 5: 1208–1221.

Wikholm R, Swett J, Torigoe Y, Blanks R (1988) Repair of severed peripheral nerve: a superior anatomic and functional recovery with a new "reconnection" technique. J Otol Head & Neck Surg 99: 353–361.

Wolf JH, English AW (2000) Muscle spindle reinnervation following phenol block. Cells Tissues Organs 166: 325–329.

Yu LM, Wosnick JH, Shoichet MS (2008) Miniaturized system of neurotrophin patterning for guided regeneration. J Neurosci Methods 171: 253–263.

Zellem R, Miller D, Kenning J, Hoenig E, Buchheit W (1989) Experimental peripheral nerve repair: environmental control directed at the cellular level. Microsurgery 10: 290–301.

Zhao Q, Dahlin L, Kanje M (1992a) Reinnervation of muscles in rats after repair of transected sciatic nerves with Y-shaped and X-shaped silicon tubes. Scand J Plast Reconstr Hand Surg 26: 265–270.

Zhao Q, Dahlin L, Kanje M, Lundborg G (1992b) Specificity of muscle reinnervation following repair of the transected sciatic nerve. J Hand Surg 17B: 257–261.

Zhao Q, Dahlin LB, Kanje M, Lundborg G, Lu S-B (1992c) Axonal projections and functional recovery following fascicular repair of the rat sciatic nerve with Y-tunnelled silicone chambers. Res Neurol Neurosci 4: 13–19.

Zheng M, Kuffler DP (2000) Guidance of regenerating motor axone in vivo by gradients of diffusible peripheral nerve-derived factors. J Neurobiol 42: 212–219.

11

SYSTEMS ORGANIZATION
AFTER NERVE REPAIR
OR TRANSFER

THE PROPERTIES of denervated muscle fibers are respecified by the activity level of the reinnervating motoneuron, and the force generated by a motor unit gradually becomes proportional to the size of its motoneuron. Postaxotomy motoneuron loss is minimal after peripheral lesions in adults, but increases in the neonatal period and after proximal lesions. Axotomized motoneurons undergo significant structural changes. Only 50–75% of muscle spindles and Golgi tendon organs are reinnervated, and many of these respond abnormally to stretch. The monosynaptic stretch reflex does not recover. Muscle afferents that reinnervate incorrect peripheral targets retain many of their central properties. When a muscle nerve is transected, its cortical representation is occupied by expansion of adjacent territories. Short-term plasticity involves unmasking of previously silent projections, whereas long-term plasticity is likely to involve long-term potentiation (LTP) and long-term depression (LTD). As a transected nerve regenerates, it reclaims only a portion of its previous cortical territory. After nerve

transfer, the control of motor output shifts from donor to recipient cortical areas, while motor input programs remain unchanged. The motor system can compensate for nerve transfer in higher primates and humans, but is unable to compensate for the disordered reinnervation that follows nerve repair even in young humans.

Cutaneous sensory receptors are reinnervated in reduced numbers and have altered receptive field properties. Collateral sprouting of intact, uninjured mechanoreceptive axons contributes little to sensory recovery. The apoptotic response of DRG neurons to axotomy is more pronounced after proximal lesions and in young animals. Misdirection of regenerating sensory axons in the periphery is mirrored by expansion and irregularity of individual nerve projections to the dorsal horn of the spinal cord. Although there is little evidence for sprouting of mechanoreceptive afferents within the dorsal horn, the receptive fields of dorsal horn neurons undergo substantial refinement. Most DRG neurons that reinnervate inappropriate targets maintain their central projections. Sensory cortex in area 3b and both the cuneate nucleus and VP nucleus of the thalamus undergo rapid changes in response to denervation in nonhuman primates. Initial reductions in GABA-mediated afferent-driven inhibition unmask existing projections from adjacent territories. More long-term changes are mediated by NMDA receptor activation. Initial cortical territories are restored after nerve crush, but digital projections remain highly disordered after nerve transection and repair. Humans undergo similar cortical plasticity after nerve injury. As the cortical territory corresponding to a cutaneous area expands, the two-point discrimination in that area improves. Temporary denervation with topical anesthetic has been used to enhance sensory retraining. The sensory and motor systems both exhibit remarkable plasticity to some challenges, but are largely unable to compensate for the lack of topographic specificity in axon regeneration.

THE MOTOR SYSTEM

The Motor Unit

As regenerating motor axons recruit denervated muscle fibers into a new motor unit, the individual properties of these fibers are respecified by the regenerating motoneuron. This was first demonstrated by cross reinnervation of the fast FDL muscle and the slow soleus muscle, after which the FDL became slowly contracting, and the soleus became rapidly contracting (Buller et al., 1960). Further investigation revealed that a range of motor unit properties were altered during this conversion (reviewed in Vrbova et al., 1995). Muscle metabolism and structure changed to reflect the new contraction speed, with adjustment of the balance between oxidative and glycolytic enzyme activity, changes in the light chain components of the myosin molecule, and alteration in the structure of both thick and thin filaments. In some instances, these changes occurred bilaterally in response to unilateral nerve cross, indicating substantial linkage of homonomous motoneuron pools across the midline (Srihari et al., 1981; Reichmann et al., 1983). Fiber type conversion is not always complete, however. Reinnervated muscle fibers may continue to express their original myosin heavy chain isoforms in addition to those acquired through conversion, and in the case of slow muscle may retain their high oxidative capacity (Gauthier et al., 1983). Additionally, there is often a dissociation of force and fatigability

characteristics (Gordon et al., 2004). As a result, it is not unusual to encounter fiber types in reinnervated muscle that do not fit the classification scheme described by Burke for normal muscle (Figure 3-3).

A series of ingenious experiments revealed that it was the relative level of motoneuronal activity that determined the fiber type within the motor unit. Contraction of the normal soleus muscle is most easily triggered by Ia muscle spindle afferents (Chapter 3). These afferents can be silenced by soleus tenotomy. The muscle is relaxed completely, the muscle spindle is no longer stretched, and Ia signaling is reduced substantially. Without most of its normal continuous activity, the soleus muscle converts from slow to fast (Vrbova, 1963a, 1963b). If the muscle is then silenced completely by spinal cord injury, its properties can either be maintained or converted by electrical stimulation at slow or high frequencies, respectively (Vrbova, 1963a; Salmons, Vrbova, 1969; Gordon et al., 1991). Similar control can be exerted by electrical stimulation of denervated muscle in otherwise normal rats (Lomo et al., 1974; Gorza et al., 1988). These results imply that, in muscle cells, gene expression must be coupled to electrical activity (Vrbova et al., 1995).

The individual muscle fibers of a normal motor unit are not contiguous, but are dispersed to varying degrees within a muscle (Figure 11-1). In the cat tibialis anterior they may occupy 8–22% of the muscle cross-section, whereas in the soleus they are spread over 41–76% of the cross-sectional area (Bodine-Fowler et al., 1993), and may overlap 15–30 other motor units when viewed on cross section (Burke et al., 1973; Roy et al., 1995). Normal muscle thus presents a mosaic of different fiber types. This intermingling results from the sequential nature of muscle fiber development (Duxson et al., 1986, 1989). As primary myotubes are being innervated by pioneering axons, each generates several secondary myotubes around its circumference. These physically separate the primary myotubes from one another. The secondary myotubes are innervated by late-arriving axons and differentiate into a variety of muscle fiber types. Intermingling of different fiber types is thus ensured by the mechanics of the developmental process. Regenerating axons, in contrast, form collaterals that reinnervate adjacent, stationary myotubes, so that fibers served by a single axon are more tightly restricted in their distribution (Kugelberg et al., 1970). This "fiber type grouping" is more prominent in fast than slow motor units (Bodine-Fowler et al., 1993),

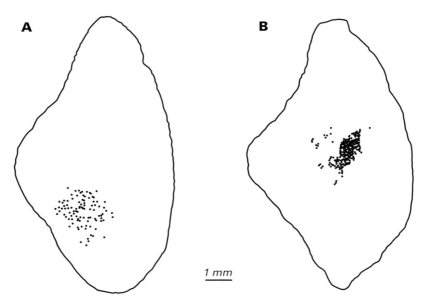

FIGURE 11-1   Distribution of fibers within a motor unit in normal (A) and reinnervated (B) rat tibialis anterior muscle. The glycogen depletion technique has been used to identify the muscle fibers corresponding to a single motor unit. The circumference of the motor units is similar, but the fibers are distributed evenly in the normal motor unit and gathered into clumps in the reinnervated unit, and thus exhibit fiber-type grouping. Reprinted with permission from Totosy de Zepetnek et al., 1992.

increases significantly as the number of reinnervating motoneurons decreases (Rafuse et al., 1996), and is more obvious in small than in large muscles (Totosy de Zepetnek et al., 1992).

During the regeneration process, large motoneurons are able to reinnervate more muscle fibers than smaller ones, and can expand to generate 5–8 times their normal force when few motor axons are available (Rafuse et al., 1992). Within each motor unit the reinnervating motoneuron establishes a dominant MHC profile, but varying degrees of fiber conversion to this type may also be represented (Bodine-Fowler et al., 1993; Unguez et al., 1995). Interestingly, although motoneurons do not selectively reinnervate individual fiber types, slow-twitch motoneurons appear to reinnervate specific areas within muscle on a selective basis (Wang, Kernell, 2002; Wang et al., 2002).

As discussed in Chapter 3, Henneman's size principle governs the integration of motor unit activity in normal muscle; the force generated by a motor unit is proportional to the size of the motoneuron. Orderly recruitment progressing from small to large motor units thus produces a continuous, smooth gradation of force (Figure 3-7). During the early months of experimental reinnervation of a muscle

by its own nerve, before the reversal of axonal and muscle atrophy and while respecification is under way, motor nerve size no longer predicts force capacity (Gordon, Stein, 1982a, 1982b). At later time periods, once atrophy is reversed and respecification of fiber type has stabilized, motor nerve size again predicts force and contraction speed. These motoneuron-driven adjustments also occur when flexor and extensor nerves are crossed (Gordon et al., 1986a, 1986b). In humans, orderly recruitment by size is restored after median nerve repair at the wrist, but not after ulnar repair at the elbow (Thomas et al., 1987). This discrepancy can be explained by the interrelationship of the muscles being reinnervated in the two circumstances. Median motor fibers at the wrist innervate muscles that power the same or closely related motions. If a motoneuron pool reinnervates several of these muscles, the forces resulting from its activation will be additive, and increments of force can be generated. Ulnar motor fibers, in contrast, innervate the antagonistic abductors and adductors of the digits. Activation of a motoneuron pool that has reinnervated both adductors and abductors will produce forces that partially cancel one another out; orderly recruitment of motor units by the size principle will not produce increments of force, and will thus be undetected in this circumstance. In situations in which it can be assessed accurately, the relationship between a given motoneuron and its muscle fibers is thus restored with remarkable fidelity after reinnervation; motoneuron size again predicts the number of fibers in the motor unit.

Motoneuron Death

The organization of the motor system will be affected to varying degrees by the death of axotomized motoneurons, depending on the age at which injury is inflicted, the location of the injury, and the opportunity for regenerating axons to contact Schwann cells in the distal nerve stump. In the rodent, peripheral axotomy in the neonatal period results in the loss of 70–90% of injured motoneurons within 1–2 weeks of the injury (Pollin et al., 1991; Li et al., 1994; Aszmann et al., 2004). In adults, nearly all motoneurons survive peripheral axotomy (Gordon et al., 1991; Pollin et al., 1991; Li et al., 1994; Xu et al., 2010) and all survive peripheral crush (Swett et al., 1991). The consequences of nerve injury are more severe, however, when the lesion is near the spinal cord. Eighty percent of motoneurons survive for 6 weeks after axotomy that leaves at least 4 mm of ventral root intact, yet only 30% will survive this long when the axotomy is adjacent to the spinal cord, eliminating all motor axon–Schwann cell contact (Gu et al., 1997). The time course of motoneuron loss is prolonged, so that an axotomy 10 mm from the spinal cord will still result in loss of 30% of motoneurons after 16 weeks (Ma et al., 2001). Motoneuron death can be minimized by providing transected axons with ready access to Schwann cells in the distal nerve stump (Tornqvist, Aldskogius, 1994; Jivan et al., 2006). After the most severe type of injury, ventral root avulsion from the spinal cord, 70–80% of rodent motoneurons will be lost by 2–3 weeks, and few if any will remain 6 weeks after the injury (Koliatsos et al., 1994; Li et al., 1995; Hoang et al., 2003). Motoneuron survival after axotomy is thus influenced by the relative trophic needs (determined by age) and supplies (determined by access to Schwann cells) in a given situation. In practical terms, motoneuron loss is unlikely to compromise the outcome of repair and reconstruction in areas distant from the spinal cord, although it is likely to play a critical role in limiting recovery potential after brachial plexus injury, especially in the neonate.

Since rodent pups are not as well developed as human babies at birth, the consequences of perinatal root injury or avulsion in humans cannot be predicted directly from rodent data.

Changes in Motoneuron Structure

Axotomized motoneurons undergo structural changes that persist long after they reinnervate muscle, and that affect their relationship with other neurons. Brannstrom and coworkers (Brannstrom et al., 1992b) calculated that, after 12 weeks of axotomy, the dendritic membrane area of α motoneurons had decreased by 36%, and the volume of these cells had been reduced by 29%. When similarly prepared motoneurons reinnervated muscle and were observed 2 years later, their dendritic volume and membrane area had returned to normal (Brannstrom et al., 1992a). The proportions of the dendritic tree were not restored, however, as the values for combined dendritic length and number of dendritic end branches were still reduced by 25%; compensation was achieved by an increase in dendritic diameters and in the number of dendrites per neuron. Motoneurons serving postural muscle in the cat cervical spine, in contrast, were found to enlarge rather than to atrophy in response to axotomy. After 11–17 weeks, their total dendritic surface area and total number of branches had increased by one-third, and the total number of branches more than doubled (Rose, Odlozinski, 1998). Differences in the function of these two motoneuron populations and in the distance between axotomy and cell body could be responsible for the discrepancy.

Axotomy results in the detachment of many synapses from the dendritic surface (Chen, 1978), a process that is mediated by nitric oxide (NO) and requires upregulation of nitric oxide synthase (NOS) (Sunico et al., 2005). Synaptic stripping and subsequent restoration after muscle reinnervation does not affect all types of boutons to the same degree. The number of excitatory S-type (spherical vesicle) boutons synapsing with the proximal dendrites of cat lumbar motoneurons nearly doubled 2 years after axotomy and reinnervation, while the number of inhibitory F-type (flat vesicle) boutons increased only slightly (Brannstrom, Kellerth, 1999). When the entire dendritic tree is considered, there is an overall loss of synapses, increasing the relative influence of synapses that are near or on the cell body.

In addition to triggering morphologic changes in the cell body and dendritic tree, axotomy provokes a reduction in the number of recurrent axon collaterals (Havton, Kellerth, 1990a). These structures synapse with Renshaw cells and provide recurrent inhibition of the motoneuron pool. Recurrent inhibition diminishes during the first 6 weeks after axotomy in parallel with collateral elimination (Havton, Kellerth, 1990b). By 12 weeks, however, it has returned to its preinjury level even though the number of collaterals is not restored. This compensation is obtained by the strengthening of remaining pathways, a change that is accompanied by alterations in synaptic ultrastructure (Havton, Kellerth, 2001). When axotomy occurs within the substance of the spinal cord (root avulsion), functional collaterals may actually emanate from the cell body or dendrites, providing an entirely new avenue for muscle reinnervation (Hoang et al., 2005).

Muscle Afferents

After nerve injury and regeneration, muscle performance will be influenced by both the number and the central connections of DRG neurons that have reinnervated muscle spindles and tendon organs. Nerve crush is followed by reinnervation of most muscle spindles and tendon organs with restoration of function in spite of abnormal receptor anatomy, demonstrating a clear lack of correspondence between receptor form and function (Hyde, Scott, 1983; Barker et al., 1986; Scott, 1987; DeSantis, Norman, 1993). Following nerve transection and repair, however, many receptors are left without afferent connections, or are reinnervated by axons that are inappropriate to their function (Koerber et al., 1994).

The complexity of normal muscle spindle innervation (Chapter 3) and the relative lack of end organ specificity during muscle afferent regeneration (Chapter 10) interact to produce a variety of abnormal innervation patterns. The morphological consequences of denervation and reinnervation after nerve transection are more pronounced than those after nerve crush. In a study of reinnervated cat soleus muscle, 3% of muscle spindles appeared normal, 43% lacked axons, and 54% had abnormal endings (Ip et al., 1988). The distribution of Ia and II afferents within the spindle was often altered, and inappropriate innervation by axons that previously served tendon organs or skin was common (Collins et al., 1986; Koerber et al., 1989; Banks, Barker, 1989; Lewin, McMahon, 1991a). Efferent input to the spindle is restored to some extent, but the

response of both β and γ fibers to stretch may be limited (Brown, Butler, 1976; Gregory et al., 1982; Scott, 1996). Approximately 50% of muscle spindles that have been reinnervated respond normally to stretch. Abnormal responses include failure to continue firing throughout the constant phase of a ramp-and-hold stretch, reduced rates of firing, and the absence of a tonic discharge (Brown, Butler, 1976; Banks et al., 1985; Banks, Barker, 1989) (Figure 11-2). The responses of muscle spindles that have been reinnervated by cutaneous afferents are even more rapidly adapting (Banks, Barker, 1989; Lewin, McMahon, 1991a). In both instances, the truncated responses provided by muscle spindles cannot accurately signal changes in the length of a muscle.

Experimental Afferent Fiber Misdirection

The extent to which lack of regeneration specificity influences Ia afferent function has been explored by redirecting gastrocnemius muscle afferents through the sural nerve to reinnervate skin in cats and rats. A complex picture has emerged in which some aspects of Ia signaling are not influenced by an inappropriate end organ, while others are modified significantly. Ia afferents that reinnervate skin respond to hair movement, and have receptive field dimensions similar to those of normal cutaneous afferents (Lewin, McMahon, 1991b). In the uninjured cat, the majority of muscle afferents are slowly adapting, in contrast to cutaneous afferents, most of which are rapidly adapting. After reinnervation of skin by the medial gastrocnemius (MG) nerve, nearly all responses to cutaneous stimulation become slowly adapting, suggesting that the axonal membrane of the regenerated muscle afferent, rather than the end organ, determines adaptation properties (Johnson et al.,1991). When similar surgery is performed in the rat, however, fewer than half of the regenerated muscle afferents are slowly adapting (Lewin, McMahon, 1991b). Although this finding was interpreted as evidence for respecification of response properties, it could also result from the normal rat MG nerve having substantially lower proportion of SA fibers to begin with (Johnson et al., 1995). Determinations of axonal conduction velocity are similarly discrepant. Stimulating proximal to the nerve repair, Johnson et al. (1995) found the conduction velocity of Ia afferents to return to 90% of normal when they reinnervated skin, providing

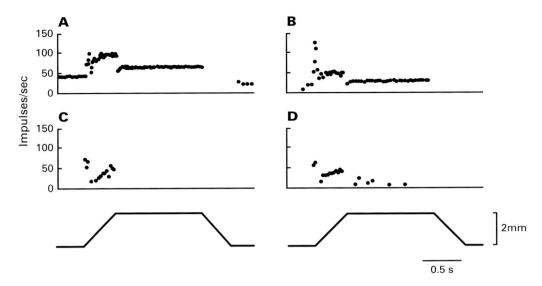

FIGURE 11-2 The response of individual muscle spindle afferents to ramp-and-hold stretch of the cat peroneus brevis muscle. The magnitude and duration of the stretch are diagrammed below the recordings. A normal (A) and reinnervated (B) spindle respond to stretch with a burst of activity followed by continued activity until the muscle is allowed to relax. Other reinnervated spindles (C, D) generate a burst of reduced amplitude and do not fire continuously throughout the stretch, and are thus unable to convey an accurate representation of muscle activity. Reprinted with permission from Barker et al., 1990.

further evidence for the durability of neuronal properties. The velocity determined in the rat was much lower, yet these studies were performed by stimulating distal to the repair, and could have been influenced by the smaller caliber and thus decreased conduction velocity of regenerated axons in the distal stump (Lewin, McMahon, 1991b; Chapter 5).

The cat gastrocnemius-sural nerve model has also been used to evaluate the effectiveness of Ia synapses on motoneurons after a variety of manipulations. In a series of experiments Mendell and coworkers applied high frequency stimuli to the gastrocnemius nerve after it had been transected and blocked off, regenerated through the sural nerve to skin, or regenerated back to the gastrocnemius muscle (Mendell et al., 1995, 1999). They found that the ability of Ia afferents to generate monosynaptic excitatory postsynaptic potentials (EPSPs) was influenced by the target of regeneration: synaptic efficacy was reduced severely when regeneration was blocked, was rescued partially by regeneration into skin, and was rescued almost completely by regeneration into muscle. The positive effects of muscle reinnervation could be duplicated and even surpassed by pumping NT-3 on the cut nerve end,

completely reversing the effects of target deprivation. Overall, these findings indicate that the effects of Ia fiber misdirection may be mitigated by the decreased effectiveness of Ia afferents that regenerate incorrectly to skin, potentially ensuring that those that do return to muscle will have the greatest effect on motoneuron firing.

Golgi Tendon Organs

Reinnervated Golgi tendon organs are also abnormal in appearance after crush injury, but function well nonetheless (Ip et al., 1977; Barker et al., 1986). After nerve repair and regeneration, only 40–45% of these tension receptors are reinnervated successfully (Banks et al., 1985; Collins et al., 1986). Of those, 50% will respond to stretch with a normal pattern of impulses but with a reduced firing rate. The remainder will exhibit phasic-only responses, or will respond only at the end and beginning of stretch, or only upon relaxation (Gregory et al., 1982; Scott et al., 1995, 1996) (Figure 11-3). The individual receptors studied by Scott and colleagues all responded normally to the muscle force developed by at least one motor unit, but abnormally to the

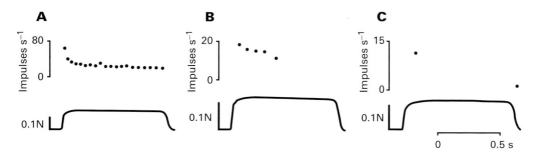

FIGURE 11-3   The response of individual Golgi tendon organs to tetanic contraction of reinnervated muscle. The magnitude and duration of the stretch are diagrammed below the recordings. (A) After nerve crush and regeneration, the receptor responds normally with an initial high-frequency burst followed by continuous firing until the contraction ceases. After nerve repair, the receptor fires an initial volley (B) or only single on-and-off impulses (C), thus failing to accurately signal the state of the muscle. Reprinted with permission from Scott et al., 1995.

force generated by others, suggesting that the abnormal responses were the result of mechanical abnormalities rather than failure of transduction. Normal Golgi tendon organs are in series with 10–20 muscle fibers that belong to many different motor units (Chapter 3). After reinnervation, however, the geometry of motor units has been revised. In the extremes, a single tendon organ could serve all of the fibers of a single motor unit on one hand, or could receive a single fiber of a motor unit, the remainder of whose fibers are anchored to tendon nearby. In the first instance, feedback would be dominated by the behavior of a single motor unit; in the second, contraction against the fixed tendon insertion would unload the tendon organ, creating the false impression of muscle relaxation (Scott, 1996).

The Stretch Reflex

The monosynaptic stretch reflex is initiated by an afferent volley from Ia muscle spindle receptors that synapse directly on motoneurons (Figure 3-10). Each Ia afferent projects collaterals to an entire motoneuron pool, as well as to a selection of motoneurons in synergistic pools. Ia synapses contact the soma or proximal dendrites of motoneurons, areas that have a relatively high impact on motoneuron firing and that exhibit good synaptic restoration after axotomy (see above). Estimates of muscle spindle reinnervation after nerve repair and regeneration vary between 50% and 75% of the population in a given muscle (Ip et al., 1988; Haftel et al., 2005). It is thus somewhat surprising that the

stretch reflex, the muscle contraction evoked in response to stretch, is not restored even after long periods of muscle reinnervation (Cope et al., 1994). Evaluation of the components of the reflex in the rat confirmed that muscle stretch evoked a robust afferent response in the dorsal root, but this rarely caused the stretched muscle to contract (Haftel et al., 2005). These same monosynaptic connections on motoneurons functioned well in response to electrical stimulation of afferents, leading the authors to conclude that centrally controlled neural circuits were actively suppressing the transmission of Ia afferent impulses. The stretch reflex contributes to muscle stiffness (Huyghues-Despointes et al., 2003), which is important for regulation of antigravity support while standing and joint coordination during locomotion (Abelew et al., 2000; Nichols, 2002; Maas et al., 2007). Understanding and eliminating the factors responsible for suppression of Ia signaling are thus important therapeutic goals.

The H Reflex

The H reflex is the electrophysiologic analog of the monosynaptic stretch reflex. Electrical stimulation of Ia afferents in peripheral nerve sends a volley of electrical activity around the reflex arc. Ia impulses travel proximally from the site of stimulation, pass through the dorsal root ganglion, and are transmitted across the Ia-motoneuron synapse. The resulting motoneuronal discharges are then propagated distally, where they can be recorded from muscle as a compound motor action potential (CMAP; Chapter 6). Because the H wave includes proximal transmission and a synaptic delay it has a greater latency than the M wave, which results from direct, anterograde stimulation of motor axons without the participation of central pathways. The vigor of the H reflex is diminished by synaptic stripping in response to axotomy, then increases as synaptic efficacy is restored, and is highly context-dependent. After repair of the rat sciatic nerve, the H reflex is robust and becomes evident at the same postoperative interval as the M wave when stimulation is performed proximal to the repair and the H reflex is recorded from gastrocnemius muscle in anaesthetized animals (Valero-Cabré, Navarro, 2001). If stimulation is performed distal to the repair in awake animals, the H reflex lags behind the first appearance of the M wave by 1 week, is briefly more prominent than in controls, then levels off at approximately 50% of control amplitude (English et al., 2007; English, personal communication). If the medial or lateral gastrocnemius nerve is transected and repaired and the intact sural nerve is stimulated in decerebrate rats without anesthesia, the H reflex is again robust (Haftel et al., 2005). This variability is consistent with variable degrees of context-dependent central suppression, as is the case for the stretch reflex itself.

Central Motor Reorganization: Experimental

The plasticity of motor cortex (MI) has been investigated most extensively by manipulating the rat facial (VII cranial) nerve. Using techniques of focal intracortical electrical stimulation, Sanes, Donoghue, and colleagues found the cortical representation of the vibrissal muscles in MI to be highly dependent on the innervation state of the muscles (Sanes et al., 1988; Donoghue et al., 1990; Sanes et al., 1990). Transection of the facial nerve led to reduction in the cortical area serving the vibrissae, with corresponding increase in the size of adjacent areas that served the forelimb and eye/eyelid. These changes occurred within hours of the injury, and could persist for months. When the facial nerve was injured in the neonatal period, the changes were similar except that the encroachment on the vibrissal territory by eye movement was greater than that seen in adults (Franchi, Veronesi, 2004). Various combinations of facial nerve (motor) and infraorbital nerve (sensory) transection revealed that alterations in sensory input were not responsible for the cortical reorganization (Franchi, Veronesi, 2006).

Further evaluation of the facial nerve system identified both an anatomic substrate and a potential mechanism for the observed plasticity. Using electrical stimulation of cortical neurons followed by labeling of the stimulated neurons with biocytin, Huntley (1997) correlated the normal projection patterns of MI neurons with their ability to participate in the reorganization induced by facial nerve transection (Figure 11-4). Vibrissal cortex that was taken over by expansion of the forelimb projection was characterized by neurons with extensive lateral projections into the normal, preinjury forelimb territory. These projections were presumably silent before the injury occurred. Vibrissal neurons that remained silent after denervation, in contrast, had no or sparse projections into the forelimb area. Rapid plasticity was thus achieved by unmasking inputs that were already present but were not normally functional. Observation of similar plasticity in response to focal blockade of the inhibitory neurotransmitter γ-aminobutyric acid (GABA) confirmed that inhibitory circuits were responsible for shaping and readjusting the functional boundaries of anatomically overlapping cortical motor representations (Jacobs, Donoghue, 1991). Mechanisms have also been proposed for shaping more permanent changes in cortical muscle representation. These are likely to result from activity-dependent long-term potentiation (LTP) and long-term depression (LTD) modulating the efficacy of synapses on the horizontal projections of cortical motor neurons (Hess et al., 1996; Hess, Donoghue, 1996a, 1996b; reviewed in Sanes, Donoghue, 2000).

The rat facial nerve model has also been used to evaluate the cortical changes resulting from facial nerve repair and regeneration (Franchi, 2000a, 2000b). Four weeks after facial nerve transection and repair, as reinnervation is just beginning, the denervated vibrissal muscles are no longer represented in the contralateral MI. There is some representation of neck and ipsilateral vibrissae muscles within the denervated area; the remainder is taken over by medial expansion of the forelimb territory and lateral expansion of the eye territory (Figure 11-5). After 4 months, the now reinnervated facial musculature is again represented in contralateral MI, but the territory remains shrunken with persistent intrusion of the forelimb and eye representation. Permanent cortical changes thus persist even after the completion of reinnervation, and can be expected to contribute to the compromise of coordinated function.

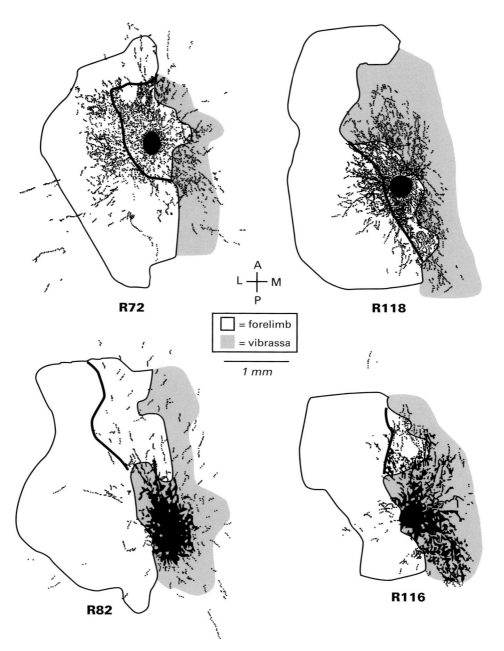

FIGURE 11-4   The surface of rat motor cortex after transection of the contralateral facial nerve. A—anterior; P—posterior; L—lateral; M—medial. The dark field on the right of each map is the residual vibrissal territory, and the light field on the left is the forelimb territory. The black line delineates the extent of the vibrissal cortex before nerve section; the light area to the right of the line has been taken over by expansion of the forelimb representation. Biocytin injection has been used to label the lateral projections from a defined area of cortex (black circle). Upper Maps: Injection within the area that has been taken over by the forelimb after facial nerve transection labels robust projections to the normal forearm territory. Lower Maps: Injection of residual vibrissal territory that has not been taken over by the forelimb representation labels few projections into forearm territory. Cortical territory thus expands readily into areas with which it shares extensive lateral projections (Upper), but not into areas with little shared innervation (Lower). Reprinted with permission from Huntley, 1997.

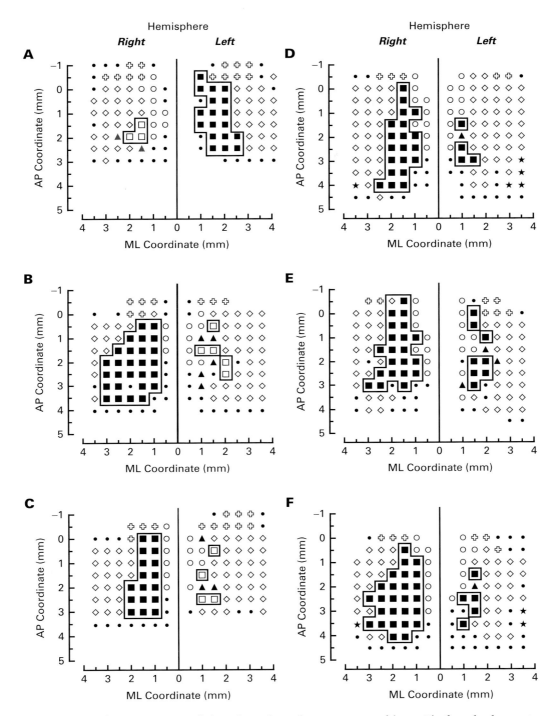

FIGURE 11-5 The representation of vibrissal muscles in the motor cortex of the rat. The frontal poles are at the bottom of each drawing. Antero-posterior coordinates are measured in millimeters from the bregma (the point at which the coronal and saggital sutures meet). Each symbol represents the muscles that respond to stimulation of the cortex at that point: Filled square—contralateral vibrissae; empty square—ipsilateral vibrissae; empty diamond—forelimb; empty cross—hindlimb; filled triangle—neck; filled star—jaw and tongue; empty circle—eye; dot—no response to stimulation. A–C: Cortical maps soon after transection of the

(Continues)

Central Motor Reorganization: Hand Replantation and Transplantation

The plasticity of human motor cortex following nerve repair has been investigated in patients who have undergone hand replantation or transplantation, or free muscle transfer to the upper extremity. The response to either immediate replantation of amputated hands or delayed hand transplantation was investigated with functional magnetic resonance imaging (fMRI), a test that localizes the increased cortical blood flow resulting from neural activity (Giraux et al., 2001; Brenneis et al., 2005; Bjorkman et al., 2007). In the cases of immediate replantation, patterns of cortical activation during finger movement were essentially normal at the earliest postoperative evaluation, and remained so thereafter. This resilience was attributed to the fact that the neuromuscular units of the long finger flexors remained intact, as only their distal tendons had been severed by the amputation. If amputation had occurred 4–6 years earlier, movement of transplanted fingers in the early postoperative period was accompanied by activation of the supplementary motor area, with the sparse M1 activation that remained occurring laterally. As the hand was reinnervated, more of M1 was activated and the center of gravity (COG) of the activity shifted medially. After free muscle transplantation, transcranial magnetic stimulation (TMS) revealed the representation of the transplanted muscle to be similar in size and location to that of the normal, intact muscle in the opposite extremity (Chen et al., 2003). Motor cortex thus remains plastic into adulthood, and is able to restore previously reassigned territory to its original use once functional connections with the periphery are restored.

Central Motor Reorganization: Intercostal Nerve Transfer

The observation that intercostal nerve transfer (ICM) could restore voluntary elbow flexion stimulated interest in learning how the CNS could effect such a remarkable transformation in motor control. In initial studies, the cortical area that activates the biceps was mapped using motor evoked potentials (MEPs) (Mano et al., 1995; Malessy et al., 1998b). These potentials are generated by magnetically stimulating motor cortex and are recorded from individual muscles in the periphery (Hallett, 2000). After intercostal nerve transfer, the area that activates the biceps initially coincides with that for intercostal muscle activation, then gradually shifts to the normal biceps location; it remains smaller than normal and is harder to stimulate. During early reinnervation, generation of MEPs is facilitated by respiration. Once voluntary control is established, facilitation is more prominent with voluntary activity than with respiration, although respiratory facilitation is never lost completely (Malessy et al., 1998a). The persistence of respiratory facilitation and its presence in the normal, contralateral biceps of patients with root avulsion has been interpreted as evidence for normal connections between the central areas that coordinate respiration, postural control, and biceps contraction (Malessy et al., 1998a) (Figure 11-6). Interestingly, trunk flexion was recently found to be an even more potent stimulus to biceps EMG activity than respiration after intercostal transfer (Chalidapong et al., 2006).

fMRI has provided further insight into the shift from respiratory to voluntary control of biceps contraction after ICM transfer (Logothetis et al., 2001). In contrast with MEP determinations, which evaluate output signal, fMRI reflects input and local intracortical processing. In the case of ICM transfer, this input is absent until muscle reinnervation occurs, then is strikingly similar to the activity that accompanies contraction of a normal biceps muscle (Malessy et al., 1998a). To summarize the effects of ICM transfer, control of motor output shifts from intercostal to biceps areas, while the motor input program remains unchanged. Malessy has hypothesized that this shift is possible because the biceps

FIGURE 11-5 (Continued)
left (A) or right (B,C) facial nerve. The denervated vibrissal muscles are no longer represented in the cortex contralateral to the injury. The large, normal representation on the opposite side of the brain corresponds to the remaining, uninjured facial nerve. The void created by reduction of the primary vibrissal motor territory has been filled by medial expansion of the forelimb representation and lateral expansion of the neck and eye representation. D–F: The right facial nerve has been transected and allowed to regenerate. The denervated and subsequently reinnervated vibrissal muscles are again represented within contralateral cortex, but within an abnormally small area. Expansions of the eye territory laterally and the forearm territory medially continue to occupy portions of the former vibrissal territory. Reprinted with permission from Franchi, 2000a.

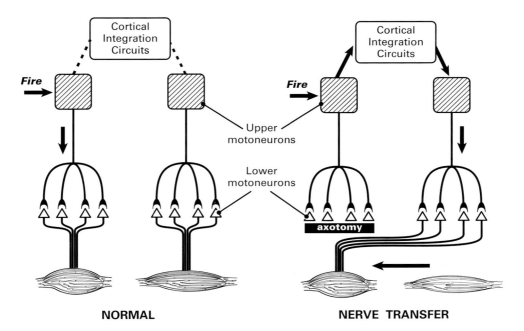

FIGURE 11-6   Central compensation for nerve transfer. On the left, normal circuitry is used to fire a specific muscle. On the right, this muscle has been denervated by traumatic axotomy, then reinnervated by transfer of a functionally related nerve. The motor cortex is able to access a given muscle through multiple, context-dependent motor programs. When a substantial portion of a motoneuron pool is reconnected to a new muscle, it can readjust its function as long as it shares one of these motor programs with the pool that controlled the muscle initially.

and intercostals are already connected through cortical circuitry responsible for coordinating elbow flexion with stabilization of the trunk (Malessy et al., 2003). Once input from the reinnervated biceps is available, these circuits are strengthened to facilitate the shift to voluntary control (Figure 11-6). This view is consistent with the lack of new, direct connections between intercostals and biceps motoneuron pools that could link their activity (Cheng et al., 1997).

Central Motor Reorganization: Nerve Transfer vs. Nerve Repair

The work described above has enhanced understanding of postoperative changes in individual components of the motor system. Although some of these have been documented at the level of individual circuits, many are more broadly descriptive. A substantial gap thus separates our understanding of mechanisms from the readily observed consequences of surgical manipulations. It is possible, however, to gain some insight by comparing the

consequences of experimental nerve repair and nerve transfer in nervous systems of varying complexity.

Nerve transfer was investigated as early as 1828, when Flourens crossed the two main nerves to the chicken wing and reported the eventual return of normal function (Flourens, 1828). In the late nineteenth and early twentieth centuries several nerve-crossing experiments, culminating in the work of Osborne and Kilvington (1910), were said to result in complete functional recovery. Upon careful review, however, many of these were found to be critically flawed (reviewed in Sperry, 1945). Subsequently, Sperry's own work demonstrated that rats were completely unable to compensate for reversal of the tibial and peroneal nerves in the leg and the musculocutaneous and radial nerves in the upper limb, even under extreme circumstances such as amputation of other extremities (Sperry, 1941, 1942). At least in rodents, it was shown conclusively that CNS plasticity could not compensate for the reassignment of major flexor and extensor motoneuron pools. A similar lack of adaptability was later found in the cat in response to both gross manipulation of muscle innervation, crossing the tibial and peroneal nerves (Gordon et al., 1986a), or the finer manipulation of crossing the buccal and zygomatic branches of the facial nerve (Gruart et al., 2003). Subhuman primates, in contrast, adapted readily to crossing the nerves to the flexors of the elbow or wrist (Sperry, 1947; Brinkman et al., 1983), an experience consistent with the remarkable adaptability to nerve transfer demonstrated clinically by human primates (Chapter 8).

As a consequence of the misdirection of axons regenerating after nerve repair, muscle can be reinnervated by motoneurons from more than one pool. Conversely, each motoneuron pool can serve more than one muscle (Brushart, Mesulam, 1980) (Figures 11-7, 7-10). In the resulting mosaic of incorrect connections, adjacent motoneurons with strong functional linkage may serve antagonistic muscles. The inability to compensate for this miswiring is readily demonstrated by EMG analysis of reinnervated muscle after experimental repair of the rat sciatic (Gramsbergen et al., 2000) and cat facial nerves (Gruart et al., 2003). Morphologically, the compromise in function parallels the degree of inappropriate reinnervation (Wikholm et al., 1988). Whereas humans are able to adjust readily to nerve transfer, they are often unable to compensate for inappropriate motor connections formed after nerve repair (Thomas et al., 1987). Similarly, co-contractions of biceps and triceps (Rollnik et al., 2000; Heise et al., 2005) or latissimus and deltoid (Gu et al., 2000) may persist for years after the misdirected regeneration that is often the consequence of perinatal brachial plexus injury.

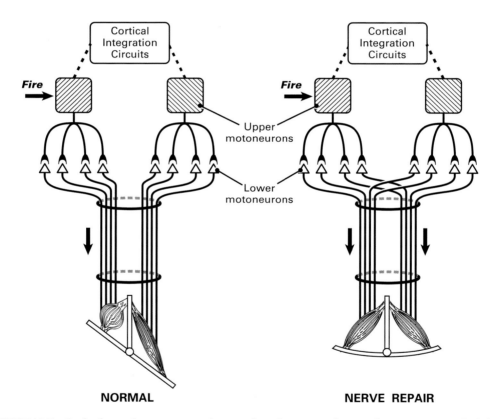

FIGURE 11-7   Lack of central compensation for axonal misdirection at the site of nerve repair. On the left, a normally innervated muscle is contracted by firing its motoneuron pool without stimulating the adjacent motoneurons that serve an antagonistic muscle. On the right, the nerve trunk has been transected and repaired. Motoneurons that once served only the target muscle now innervate both that muscle and its antagonist. The motoneuron pool is a relatively inflexible unit of function and is wired to fire as a unit. An attempt to fire one muscle will now result in the contraction of both that muscle and its antagonist, resulting in a significant degradation of function.

Higher primates and humans, even babies, are unable to compensate for the peripheral miswiring imposed on the nervous system by nerve injury and repair. This observation is consistent with the hypothesis proposed in Chapter 3: the motoneuron pool, not the motor unit, is the quantum of motor organization. There is apparently no circuitry capable of reorganizing projections to individual motoneurons so that each reinnervated muscle is again served by a discrete motoneuron pool. It is still possible, however, that activity-dependent modifications of synaptic efficiency could modulate the activation of inappropriate connections. The inability of the human motor system to compensate for miswiring within a motoneuron pool (nerve repair) thus contrasts dramatically with the excellent results often obtained by transfer of part or all of an intact motoneuron pool along with its afferent circuits (nerve transfer) (Chapter 8). Phylogenetically, the ability to compensate readily for nerve transfer parallels the development of direct corticomotoneuronal projections. If these projections can be shown to play a critical role in plasticity, it may be possible to selectively strengthen them in order to speed the often delayed response to nerve transfer.

THE SENSORY SYSTEM

End Organ Reinnervation

The reinnervation and function of cutaneous mechanoreceptors in nonhuman and human primates has been studied histologically with skin biopsies, and electrophysiologically with neurography in humans and single fiber recordings in other primates. The Pacinian (PC) and Meissner (RA) corpuscles are the two rapidly adapting receptors in primate glabrous skin (see Chapter 2, Table 2-1 for summary of receptor properties). Fewer than 50% of primate Pacinian corpuscles show histologic evidence of reinnervation after nerve crush or repair, and in those that are reinnervated the axon is often misplaced (Wong, Kanagasuntheram, 1971; Archibald et al., 1995). Only 3 of 79 regenerated single fibers studied in the baboon and none of 65 in a human study could be identified as Pacinian afferents (Terzis, Dykes, 1980; Mackel et al., 1983). As a consequence of infrequent reinnervation of Pacinian corpuscles, the perception of high frequency vibrations that is critical to sensing through a tool (Chapter 2) will be compromised in reinnervated skin. Fortunately, the receptive field of the Pacinian corpuscle is so large that this function might still be provided by corpuscles in adjacent, normally innervated skin. The other rapidly adapting sensory ending, the Meissner corpuscle, has also been studied in detail. Biopsy of reinnervated human fingers revealed that Meissner corpuscles were innervated in 12/17 patients (16/23 fingers); in these cases, histology did not predict function (Jabaley et al., 1976). When larger areas of skin were excised in the process of recontouring toes transplanted to the hand, the density of Meissner corpuscles was found to be reduced by nearly two-thirds from values in normal skin (Wei et al., 2000). In these patients, perhaps because a larger, more representative sample was obtained, receptor density did predict function. In both primates and humans, Meissner corpuscles were reinnervated in reduced numbers, but gradually regained near-normal thresholds and receptive field size and contour (Terzis, Dykes, 1980; Mackel et al., 1983). The ability to perceive skin motion is thus preserved to some degree, although localization of stimuli could still be compromised by misdirected regeneration.

The Merkel cell (SAI) and SAII (possible Ruffini organ) are the slowly adapting receptors in glabrous skin. In cats and rats, denervation reduces the Merkel cell population by approximately two-thirds within 2–3 months (English et al., 1983; Nurse et al., 1984). In primates, reinnervated receptors characterized only as SA had increased thresholds and were saturated at lower indentation depths, significantly reducing the range of stimuli to which they could respond (Terzis, Dykes, 1980). In humans, the receptive fields of reinnervated SAI receptors were also reduced in size (Mackel et al., 1983). These abnormalities are likely to compromise perception of form and texture. Recently, the performance of SAI receptors was shown to be enhanced in animals overexpressing NT-3, a finding associated with an increase in the expression of acid-sensing ion channels (McIlwrath et al., 2007; Lawson et al., 2008). The morphologically elusive SAII receptor is reinnervated in proportion to its normal density after human nerve repair, and regains relatively normal threshold and discharge rates (Mackel et al., 1983). The basis for perceiving hand conformation and of forces acting on the hand should thus be at least partially restored.

Collateral Sprouting

Although this discussion has focused on reinnervation of skin by regenerating axons, it is important to recognize that collateral sprouting from intact, adjacent skin may also occur. This has been documented repeatedly in adult rats for both polymodal nociceptor C fibers (Brenan, 1986; Wiesenfeld-Hallin et al., 1989; Doubleday, Robinson, 1992) and sharp pain–conducting Aδ fibers (Devor et al., 1979; Diamond et al., 1987). Similar sprouting of low-threshold mechanoreceptor fibers has been found in neonatal animals, but not in adults (Horch, 1981; Jackson, Diamond, 1981; Kinnman et al., 1992). Clinical evidence of collateral sprouting from human low threshold mechanoreceptors has been reported and occasionally confirmed by block of adjacent nerves (e.g., Aszmann et al., 1996; Jaaskelainen, Peltola, 1996). The basis for these and similar findings is likely to involve complex interactions of several factors (Inbal et al., 1987). In the largest uniform clinical series, consisting of patients who had previously undergone extensive harvest of the medial or posterior cutaneous nerves of the forearm for nerve graft, the margins of light touch sensibility had encroached on the denervated area by a mean of only 6 mm (Healy et al., 1996). Although collateral sprouting of low threshold mechanoreceptor fibers may thus occur in some cases, it certainly cannot be relied on for any consistent sensory improvement.

Afferent Neuron Death

Primary afferent neurons are more sensitive than motoneurons to the effects of axotomy. The magnitude of these effects differs significantly among studies, due primarily to the use of several different counting techniques. As a general rule, however, more neurons are lost after transection than after crush, when the lesion is proximal rather than distal, and in neonates rather than in adults. Axotomy 10 mm distal to the C7 DRG results in loss of 50% of neurons prelabeled with Fast Blue by 4 months, an effect that is not ameliorated by nerve repair (Ma et al., 2001; Ma et al., 2003, Jivan et al., 2006). A similar distance from the L5 DRG, axotomy reduced the neuron count by 35% at 45 days, while crush reduced it by only 30% (Vestergaard et al., 1997; Degn et al., 1999). In both instances, small dark cells were more vulnerable than large light cells.

When axotomy is performed more distally, at the level of the sciatic nerve, neuronal loss as estimated by corrected neuron counts is 20% in adults, rising to 70–75% in neonates (Schmalbruch, 1987). If stereological techniques are applied, sciatic axotomy is seen to result in progressive neuronal loss from the L5 DRG, with a 14% reduction by 8 weeks that increases to 37% at 32 weeks (Tandrup et al., 2000). Again, small dark cells were more sensitive to axotomy than were their larger counterparts; these were subsequently found to be cutaneous afferents, with little death within the muscle afferent population (Welin et al., 2008). When both L4 and L5 were analyzed in a similar study, the overall loss was already 35% by 8 weeks, and stabilized at this level to 26 weeks (Hart et al., 2002). Neuron loss after peripheral axotomy may thus compromise sensory input from skin to a significant degree, though critical mechanoreceptive input should be relatively unaffected.

Dorsal Horn Reinnervation

The loss of topographic specificity during the regeneration of afferent fibers degrades the somatotopic mapping of the limbs to the dorsal horn. As was illustrated by Figure 10-10, after repair of the rat peroneal nerve the normally narrow projection of afferents from the tibialis anterior muscle (innervated by the peroneal nerve) to the dorsal horn expands to include dorsal horn territory that normally serves peroneal-innervated skin; both cutaneous and muscle afferents have reinnervated muscle (Brushart et al., 1981). When the entire sciatic nerve is repaired, the dorsal horn territory serving the tibialis anterior becomes even larger, indicating that afferents from the tibial nerve have entered the peroneal nerve at the repair site, and have then reinnervated the tibialis anterior. Similar tracing studies from the digits of primates with regenerated median nerves reveal both transverse and longitudinal spread of the digital projection (Florence et al., 1994). In the cat, the receptive fields of dorsal horn neurons return to normal after nerve crush, but are topographically disordered after recovering from nerve transection (Lisney, 1983a, 1983b). Without compensatory changes at more proximal levels, mechanosensitive information that reaches the cortex will thus be mapped incorrectly.

Dorsal Horn Plasticity

Current evidence suggests that dorsal horn collaterals of low-threshold mechanoreceptive afferents (LTMRs) do not undergo significant sprouting in response to injury. Until recently, however, this was not the predominant view. These afferents were not found to project to lamina II of the dorsal horn (the substantia gelatinosa, an area thought to receive only unmyelinated pain afferents) in early studies performed with HRP (Light, Perl, 1979). After peripheral nerve injury, in contrast, bulk labeling with Choleragenoid-horseradish peroxidase (B-HRP) revealed substantial projections to lamina II (Woolf et al., 1992, 1995). Since B-HRP was then thought to label A-fiber projections selectively, the assumption was made that myelinated afferents, including those of LTMRs, had sprouted into lamina II, where they could now be responsible for mechanical allodynia. Single fiber studies obtained by injecting identified A-β collaterals within the dorsal columns with HRP confirmed that some of these fibers projected into lamina II after peripheral axotomy and regeneration (Koerber et al., 1994).

As the ramifications of dorsal horn plasticity were explored, the selectivity of B-HRP for A fibers came into question (discussed in Woodbury et al., 2008). Tracing with neurobiotin and introduction of a new, in vitro preparation that facilitated labeling the entire peripheral and most of the central arbor of an identified neuron provided a revised view of normal dorsal horn projections; what were previously thought to be the sprouts of low-threshold mechanoreceptors were, in fact, shown to be normal terminations of myelinated axons within lamina II (Hughes et al., 2003; Boada, Woodbury, 2008). Many of these were Aβ nociceptors, the most rapidly conducting nociceptive fibers and thus the first to signal pain to the CNS, and others were down hair follicle afferents (Boada, Woodbury, 2008). Application of this technique to regenerated nerve revealed that low-threshold mechanoreceptors had not sprouted into lamina II. (Woodbury et al., 2008). In retrospect, it appears that injury enhanced the labeling of lamina II collaterals that were already there, and that were labeled readily by single fiber HRP injections in the dorsal columns, but not from the periphery with B-HRP.

Although there now appears to be little structural plasticity within the dorsal horn, there is ample evidence for physiologic plasticity. This has been explored in cats that previously underwent tibial and sural nerve repair (Koerber et al., 1995; Koerber, Mirnics, 1996; Koerber et al., 2006). Soon after afferent axons had reinnervated the skin, the receptive fields of dorsal horn neurons were abnormally large, often discontinuous, and sometimes included adjacent skin that had never been denervated (Figure 11-8). Within these receptive fields, sensitivity to stimuli was variable, so that occasional "hot spots" could be identified. Many of the properties exhibited by dorsal horn neurons mirror abnormalities in the newly established peripheral receptive fields of their synaptic partners in the DRG: fragmentation into multiple islands, often with irregular borders, and variable sensitivity throughout the field with occasional "hot spots" (Terzis, Dykes, 1980; Horch, Lisney, 1981).

In normal animals, all the fibers activated by stimulating the skin within the receptive field of a dorsal horn neuron are synaptically coupled to that neuron. This connectivity was evaluated in a longitudinal series of cat nerve repairs by recording from individual dorsal horn neurons while electrically stimulating the skin within their receptive fields (Koerber et al., 2006). Six months after nerve repair, only 35% of the stimulus sites were innervated by fibers with synaptic inputs to the dorsal horn neuron that defined the receptive field under study. This finding is consistent with a lack of topographic specificity in sensory axon regeneration (Figure 11-8); peripheral axons that normally subserved the receptive field of a single dorsal horn neuron have been misdirected at the repair site, and have reinnervated patches of skin in multiple areas. Conversely, during the regeneration process any given receptive field is overlapped by axons that have wandered in from distant areas, and would thus not be synaptically coupled to the reference neuron. By 9–12 months, 86% of afferents sampled within a receptive field were coupled to the reference neuron, and the receptive field itself was reduced in size. These changes are coincident with alterations in the efficacy of synapses between the arbors of afferent axons and dorsal horn neurons (Figure 11-9). As a result, dorsal horn neurons will once again represent discrete receptive fields. Clearly, however, this plasticity is driven by individual receptive fields, and cannot be expected to influence large-scale topographic organization.

Not only does sensory axon regeneration lack inherent topographic specificity, it also lacks end organ specificity (Chapter 10). As a result, there are frequent mismatches between peripheral receptors on the one hand and DRG neurons and their central processes on the other. Examination of both naturally occurring and intentional mismatches in the cat produced little evidence of respecification of central synaptic connections (Nishimura et al., 1993; Koerber et al., 1994). In the rat, in contrast, sural neurons redirected to the gastrocnemius muscle were found to adjust both their physiologic properties and the somatotopy of their dorsal horn representation toward those of the original gastrocnemius afferents (Lewin, McMahon, 1991c, 1993).

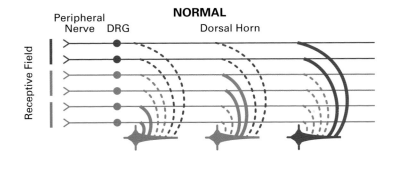

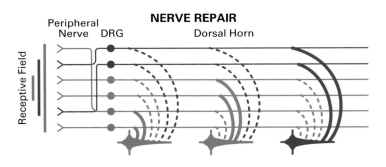

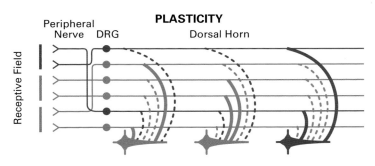

FIGURE 11-8   Dorsal horn compensation for misdirected sensory axon regeneration. Top: Three dorsal horn neurons each receive active projections (thick solid lines) from 2 DRG neurons with overlapping receptive fields. The dorsal horn neurons also receive latent projections (dotted lines) from other DRG neurons with distant receptive fields. Middle: After transection and misdirected regeneration of peripheral axons, the receptive fields of dorsal horn neurons are enlarged and irregular, and will contain projections that are not electrically coupled to (synapse on) the reference DRG neuron. Bottom: As a result of dorsal horn plasticity, incorrect projections are weakened and appropriate latent connections are strengthened. Receptive fields are reduced in size and their constituent neurons are again coupled electrically.

Cortical Changes in Response to Experimental Nerve Injury and Regeneration

False sensory localization, long recognized as the hallmark of posttraumatic sensory axon regeneration (Chapter 5), was the starting point for investigation

of cortical organization after nerve repair (Paul et al., 1972). These authors reasoned that:

> there is a kind of "fixed locus" of reference intrinsic in the cortical somatotopic skin representation. Derangement of this basic organization is compatible with return of function

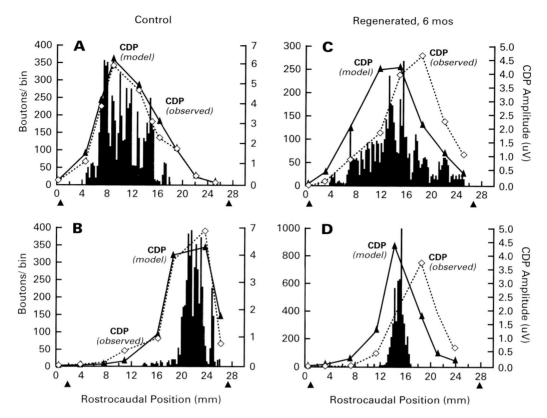

FIGURE 11-9   Evaluating dorsal horn plasticity by comparing the density of boutons on labeled dorsal column axons with the cord dorsum potentials (CDPs) that result from their stimulation. The solid line represents the expected potential at each level of the dorsal horn calculated from the bouton distribution, and the dotted line represents the actual cord dorsum potential at each level. In controls (A,B) the two curves are nearly identical; the boutons are functioning as expected. After nerve repair (C,D) the curves do not match; as a result of plasticity, some boutons are contributing more than others to the CDP. Reprinted with permission from Koerber et al., 2006.

of the basic modalities of sensation, but disruption of the spatial relationships of the body part projections to the cortex may result in misinterpretation of tactile localization. Thus, if neuron A originally innervated point B on the index finger, and following regeneration now innervates point C on another digit, central activity resulting from stimulation of nerve ending A will now be interpreted as originating from its original location.(p2)

Rhesus monkeys were studied 6.5–7.5 months after transection and repair of their median nerves. The receptive fields of neurons in sensory cortex were mapped by inserting a microelectrode into the cortical surface at 0.5 mm intervals on a two-dimensional

grid while stimulating the surface of the reinnervated skin. The investigators found marked disorganization of the normal somatotopic organization of cortical areas 1 and 3b (Chapter 2). Additionally, the normally homogeneous input to cortical columns now included more than one sensory modality, and the overall distribution of SA afferents across the sensory cortex was altered. All of these findings were readily attributable to disordered regeneration of cutaneous afferents, strengthening the original hypothesis.

A decade later, the next major investigation of primate cortical reorganization was also designed to explore the central consequences of peripheral nerve damage. In a series of experiments, Merzenich, Wall, Kaas, and coworkers performed detailed cortical mapping after transection, crush, or transection and repair of the median nerve (Merzenich et al., 1983a, 1983b; Wall et al., 1983, 1986). Owl monkeys were used for many of these preparations, as the sensory cortex is superficial and relatively easy to study; Paul and coworkers (Paul et al., 1972) had to cut away frontal lobe to access areas 1 and 3b because, in the rhesus monkey, these areas are partially concealed within the central sulcus.

Transection of the median nerve is followed immediately by silencing of the cortical surface that normally receives median inputs (Merzenich et al., 1983a, 1983b) (Figure 11-10). This silent area is

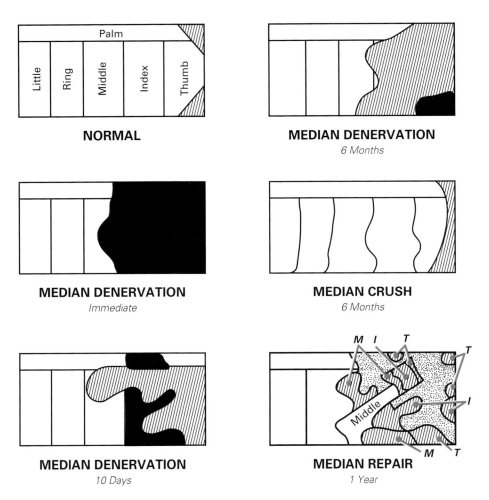

FIGURE 11-10 Plasticity of cortical area 3b in the primate. Dark areas are silent, hatched areas represent hairy skin on the dorsum of the hand. Normally, the digits are represented in an orderly fashion, with more territory assigned to the radial side of the hand than to the ulnar side. Immediately after transection of the median nerve, the median territory becomes silent. In the ensuing days, the dorsal hand territory undergoes dramatic expansion to occupy much of the previously median territory, which is also occupied partly by an expansion of the ulnar hand territory. After 6 months of continuous denervation, the majority of the previously median territory now represents hairy skin on the dorsum of the hand. Regeneration after nerve crush restores somatotopy that is nearly normal. Even 1 year after nerve repair, however, the area serving the median nerve (stippled) is grossly irregular and is interrupted by many islands of residual dorsal hand representation (T = thumb, I = index finger, M = middle finger). These diagrams are conceptual simplifications of data from Merzenich et al., 1983a,1983b and Wall et al., 1983, 1986.

then subsumed by expansion of adjacent territories, predominantly radial-innervated dorsal skin, but also ulnar-innervated glabrous skin. Although the facial representation is also adjacent to the median nerve territory, it does not expand under these conditions. The expansions are topographically crude at the outset and become more organized and well-delineated with time, yet their boundaries remain plastic for months after denervation. The expansion of the radial nerve territory is still organized by digit, so that each dorsal territory extends to occupy what was previously the volar territory of the same finger. The more a given topographic projection expands, the smaller individual receptive fields become. These observations led the investigators to conclude that, in the absence of a permanently embedded perceptual map, somatosensory cortex is subject to ongoing territorial competition. They also predicted a treatment strategy that has only recently been investigated:

> It is of special interest that over at least much of reorganized cortex, receptive field areas are a reciprocal function of the "magnification" of "new" and expanded representations. This indicates, at the first level, that improvements in tactile acuity might be expected over skin surfaces bordering the median nerve field. Such changes have never been reported in humans but should be sought. (Merzenich et al., 1983b)

Crush of the median nerve at the wrist allows the majority of afferent fibers to regenerate, and to return to the cutaneous territories that they served initially. Under these conditions, cortical reorganization occurs in two distinct phases (Figure 11-10). The early stages of recovery are similar to those that follow nerve transection, with initial silencing of the median territory, followed by expansion of adjacent territories to fill the void left by median denervation. In the second phase, reinnervated tissues reclaim the former median territory. The subsequent reoccupation of median cortex is not an all-or-nothing phenomenon, but a gradual process that mirrors the reinnervation of the skin from proximal in the palm to the digit tip distally (Wall et al., 1983).

The cortical reorganization that follows nerve transection and repair, in contrast, is far less orderly (Wall et al., 1986) (Figure 11-10). Although the receptive fields of cortical neurons could be single and discrete, many neurons were encountered that responded to stimulation of multiple cutaneous areas, that responded to stimulation of a large area (Pacinian-like), or that did not respond to cutaneous stimulation at all. The overall topography of the median nerve projection was characterized by discontinuous, patchy digital representations in both correct and incorrect locations, and by extensive overlap of the representations of both adjacent and nonadjacent surfaces. These features could all be explained as the cortical manifestations of axonal sprouting and disorganization at the site of nerve repair.

Thalamic and Brainstem Nuclei

Most early efforts to determine the central consequences of peripheral nerve injury focused on the cerebral cortex, as this was the easiest area to access surgically and electrophysiologically. It soon became apparent, however, that both the cuneate nucleus and ventroposterior (VP) nucleus of the thalamus also exhibited substantial plasticity. The long-term effects of median nerve transection and repair were evaluated by comparing the HRP-labeled projections of digital skin to the cuneate nucleus with projections of the same area to cortex as determined electrophysiologically (Florence et al., 1994) (Figures 11-11, 11-12). The wide distribution of label in the cuneate nucleus corresponded to an enlarged representation of the corresponding digit in area 3b. The patterns of cuneate and cortical representations were not necessarily the same, however, as one could be continuous and the other fragmented, indicating the lack of precise mapping from one to the other.

Further work disclosed that both cortical and cuneate changes occurred immediately after peripheral nerve injury (Kolarik et al., 1994; Xu, Wall, 1997, 1999). In both areas, neurons that lost cutaneous input rapidly acquired receptive fields on the radial-innervated dorsal hand, and the map of this area expanded accordingly. Since area 3b is driven largely by dorsal column inputs that synapse in the cuneate and gracile nuclei (Chapter 2), cortical changes appear to reflect, at least in part, plasticity within the cuneate nucleus. Additionally, however, there are differences in cuneate and cortical responses that suggest that both are shaped by mechanisms that act concurrently but separately: the dorsal hand projection expands to occupy 60% of the cuneate hand territory and only 40% of the hand cortex in area 3b, cuneate projections are

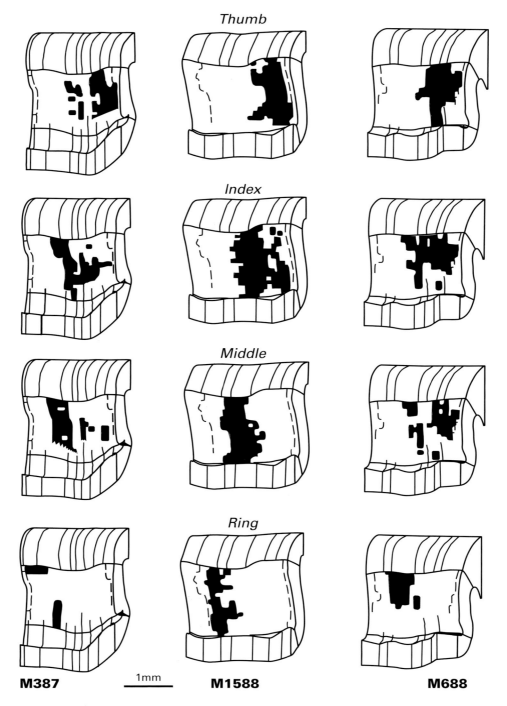

Thumb

Index

Middle

Ring

M387   1mm   **M1588**   **M688**

FIGURE 11-11   The area representing individual digits in cortical area 3b after recovery from median nerve repair in 3 adult macaque monkeys. Digits are represented in sequence from the thumb (above) to the ring finger (below). Each vertical column represents the digits of the monkey identified at the bottom. By separating the digital representations it is possible to appreciate the substantial overlap among digits and the marked irregularity of each projection. Reprinted with permission from Florence et al., 1994.

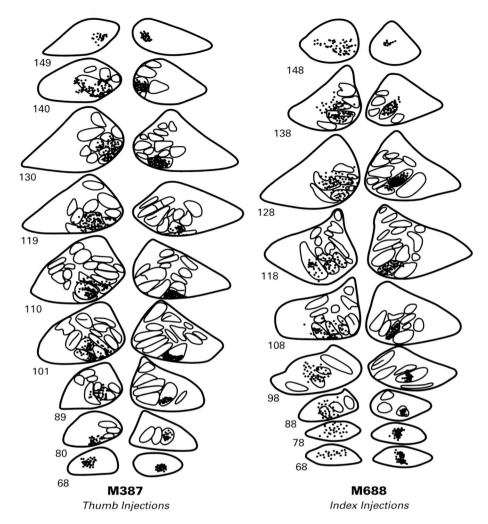

149

140

130

119

110

101

89

80

68

M387
Thumb Injections

148

138

128

118

108

98

88

78

68

M688
Index Injections

FIGURE 11-12   In animals M387 and M688 of Figure 11-11, digital projections to the cuneate nucleus were mapped by injecting conjugates of HRP into the tips of the thumb (M387) or middle finger (M688) after recovery from left median nerve repair. The corresponding normal digit was injected on the right. Rostral-superior, caudal-inferior. Numbers refer to individual tissue sections. The cuneate somatotopy is best appreciated on section 101, left side, where the thumb is represented on the lateral aspect of the digital row, and on section 118, right side, where the index finger is represented just medial to the thumb location. The topographic disorganization of both projections is readily apparent on the left side of each section. Reprinted with permission from Florence et al., 1994.

continuous while cortical projections are often discontinuous, and cuneate receptive fields are larger than those in area 3b (Wall et al., 2002).

The VP nucleus of the thalamus, the relay between the cuneate nucleus and cortex (Chapter 2), was found to have somatotopic alterations consistent with those described for the other areas (Jones, Pons, 1998; Churchill et al., 2001). These changes were also found to occur rapidly, and to be modified

by both descending and ascending inputs. In spite of the complex interdependency of the relay nuclei and cortex in determining the organization of projections at each level, the greatest capacity for plasticity resides within cortex: cortical receptive fields are refined by both the passage of time and by interaction with an enriched environment, whereas those in the cuneate and VPL are little changed by these circumstances (Florence et al., 2001; Churchill,

Garraghty, 2006). The cortex is also the site of marked plasticity after perinatal nerve injury and repair. Nearly normal response properties and somatotopy are restored within area 3b, yet abnormalities persist in cuneate and VPL that mirror those resulting from nerve repair in adult animals (Florence et al., 1996).

Mechanisms of Cortical Plasticity

Current evidence suggests that cortical reorganization in response to nerve injury occurs in at least two and perhaps three stages. As described above, the initial changes occur within minutes of injury. Although median nerve transection silences most of the previously median territory, approximately 25% responds immediately to stimulation of dorsal skin (Garraghty, Muja, 1996). This rapid plasticity is achieved by unmasking inputs that are already present but not normally functional (Schroeder et al., 1995). GABA has been found to constrain the receptive fields of cortical neurons, and is rapidly depleted in layer IV of de-afferented cortex (Hicks, Dykes, 1983; Wellman et al., 2002; Garraghty et al., 2006). It is currently thought that de-afferentation reduces local GABA concentrations, thereby eliminating the afferent-driven inhibition that normally constrains latent connections. The second phase of reorganization fills in the initially unresponsive areas of cortex in the ensuing weeks and requires activation of NMDA receptors (Garraghty, Muja, 1996). The final reorganization of somatotopy, which is achieved by one year after injury, may also result from an increase of the lateral projections of cortical neurons, although this mode of expansion requires confirmation (Florence et al., 1998).

Human Cortical Plasticity

The CNS response to nerve injury and repair has also been studied in humans. Patients with chronic carpal tunnel syndrome were evaluated with magnetoencephalography and found indirectly to have a decrease in the cortical area devoted to the median nerve (Druschky et al., 2000, Diesch et al., 2001). Similarly, the potentials evoked by stimulation of the ulnar nerve adjacent to compressed median nerves were greater than those in controls at spinal cord, brainstem, and cortical levels, suggesting compensatory expansion of the ulnar territory (Diesch et al., 2001). The most direct evidence has been obtained in a combined fMRI and somatosensory

evoked potential (SSEP) study of patients at various stages of recovery after median nerve repair (Hansson, Brismar, 2003). Median digital territories were enlarged by over 40% yet normal SSEP data were obtained by stimulating the median nerve proximal to the injury. These findings are consistent with the enlarged, overlapping digital territories mapped by Wall et al. (1986) in area 3b (Figure 11-11).

Recently, exploration of the immediate consequences of human nerve dysfunction has revealed a potential treatment modality. In the context of an SSEP study of cortical map boundaries, Waberski et al. (2003) found that local anesthetic block of the thumb was sufficient to move the index and middle finger territories toward that of the thumb. Similarly, when the entire radial and median nerves were blocked, the cortical territories on either side, the ulnar and lip, moved closer together (Weiss et al., 2004). This migration was accompanied by increased two-point discrimination in the lip, as predicted by Merzenich et al. (1983b), and mislocalization of touch of ulnar-innervated skin to the median-innervated digits, consistent with expansion of the cortical area devoted to the ulnar nerve. Bjorkman et al. (2004) approached the issue from a more clinical perspective, demonstrating that a topical anesthetic block of forearm skin increased two-point discrimination in the digits, a change that they found to correlate with fMRI evidence of expansion of the cortical hand territory into that of the forearm (Bjorkman et al., 2009). This is one of the few instances in which a series of basic science investigations has led directly to an intervention that effectively modifies the consequences of nerve injury (Rosen et al., 2006).

CONCLUSIONS

The functional consequences of nerve injury and repair for the sensory and motor systems have been reviewed and correlated with current knowledge of the underlying neuropathology. In both instances, the organizational changes that have been documented are largely consistent with the clinical findings. Furthermore, in each system the nature of the clinical deficits can be explained by the system's unique organizational characteristics.

In the motor system, individual motoneurons respecify muscle fiber properties to reconstruct functional motor units. At the central end of the system, cortical neurons are able to access motoneurons through a variety of contextual circuits, suggesting the potential for great plasticity. Lodged between these plastic areas, however, lies the motoneuron pool. Analysis of the local spinal cord circuitry suggests that motoneuron pools are addressed as a unit. Higher primates and humans, those with direct cortico-motoneuronal connections, are able to reassign the function of an intact motoneuron pool after nerve transfer, often with great facility. They are not, however, even as infants, able to compensate for the reinnervation of several muscles by motoneurons from a single pool after nerve repair. In the sensory system, in contrast, sensory channels are normally tightly focused, with a high level of correspondence between individual end organs and area 3b somatosensory cortical neurons. During reinnervation of the skin, receptive fields are gradually sharpened and multiple receptive fields are eliminated. Some degree of plasticity is thus able to effect short-range changes to refine the sensory channel, consistent with the paucity of faulty sensory localization between areas close to one another. The greatest challenge for the sensory system is posed by the topographic irregularities that arise from misdirection of regenerating cutaneous axons to inappropriate areas of skin. The cortex and relay nuclei are remarkably plastic in responding to the elimination of inputs from an injured nerve, and are able to expand existing territories to re-occupy a denervated area with great alacrity. When inputs return in topographic disarray, in contrast, the tight organization of the original projections allows little compensation, resulting in false sensory localization. The ability of the developing sensory system to restore cortical order, even in the face of continued disorder in the relay nuclei, is consistent with the near-normal recovery often observed after major nerve injury in the very young. In the adult, promotion of topographically specific regeneration remains one of the primary challenges of nerve repair.

REFERENCES

Abelew TA, Miller MD, Cope TC, Nichols TR (2000) Local loss of proprioception results in disruption of interjoint coordination during locomotion in the cat. J Neurophysiol 84: 2709–2714.

Archibald SJ, Shefner J, Krarup C, Madison RD (1995) Monkey median nerve repaired by nerve graft or collagen nerve guide tube. J Neurosci 15: 4109–4123.

Aszmann OC, Muse V, Dellon AL (1996) Evidence in support of collateral sprouting after sensory nerve resection. Ann Plast Surg 37: 520–525.

Aszmann OC, Winkler T, Korak K, Lassmann H, Frey M (2004) The influence of GDNF on the timecourse and extent of motoneuron loss in the cervical spinal cord after brachial plexus injury in the neonate. Neurol Res 26: 211–217.

Banks RW, Barker D, Brown HG (1985) Sensory reinnervation of muscles following nerve section and suture in cats. J Hand Surg 10B: 340–344.

Banks RW, Barker D (1989) Specificities of afferents reinnervating cat muscle spindles after nerve section. J Physiol 408: 345–372.

Barker D, Scott JJ, Stacey MJ (1986) Reinnervation and recovery of cat muscle receptors after long-term denervation. Exp Neurol 94: 184–202.

Barker D, Berry RB, Scott JJ (1990) The sensory reinnervation of muscles following immediate and delayed nerve repair in the cat. Br J Plast Surg 43(1): 107–111.

Bjorkman A, Rosen B, Lundborg G (2004) Acute improvement of hand sensibility after selective ipsilateral cutaneous forearm anaesthesia. Eur J Neurosci 20: 2733–2736.

Bjorkman A, Waites A, Rosen B, Larsson EM, Lundborg G (2007) Cortical reintegration of a replanted hand and an osseointegrated thumb prosthesis. Acta Neurochir Suppl 100: 109–112.

Bjorkman A, Weibull A, Rosen B, Svensson J, Lundborg G (2009) Rapid cortical reorganisation and improved sensitivity of the hand following cutaneous anaesthesia of the forearm. Eur J Neurosci 29: 837–844.

Boada MD, Woodbury CJ (2008) Myelinated skin sensory neurons project extensively throughout adult mouse substantia gelatinosa. J Neurosci 28: 2006–2014.

Bodine-Fowler SC, Unguez GA, Roy RR, Armstrong AN, Edgerton VR (1993) Innervation patterns in the cat tibialis anterior six months after self-reinnervation. Muscle & Nerve 16: 379–391.

Brannstrom T, Havton L, Kellerth JO (1992a) Restorative effects of reinnervation on the size and dendritic arborization patterns of axotomized cat spinal alpha-motoneurons. J Comp Neurol 318: 452–461.

Brannstrom T, Havton L, Kellerth JO (1992b) Changes in size and dendritic arborization patterns of adult cat spinal alpha-motoneurons following permanent axotomy. J Comp Neurol 318: 439–451.

Brannstrom T, Kellerth JO (1999) Recovery of synapses in axotomized adult cat spinal motoneurons after reinnervation into muscle. Exp Brain Res 125: 19–27.

Brenan A (1986) Collateral reinnervation of skin by C-fibres following nerve injury in the rat. Brain Res 385: 152–155.

Brenneis C, Loscher WN, Egger KE, Benke T, Schocke M, Gabl MF, Wechselberger G, Felber S, Pechlaner S, Margreiter R, Piza-Katzer H, Poewe W (2005) Cortical motor activation patterns following hand transplantation and replantation. J Hand Surg Br 30: 530–533.

Brinkman C, Porter R, Norman J (1983) Plasticity of motor behavior in monkeys with crossed forelimb nerves. Science 220: 438–440.

Brown MC, Butler RG (1976) Regeneration of afferent and efferent fibres to muscle spindles after nerve injury in adults cats. J Physiol 260: 253–266.

Brushart TM, Mesulam MM (1980) Alteration in connections between muscle and anterior horn motoneurons after peripheral nerve repair. Science 208: 603–605.

Brushart TM, Henry EW, Mesulam MM (1981) Reorganization of muscle afferent projections accompanies peripheral nerve regeneration. Neuroscience 6: 2053–2061.

Buller AJ, Eccles JC, Eccles RM (1960) Interactions between motoneurones and muscles in respect of the characteristic speeds of their responses. J Physiol 150: 417–439.

Burke RE, Levine DN, Tsairis P, Zajac FE (1973) Physiological types and histochemical profiles in motor units of the cat gastrocnemius. J Physiol 234: 723–748.

Chalidapong P, Sananpanich K, Klaphajone J (2006) Electromyographic comparison of various exercises to improve elbow flexion following intercostal nerve transfer. J Bone Joint Surg Br 88: 620–622.

Chen DH (1978) Qualitative and quantitative study of synaptic displacement in chromatolyzed spinal motoneurons of the cat. J Comp Neurol 177: 635–664.

Chen R, Anastakis DJ, Haywood CT, Mikulis DJ, Manktelow RT (2003) Plasticity of the human motor system following muscle reconstruction: a magnetic stimulation and functional magnetic resonance imaging study. Clin Neurophysiol 114: 2434–2446.

Cheng H, Shoung HM, Wu ZA, Chen KC, Lee LS (1997) Functional connectivity of the transected brachial plexus after intercostal neurotization in monkeys. J Comp Neurol 380: 155–163.

Churchill JD, Arnold LL, Garraghty PE (2001) Somatotopic reorganization in the brainstem and thalamus following peripheral nerve injury in adult primates. Brain Res 910: 142–152.

Churchill JD, Garraghty PE (2006) The influence of post-nerve injury survival duration on receptive field size: location, location, location. Neurosci Lett 405: 10–13.

Collins WF, Mendell LM, Munson JB (1986) On the specificity of sensory reinnervation of cat skeletal muscle. J Physiol 375: 587–609.

Cope TC, Bonasera SJ, Nichols TR (1994) Reinnervated muscles fail to produce stretch reflexes. J Neurophysiol 71: 817–820.

Degn J, Tandrup T, Jakobsen J (1999) Effect of nerve crush on perikaryal number and volume of neurons in adult rat dorsal root ganglion. J Comp Neurol 412: 186–192.

DeSantis M, Norman WP (1993) Location and completeness of reinnervation by two types of neurons at a single target: the feline muscle spindle. J Comp Neurol 336: 66–76.

Devor M, Schonfeld D, Seltzer Z, Wall PD (1979) Two modes of cutaneous reinnervation following peripheral nerve injury. J Comp Neurol 185: 211–220.

Diamond J, Coughlin M, Macintyre L, Holmes M, Visheau B (1987) Evidence that endogenous beta nerve growth factor is responsible for the collateral sprouting, but not the regeneration, of nociceptive axons in adult rats. Proc Natl Acad Sci USA 84: 6596–6600.

Diesch E, Preissl H, Haerle M, Schaller HE, Birbaumer N (2001) Multiple frequency steady-state evoked magnetic field mapping of digit representation in primary somatosensory cortex. Somatosens Mot Res 18: 10–18.

Donoghue JP, Suner S, Sanes JN (1990) Dynamic organization of primary motor cortex output to target muscles in adult rats. II. Rapid reorganization following motor nerve lesions. Exp Brain Res 79: 492–503.

Doubleday B, Robinson PP (1992) The role of nerve growth factor in collateral reinnervation by cutaneous C-fibres in the rat. Brain Res 593: 179–184.

Druschky K, Kaltenhauser M, Hummel C, Druschky A, Huk WJ, Stefan H, Neundirfer B (2000) Alteration of the somatosensory cortical map in peripheral mononeuropathy due to carpal tunnel syndrome. Neuroreport 11: 3925–3930.

Duxson MJ, Ross JJ, Harris AJ (1986) Transfer of differentiated synaptic terminals from primary myotubes to new-formed muscle cells during embryonic development in the rat. Neurosci Lett 71: 147–152.

Duxson MJ, Usson Y, Harris AJ (1989) The origin of secondary myotubes in mammalian skeletal muscles: ultrastructural studies. Development 107: 743–750.

English AW, Chen Y, Carp J, Wolpaw JR, Chen XY (2007) Recovery of electromyographic activity after transection and surgical repair of the rat sciatic nerve. J Neurophysiol 97: 1127–1134.

English KB, Kavka-Van Norman D, Horch K (1983) Effects of chronic denervation in type I cutaneous mechanoreceptors (Haarscheiben). Anat Rec 207: 79–88.

Florence SL, Garraghty PE, Wall JT, Kaas JH (1994) Sensory afferent projections and area 3b somatotopy following median nerve cut and repair in macaque monkeys. Cereb Cortex 4: 391–407.

Florence SL, Jain N, Pospichal MW, Beck PD, Sly DL, Kaas JH (1996) Central reorganization of sensory pathways following peripheral nerve regeneration in fetal monkeys. Nature 381: 69–71.

Florence SL, Taub HB, Kaas JH (1998) Large-scale sprouting of cortical connections after peripheral injury in adult macaque monkeys. Science 282: 1117–1121.

Florence SL, Boydston LA, Hackett TA, Lachoff HT, Strata F, Niblock MM (2001) Sensory enrichment after peripheral nerve injury restores cortical, not thalamic, receptive field organization. Eur J Neurosci 13: 1755–1766.

Flourens MP (1828) Experiences sur la reunion ou cicatrisation des plaies de la Moelle epiniere et des nerfs. Ann Sci Natur ser.1, 13: 113–122.

Franchi G (2000a) Changes in motor representation related to facial nerve damage and regeneration in adult rats. Exp Brain Res 135: 53–65.

Franchi G (2000b) Reorganization of vibrissal motor representation following severing and repair of the facial nerve in adult rats. Exp Brain Res 131: 33–43.

Franchi G, Veronesi C (2004) Long-term motor cortex reorganization after facial nerve severing in newborn rats. Eur J Neurosci 20: 1885–1896.

Franchi G, Veronesi C (2006) Short-term reorganization of input-deprived motor vibrissae representation following motor disconnection in adult rats. J Physiol 574: 457–476.

Garraghty PE, Muja N (1996) NMDA receptors and plasticity in adult primate somatosensory cortex. J Comp Neurol 367: 319–326.

Garraghty PE, Arnold LL, Wellman CL, Mowery TM (2006) Receptor autoradiographic correlates of deafferentation-induced reorganization in adult primate somatosensory cortex. J Comp Neurol 497: 636–645.

Gauthier GF, Burke RE, Lowey S, Hobbs AW (1983) Myosin isozymes in normal and cross-reinnervated cat skeletal muscle fibers. J Cell Biol 97: 756–771.

Giraux P, Sirigu A, Schneider F, Dubernard JM (2001) Cortical reorganization in motor cortex after graft of both hands. Nat Neurosci 4: 691–692.

Gordon T, Stein RB (1982a) Reorganization of motor-unit properties in reinnervated muscles of the cat. J Neurophysiol 48: 1175–1190.

Gordon T, Stein R (1982b) Time course and extent of recovery in reinnervated motor units of cat triceps surae muscles. J Physiol 323: 307–323.

Gordon T, Stein RB, Thomas CK (1986a) Innervation and function of hind-limb muscles in the cat after cross-union of the tibial and peroneal nerves. J Physiol 374: 429–441.

Gordon T, Stein RB, Thomas CK (1986b) Organization of motor units following cross-reinnervation of antagonistic muscles in the cat hind limb. J Physiol 374: 443–456.

Gordon T, Gillespie J, Orozco R, Davis L (1991) Axotomy-induced changes in rabbit hindlimb nerves and the effects of chronic electrical stimulation. J Neurosci 11: 2157–2169.

Gordon T, Thomas CK, Munson JB, Stein RB (2004) The resilience of the size principle in the organization of motor unit properties in normal and reinnervated adult skeletal muscles. Can J Physiol Pharmacol 82: 645–661.

Gorza L, Gundersen K, Lomo T, Schiaffino S, Westgaard RH (1988) Slow-to-fast transformation of denervated soleus muscles by chronic high-frequency stimulation in the rat. J Physiol 402: 627–649.

Gramsbergen A, Ijkema-Paassen J, Meek MF (2000) Sciatic nerve transection in the adult rat: abnormal EMG patterns during locomotion by aberrant innervation of hindleg muscles. Exp Neurol 161: 183–193.

Gregory JE, Luff AR, Proske U (1982) Muscle receptors in the cross-reinnervated soleus muscle of the cat. J Physiol 331: 367–383.

Gruart A, Streppel M, Guntinas-Lichius O, Angelov DN, Neiss WF, Delgado-García JM (2003) Motoneuron adaptability to new motor tasks following two types of facial-facial anastomosis in cats. Brain 126: 115–133.

Gu YD, Chen L, Shen LY (2000) Classification of impairment of shoulder abduction in obstetric brachial plexus palsy and its clinical significance. J Hand Surg [Br Eur] 25B: 46–48.

Gu YM, Spasic Z, Wu WT (1997) The effects of remaining axons on motoneuron survival and NOS expression following axotomy in the adult rat. Dev Neurosci 19: 255–259.

Haftel VK, Bichler EK, Wang QB, Prather JF, Pinter MJ, Cope TC (2005) Central suppression of regenerated proprioceptive afferents. J Neurosci 25: 4733–4742.

Hallett M (2000) Transcranial magnetic stimulation and the human brain. Nature 406: 147–150.

Hansson T, Brismar T (2003) Loss of sensory discrimination after median nerve injury and activation in the primary somatosensory cortex on functional magnetic resonance imaging. J Neurosurg 99: 100–105.

Hart AM, Brannstrom T, Wiberg M, Terenghi G (2002) Primary sensory neurons and satellite cells after peripheral axotomy in the adult rat: timecourse of cell death and elimination. Exp Brain Res 142: 308–318.

Havton L, Kellerth JO (1990a) Elimination of intramedullary axon collaterals of cat spinal alpha-motoneurons following peripheral nerve injury. Exp Brain Res 79: 65–74.

Havton L, Kellerth JO (1990b) Plasticity of recurrent inhibitory reflexes in cat spinal motoneurons following peripheral nerve injury. Exp Brain Res 79: 75–82.

Havton LA, Kellerth JO (2001) Transformation of synaptic vesicle phenotype in the intramedullary axonal arbors of cat spinal motoneurons following peripheral nerve injury. Exp Brain Res 139: 297–302.

Healy C, LeQuesne PM, Lynn B (1996) Collateral sprouting of cutaneous nerves in man. Brain 119: 2063–2072.

Heise CO, Goncalves LR, Barbosa ER, Gherpelli JL (2005) Botulinum toxin for treatment of cocontractions related to obstetrical brachial plexopathy. Arq Neuropsiquiatr 63: 588–591.

Hess G, Aizenman CD, Donoghue JP (1996) Conditions for the induction of long-term potentiation in layer II/III horizontal connections of the rat motor cortex. J Neurophysiol 75: 1765–1778.

Hess G, Donoghue JP (1996a) Long-term depression of horizontal connections in rat motor cortex. Eur J Neurosci 8: 658–665.

Hess G, Donoghue JP (1996b) Long-term potentiation and long-term depression of horizontal connections in rat motor cortex. Acta Neurobiol Exp (Wars) 56: 397–405.

Hicks TP, Dykes RW (1983) Receptive field size for certain neurons in primary somatosensory cortex is determined by GABA-mediated intracortical inhibition. Brain Res 274: 160–164.

Hoang TX, Nieto JH, Tillakaratne NJK, Havton LA (2003) Autonomic and motor neuron death is progressive and parallel in a lumbosacral ventral root avulsion model of cauda equina injury. J Comp Neurol 467: 477–486.

Hoang TX, Nieto JH, Havton LA (2005) Regenerating supernumerary axons are cholinergic and emerge from both autonomic and motor neurons in the rat spinal cord. Neuroscience 136(2): 417–423.

Horch K (1981) Absence of functional collateral sprouting of mechanoreceptor axons into denervated areas of mammalian skin. Exp Neurol 74: 313–317.

Horch KW, Lisney SJW (1981) On the number and nature of regenerating myelinated axons after lesions of cutaneous nerves in the cat. J Physiol 313: 275–286.

Hughes DI, Scott DT, Todd AJ, Riddell JS (2003) Lack of evidence for sprouting of Aβ afferents into the superficial laminas of the spinal cord dorsal horn after nerve section. J Neurosci 23: 9491–9499.

Huntley GW (1997) Correlation between patterns of horizontal connectivity and the extend of short-term representational plasticity in rat motor cortex. Cereb Cortex 7: 143–156.

Huyghues-Despointes CM, Cope TC, Nichols TR (2003) Intrinsic properties and reflex compensation in reinnervated triceps surae muscles of the cat: effect of activation level. J Neurophysiol 90: 1537–1546.

Hyde D, Scott JJ (1983) Responses of cat peroneus brevis muscle spindle afferents during recovery from nerve-crush injury. J Neurophysiol 50: 344–357.

Inbal R, Rousso M, Ashur H, Wall PD, Devor M (1987) Collateral sprouting in skin and sensory recovery after nerve injury in man. Pain 28: 141–154.

Ip MC, Vrbova G, Westbury DR (1977) The sensory reinnervation of hind limb muscles of the cat following denervation and de-efferentation. Neuroscience 2: 423–434.

Ip MC, Luff AR, Proske U (1988) Innervation of muscle receptors in the cross-reinnervated soleus muscle of the cat. Anat Rec 220: 212–218.

Jaaskelainen SK, Peltola JK (1996) Electrophysiologic evidence for extremely late sensory collateral reinnervation in humans. Neurology 46: 1703–1705.

Jabaley ME, Burns JE, Orcutt BA, Bryant WM (1976) Comparison of histologic and functional recovery after peripheral nerve repair. J Hand Surg 1: 119–130.

Jackson PC, Diamond J (1981) Regenerating axons reclaim sensory targets from collateral nerve sprouts. Science 214: 926–928.

Jacobs KM, Donoghue JP (1991) Reshaping the cortical motor map by unmasking latent intracortical connections. Science 251: 944–947.

Jivan S, Novikova LN, Wiberg M, Novikov LN (2006) The effects of delayed nerve repair on neuronal survival and axonal regeneration after seventh cervical spinal nerve axotomy in adult rats. Exp Brain Res 170: 245–254.

Johnson RD, Munson JB (1991) Regenerating sprouts of axotomized cat muscle afferents express characteristic firing patterns to mechanical stimulation. J Neurophysiol 66: 2155–2158.

Johnson RD, Taylor JS, Mendell LM, Munson JB (1995) Rescue of motoneuron and muscle afferent function in cats by regeneration into skin. I. Properties of afferents. J Neurophysiol 73: 651–661.

Jones EG, Pons TP (1998) Thalamic and brainstem contributions to large-scale plasticity of primate somatosensory cortex. Science 282: 1121–1125.

Kinnman E, Aldskogius H, Johansson O, Wiesenfeld-Hallin Z (1992) Collateral reinnervation and expansive regenerative reinnervation by sensory axons into "foreign" denervated skin: an immunohistochemical study in the rat. Exp Brain Res 91: 61–72.

Koerber H, Mirnics K, Brown P, Mendell L (1994) Central sprouting and functional plasticity of regenerated primary afferents. J Neurosci 14: 3655–3671.

Koerber HR, Mirnics K (1996) Plasticity of dorsal horn cell receptive fields after peripheral nerve regeneration. J Neurophysiol 75: 2255–2267.

Koerber HR, Seymour AW, Mendell LM (1989) Mismatches between peripheral receptor type and central projections after peripheral nerve regeneration. Neurosci Lett 99: 67–72.

Koerber HR, Mirnics K, Mendell LM (1995) Properties of regenerated primary afferents and their functional connections. J Neurophysiol 73: 693–702.

Koerber HR, Mirnics K, Lawson JJ (2006) Synaptic plasticity in the adult spinal dorsal horn: the appearance of new functional connections following peripheral nerve regeneration. Exp Neurol 200: 468–479.

Kolarik RC, Rasey SK, Wall JT (1994) The consistency, extent, and locations of early-onset changes in cortical nerve dominance aggregates following injury of nerves to primate hands. J Neurosci 14: 4269–4288.

Koliatsos VE, Price WL, Pardo CA, Price DL (1994) Ventral root avulsion: an experimental model of death of adult motor neurons. J Comp Neurol 342: 35–44.

Kugelberg E, Edstrom L, Abbruzzese M (1970) Mapping of motor units in experimentally reinnervated rat muscle: interpretation of histochemical and atrophic fibre patterns in neurogenic lesions. J Neurol Neurosurg Psychiatry 33: 319–329.

Lawson J, McIlwrath SL, Koerber HR (2008) Changes in skin levels of two neurotrophins (glial cell line derived neurotrophic factor and neurotrophin-3) cause alterations in cutaneous neuron responses to mechanical stimuli. Sheng Li Xue Bao 60: 584–596.

Lewin GR, McMahon SB (1991a) Physiological properties of primary sensory neurons appropriately and inappropriately innervating skeletal muscle in adult rats. J Neurophysiol 66: 1218–1230.

Lewin GR, McMahon SB (1991b) Physiological properties of primary sensory neurons appropriately and inappropriately innervating skin in the adult rat. J Neurophysiol 66: 1205–1217.

Lewin GR, McMahon SB (1991c) Dorsal horn plasticity following re-routing of peripheral nerves: evidence for tissue-specific neurotrophic influences from the periphery. Eur J Neurosci 3: 1112–1122.

Lewin GR, McMahon SB (1993) Muscle afferents innervating skin form somatotopically appropriate connections in the adult rat dorsal horn. Eur J Neurosci 5: 1083–1092.

Li L, Oppenheim RW, Lei M, Houenou LJ (1994) Neurotrophic agents prevent motoneuron death following sciatic nerve section in the neonatal mouse. J Neurobiol 25: 759–766.

Li LX, Wu WT, Lin LFH, Lei M, Oppenheim RW, Houenou LJ (1995) Rescue of adult mouse motoneurons from injury-induced cell death by glial cell line-derived neurotrophic factor. PNAS 92: 9771–9775.

Light AR, Perl ER (1979) Spinal termination of functionally identified primary afferent neurons with slowly conducting myelinated fibers. J Comp Neurol 186: 133–150.

Lisney SJ (1983a) Changes in the somatotopic organization of the cat lumbar spinal cord following peripheral nerve transection and regeneration. Brain Res 259: 31–39.

Lisney SJ (1983b) The cat lumbar spinal cord somatotopic map is unchanged after peripheral nerve crush and regeneration. Brain Res 271: 166–169.

Logothetis NK, Pauls J, Augath M, Trinath T, Oeltermann A (2001) Neurophysiological investigation of the basis of the fMRI signal. Nature 412: 150–157.

Lomo T, Westgaard RH, Dahl HA (1974) Contractile properties of muscle: control by pattern of muscle activity in the rat. Proc R Soc Lond B Biol Sci 187: 99–103.

Ma JJ, Novikov LN, Wiberg M, Kellerth JO (2001) Delayed loss of spinal motoneurons after peripheral nerve injury in adult rats: a quantitative morphological study. Exp Brain Res 139: 216–223.

Ma JJ, Novikov LN, Kellerth JO, Wiberg M (2003) Early nerve repair after injury to the postganglionic plexus: an experimental study of sensory and motor neuronal survival in adult rats. Scand J Plast Reconstr Surg Hand Surg 37: 1–9.

Maas H, Prilutsky BI, Nichols TR, Gregor RJ (2007) The effects of self-reinnervation of cat medial and lateral gastrocnemius muscles on hindlimb kinematics in slope walking. Exp Brain Res 181: 377–393.

Mackel R, Kunesch E, Waldhor F, Struppler A (1983) Reinnervation of mechanoreceptors in the human glabrous skin following peripheral nerve repair. Brain Res 268: 49–65.

Malessy MJA, Thomeer RTWM, Van Dijk JG (1998a) Changing central nervous system control following intercostal nerve transfer. J Neurosurg 89: 568–574.

Malessy MJA, Van der Kamp W, Thomeer RTWM, Van Dijk JG (1998b) Cortical excitability of the biceps muscle after intercostal-to-musculocutaneous nerve transfer. Neurosurgery 42: 787–794.

Malessy MJA, Bakker D, Dekker J, Van Dijk JG, Thomeer RTWM (2003) Functional magnetic resonance imaging and control over the biceps muscle after intercostal-musculocutaneous nerve transfer. J Neurosurg 98: 261–268.

Mano Y, Nakamuro T, Tamura R, Takayanagi T, Kawanishi K, Tamai S, Mayer RF (1995) Central motor reorganization after anastomosis of the musculocutaneous and intercostal nerves following cervical root avulsion. Ann Neurol 38: 15–20.

McIlwrath SL, Lawson JJ, Anderson CE, Albers KM, Koerber HR (2007) Overexpression of neurotrophin-3 enhances the mechanical response properties of slowly adapting type 1 afferents and myelinated nociceptors. Eur J Neurosci 26: 1801–1812.

Mendell LM, Taylor JS, Johnson RD, Munson JB (1995) Rescue of motoneuron and muscle afferent function in cats by regeneration into skin. II. Ia-motoneuron synapse. J Neurophysiol 73: 662–673.

Mendell LM, Johnson RD, Munson JB (1999) Neurotrophin modulation of the monosynaptic reflex after peripheral nerve transection. J Neurosci 19: 3162–3170.

Merzenich MM, Kaas JH, Wall JT, Sur M, Nelson RJ, Felleman DJ (1983a) Progression of change following median nerve section in the cortical representation of the hand in areas 3b and 1 in adult owl and squirrel monkeys. Neuroscience 10: 639–665.

Merzenich MM, Kaas JH, Wall J, Nelson RJ, Sur M, Felleman D (1983b) Topographic reorganization of somatosensory cortical areas 3b and 1 in adult monkeys following restricted deafferentation. Neuroscience 8: 33–55.

Nichols TR (2002) The contributions of muscles and reflexes to the regulation of joint and limb mechanics. Clin Orthop Relat Res, no. 403 (Suppl):S43–S50.

Nishimura H, Johnson RD, Munson JB (1993) Rescue of neuronal function by cross-regeneration of cutaneous afferents into muscle in cats. J Neurophysiol 70: 213–222.

Nurse CA, Macintyre L, Diamond J (1984) A quantitative study of the time course of the reduction in Merkel cell number within denervated rat touch domes. Neuroscience 11: 521–533.

Osborne WA, Kilvington B (1910) Central nervous response to peripheral nerve distortion. Part II. Brain 33: 288–292.

Paul RL, Goodman H, Merzenich M (1972) Alterations in mechanoreceptor input to Brodmann's areas 1 and 3 of the postcentral hand area of Macaca mulatta after nerve section and regeneration. Brain Res 39: 1–19.

Pollin M, McHanwell S, Slater C (1991) The effect of age on motor neurone death following axotomy in the mouse. Development 112: 83–89.

Rafuse VF, Gordon T, Orozco R (1992) Proportional enlargement of motor units after partial denervation of cat triceps surae muscles. J Neurophysiol 68: 1261–1276.

Rafuse VF, Gordon T (1996) Self-reinnervated cat medial gastrocnemius muscles .1. Comparisons of the capacity for regenerating nerves to form enlarged motor units after extensive peripheral nerve injuries. J Neurophysiol 75: 268–281.

Reichmann H, Srihari T, Pette D (1983) Ipsi- and contralateral fibre transformations by cross-reinnervation: a principle of symmetry. Pflugers Arch 397: 202–208.

Rollnik JD, Hierner R, Schubert M, Shen ZL, Johannes S, Triger M, Wohlfarth K, Berger AC, Dengler R (2000) Botulinum toxin treatment of cocontractions after birth-related brachial plexus lesions. Neurology 55: 112–114.

Rose PK, Odlozinski M (1998) Expansion of the dendritic tree of motoneurons innervating neck muscles of the adult cat after permanent axotomy. J Comp Neurol 390: 392–411.

Rosen B, Bjorkman A, Lundborg G (2006) Improved sensory relearning after nerve repair induced by selective temporary anaesthesia: a new concept in hand rehabilitation. J Hand Surg Br 31: 126–132.

Roy RR, Garfinkel A, Ounjian M, Payne J, Hirahara A, Hsu E, Edgerton VR (1995) Three-dimensional structure of cat tibialis anterior motor units. Muscle & Nerve 18: 1187–1195.

Salmons S, Vrbova G (1969) The influence of activity on some contractile characteristics of mammalian fast and slow muscles. J Physiol 201: 535–549.

Sanes JN, Donoghue JP (2000) Plasticity and primary motor cortex. Annu Rev Neurosci 23: 393–415.

Sanes JN, Suner S, Donoghue JP (1990) Dynamic organization of primary motor cortex output to target muscles in adult rats. I. Long-term patterns of reorganization following motor or mixed peripheral nerve lesions. Exp Brain Res 79: 479–491.

Sanes JN, Suner S, Lando JF, Donoghue JP (1988) Rapid reorganization of adult rat motor cortex somatic representation patterns after motor nerve injury. Proc Natl Acad Sci USA 85: 2003–2007.

Schmalbruch H (1987) Loss of sensory neurons after sciatic nerve section in the rat. Anat Rec 219: 323–329.

Schroeder CE, Seto S, Arezzo JC, Garraghty PE (1995) Electrophysiological evidence for overlapping dominant and latent inputs to somatosensory cortex in squirrel monkeys. J Neurophysiol 74: 722–732.

Scott JJ (1996) The functional recovery of muscle proprioceptors after peripheral nerve lesions. J Peripher Nerv Syst 1: 19–27.

Scott JJ, Petit J, Davies P (1996) The dynamic response of feline Golgi tendon organs during recovery from nerve injury. Neurosci Lett 207: 179–182.

Scott JJA (1987) The reinnervation of cat muscle spindles by skeletofusimotor axons. Brain Res 401: 152–154.

Scott JJA, Davies P, Petit J (1995) The static sensitivity of tendon organs during recovery from nerve injury. Brain Res 697: 225–234.

Sperry RW (1941) The effect of crossing nerves to antagonistic muscles in the hind limb of the rat. J Comp Neurol 75: 1–19.

Sperry RW (1942) Transplantation of motor nerves and muscles in the forelimb of the rat. J Comp Neurol 76: 283–321.

Sperry RW (1945) The problem of central nervous reorganization and muscle transposition. Quart Rev Biol 20: 311–369.

Sperry RW (1947) Effect of crossing nerves to antagonistic limb muscles in the monkey. Arch Neurol Psychiatry 58: 452–473.

Srihari T, Seedorf U, Pette D (1981) Ipsi- and contralateral changes in rabbit soleus myosins by cross-reinnervation. Pflugers Arch 390: 246–249.

Sunico CR, Portillo F, Gonzalez-Forero D, Moreno-Lopez B (2005) Nitric-oxide-directed synaptic remodeling in the adult mammal CNS. J Neurosci 25: 1448–1458.

Swett JE, Hong CZ, Miller PG (1991) All peroneal motoneurons of the rat survive crush injury but some fail to reinnervate their original targets. J Comp Neurol 304: 234–252.

Tandrup T, Woolf CJ, Coggeshall RE (2000) Delayed loss of small dorsal root ganglion cells after transection of the rat sciatic nerve. J Comp Neurol 422: 172–180.

Terzis JK, Dykes RW (1980) Reinnervation of glabrous skin in baboons: properties of cutaneous mechanoreceptors subsequent to nerve transection. J Neurophysiol 44: 1214–1225.

Thomas CK, Stein RB, Gordon T, Lee RG, Elleker MG (1987) Patterns of reinnervation and motor unit recruitment in human hand muscles after complete ulnar and median nerve section and resuture. J Neurol Neurosurg Psychiatry 50: 259–268.

Tornqvist E, Aldskogius H (1994) Motoneuron survival is not affected by the proximo-distal level of axotomy but by the possibility of regenerating axons to gain access to the distal nerve stump. J Neurosci Res 39: 159–165.

Totosy de Zepetnek J, Zung H, Erdebil S, Gordon T (1992) Innervation ratio is an important determinant of force in normal and reinnervated rat tibialis anterior muscle. J Neurophysiol 67: 1385–1403.

Unguez GA, Roy RR, Pierotti DJ, Bodine-Fowler S, Edgerton VR (1995) Further evidence of incomplete neural control of muscle properties in cat tibialis anterior motor units. Am J Physiol Cell Physiol 268: C527–C534.

Valero-Cabré A, Navarro X (2001) H reflex restitution and facilitation after different types of peripheral nerve injury and repair. Brain Res 919: 302–312.

Vestergaard S, Tandrup T, Jakobsen J (1997) Effect of permanent axotomy on number and volume of dorsal root ganglion cell bodies. J Comp Neurol 388: 307–312.

Vrbova G (1963a) The effect of motoneurone activity on the speed of contraction of striated muscle. J Physiol 169: 513–526.

Vrbova G (1963b) Changes in the motor reflexes produced by tenotomy. J Physiol 166: 241–250.

Vrbova, G., T. Gordon and R. Jones (1995) Plasticity of muscles and their motor units. In: *Nerve-Muscle Interaction*, 2nd ed., pp 109–136, London: Chapman & Hall.

Waberski TD, Gobbele R, Kawohl W, Cordes C, Buchner H (2003) Immediate cortical reorganization after local anesthetic block of the thumb: source localization of somatosensory evoked potentials in human subjects. Neurosci Lett 347: 151–154.

Wall JT, Felleman DJ, Kaas JH (1983) Recovery of normal topography in the somatosensory cortex of monkeys after nerve crush and regeneration. Science 221: 771–773.

Wall JT, Kaas JH, Sur M, Nelson RJ, Felleman DJ, Merzenich MM (1986) Functional reorganization in somatosensory cortical areas 3b and 1 of adult monkeys after median nerve repair: possible relationships to sensory recovery in humans. J Neurosci 6: 218–233.

Wall JT, Xu J, Wang X (2002) Human brain plasticity: an emerging view of the multiple substrates and mechanisms that cause cortical changes and related sensory dysfunctions after injuries of sensory inputs from the body. Brain Res Brain Res Rev 39: 181–215.

Wang LC, Copray S, Brouwer N, Meek MF, Kernell D (2002) Regional distribution of slow-twitch muscle fibers after reinnervation in adult rat hindlimb muscles. Muscle Nerve 25: 805–815.

Wang LC, Kernell D (2002) Recovery of type I fiber regionalization in gastrocnemius medialis of the rat after reinnervation along original and foreign paths, with and without muscle rotation. Neuroscience 114: 629–640.

Wei FC, Carver N, Lee YH, Chuang DCC, Cheng SL (2000) Sensory recovery and Meissner corpuscle number after toe-to-hand transplantation. Plast Reconstr Surg 105: 2405–2411.

Weiss T, Miltner WH, Liepert J, Meissner W, Taub E (2004) Rapid functional plasticity in the primary somatomotor cortex and perceptual changes after nerve block. Eur J Neurosci 20: 3413–3423.

Welin D, Novikova LN, Wiberg M, Kellerth JO, Novikov LN (2008) Survival and regeneration of cutaneous and muscular afferent neurons after peripheral nerve injury in adult rats. Exp Brain Res 186: 315–323.

Wellman CL, Arnold LL, Garman EE, Garraghty PE (2002) Acute reductions in GABAA receptor binding in layer IV of adult primate somatosensory cortex after peripheral nerve injury. Brain Res 954: 68–72.

Wiesenfeld-Hallin Z, Kinnman E, Aldskogius H (1989) Expansion of innervation territory by afferents involved in plasma extravasation after nerve regeneration in adult and neonatal rats. Exp Brain Res 76: 88–96.

Wikholm R, Swett J, Torigoe Y, Blanks R (1988) Repair of severed peripheral nerve: a superior anatomic and functional recovery with a new "reconnection" technique. J Otol Head & Neck Surg 99: 353–361.

Wong WC, Kanagasuntheram R (1971) Early and late effects of median nerve injury on Meissner's and Pacinian corpuscles of the hand of the macaque (M. fascicularis). J Anat 109: 135–142.

Woodbury CJ, Kullmann FA, McIlwrath SL, Koerber HR (2008) Identity of myelinated cutaneous sensory neurons projecting to nocireceptive laminae following nerve injury in adult mice. J Comp Neurol 508: 500–509.

Woolf CJ, Shortland P, Coggeshall RE (1992) Peripheral nerve injury triggers central sprouting of myelinated afferents. Nature 355: 75–78.

Woolf CJ, Shortland P, Reynolds M, Ridings J, Doubell T, Coggeshall RE (1995) Reorganization of central terminals of myelinated primary afferents in the rat dorsal horn following peripheral axotomy. J Comp Neurol 360: 121–134.

Xu J, Wall JT (1997) Rapid changes in brainstem maps of adult primates after peripheral injury. Brain Res 774: 211–215.

Xu J, Wall JT (1999) Evidence for brainstem and supra-brainstem contributions to rapid cortical plasticity in adult monkeys. J Neurosci 19: 7578–7590.

Xu QG, Forden J, Walsh SK, Gordon T, Midha R (2010) Motoneuron survival after chronic and sequential peripheral nerve injuries in the rat. J Neurosurg 112: 890–899.

12

TREATMENT STRATEGIES

NERVE REGENERATION depends on multiple coordinated events for its success, each of which could be manipulated to enhance functional restoration. The physiology of axotomized neurons may be influenced through retrograde transport or electrical conduction, and by small molecules that pass the blood-brain barrier. The distal pathway is more difficult to access, as it is physically widespread and is deprived of axoplasmic transport soon after axotomy. The CNS response to input that has been modified by nerve regeneration can be improved by sensory re-education. This process has been enhanced by substituting hearing for touch and by using anesthetics to increase the cortical area corresponding to the injured nerve. Promoting neural plasticity by dissolving the perineuronal nets that stabilize synapses has also been found to improve function after experimental nerve repair. Axotomy-induced loss of DRG neurons may be prevented, although an impact on function has not been demonstrated. Neural regeneration state is enhanced by brief electrical stimulation at the time of nerve repair.

Stimulation upregulates neuronal BDNF, TrkB, GAP-43, actin, and Tα1 tubulin, and hastens reinnervation of the distal stump by regenerating axons. It provides central but not peripheral conditioning, and does not appear to increase the speed of axon regeneration. Stimulation enhanced function in a mouse gait model and improved muscle reinnervation and nerve conduction properties after carpal tunnel release. Regeneration may also be enhanced in a similar manner by exercise. At the molecular level, neuronal regeneration state may be raised by increasing intracellular cAMP, by modifying ligand-receptor interactions, and by increasing the activation of transcription factors. Chronic axotomy reduces the ability of neurons to regenerate, and has been reversed with growth factors and FK506.

Substitution of biologic glue for sutures has been explored for nearly a century and is a time-saving option when nerve ends can be joined without tension. Techniques of wrapping the repair site to isolate it and confine axons to specific fascicles have been intermittently popular, yet have not improved clinical outcome. Fusion of individual transected axons has been performed and may one day circumvent the secondary consequences of nerve injury once the problems associated with scaling up to fuse thousands of axons are addressed. In spite of substantial investigation, there is no clear consensus regarding the use of pulsed electromagnetic fields (PEMF) to enhance regeneration. Some pathway-derived growth factors support regeneration, yet increasing their concentrations above normal levels does not consistently improve regeneration. Gene therapy, currently delivered with viral vectors, is likely to be a mainstay of therapy once the extent and duration of expression can be controlled. Electroporation of nerve in vivo is a nonviral technique of gene therapy that results in transient gene expression and thus avoids the problem of trapping axons in long-standing growth factor concentrations. Thyroid hormone and testosterone, both found to promote experimental regeneration, are limited in their clinical usefulness by side effects and dosing requirements. Gradient-based constructs, harbingers of a truly biologic approach to nerve repair, are being applied to the challenge of axon sorting. Removal of inhibitory components from the repair site enhances regeneration at the potential expense of compromising regeneration specificity. Attention must also be paid to preserving the viability and responsiveness of distal stump Schwann cells that may remain denervated for months. Temporary reinnervation with axons from other nerves, treatment of Schwann cells with growth factors, and augmentation of the Schwann cell population with stem cells are all under investigation.

Prolonged denervation limits the potential for muscle to be reinnervated when axons arrive. Electrical stimulation and temporary ingrowth of sensory axons improve muscle morphology, but improved function has only been demonstrated intermittently. Protease inhibition has shown promise in primate experiments, but has not been subject to clinical trial. Creation of new motoneuron pools within distal portions of denervated nerve may prove useful in preserving muscle when long periods of denervation are anticipated, such as proximal ulnar nerve or brachial plexus injury.

THE CHALLENGE

To maximize clinical improvement after peripheral nerve injury, a treatment strategy must accomplish the following: (1) Enhance and maintain the neuronal growth state to promote axons across the inhibitory milieu of the repair site and speed regeneration, (2) Increase regeneration specificity by guiding axons to functionally appropriate Schwann cell tubes in the distal stump, (3) Maintain the ability of chronically denervated Schwann cells to support regeneration, (4) Sustain the viability of denervated end organs, and (5) Maximize the CNS compensation for peripheral miswiring. Other goals, such as preventing the death of axotomized neurons, may be important in some settings but not in others. The consequences of failure in each of these categories have been described in earlier chapters. Chapter 12 will present many of the solutions that have been devised for these challenges. Its organization mirrors that of Chapter 9, focusing on specific anatomical areas and the events that occur there rather than on treatment modalities per se.

The peripheral nervous system poses unique challenges to therapy. Its neurons lie within the blood-brain barrier, which limits access to circulating medications. Molecules that do not pass the barrier, including genes that code for desired molecules, can only be introduced by direct injection into the DRG or spinal cord, or by infusion into the CSF, techniques unlikely to be employed clinically. The primary window of access is at the site of nerve transection, where injured neurons can be reached directly through electrical stimulation or axoplasmic transport. The distal stump poses an even more difficult problem, since axoplasmic transport within denervated nerve ceases within hours of injury. Exposure of the cut end of the distal stump at the time of nerve repair thus fails to provide a means of delivering treatments to the majority of Schwann cells that have been denervated. Furthermore, these cells are arrayed along lengthy nerves that can only be accessed directly by extensive surgical exposure, a clinically unacceptable option. Therapy for denervated Schwann cells after nerve transection and repair must therefore take advantage of the long-standing breakdown of the blood-brain barrier in denervated nerve, and is thus likely to be limited to molecules that can be delivered through the circulation. Theoretically, it might also be possible to use blood-borne macrophages or targeted stem cells to deliver drugs or genes to Schwann cells during the process of Wallerian degeneration. Direct treatment of Schwann cells is possible, however, in situations where nerve graft is harvested, and thus completely exposed, before it is used to bridge a nerve gap.

PROMOTING CNS PLASTICITY

Sensory Re-education

At a time when many were attempting to improve the outcomes of nerve repair by refining surgical technique, others, spurred on by growing awareness of plasticity within the CNS, sought to modify perception of the signals transmitted from newly reinnervated skin. This approach was devised by Wynn Parry (Wynn Parry, 1966; Wynn Parry, Salter, 1976), who introduced a progressive series of exercises that trained patients to recognize shapes, textures, and common objects, and to localize stimuli correctly. In spite of relatively poor recovery of two-point discrimination (2-PD), many patients rehabilitated with this technique regained excellent use of their hands as evidenced by successful return to trades that required manual dexterity.

Soon after Wynn Parry introduced the concept of sensory re-education, Dellon and colleagues refined the protocol by separating it into early and late phases and by recommending separate stimulus patterns for slowly- and rapidly adapting receptor populations, ending with repeated testing of 2-PD as part of the training process (Dellon et al., 1974). Patients treated in this way lowered their 2-PD dramatically over short periods; one patient improved from 45 mm to 6 mm over 3 weeks and another from 25 mm to 2 mm over 3 weeks. Interestingly, 2-PD in the normal digits of these patients also improved during the training period. As discussed in Chapter 4, testing 2-PD generates perceptions arrayed along a continuum of sensations, rather than two completely different sensations that correspond to one or two points. The decrease in 2-PD seen with repeated testing can thus result from increasing familiarity with this continuum, manifested as shifting criteria for one vs. two points. When testing 2-PD is used both as a training technique and as the tool for final evaluation, it is thus possible that a substantial part of the measured recovery is the result of learning rather than of true physiologic change.

Sensory re-education was rapidly embraced as a treatment modality, at least in part because it seemed intrinsically obvious that it should work. Although the technique is now used in many centers, there have been few comparative evaluations of its effectiveness after primary nerve repair (Oud et al., 2007). The only prospective, randomized trial of classical sensory re-education was limited to digital nerve repairs (Cheng et al., 2001). In this study, repeated tactile stimulation with a ridged device improved 2-PD 6 months after nerve repair. The effectiveness of sensory re-education after median nerve repair was evaluated in a prospective study in which the most motivated and cooperative patients were picked for the treatment group, potentially biasing the outcome (Mavrogenis et al., 2009). Rehabilitation that included object identification and training in the localization of stimuli (locognosia) resulted in significant improvement in locognosia, but not in static or moving 2-PD after 18 months. An additional study of median nerve repair found that sensory re-education with graded textures and object recognition training improved object recognition in comparison to historical controls, but did not improve 2-PD (Imai et al., 1996). A prospective, randomized trial of sensory re-education evaluated with tests of both sensibility and function would thus be a significant contribution.

Lundborg, Rosen and colleagues have devised two ingenious strategies to enhance sensory re-education. In the first, they cover the denervated hand with a sensor glove that translates friction sounds into audible signals, in effect substituting hearing for touch until cutaneous sensibility returns (Rosen, Lundborg, 2003). This sensory substitution approach is based on the hypothesis that afferent input from the hand, even though of a novel modality, can preserve the hand's original cortical representation after injury (Chapters 2 and 11). In a prospective study of median nerve repair, they found that use of the sensor glove resulted in improved tactile gnosis as measured by the STI test (Rosen, Lundborg, 2007) (Chapter 4, Table 4-3). Functional MRI (fMRI) studies demonstrated that normal subjects could be trained with the sensor glove to activate their somatosensory cortex in response to auditory stimuli, findings consistent with the operating hypothesis (Lundborg et al., 2005).

The second strategy for improving the results of sensory re-education was based on an earlier prediction by Merzenich et al. (1983) that was quoted in Chapter 11. They observed that interruption of afferent input from one area of skin resulted in expansion of the cortical area serving adjacent skin, and predicted that tactile acuity in this area should increase in proportion to the expansion of its cortical representation (Chapter 11). This proved to be the case, as axillary anesthesia of one upper extremity induced a rapid, significant improvement in both 2-PD and pressure thresholds in the opposite hand (Bjorkman et al., 2005). Similar changes were found to result from application of topical anesthetic to the ipsilateral wrist and forearm (Bjorkman et al., 2004). A subsequent prospective, randomized, double-blind study found that repeated application of topical anesthetic to the forearm during sensory re-education of the ipsilateral hand improved both perception of touch and tactile gnosis as measured 1 month after the last anesthetic application, although this effect could no longer be demonstrated 8 months after the intervention (Rosen et al., 2006; Lundborg et al., 2007) (Figure 12-1). Through these innovations Lundborg, Rosen, and their colleagues have introduced new paradigms that are certain to influence our approach to nerve injuries in the future.

Manual Stimulation of Target Muscles

Rats do not regain normal patterns of whisker movement (whisking) after transection and repair of the facial nerve (Figure 6-9; Chapter 7). A normal whisking pattern is restored, however, if the whiskers are manually stimulated during the recovery period (Angelov et al., 2007). This treatment also improves functional outcomes after experimental facial nerve grafting and hypoglossal-facial nerve transfer, but to a lesser degree (Guntinas-Lichius et al., 2007). Manual whisker stimulation is effective only when whisker afferents remain intact, and has been found to reduce polyneuronal innervation of motor endplates and to restore synaptic input to motoneurons without altering regeneration specificity (Angelov et al., 2007; Pavlov et al., 2008). It is not clear how this strategy could be applied to denervated extremity muscles, as both efferent and afferent innervation travel together and are disrupted by peripheral nerve injury.

Intraspinal Chondroitinase Injection

Plasticity within the spinal cord is normally kept in check by perineuronal nets, coatings of inhibitory

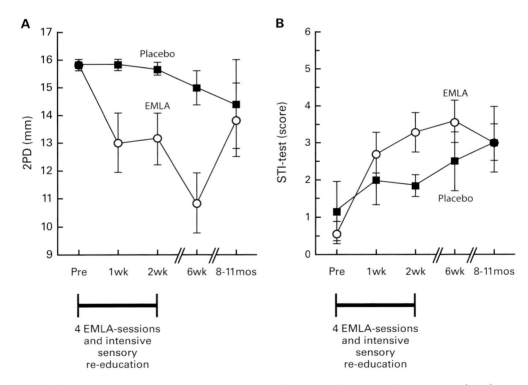

FIGURE 12-1   A new approach to sensory re-education. The results of two-point discrimination (2PD) (A) and shape/texture identification test (STI) (B) testing in patients who have undergone intensive sensory re-education with or without forearm anesthesia resulting from application of EMLA cream. This approach is based on the finding of Merzenich et al. (1983) that the volume of cortex devoted to a given area of skin can be increased by blocking afferent input from adjacent areas. Improvement in sensibility in the digits was rapid and was maintained for 6 weeks, but was lost by 8–11 months. Reprinted from Lundborg et al., 2007 with permission.

chondroitin sulfate proteoglycans that stabilize synapses on dendrites and cell bodies (Deepa et al., 2006). Dissolving these nets by injection of chondroitinase ABC (Ch ABC) destabilizes synapses and promotes axonal sprouting (Massey et al., 2006). In a landmark series of experiments Galtrey and colleagues repaired the median and ulnar nerves of rats, a procedure that reduces skilled paw reaching (Galtrey et al., 2007). Animals that received intraspinal injections of Ch ABC 4 weeks after repair went on to have increased axon sprouting and improved functional recovery (Figure 12-2). This treatment has been applied successfully to afferent sensory projections and to the injured spinal cord (Cafferty et al., 2008; Tester, Howland, 2008; Garcia-Alias et al., 2009). Although the current procedure is quite invasive, the overall strategy holds promise as a means of compensating for the axonal misdirection that accompanies nerve regeneration.

NEURONAL RESCUE

Motoneurons

As discussed in chapter 11, the motoneuron response to axotomy depends on the age of the animal and the proximity of the injury to the spinal cord. The majority of motoneurons may be lost after proximal injury in neonates, whereas little or no loss occurs after peripheral injury in adults. Motoneuron rescue is thus not a critical issue for most peripheral nerve repairs. Strategies to rescue motoneurons after very proximal injuries such as root avulsion are discussed in Chapter 8.

DRG Neurons

Unlike motoneurons, substantial numbers of adult DRG neurons may be lost as a consequence of peripheral axotomy (Ranson, 1906). Estimates of the percentage of DRG neurons that die vary according to both the anatomical model and the counting technique used, ranging from 20 to 50% (Chapter 11). Cutaneous afferent neurons appear to be more susceptible to axotomy than muscle afferents (Welin et al., 2008). Postaxotomy neuron loss is a gradual process that continues for 3–4 months after injury (Tandrup et al., 2000; Ma et al., 2001), providing an ample window for treatments aimed at the prevention of cell death.

The survival effect of NGF on developing and postnatal DRG neurons and its ability to support

the phenotype of these neurons in adulthood suggested that NGF might also be effective in preventing the death of adult neurons in response to axotomy (Rich et al., 1987). This proved to be the case, as application of NGF to the proximal stump of the transected rat sciatic nerve prevented neuron loss for up to 6 weeks (Otto et al., 1987; Rich et al., 1987). Subsequent work suggested that NT-3 and thyroid hormone were also effective in preserving axotomized DRG neurons, whereas BDNF and CNTF were not (Groves et al., 1999; Ljungberg et al., 1999; Schenker et al., 2003). Nothing about the DRG is quite this straightforward, however, as further careful investigation revealed that NT-3 was not preventing apoptosis of DRG neurons, but instead was stimulating the differentiation of non-neuronal cells into neurons (Groves et al., 2003; Kuo et al., 2005, 2007).

Other strategies for neural protection have been investigated to avoid the potential side effects of growth factors and hormones. Mitochondrial protection with acetyl-L-carnitine and N-acetylcysteine have both been found to protect DRG neurons from the effects of axotomy in a dose-dependent fashion; N-acetylcysteine treatment has also increased the number of DRG neurons that regenerate through a rat sciatic nerve graft (Hart et al., 2002; Wilson et al., 2003; Hart et al., 2004; Welin et al., 2009).

ENHANCING NEURONAL REGENERATION STATE

Brief Electrical Stimulation

The conditioning effect, described in Chapter 9, was the first concrete indication that neuron biology could be manipulated to accelerate axon regeneration. Once this threshold was crossed, investigators sought means of achieving the same result without the need for a preinjury. The possible efficacy of electrical stimulation was suggested by experiments in which the entire rat leg was stimulated percutaneously after freeze lesions at various levels of the sciatic and peroneal nerves (Sebille, Bondoux-Jahan, 1980). In this preparation stimulation reduced the latency between injury and the onset of regeneration, but did not speed regeneration once it had begun. Subsequent experiments in which nerve was stimulated directly revealed that as little as 15 minutes of stimulation could accelerate the return of distal motor function after rat sciatic and soleus muscle nerve lesions (Nix, Hopf, 1983; Pockett, Gavin, 1985).

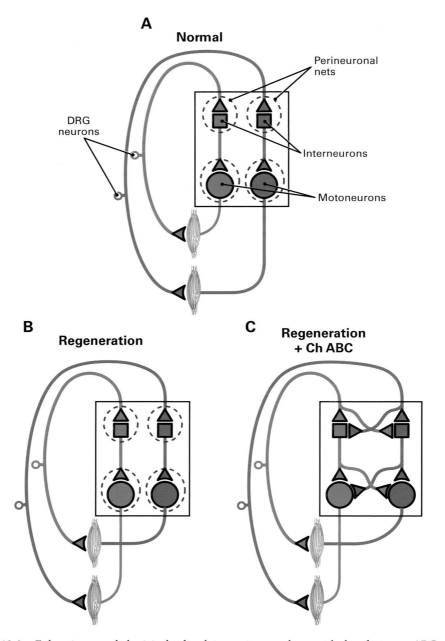

A
Normal

Perineuronal nets

DRG neurons

Interneurons

Motoneurons

B
Regeneration

C
Regeneration + Ch ABC

FIGURE 12-2 Enhancing neural plasticity by dissolving perineuronal nets with chondroitinase ABC (Ch ABC). A. A simple reflex arc. B. After nerve transection and repair, muscles have been reinnervated by inappropriate motoneurons, compromising function. C. Intraspinal injection of Ch ABC dissolves the perineuronal nets that stabilize synapses, permitting axons to sprout and compensate centrally for the peripheral miswiring. Based on a concept described by Galtrey et al., 2007.

In spite of their early success, however, these investigators published no further work on the use of electrical stimulation to enhance peripheral nerve regeneration.

The first systematic attempts to promote axon regeneration with electrical stimulation were undertaken by Gordon and colleagues, who found that 1 hour of 20 Hz stimulation daily for 2 weeks nearly doubled the number of motoneurons that projected axons to the muscle branch 3 weeks after rat femoral nerve transection and repair (Figure 12-3) (Al-Majed et al., 2000b). Stimulation was later shown to enhance sensory axon regeneration in a similar manner (Brushart et al., 2005; Geremia et al., 2007). Varying the duration of stimulation revealed that 1 hour produced maximal effects on both sensory and motor regeneration, with longer periods resulting in no added benefit to motoneurons and a reduced effect for DRG neurons (Figure 12-4) (Al-Majed et al., 2000b; Geremia et al., 2007). This protocol was designed to fire the axotomized motoneurons at a physiologic rate, and is conceptually distinct from attempts to manipulate the growth cone with constant currents that are too low to provoke an action potential (see below). Functional improvement in response to stimulation of femoral nerve repairs evaded detection when gait parameters were evaluated viewing animals from the side (Brushart, unpublished data), but was readily apparent when a new technique was developed to quantify gait from the rear (Irintchev et al., 2005; Eberhardt et al., 2006).

The molecular consequences of brief electrical stimulation at the time of nerve repair have been studied in both central neurons and the distal nerve pathway. It was appreciated early on that the effects of stimulation can be abolished by blocking central conduction during the stimulation process, establishing the primacy of events within the neuron (Al-Majed et al., 2000b; Geremia et al., 2007). These include accelerated and enhanced upregulation of BDNF, its TrkB receptor, and the regeneration-associated gene GAP-43 by both DRG and motor neurons (Al-Majed et al., 2000a; Al-Majed et al., 2004; English et al., 2007; Geremia et al., 2007), and accelerated upregulation of the regeneration-associated gene Tα1 tubulin in concert with reduced expression of medium-molecular-weight neurofilament (NFM) in motoneurons (Al-Majed et al., 2004). Notably, however, stimulation does not affect the behavior of all motoneurons equally; only those capable of upregulating polysialic acid (PSA) respond to stimulation with enhanced PMR (Franz et al., 2008). In the periphery, stimulation was found to increase expression of the HNK-1 carbohydrate within motor pathways and to increase the concentration of

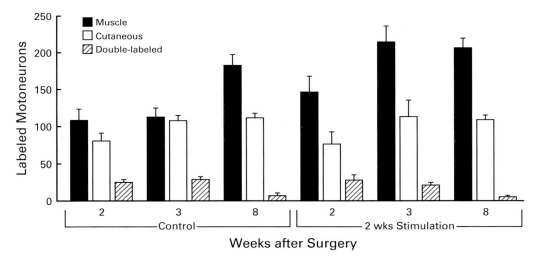

FIGURE 12-3   The development of preferential motor reinnervation (PMR) after transection and repair of the rat femoral nerve. The animals represented on the right received one hour of electrical stimulation/day for 2 weeks; those on the left were not stimulated. At 2, 3, or 8 weeks after surgery the femoral cutaneous and muscle branches were exposed to different fluorescent tracers to identify motoneurons that had correctly reinnervated the muscle branch (solid bars), incorrectly reinnervated the cutaneous branch (open bars), or that had sent collateral sprouts down both pathways (hatched bars). In unstimulated animals equal numbers of motoneurons projected correctly to muscle and incorrectly to skin at both 2 and 3 week intervals; PMR was generated between 3 and 8 weeks. Animals receiving stimulation already demonstrated PMR at 2 weeks, and by 3 weeks twice as many motoneurons projected to muscle as to skin. Stimulation thus sped the development of PMR. From Al-Majed et al., 2000b.

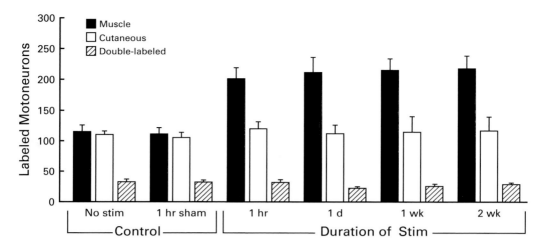

FIGURE 12-4   Influence of the duration of stimulation on the development of PMR as determined 3 weeks after rat femoral nerve repair (see Figure 12-3 for experimental details). Stimulation could be performed for as little as one hour and still enhance PMR markedly (right). In control animals (left) placing the stimulation wires (sham stimulation) did not modify the normal course of regeneration. From Al-Majed et al., 2000b.

several growth factors (Eberhardt et al., 2006; Wang et al., 2009). Although these effects could result directly from stimulation of the distal pathway, it is also possible that they are the secondary consequence of accelerated contact between Schwann cells and axons that reach the periphery in greater numbers in response to stimulation.

The observation that electrical stimulation at the time of nerve repair hastens distal pathway and/or end organ reinnervation has been confirmed by several investigators (Franz et al., 2008; Wang et al., 2009; Asensio-Pinilla et al., 2010). Additional potential effects include an increase in the total volume of regeneration and/or an increase in regeneration specificity. Initial quantification of motoneuron regeneration with retrograde tracing indicated that stimulation increased the total number of motoneurons that reached distal pathways at 8 weeks, though

---

FIGURE 12-5   Sequential double-labeling experiments in the rat femoral nerve to evaluate the effects of electrical stimulation on the specificity of sensory axon regeneration. A. Sequence of experimental manipulations. DRG neurons projecting to the femoral muscle branch were prelabeled with Fluoro-Gold. Two weeks later the proximal femoral nerve was transected and repaired with (below) or without (above) 1 hour of 20 Hz electrical stimulation. After 3 weeks of regeneration the muscle branch was again labeled with Fluoro-Ruby to identify DRG neurons that had reinnervated the muscle branch. B. Three labeling patterns may result from sequential double-labeling of the femoral muscle branch. Neurons labeled only with Fluoro-Gold originally projected to the muscle branch where they picked up the Fluoro-Gold prelabel. After the nerve repair, they either failed to regenerate or regenerated down the femoral cutaneous branch; in both instances they would not be exposed to Fluoro-Ruby. Neurons labeled with only Fluoro-Ruby regenerated into the muscle branch, but did not project to this branch initially, and thus had no opportunity to pick up Fluoro-Gold at the beginning of the experiment. Double-labeled neurons, those containing both tracers, originated in the muscle branch and returned there after nerve repair. Double-labeled neurons have thus demonstrated regeneration specificity. C. Counts of labeled DRG neurons in unstimulated (left) and stimulated (right) groups. Stimulation significantly decreased both single-labeled populations, those that projected to the muscle nerve initially but did not return there (pre only) and those that grew into the muscle nerve from an inappropriate source (post only). The population of double-labeled neurons (double), those that innervated muscle originally and regenerated back to the muscle branch, was increased significantly, indicating that regeneration specificity was enhanced. The total number of neurons labeled at the beginning (total pre) and end (total regen) of the experiment was not influenced by stimulation. From Brushart et al., 2005.

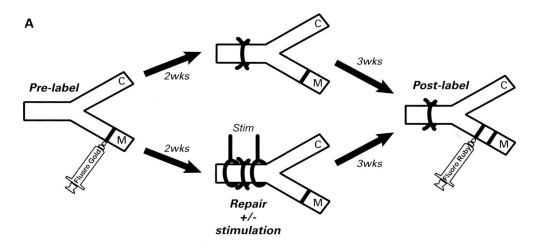

A

Pre-label

2wks → C, M

3wks → Post-label

Fluoro Gold

Stim

Repair +/- stimulation

2wks

3wks

Fluoro Ruby

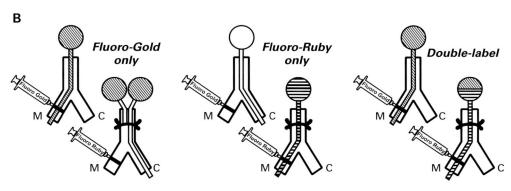

B

Fluoro-Gold only

Fluoro-Ruby only

Double-label

Fluoro Gold

Fluoro Ruby

M   C

M   C

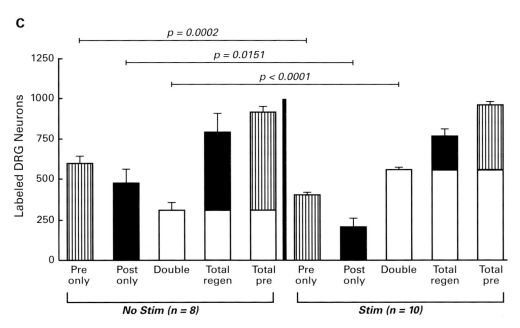

C

p = 0.0002

p = 0.0151

p < 0.0001

Labeled DRG Neurons

1250
1000
750
500
250
0

Pre only | Post only | Double | Total regen | Total pre

No Stim (n = 8)

Pre only | Post only | Double | Total regen | Total pre

Stim (n = 10)

413

statistical significance was not determined (Al-Majed et al., 2000b). Later experiments that were evaluated after 3 weeks, the time at which preferential reinnervation of the femoral muscle branch by motoneurons (PMR) is evident after stimulation but not in controls, do not provide information about long-term reinnervation. In two groups of experiments that were followed for 6–10 weeks there was no indication that the total number of motoneurons innervating the periphery was increased by stimulation (Franz et al., 2008; Wang et al., 2009). These experiments did, however, confirm that stimulation-induced enhancement of PMR increases throughout the reinnervation period. In the sensory system, regeneration specificity was found to be enhanced substantially by stimulation when evaluated 3 weeks after nerve repair, and the data support the conclusion that this enhancement must carry through to the completion of regeneration (Figure 12-5) (Brushart et al., 2005). These experiments all evaluated sensory/motor specificity, which is known to shape regeneration under normal circumstances. Evaluation of the effects of stimulation on topographic specificity at the fascicular level, in contrast, revealed that stimulation actually increased inappropriate reinnervation of the tibial fascicle by peroneal axons (English, 2005). This is not surprising, as there is no evidence for an intrinsic mechanism to correct topographic projection errors.

Electrical stimulation could hasten reinnervation of distal motor nerve by increasing the speed of axon regeneration, by reducing the delay in crossing the repair site, or by a combination of the two. Precise quantification of regeneration speed by using radiotracers (Chapter 6) revealed that stimulation did not increase the speed of early motor axon regeneration in either nerve crush or nerve transection models (Brushart et al., 2002) (Figure 12-6). Applying fluorescent tracers just distal to the repair site to identify regenerating motor axons as soon as they entered the distal stump demonstrated that stimulation did recruit motor axons to cross the repair gap, effectively reducing regeneration stagger (Brushart et al., 2002) (Figure 12-7). That stimulation should act by increasing the number of neurons regenerating rather than regeneration speed is consistent with the experimental results cited previously (Figures 12-3, 12-4); approximately 100 motoneurons are labeled from the muscle branch at 3 weeks even without stimulation, and have thus regenerated with sufficient speed to reach the site of tracer application. To increase this number it is necessary to increase the number of motoneurons regenerating within the distal stump rather than to make the ones already there grow more rapidly.

The effects of electrical stimulation on regeneration speed can also be deduced from experiments in mice that express fluorescent proteins in their axons (English et al., 2007). In this model, stimulation did not increase the distance reached by the fastest axons (regeneration speed), but did increase the numbers of axons that entered the distal stump and progressed for intermediate distances (reduced regeneration stagger). In the one human study to date, electrical stimulation at the time of carpal tunnel release hastened muscle reinnervation and the return of sensory conduction velocity, although the relative contributions of early neuron recruitment and enhanced regeneration speed cannot be determined in this setting (Gordon et al., 2010).

A phenomenological question that is raised by the study of regeneration speed is whether or not electrical stimulation can duplicate the conditioning effect. As was discussed in Chapter 9, conditioning can be broken down into classical (peripheral) conditioning and central conditioning. Classical conditioning requires a peripheral "priming" lesion and is manifest as an increase in peripheral regeneration speed after a second peripheral injury. Central conditioning, in contrast, has been described in response to a range of stimuli and can be manifest in a variety of ways: enhanced outgrowth of DRG neurites in vitro, increased penetration of the DREZ by regenerating dorsal root axons, or increased growth of the central continuation of these axons when they are injured within the dorsal columns. The possibility of peripheral conditioning was investigated using the same radiotracer technique that was used to quantify the conditioning effect initially (Figure 12-8) (McQuarrie, 1978). Regeneration speed was not enhanced when nerve crush was preceded by 1 hour of 20 Hz electrical stimulation delivered 1 week before the crush, ruling out the possibility of a peripheral conditioning effect (Brushart et al., 2002). Similarly, stimulation 1 week before nerve transection and nerve repair did not enhance PMR (Figure 12-9).

A closely related and clinically relevant question is whether electrical stimulation can enhance regeneration when nerve repair is delayed for several days after the nerve is injured. Under these circumstances the neuron has been conditioned by the initial injury and the distal pathway has been predegenerated, both conditions favorable to regeneration (Brushart et al., 1998). When femoral nerve transection was followed

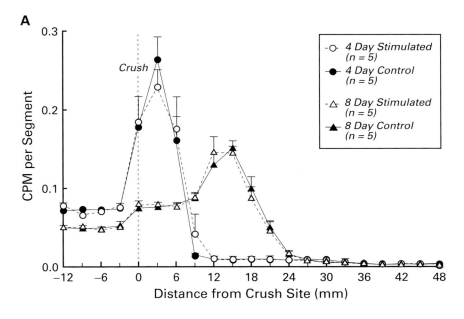

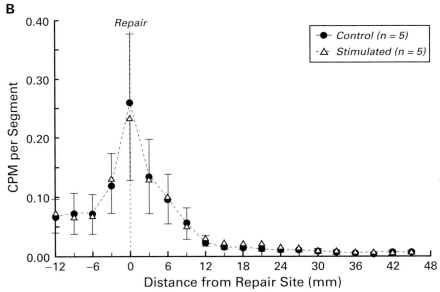

FIGURE 12-6   Electrical stimulation does not increase regeneration speed after either nerve crush or transection. A. Use of radiolabel to measure the speed of axon regeneration as described in Figure 9-6. A. At both 4 and 8 days after nerve crush the distribution of radiolabel is nearly identical in stimulated and nonstimulated nerves. Stimulation has not increased the distance between the fronts of regenerating axons, and has therefore not increased regeneration speed. B. Eight days after nerve transection and repair the bulk of radioactivity, and thus the highest concentration of growth cones, remains at the repair site. Comparison of this curve with those in A emphasizes the magnitude of staggered regeneration after nerve repair. The fastest axons have covered the same distance in stimulated and nonstimulated groups, indicating that stimulation has not increased regeneration speed after nerve repair. From Brushart et al., 2002.

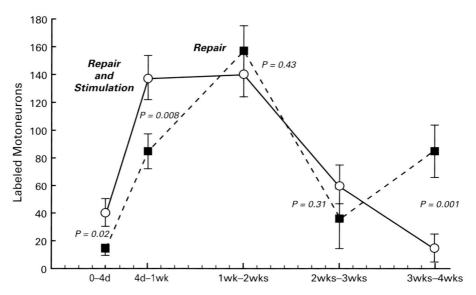

FIGURE 12-7   The magnitude of regeneration stagger is diminished by electrical stimulation. Nerve 2 mm distal to the site of repair was labeled with fluorescent tracer to identify motoneurons as soon as possible after they entered the distal nerve stump. Plots represent the number of motoneurons that have crossed the repair for the first time during the intervals 0–4 days, 4 days–1 week, 1 week–2 weeks, 2 weeks–3 weeks, and 3 weeks–4 weeks. Without stimulation, the greatest number of motor neurons cross the repair between 1 and 2 weeks, with a second wave of crossings between 3 and 4 weeks. Stimulation shifts this curve to the left, so that equal numbers of motoneurons cross in the 4 days–1 week and the 1 week–2 week intervals, and the peak of delayed reinnervation is eliminated. From Brushart et al., 2002

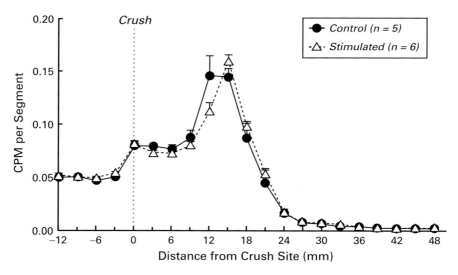

FIGURE 12-8   Electrical stimulation does not result in classical (peripheral) conditioning of motoneurons. Nerves were either exposed or exposed and stimulated, then crushed 1 week later. After 8 days of regeneration, the distribution of radiolabel within motor axons and growth cones has not been altered by stimulation. Had the neurons been conditioned by the stimulation, their axons would have grown farther than the control axons. From Brushart et al., 2002.

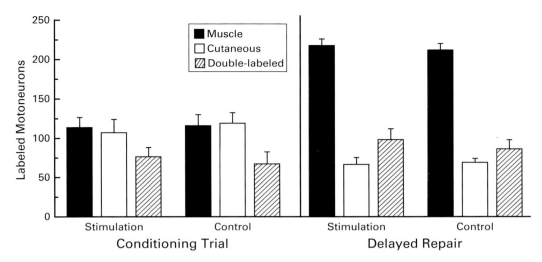

FIGURE 12-9 The effects of brief electrical stimulation on PMR when delivered 1 week before femoral nerve injury (conditioning trial, n = 11) or at the time of delayed repair 1 week after crush injury (delayed repair, n = 10). Stimulating 1 week before nerve repair did not increase the number of motoneurons labeled from the femoral branches after 3 weeks of regeneration and did not influence PMR. Specificity was enhanced in unstimulated animals after delayed repair, and was not increased by stimulation. In the interval between the initial crush injury and the repair motoneurons were conditioned and pathway support for regeneration was enhanced by Wallerian degeneration. Three times as many motoneurons projected to the muscle branch as to the cutaneous branch after 3 weeks of regeneration, a degree of specificity that could not be enhanced further by stimulation. Brushart, unpublished data.

in 1 week by repair with or without stimulation, PMR after 3 weeks of regeneration was already dramatic in control animals and was not enhanced further by stimulation (Figure 12-9). This result is consistent with the hypothesis that stimulation enhances the growth state of neurons, empowering them to cross the inhibitory milieu of the repair site. When neurons are preconditioned their growth state is already enhanced, and when the pathway is predegenerated many of the inhibitory components have been removed. Evidence to date suggests that there is a limit to the positive effects of preconditioning and reducing inhibition, and the addition of stimulation does not appear to exceed that limit. In an analogous situation, elevation of neuronal cAMP with rolipram and removal of inhibitory chondroitin sulfate proteoglycans with ChABC both enhanced regeneration, but the effects were not additive (Udina et al., 2010).

In contradistinction to its effects in the periphery, stimulation has been found to provide some components of central conditioning. Outgrowth from cultured DRG neurons is enhanced when their

peripheral processes are stimulated 1 week before they are harvested (Udina et al., 2008). Similarly, the dorsal column projections of neurons that have been stimulated from the periphery respond to transection with increased outgrowth into the lesion site, but not with improved long-distance regeneration. This behavior mirrors that in the periphery, where stimulation has been shown to promote axons across the inhibitory milieu of the repair site irrespective of its effects on long-term regeneration. Interestingly, although stimulation elevated levels of cAMP within DRG neurons to a degree equal to that of peripheral conditioning, it did not promote the growth of injured dorsal column axons to the same degree (Udina et al., 2008), emphasizing the complexity of regulation that must distinguish central and peripheral conditioning from one another.

Electrical stimulation has the potential to be an effective adjunct to peripheral nerve repair. It can be performed with equipment that is readily available in the operating rooms of many peripheral nerve surgeons, involves minimal risk, and does not require implantation of devices or the use of medications with their potential side effects. Recent evidence has also demonstrated that stimulation can be scaled up from small animal models to the treatment of human nerves after the release of nerve compression (Gordon et al., 2010). It remains to be seen if the considerable success in small animal transection models can also be translated to the clinic.

Exercise

The effects of exercise on axon regeneration after nerve transection and repair have received little attention until recently. In early studies, muscle reinnervation after cross-repair of the guinea pig soleus and flexor hallucis muscles was not affected by exercise (Crockett, Edgerton, 1975), whereas access to a running wheel was associated with a delay in reinnervation of the mouse soleus muscle after tibial nerve repair (Badke et al., 1989). More recent work has shown that treadmill running after nerve repair enhances muscle afferent reinnervation (Marqueste et al., 2004), increases the amplitude of the M wave and the number of myelinated axons in distal portions of the repaired nerve (Asensio-Pinilla et al., 2010), and promotes early axon regeneration without a negative impact on regeneration specificity (Sabatier et al., 2008; English et al., 2009).

The mechanisms through which exercise may influence axon regeneration have been studied after nerve crush rather than after transection and repair. In the rat sciatic nerve crush model treadmill exercise was found to increase the speed of functional recovery, the maturation of myelinated fibers, and motor nerve conduction velocity (van Meeteren et al., 1997; Ilha et al., 2008). Similar exercise programs increased the expression of BDNF and resulting BDNF protein levels in both motoneurons and muscle (Gómez-Pinilla et al., 2001). NT-3 expression, in contrast, was initially downregulated by exercise, but was then upregulated by the fifth day of training (Gómez-Pinilla et al., 2001). NT-3 protein was most concentrated in the dorsal horn, suggesting a role in afferent plasticity (Ying et al., 2003). Within the DRG, enhanced outgrowth of DRG neurons cultured from animals that had been exercised previously was associated with increased expression of BDNF, NT-3 synapsin 1, and GAP43 (Molteni et al., 2004). Exercise thus upregulates factors that have been associated with both motor axon regeneration and afferent plasticity, suggesting a potential for exercise as an adjunct to nerve repair.

Targeted Modification of Neuronal Signaling

The positive effects of electrical stimulation and exercise have already been demonstrated in vivo; most current research in these areas has sought to elucidate underlying mechanisms. As illustrated in Chapter 9, in contrast, a great deal of recent research has taken as its starting point specific components of known signaling pathways, and has explored the consequences of their manipulation. One of the first examples of this approach involved increasing the intracellular concentration of the second messenger cyclic adenosine monophosphate (cAMP). During the initial investigations of growth factor signaling, when nerve growth factor (NGF) was the only known neurotrophin, it was hypothesized that NGF might signal through cAMP to promote regeneration (Pichichero et al., 1973). In early experiments, intramuscular injection of the cAMP analog dibutyryl cAMP (50 mg/Kg) was found to speed the recovery of withdrawal from painful stimuli after sciatic nerve crush in rats (Pichichero et al., 1973). Although this behavioral observation was confirmed (Gershenbaum, Roisen, 1980), others found that regeneration speed as measured by the pinch test (Chapter 6) was not enhanced by an identical protocol (McQuarrie et al., 1977).

Intracellular cAMP levels may also be enhanced by specific measures that increase its production or reduce its degradation. Use of forskolin to increase cAMP concentrations by activating adenylate cyclase was found to enhance the speed of peripheral nerve regeneration in the frog by as much as 40% (Kilmer, Carlsen, 1984). Conversely, inhibition of cAMP breakdown with the drug rolipram increased the number of motoneurons that crossed a site of nerve transection after both 1 and 2 weeks, and increased the number of DRG neurons that crossed at 2 weeks (Udina et al., 2010). The bulk of evidence thus suggests that regeneration can be speeded by increasing intracellular cAMP concentrations (see Chapter 9).

Recent attempts to enhance neuronal regeneration state have included manipulation of ligand-receptor interactions and transcription factors. Integrin signaling has already been shown to play a pivotal role in determining the fate of injured axons (Figure 9-32). DRG neurons upregulate α7β1 integrin after peripheral but not central axotomy, require α7β1 integrin for the conditioning effect both in vitro and in vivo, and can have their regenerative performance in vitro enhanced to equal that of young neurons by transgenic overexpression of integrin (Condic, 2001; Ekstrom et al., 2003; Wallquist et al., 2004). It is thus reasonable to anticipate that overexpression of $\alpha7\beta1$ integrin in vivo could enhance peripheral regeneration. More direct evidence is available for activation of the translocator protein (TSPO) by the ligand Ro5-4864 (Mills et al., 2008). TSPO, initially known as the peripheral benzodiazepine receptor, is an outer mitochondrial membrane protein that regulates steroid synthesis and is upregulated by facial motoneurons and small DRG neurons after axotomy (Gehlert et al., 1997; Casellas et al., 2002; Mills et al., 2005). Treatment with Ro5-4864 enhanced whisker motion 4 weeks after facial nerve transection and increased the early regeneration distance of axotomized sensory axons as measured by the pinch test (Mills et al., 2005; Mills et al., 2008), indicating a potential role for Ro5-4864 as an adjunct to nerve repair.

Elucidation of the critical role played by transcription factors in determining the response to nerve injury (Chapter 9) suggests that modification of signaling at this level may be a powerful strategy to promote nerve regeneration. A primary example is the transcription factor cJun. A critical role for cJun in signaling peripheral axon regeneration is indicated by: (1) upregulation in the adult DRG soon after injury (Kenney, Kocsis, 1998), (2) Upregulation by axotomized adult DRG neurons but not by axotomized CNS neurons or developing PNS neurons (Broude et al., 1997; Raivich et al., 2004), (3) Activation by peripheral but not by central axotomy (Broude et al., 1997), and (4) Reduction of axonal outgrowth from cultured DRG neurons by inhibition of cJun phosphorylation (Lindwall et al., 2004). Several aspects of facial nerve regeneration in cJun knockout mice were found to be defective (Raivich et al., 2004), strongly suggesting that therapeutic upregulation of cJUN could potentially enhance regeneration. Similarly, activating transcription factor-3 (ATF-3) is upregulated in response to peripheral but not to central axotomy, is differentially regulated within subpopulations of DRG neurons, and the extent of its expression within neurons correlates with their relative ability to regenerate (Averill et al., 2004; Seijffers et al., 2006; Reid et al., 2010). Virally induced overexpression of ATF-3 in cultured DRG neurons promotes neurite outgrowth (Seijffers et al., 2006), suggesting that selective upregulation of ATF-3 in vivo might enhance sensory axon regeneration.

Counteracting Chronic Axotomy

Chronic neuronal axotomy is a major factor limiting recovery after experimental nerve transection and repair; after only 2 months of axotomy 50% of rat motoneurons lose their ability to regenerate (Fu, Gordon, 1995) (Chapter 9). Gordon and coworkers have investigated two strategies to overcome this deficit. In both sets of experiments the rat tibial nerve was transected and prevented from regenerating for 2 months, then joined to the freshly transected peroneal nerve. The number of tibial motoneurons regenerating into the peroneal nerve was increased by 20–25% by continuously pumping GDNF or BDNF onto the site of nerve repair (Boyd, Gordon, 2003). When the factors were applied together the effects were additive, so that the volume of regeneration approached that seen after immediate nerve repair. A similar effect could be produced by systemic administration of FK506 (Sulaiman et al., 2002a). Treatment of chronic axotomy may prove to be one of the most effective means of improving the outcome of nerve repair. Axotomized motoneurons remain viable after they lose their ability to regenerate (Xu et al., 2009), so once reactivated they can still regenerate and contribute to function. Few other maneuvers have the potential to double the number of motoneurons that regenerate after a transection injury.

THE REPAIR SITE

Modifications of Repair Technique

NERVE WRAPPING

Enclosing the site of nerve repair within a mechanical sleeve has been practiced intermittently since the nineteenth century (von Bungner, 1891). Sleeving techniques have been pursued in order to minimize ingrowth of scar and outwandering of axons, to promote longitudinal alignment of regenerating axons, and to provide mechanical stability to the repair. Between the early experience of von Bungner and the outset of World War II (WWII), sleeving had been performed with artery, vein, decalcified bone, fascia, muscle, fat, parchment, agar, and rubber, all with little clear evidence of success (reviewed by Ducker, Hayes, 1968). Enthusiasm for the concept persisted nonetheless, resulting in the application of tantalum foil to over a thousand nerve repairs during WWII. In their extensive follow-up of WWII nerve injuries, Woodhall and Beebe found that this practice improved both the mean relative power of muscle contraction and the number of muscles contracting by 20–25%, yet also necessitated a second surgery for removal of fragmented tantalum in 25% of cases (Woodhall, Beebe, 1956). Millipore filter was applied with equal enthusiasm during the 1950s, but was later found to calcify, again requiring a second surgery in many patients (Bassett et al., 1959).

The complications of tantalum foil and Millipore wrapping techniques stimulated experimentation with more modern materials as they became available. A thin silicon wrap enhanced the structural appearance of repairs performed in the chimpanzee (Ducker, Hayes, 1968), wrapping with a collagen sheet increased the number of mechanoreceptors that were reinnervated after repair of cat cutaneous nerves (Gibby et al., 1983), and a Gore-tex wrap prevented axon exchange between adjacent repairs in the cat (Young et al., 1984). From a more technical perspective, wrapping with a sheet of biodegradable glass fiber was found to speed the process of sheep median nerve repair without compromising outcome by a variety of criteria (Jeans et al., 2007).

Recently, two novel approaches to nerve wrapping have been investigated. The first has utilized the technique of photochemical bonding to seal the site of nerve repair with amniotic membrane. In the rat and rabbit this technique has resulted in improvement in the morphology and electrophysiologic performance of regenerated axons as well as in statistically significant but modest improvement in SFI (Henry et al., 2009; O'Neill et al., 2009). The disadvantages of amniotic photobonding are that it requires suture repair of the nerve before application of the amniotic sleeve, and a laser is required for the photobonding procedure. The second approach involves wrapping the repair site with a sheet of poly-3-hydroxybutyrate (PHB), a biodegradable polymer synthesized by bacteria (Hazari et al., 1999; Aberg et al., 2009). Wrapping cat superficial radial nerve repairs increased mean fiber diameters in the distal stump after 1 year, and a prospective, randomized trial of wrapping median and/or ulnar nerve repairs in 12 patients revealed no adverse consequences and a tendency toward improved sensory and motor function. On the basis of this preliminary experience, it is certainly possible that enclosing nerve repairs within a nonreactive, biodegradable membrane could result in incremental improvements in clinical outcome. Furthermore, individual wrapping of fascicular groups might reduce axonal outwandering and thus the number of projection errors.

LASER REPAIR

The laser was first applied to the nervous system as a cutting tool (Fischer et al., 1983), but its actions in coagulating and bonding tissue were exploited soon thereafter as a means of resealing the epineurium during nerve repair (Almquist et al., 1984; Schober et al., 1986). Early investigators used the argon laser to coagulate a "blood patch" applied to the nerve, and were able to demonstrate improvements in axonal organization at the repair site, in the caliber of regenerated axons, and in muscle function after laser repair of the rabbit peroneal nerve (Campion et al., 1990).

The majority of subsequent experiments have been performed with the CO_2 laser by using power in the 90–100 milliwatt range and pulse durations of 1 second or less, as more prolonged or intense exposure was found to damage intact nerve (Menovsky et al., 1996, 2000). Although morphologic and functional results of laser-assisted nerve repair were found to be comparable or superior to those of suture repair, 12–41% of repairs dehisced spontaneously, indicating that the tissue bond could not reliably withstand the tensile forces that act on a routine end-to-end nerve repair (Maragh et al., 1988; Huang et al., 1992). This problem could be overcome by laser-welding soft tissue over the repair site to increase its strength, by supplementing the repair with "protein solder" such as albumin, or by performing tension-free nerve grafting (Bailes et al., 1989; Kim, Kline, 1990; Menovsky, Beek, 2001). Application of these techniques produced results that were comparable but not clearly superior to those of suture repair, and they have yet to be evaluated in a clinical setting.

FROM PLASMA CLOT TO FIBRIN GLUE

To reduce the difficulties of nerve suture and to minimize the disorganisation of the fibers which is apt to be produced by stitches, even if restricted as far as possible to the epineurium, a method has been devised by which stumps can be held together with concentrated coagulated blood plasma. (Young, Medawar, 1940)

The first plasma clot sutures were performed in the rabbit with cockerel (young rooster) plasma that congealed when chick embryo extract was added to the mixture (Young, Medawar, 1940). The procedure was soon modified by substitution of autologous plasma to reduce the inflammatory reaction and use of a special mold that ensured circumferential bonding to prevent disruption of the repair (Tarlov, Benjamin, 1942, 1943). A modified technique with silk stay sutures was applied during WWII with subjective improvement of outcomes in 350 patients (Bateman, 1948).

The initial plasma clot technique was abandoned after the war because of its poor reliability without additional support and because of the effort required to prepare autologous plasma. Interest was then revived in the 1970s when it was shown that the strength of the repair could be enhanced by the addition of concentrated fibrinogen to the mix (Matras et al., 1973), and was bolstered further by the introduction of a convenient off-the-shelf product in Europe. Soon thereafter Narakas reported on a large series of clinical nerve repairs with fibrin glue, often supplemented with additional sutures (Egloff, Narakas, 1983; Narakas, 1988). He believed that glueing could be performed in one-third of the time required for suture of an equivalent structure, and estimated that outcomes were improved by 15% (Narakas, 1988).

The effectiveness of a variety of commercially available fibrin glues has been evaluated experimentally. Early studies in the rat sciatic model found nerve conduction properties to be similar after suture vs. fibrin glue + stay suture repairs, but inferior after glueing if no stay sutures were used (Smahel et al., 1987; Maragh et al., 1990). Recent studies have found more rapid return of toe spread, enhanced conduction parameters, and improved histologic appearance with fibrin glue alone as opposed to microsutures alone (Martins et al., 2005; Ornelas et al., 2006a, 2006b). The tensile strength of repairs has been tested immediately after repair in specimens of human cadaveric and rabbit sciatic nerve, and at several time intervals after repair in the rat sciatic nerve (Temple et al., 2004; Isaacs et al., 2008; Nishimura et al., 2008). Suture repairs were always stronger than fibrin glue repair initially, a difference that persisted for the first postoperative week but was not seen after 2 weeks.

Clinically, fibrin glue nerve repair has proven to be an attractive alternative to microsuture in situations where tension-free juncture can be performed. Fibrin glueing has become the technique of choice for several brachial plexus surgeons (e.g., Malessy et al., 2004, Lin et al., 2009), although this transition

has occurred with little fanfare and without comparative clinical studies. It has also proven useful for facial nerve repair and reconstruction because of its relative ease of application in confined spaces and because of the mechanical stability of the facial nerve in its intraosseous portions. In two series of facial nerve repairs and grafts, Grade 3 recovery as measured on the House-Brackman scale (Chapter 5) was obtained in 60–80% of patients, results comparable to those obtained with sutures (Sterkers et al., 1990; Bozorg Grayeli et al., 2005.)

AXON FUSION

Many of the negative consequences of a lengthy period of axon degeneration and regeneration could be overcome by immediate reconnection of severed axons. Theoretically, such a technique could prevent Wallerian degeneration of the distal pathway and restore function quite rapidly. The goal of fusing axonal segments in the proximal and distal stumps has been pursued by Bittner and colleagues for many years. Their work was stimulated by early observations of regeneration in the earthworm and crayfish, in which the distal portion of transected axons remain intact for several months after they have been disconnected from the cell body (Birse, Bittner, 1981; Bouton, Bittner, 1981). As a result of their relative stability, segments of these axons could be rejoined with polyethylene glycol (PEG), a chemical used previously to fuse cells in vitro (Anders et al., 1978). In early experiments, axoplasmic continuity and conduction were restored in a small percentage of crayfish axons that were reconnected with PEG in vitro (Bittner et al., 1986). With improvements in technique, it became possible to restore functional connectivity of severed earthworm giant axons in vivo (Lore et al., 1999). Fusion of earthworm axons has also been achieved using electric fields and laser light (Yogev et al., 1991; Todorov et al., 1992).

Were it possible to restore the functional continuity of severed mammalian axons in vivo, several challenges would need to be addressed before the technique could be applied to peripheral nerve repair. First and foremost, it would be necessary to prevent Wallerian degeneration. Given the substantial delay before the onset of Wallerian degeneration in the C57Wld^s mouse (Chapter 9: Wallerian degeneration), this no longer seems impossible. Secondly, it would be imperative that axons in the proximal stump be joined to functionally homologous axons in the distal stump. Currently, there is no practical way to functionally identify individual transected axons in vivo. Additional challenges include the obligate delay between injury and treatment in the clinical setting, the need to provide a tension-free environment for the repair, and the difficulty of addressing several thousand axons in a timely fashion. Recent work has begun to address these problems, so that axon fusion could conceivably be a treatment modality in the indeterminate future (Sretavan et al., 2005; Britt et al., 2010).

CELLULAR AUGMENTATION

The olfactory neuroepithelium retains the embryonic capacity to produce new olfactory receptor neurons throughout life (summarized in Li et al., 2007). These neurons sprout axons that are then able to reenter the brain from the periphery, growing through channels provided by olfactory ensheathing cells (OECs). When OECs are transplanted into crushed peripheral nerve, they form peripheral myelin and restore appropriate sodium channel organization at nodes of Ranvier (Dombrowski et al., 2006). Addition of fluorescence-tagged OECs to the site of sciatic nerve repair resulted in remyelination of axons by labeled cells, increased distal axon numbers and conduction velocities, and improved SFI when compared with control repairs in which only medium was added (Radtke et al., 2009) (Figure 12-10). In the facial nerve model, application of OECs to the site of nerve repair hastened the return of whisking without influencing the accuracy of regeneration in one study (Podhajsky et al., 2005), whereas wrapping the repair with intact olfactory epithelium was found to improve both the specificity of regeneration and ultimate function in another (Guntinas-Lichius et al., 2002). It remains to be seen whether these unique cells offer significant advantages over Schwann cells in the setting of end-to-end nerve repair.

THE REPAIR SITE AND/OR DISTAL PATHWAY

Promoting Regeneration

MANIPULATING GROWTH CONES WITH ELECTRIC FIELDS

Modification of neurite growth by weak electric currents was observed soon after the invention by

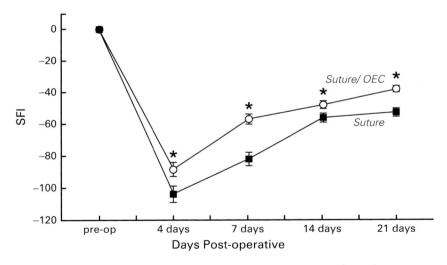

FIGURE 12-10   The sciatic functional index (SFI) after transection and suture (suture) or suture with the addition of olfactory ensheathing cells (suture/OEC). This graph was interpreted as showing that animals with OEC transplantation showed greater functional recovery. It should be noted, however, that at day 4 the SFI had not decreased as much in the OEC group as it had in controls; the percentage of functional recovery from baseline was equal in the two groups. Similarly, OEC improved SFI at 7 days, before any muscle reinnervation could have occurred. The benefits of engrafting OEC in these experiments are thus due, at least in part, to mechanisms that do not require regeneration, such as the reduction of neuroma pain. Reprinted from Radtke et al., 2009, with permission.

Harrison of the tissue culture technique (Ingvar, 1920). Subsequent work established that both the direction and speed of neurite extension could be influenced, with enhanced growth occurring toward the cathode (the electrode through which current enters the medium) (Marsh, Beams, 1946; Sisken, Smith, 1975; Jaffe, Poo, 1979; Patel, Poo, 1982). On the basis of these findings, the effects of weak electric current were evaluated in vivo. In the rat model, 10-μA currents were found to stimulate collateral sprouting from intact sensory axons and to increase the speed of muscle reinnervation after sciatic nerve transection and repair (Pomeranz et al., 1984; McDevitt et al., 1987).

Interpretation of the results of subsequent studies is complicated by the use of different currents and evaluation techniques in each laboratory. A constant current of 0.6 μA increased regeneration distance 1 week after rat sciatic nerve repair as measured by the distal propagation of current density (Kerns et al., 1991); a current of 1.5 μA increased neurofilament antibody staining in the distal stump at 6, 12, and 18 days after surgery (Politis et al., 1988); a current of 10 μA did not have a significant influence on development of twitch tension (Kerns et al., 1994); and a current of 20 μA had no impact on return of the toe spread reflex, muscle force, or number of myelinated fibers (McGinnis, Murphy, 1992). The fragmentary evidence available thus suggests that lower currents are more effective in promoting early regeneration events, but long-term studies are needed.

PULSED ELECTROMAGNETIC FIELDS

An alternative to the direct application of weak electric currents, an invasive procedure, is noninvasive treatment with pulsed electromagnetic fields (PEMF). Rapid changes in a magnetic field produce current in a conductor that passes through it, in this case a peripheral nerve. This approach originated in the clinical observation that patients undergoing treatment for tibial nonunion with PEMF appeared to heal their adjacent nerve injuries more readily than did patients without stimulation (Bassett et al., 1981). Initial results of PEMF treatment after experimental nerve repair were promising, with earlier and more substantial return of muscle force and higher numbers of well-myelinated axons in animals receiving stimulation (Ito, Bassett, 1983).

The year after the Ito and Bassett study, two other laboratories also reported on the use of PEMF to promote nerve regeneration after transection

and suture. Stimulation of the repaired cat peroneal nerve increased the number of motoneurons that reinnervated the tibialis anterior muscle, and stimulation of the repaired rat peroneal nerve hastened the return of the toe spread reflex and increased the number of myelinated axons in the distal nerve stump (Orgel et al., 1984; Raji, 1984). Subsequent studies of PEMF and nerve repair demonstrated more rapid return of whisker function after repair of the rat facial nerve and a decrease in NGF activity within DRG neurons in response to stimulation (Byers et al., 1998; Longo et al., 1999). The latter finding suggested that PEMF might amplify the injury signal provided by a loss of NGF transport (Chapter 9). After nerve repair and transection, the available evidence thus indicates that PEMF can promote peripheral nerve regeneration.

The majority of experiments with PEMF have been performed on nerves injured by crush rather than transection, and have provided evidence both for (Sisken et al., 1989; Rusovan et al., 1992; Walker et al., 1994) and against (Guven et al., 2005; Walker et al., 2007; Baptista et al., 2009) a positive PEMF effect on axon regeneration. A possible reason for this inconsistency may be the differences in signal configurations that were used in the various experiments (Walker et al., 2007). It will thus be important to use a single model to compare the effects of PEMF on regeneration after crush and transection and to analyze the regeneration effects of various wave configurations.

ULTRASOUND

Therapeutic ultrasound has been found to speed the recovery of SFI and toe spread after sciatic nerve crush (Mourad et al., 2001; Raso et al., 2005; Chen et al., 2010), but its effect on regeneration after end-to-end nerve repair or nerve grafting has not been evaluated.

HYPERBARIC OXYGEN

The effects of hyperbaric oxygen on nerve regeneration have been evaluated in a variety of models (reviewed in Sanchez, 2007). Although hyperbaric oxygen has been found to enhance regeneration under some circumstances, the need for treatment within hours of injury and the limited availability of hyperbaric chambers severely limit the practicality of this therapeutic option.

PHOTOTHERAPY

In addition to its use as a cutting and welding tool, the laser has also been applied to peripheral nerve to enhance regeneration. In initial experiments, laser treatment of crushed rat sciatic nerve was found to maintain conduction of action potentials in treated nerves similar to those in controls from the first day after injury (Rochkind et al., 1987), indicating that Wallerian degeneration had not occurred. Subsequent studies in the rat sciatic model have demonstrated an increase in the number and myelination of axons distal to the repair site at 3 and 10 weeks after repair without improvement in SFI (Shamir et al., 2001; dos Reis et al., 2009). In the facial nerve model, laser treatment was found to increase the number of motoneurons regenerating soon after crush and to promote elevation of calcitonin gene-related peptide (CGRP) and motoneuron survival after transection (Anders et al., 1993; Snyder et al., 2002). There is currently no consensus regarding the mechanism through which laser treatment influences nerve regeneration (discussed in dos Reis et al., 2009).

GROWTH FACTORS

Attempts to promote axon regeneration with growth factors have been discussed in Chapter 8 (nerve gaps) and Chapter 9 (end-to-end repair). These chapters describe a range of environments in which application of exogenous growth factors has enhanced regeneration. In most of these situations regenerating axons must not only cross a defect in the basal lamina, but must also traverse inhibitory terrain to cross an unstructured gap, to reinnervate various acellular scaffolds, or to enter or leave the CNS.

The following discussion is limited to the effects of exogenous growth factors on end-to-end nerve repair. In this setting the results of treatment with growth factors have often been more modest than those achieved when regenerating axons were challenged by more inhibitory environments.

NERVE GROWTH FACTOR (NGF)

Long-term delivery of NGF to rat sciatic nerve repair sites or into short intraneural gaps increased distal axon numbers in the former case, but enhanced neither axon numbers nor function as measured by SFI in the latter (Santos et al., 1998; Young et al., 2001). Similarly, overexpression of NGF in the distal sciatic stump did not increase the number of DRG neurons that reinnervated nerve 1 cm distal to the repair (Tannemaat et al., 2008); overexpression of NGF within the femoral cutaneous branch enhanced its selective reinnervation by DRG neurons without increasing the total number of neurons that regenerated their axons (Hu et al., 2010). Application of NGF to nerve repair sites in fibrin glue resulted in a modest but significant increase in the number of motoneurons reinnervating the distal stump at 12 weeks but did not improve motor function (Jubran, Widenfalk, 2003).

BRAIN-DERIVED NEUROTROPHIC FACTOR (BDNF)

Sensory function was not enhanced by adding BDNF to a short (0.5-mm) gap repair of the cat lingual nerve (Yates et al., 2004). Slow release of BDNF from collagen matrices in the rat hastened the onset of facial nerve regeneration by 3 days without influencing ultimate function, and improved SFI from about −70 to −60, still a poor outcome (Utley et al., 1996; Kohmura et al., 1999). Low doses of BDNF (0.5–2 µg/day by osmotic pump) did not influence motoneuron regeneration, whereas higher doses (12–20 µg/day) inhibited regeneration by signaling through the p75NTR (Boyd, Gordon, 2002). Recently, an intermediate dose of 6 µg/day was found to increase the number of motoneurons that regenerated through a 20-mm rat tibial nerve graft (Hontanilla et al., 2007).

NEUROTROPHIN-3 (NT-3)

After nerve repair with a short (1–2 mm) gap, application of exogenous NT-3 had no effect on recovery of SFI in the rat and negatively influenced lingual nerve regeneration in the cat (Young et al., 2001; Robinson et al., 2004).

NEUROTROPHIN 4/5 (NT-4/5)

When applied to the site of nerve repair in a fibrin gel, NT-4/5 increased both the early reinnervation of the distal stump (English et al., 2005) and the number and size of regenerating axons, resulting in statistically significant improvement in SFI (Yin et al., 2001).

GLIAL-DERIVED NEUROTROPHIC FACTOR (GDNF)

Sensory recovery is hastened by application of GDNF to nerve repairs in fibrin gel, although neuropathic pain may result (Jubran, Widenfalk, 2003). The number of motoneurons that reinnervate the distal stump after immediate nerve repair, as determined by retrograde labeling, is not enhanced by GDNF application by either fibrin gel or osmotic pump (Boyd, Gordon, 2003; Jubran, Widenfalk, 2003).

INSULIN-LIKE GROWTH FACTOR-1 (IGF-1)

When applied to sciatic nerve grafts, IGF-1 enhanced muscle weight, axon number, and g-ratio (Chapter 1) (Fansa et al., 2002). In the rat cross-facial nerve graft model, local infusion of IGF-1 hastened the return of blinking and improved both muscle and axon morphology (Thanos et al., 1999, 2001). Systemic infusion of IGF-1 did not influence ultimate function after repair of the rat median nerve (Lutz et al., 1999).

FIBROBLAST GROWTH FACTORS (FGF-1,2)

There was no improvement in sensory or motor function when glue containing FGF-1 was placed around sciatic nerve repairs (Jubran, Widenfalk, 2003). Similarly, adding Schwann cells that overexpressed FGF-2 to rat facial nerve repair did not modify axon branching or improve ultimate function (Haastert et al., 2009).

Many of the growth factors listed above are upregulated within the distal nerve stump after axotomy, often differentially within sensory and motor pathways (Chapter 9). At least some must play a direct role in promoting nerve regeneration as evidenced by the profound effect of their removal. For instance, systemic treatment of mice with BDNF antibody after nerve crush reduced the length of the regenerate by 25% and the number of axons in the distal stump by 83% (Zhang et al., 2000). Provision of further BDNF, as discussed above, has not been found to enhance regeneration to a proportional degree in rodent models. It is thus likely, at least for growth factors such as BDNF, that the distal stump already provides the factor in sufficient quantities. In reaching this conclusion, however, it is important to keep the context in mind. The majority of these experiments have been performed in rodent models in which regenerating axons may contact their end organs within a matter of weeks. During the brief period in which axons are growing through distal pathways, these pathways are optimized for

regeneration by substantial growth factor upregulation. In the clinical setting, in contrast, pathways may remain denervated for long periods, so that augmentation of pathway growth factors may be essential for effective regeneration (see below).

The greatest challenges in using exogenous growth factors are to deliver them at the dose and time that they are needed. This point has been emphasized by recent experiments in which viral vectors were used to upregulate growth factor expression in peripheral nerve. GDNF overexpressed by previously avulsed ventral roots that were inserted back in the spinal cord was able to prevent motoneuron atrophy and stimulate nerve regeneration, but only as far as the area injected with virus (Eggers et al., 2008). Motoneurons were trapped by high concentrations of GDNF, and were apparently unable to regenerate against a strong GDNF gradient to proceed into untreated portions of nerve. A similar phenomenon was observed and found to be factor-specific during trials of gene therapy to augment nerve repair (Tannemaat et al., 2008); motor axons were trapped in areas of elevated GDNF expression, forming "axon coils," yet were unaffected by high concentrations of NGF. Whereas elevated GDNF levels do not in themselves interfere with nerve regeneration, high doses of other factors such as BDNF actually hinder the process (Boyd, Gordon, 2002), again emphasizing the importance of precise dosing. These experiments also illustrate the importance of controlling the duration of gene expression. Were GDNF overexpression transient, even at high levels, axons would still be able to move on into distal portions of the pathway once the levels had decreased. In retrospect, it was perhaps fortuitous that early attempts to augment nerve repair with growth factors involved treatment for short periods. The effects on promoting axons across the repair site could be observed, yet local growth factor concentrations would decrease rapidly enough to let axons proceed distally.

Gene therapy to deliver growth factors during nerve regeneration is likely to become a mainstay of therapy for peripheral nerve injury. Further use of viral vectors to deliver genes will obviously require the use of promoters that can be turned off and on when required (Blesch, Tuszynski, 2007), and ultimately regulated by the presence or absence of axon contact. Gene transfer is not without risk, however, as iatrogenic leukemia and death have resulted from virus-mediated gene transfer in clinical trials (Marshall, 1999; Raper et al., 2003). In order to

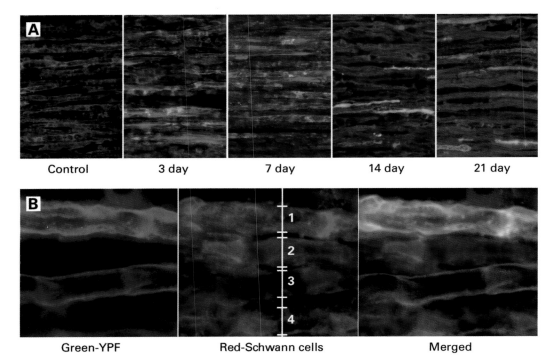

| Control | 3 day | 7 day | 14 day | 21 day |

| Green-YPF | Red-Schwann cells | Merged |

FIGURE 12-11   A. The time course of gene expression after electroporation of the gene for green fluorescent protein (GFP) into intact peripheral nerve. Ten micrometer longitudinal peripheral nerve sections viewed at 20x. Schwann cells are labeled with antibodies to S-100 (red) and cells expressing the electroporated gene are green. Expression is robust during the first week posttreatment, but then declines. B. The green channel (left), red channel (center), and merged image (right) of a fluorescent photograph of intact nerve 3 days after electroporation. Ten micrometer section longitudinal section, original magnification 40x. GFP expression (green) overlaps the distribution of S-100 positive (red) Schwann cells, indicating that the electroporated gene is being expressed by Schwann cells. The center image is marked to delineate individual Schwann cell tubes. From Aspalter et al., 2008.

avoid the potential complications of viral use, Aspalter et al. developed a procedure for electroporating peripheral nerve in vivo (Aspalter et al., 2008) (Figure 12-11). This technique is rapid, relatively atraumatic, and results in expression of the target gene in 28% of treated Schwann cells. Expression drops off rapidly after 1 week, so this is an excellent technique for providing a short burst of growth factor expression. Electroporation and current techniques of viral gene transfer can both be applied to nerve graft between harvest and reimplantation, but their application to nerve repair is limited by the need to expose the nerve surgically before it can be treated.

HORMONES

Thyroid hormone and testosterone have both been investigated as potential regeneration enhancers.

Interest in the functions of the thyroid gland was heightened by the publication in 1891 of the first successful treatment of hypothyroidism with thyroid extract (Murray, 1891). Soon thereafter Marinesco, a colleague of Ramon y Cajal, found that peripheral nerve regeneration was impaired by removal of the thyroid gland (Marinesco, 1910). The first quantitative studies were performed by Cockett, who introduced the technique of analyzing longitudinal nerve sections to measure regeneration speed (Cockett, 1972). She found that the front of regenerating axons proceeded more rapidly when rats were treated with triiodothyronine (T3), an effect that was dose-dependent (Cockett, Kiernan, 1973). These positive effects on regeneration speed could not, however, be confirmed with the radiotracer technique (Berenberg et al., 1977), even though hypothyroidism was found with this technique to slow regeneration (Talman, 1979). More recently exogenous T3 has been found to promote regeneration across nerve gaps, where it can be applied locally, but has not been used to treat end-to-end suture (Danielsen et al., 1986; Barakat-Walter et al., 2007).

Regeneration after hypoglossal nerve crush proceeds more rapidly in male than in female rats, suggesting that male sex hormones might promote regeneration (Yu, 1982). This conjecture was confirmed when it was found that exogenous androgen enhanced regeneration in both sexes (Yu, Srinivasan, 1981; Yu, 1982). Later exploration of androgen treatment in the hamster facial nerve revealed that testosterone hastened the return of facial motor function and increased regeneration speed by 13% as measured with radiotracers (Kujawa et al., 1989; Kujawa et al., 1993). To produce these effects, however, treatment must be administered within 6 hours of injury (Tanzer, Jones, 2004). Testosterone has also been shown to enhance regeneration of the crushed sciatic nerve (Kujawa et al., 1993; Brown et al., 1999), though no studies of end-to-end repair have been published to date.

Bioengineering to Sort Axon Populations

The field of biomedical engineering has recently influenced peripheral nerve regeneration studies through the introduction of techniques for the fabrication of bioactive prosthetic nerve guides. Considerable effort has been expended to promote the growth of increased numbers of axons over greater distances (Chapter 8). For these devices to exceed the performance of autologous nerve graft, however, they will need to do what nerve graft cannot: to sort a mixed population of axons into topographic and/or functional subsets that can be directed to individual fascicles in the distal nerve stump.

The prerequisites for axon sorting are that the direction of axon growth be responsive to guidance cues, and that discrete axon populations respond to different cues, or respond to the same cues differently. The guidance of regenerating peripheral axons by diffusible factors, termed neurotropism, was observed by Ramon y Cajal (1928) (Figure 12-12) and confirmed in the modern era by the experiments of Gunderson and Barrett in vitro (Gunderson, Barrett, 1979) and those of Kuffler in vivo (Kuffler, 1996). A differential directional response to the

neurotrophins has been observed in embryonic neurons both at the sensory-motor level and among different populations of DRG neurons (Paves, Saarma, 1997; Tucker et al., 2001). In adult tissue, NGF and NT-3 have been shown to direct regeneration of discrete neuron populations (Webber et al., 2008; Alto et al., 2009). On the basis of these promising results, a comprehensive exploration of the sensitivity of discrete neuron populations to the range of defined factors could be extremely helpful.

Guidance cues may be presented to regenerating axons in two ways: as soluble diffusion gradients or as fixed substrate-bound patterns. Although undefined diffusion gradients emanating from point sources of growth factor (beads) or focal overexpression of the factor have been effective in guiding regeneration in vitro (Tucker et al., 2001; Alto et al., 2009), it is considerably more difficult to construct and maintain soluble gradients with defined properties. Inroads have been made in vitro by using gels to slow diffusion and stabilize gradients at least temporarily (Cao, Shoichet, 2001; Rosoff et al., 2004). Initial experiments in vivo have succeeded in generating gradients of NGF that persist within an enclosed tube for as long as 30 minutes, but are lost by 45 minutes (Kemp et al., 2007).

An alternative to the laborious process of maintaining a dynamic gradient is to present axons with a predetermined gradient of a growth factor that is substrate-bound and thus is relatively permanent. Recent studies have shown that immobilized NGF maintains its ability to promote neuron survival and neurite extension, indicating the potential utility of this approach (MacInnis, Campenot, 2002; Gomez, Schmidt, 2007). The technology for producing bound protein gradients is evolving rapidly (Yu et al., 2008; Mai et al., 2009) and should become one of the more fruitful applications of biotechnology to nerve regeneration.

Removal of Inhibitory Components

Elements of the regeneration environment that are potentially inhibitory to regeneration include the myelin-associated glycoprotein (MAG), the chondroitin sulfate proteoglycans (CSPGs), and collagen scar. MAG is normally concentrated on the inner, adaxonal membrane of myelinating Schwann cells (Figure 1-2). In mice with delayed Wallerian degeneration (C57BL/Wld^s), distal stump reinnervation is enhanced by eliminating MAG, suggesting an inhibitory role for MAG in peripheral nerve

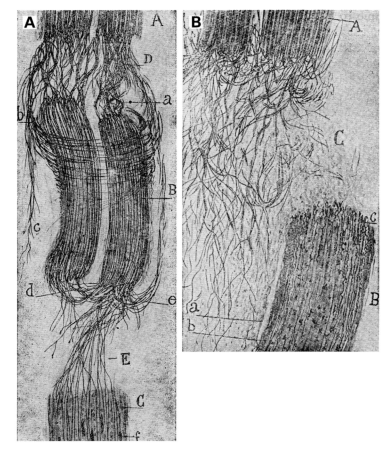

FIGURE 12-12   Drawings of silver-stained peripheral nerve sections prepared by Ramon y Cajal to illustrate the action of neurotropism. A-Left. Axons grow from the proximal nerve stump (A) and cross a gap before they reinnervate two segments of nerve graft (B). Many axons grow through the grafts, out the other ends of the grafts (E), and across an even larger gap to reinnervate an additional nerve segment (C). B-Right. Axons regenerating from a transected nerve (A) are not drawn to nerve graft B, which has been treated with chloroform to kill all cellular elements. From these and similar observations Ramon y Cajal concluded that regenerating axons were guided to other nerve by a diffusible substance that required cellular activity for its elaboration. Reprinted from Ramon y Cajal, 1928.

regeneration (Schafer et al., 1996). MAG function has been manipulated in two studies of end-to-end nerve repair, with enhanced outcomes resulting from both increased and decreased MAG activity. Application of MAG to sciatic nerve repair in fibrin glue reduced axon branching by activation of RhoA, increased topographically specific reinnervation of the tibial and peroneal sciatic branches, and improved SFI (Tomita et al., 2007). In the femoral nerve model, long-term administration of MAG antibodies enhanced PMR both 4 and 6 weeks after nerve repair (Mears et al., 2003) (Figure 12-13). These experiments differ both in the timing of

treatment and in the surgical model, so further work will be needed to define the role of MAG in specific settings. Similarly, it will be important to determine whether inhibiting RhoA, a component of the MAG signaling pathway (Figure 9-1), might promote peripheral axon regeneration in vivo. RhoA inhibition with nonsteroidal anti-inflammatory drugs (NSAIDs) has recently been found to promote CNS regeneration (Fu et al., 2007), and the drugs are already in common use.

Local inactivation of CSPGs with chondroitinase more than doubles the number of axons that reinnervate the distal stump 4 days after nerve repair

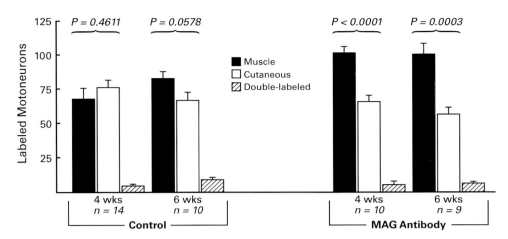

FIGURE 12-13   The effects of daily administration of MAG antibodies to mice after transection and repair of their femoral nerves. Motoneurons have been labeled from the femoral muscle branch (solid bars), the femoral cutaneous branch (open bars), or from both (hatched bars). In untreated mice there is no evidence for PMR after 4 weeks, and an insignificant trend toward PMR after 6 weeks. With daily antibody treatment, in contrast, PMR is already pronounced after 4 weeks. Reducing or eliminating MAG function with blocking antibodies thus increases both the number of motoneurons regenerating and their target specificity. From Mears et al., 2003.

(Zuo et al., 2002) and substantially increases the number of motoneurons and DRG neurons labeled from the distal stump after 2 weeks (Udina et al., 2010).

In the longer term, retrograde regeneration of axons into the extrafascicular compartment of the proximal sciatic stump is reduced significantly and hindpaw grip strength is enhanced by 8% over saline-treated controls (Graham et al., 2007). Inactivation of heparin-sulfate proteoglycans has also been found to promote early regeneration (Groves et al., 2005). Proteoglycan removal may, however, have deleterious effects. In a recent series of mouse sciatic nerve repairs, inappropriate reinnervation of the peroneal nerve by tibial axons was increased by chondroitinase treatment (English, 2005), raising the possibility that proteoglycans may function normally to restrict outwandering of axons and thus serve to minimize reinnervation of inappropriate targets. Although proteoglycan degradation is clearly useful in promoting axons through acellular nerve grafts (Krekoski et al., 2001; Neubauer et al., 2007) application of this strategy to end-to-end nerve repair cannot be recommended until its consequences for regeneration specificity are defined more clearly.

Reduction of scarring at the site of nerve repair has been revisited periodically as a means of enhancing nerve regeneration (Chapter 9). Reduction of local scarring with collagenase was not found to speed regeneration as measured by the pinch test or to enhance muscle tetanic contraction force (Rydevik et al., 2002). Local treatment with Interleukin-10, however, reduced collagen deposition and enhanced conduction across the repair site (Atkins et al., 2007). Scar reduction and inactivation of MAG and CSPGs may thus be helpful at some times and if obtained through particular mechanisms, but are not yet blanket strategies for improving outcome after end-to-end nerve repair.

Supporting Chronically Denervated Schwann Cells

In the rodent model, pathway support of axon regeneration diminishes rapidly with increasing periods of Schwann cell denervation. Expression of growth factors subsides, many Schwann cell markers are downregulated, the basal lamina deteriorates, and the nerve environment becomes hypoperfused (Chapter 9). Maintaining the viability and responsiveness of denervated Schwann cells is thus an important component of maximizing recovery after nerve repair.

Three techniques of maintaining pathway viability have been explored: temporary reinnervation with axons from other nerves, treatment of Schwann cells with growth factors, and augmentation of the Schwann cell population with stem cells. The possibility of protecting Schwann cells with locally available axons has been explored in the rat femoral nerve model (Sulaiman et al., 2002b; Midha et al., 2005). The cutaneous (saphenous) branch was transected and reinnervated from the muscle branch, the cutaneous branch, or left denervated. Eight weeks later it was again transected and reinnervated from the muscle branch for 6 weeks, then backlabeled with fluorescent tracer. Significantly more motoneurons reinnervated cutaneous nerves that had been occupied by motor axons for 8 weeks than those that had been temporarily reinnervated with cutaneous axons or left denervated. The receptiveness of the pathway to motor axons can thus be maintained with motor axons, but not with cutaneous axons. These findings are consistent with later work demonstrating that the growth factor expression by Schwann cells in a nerve graft can be modified by reinnervating the graft with axons of a different modality (Hoke et al., 2006). Although temporary reinnervation is appealing in its simplicity, protection of motor nerve would require the sacrifice of motor axons that could just as well be used for a nerve transfer. It does suggest, however, that strategies to duplicate signaling from axon to Schwann cell could effectively preserve Schwann cell viability and function.

Chronically denervated Schwann cells have been resuscitated with neuregulin (originally named glial growth factor, or GGF) and transforming growth factor-β (TGF-β). Schwann cells that had been denervated for 2–6 months in vivo responded to neuregulin with cellular proliferation and reexpression of the neural cell adhesion molecule (N-CAM) and N-cadherin, adhesion molecules that are downregulated progressively by increasing periods of denervation (Li et al., 1998). In vivo, the ability of Schwann cells denervated for 6 months to support regeneration across a nerve gap was enhanced significantly by incubating them with TGF-β and forskolin for 48 hours before placing them in the gap (Sulaiman, Gordon, 2002). Although neither of these treatments has been applied to Schwann cells that have been chronically denervated distal to a nerve repair, reactivation or maintenance of denervated Schwann cells in situ would be expected to enhance regeneration dramatically, especially in the clinical setting where Schwann cells remain denervated for months to years because of the long distances involved.

In addition to preserving and/or rescuing Schwann cells that are already present within chronically denervated nerve, it is also possible to enhance the cellular population by adding stem cells. In initial experiments, neural stem cells derived from neonatal cerebellar granule cells were injected into nerve that had been axotomized 6 months previously (Heine et al., 2004). Freshly cut motor axons were able to regenerate through these nerves to restore function, but could not regenerate through untreated nerve (Figure 12-14). Exploration of alternative stem cell sources revealed that skin-derived precursors (SDPs), cells of neural crest origin, can be differentiated into Schwann cells under appropriate conditions (Toma et al., 2001). These cells upregulate myelin proteins when cultured with sensory neurons and have been shown to myelinate previously demyelinated axons in vivo (McKenzie et al., 2006). When injected into chronically denervated nerve they promote the regeneration of increased numbers of motoneurons and enhance muscle reinnervation by morphologic and electrophysiologic criteria (Walsh et al., 2010). In addition to their direct role in myelinating axons, these cells could also be providing growth factors, producing matrix metalloproteinases that degrade inhibitory chondroitin sulfate proteoglycans, or interacting with Schwann cells to modify their phenotype (Walsh et al., 2010). This strategy is currently limited by the need for direct access to the nerve undergoing treatment, but could be enhanced by developing stem cells capable of targeting denervated Schwann cells from the circulation or of migrating aggressively from the repair site down the distal nerve stump.

SUPPORTING DENERVATED MUSCLE

Electrical Stimulation

Electrical stimulation to minimize the atrophy of denervated muscle has been in and out of vogue several times since it was described by Duchenne in 1855 (Duchenne de Boulogne, 1855). He treated several cases of upper extremity paralysis resulting from closed nerve injury, such as stretch during shoulder dislocation, and reported uniformly favorable outcomes (Figure 12-15). In the interim, it has become clear that electrical stimulation can maintain the bulk and contractile properties of denervated muscle to varying degrees depending on the animal model and the stimulation parameters

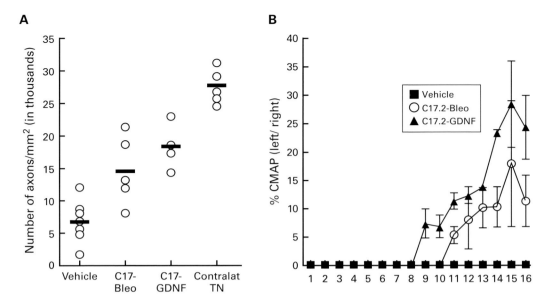

FIGURE 12-14   Neural stem cells enhance regeneration through chronically denervated peripheral nerves. In these experiments, rat tibial nerves that had been maintained in a denervated state for 6 months were injected with C17.2 neural stem cells engineered to express GDNF (C17.2-GDNF), C17.2 neural stem cells engineered with bleomycin resistance gene (C17.2-Bleo), or vehicle, then reinnervated with freshly transected peroneal nerve axons for 4 months. A. The density of axons in the distal tibial nerve was enhanced significantly in both groups treated with stem cells. B. The return of compound motor action potentials (CMAPs) in the foot muscles innervated by the tibial nerve. CMAPs returned earlier and to a significantly greater degree in animals transplanted with C17.2-GDNF stem cells. There was no reinnervation in animals that did not receive stem cells. Reprinted with permission from Heine et al., 2004.

(Dow et al., 2004; Kern et al., 2004; Ashley et al., 2007, 2008). Whether these benefits can be maintained after stimulated muscle is reinnervated, however, remains controversial.

Ultimate muscle mass and contractile properties have been enhanced by stimulation in experiments in which nerves have been crushed or transected and sutured relatively near target muscles (Cole, Gardiner, 1984; Salerno et al., 1990; Marqueste et al., 2006). These muscles have not been denervated for prolonged periods, and have been stimulated both while denervated and during the reinnervation process.

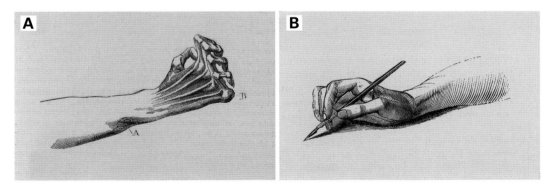

FIGURE 12-15   The ideal result of preserving denervated muscle with electrical stimulation. This patient received a closed proximal ulnar nerve injury that resulted in severe intrinsic muscle atrophy and secondary deformity (A). His dramatic recovery (B) was attributed to electrical stimulation of the denervated muscles until they were reinnervated. The actual utility of this technique continues to be debated. From Duchenne, 1855.

Benefits were also seen in a larger dog model of immediate repair 12 cm proximal to the stimulated muscle (Williams, 1996). This work culminated in an uncontrolled clinical trial that produced encouraging results (Nicolaidis, Williams, 2001). The effectiveness of electrical stimulation could not be confirmed, however, when muscle was experimentally denervated for prolonged periods (Dow et al., 2007). Stimulation of the rat extensor digitorum longus (EDL) muscle during a 3.5-month denervation period preceding nerve repair did not improve muscle mass, maximum tetanic tension, or walking track parameters when measured 6.5 months after repair. As was discussed in Chapter 9 (Part 1, "Chronic Axotomy"; Part 3, "Chronic Denervation"), prolonged axotomy reduces the proportion of motoneurons that regenerate and chronic denervation reduces pathway support for regeneration, making it difficult to isolate muscle effects in this model. A crossed nerve paradigm in which a freshly axotomized nerve is used to reinnervate muscle that has been denervated and stimulated for several months could provide a more realistic appraisal of efficacy.

Sensory Protection

The consequences of experimentally misdirecting sensory axons into muscle were studied extensively in the early twentieth century. The pertinent questions at that time were: (1) Is the nature and function of axon–end organ connections determined by the regenerating neuron or by the recipient end organ? and (2) Can sensory axons provide trophic support for denervated muscle? Although many experiments addressed these issues with varying degrees of rigor (summarized in Kilvington, 1912), two in particular provided definitive results with relatively modern techniques (Gutmann, 1945; Weiss, Edds, 1945). In both instances, sensory axons were shown to ramify extensively within muscle, but without restoring functional connections or providing trophic support.

Motivated by in vitro evidence that DRG neurons could provide at least some support to muscle fibers (e.g., Peterson, Crain, 1972), Ochi and colleagues grafted DRGs onto the cut peroneal nerve in the rat (Ochi et al., 1992, 1996). In these preparations muscle wet weight and contraction properties were enhanced by sensory reinnervation, but ultimate function after reinnervation by motor axons was not evaluated. Subsequent experiments confirmed that sensory reinnervation was effective in delaying muscle atrophy (Hynes et al., 1997; Wang et al., 2001; Zuijdendorp et al., 2010). As noted in the previous discussion of electrical stimulation, however, preservation of muscle morphology does not automatically translate to improved function once the muscle is reinnervated. Two recent groups of experiments have addressed this issue. Using a nerve-crossing paradigm, Bain et al. showed that after 4 or 6 months of tibial nerve axotomy, gastrocnemius twitch and tetanic isometric contraction force were significantly greater when saphenous nerve axons had been used to "protect" the muscle before it was reinnervated by freshly axotomized peroneal motor axons (Bain et al., 2001). After 6 months of musculocutaneous nerve axotomy, sensory protection enhanced muscle weight but did not improve grooming function as determined 1 month after muscle reinnervation by the freshly transected medial pectoral nerve (Papakonstantinou et al., 2002). Although sensory protection has been applied in one clinical case with apparent success (Bain et al., 2008), there is still no consensus regarding its clinical potential. In a related procedure that has been used more often, ipsilateral hypoglossal to facial nerve transfer has been used to "babysit" denervated facial musculature while additional motor axons regenerate through grafts from the opposite facial nerve (Terzis, Tzafetta, 2009). The hypoglossal axons are never transected, however, so this procedure is in fact a permanent nerve transfer rather than a temporary protective maneuver.

Protease Inhibition

Protease inhibition, first explored as a strategy for treating muscular dystrophy, was also found to reduce the atrophy of denervated muscle (Stracher et al., 1978, 1979). Calcium-activated neutral protease (CANP), one of the enzymes that breaks down muscle fibers, is found in multiple intra- and extracellular locations within both nerve and muscle and can be inactivated by the protease inhibitor leupeptin (Badalamente et al., 1987). These observations suggested that administration of leupeptin might improve the results of nerve repair by reducing muscle atrophy during the denervation period (Hurst et al., 1984; Badalamente et al., 1989). In a series of primate experiments long-term administration of leupeptin increased the speed of conduction across nerve repairs performed 2 months previously, and increased the size of myofibers and the number of myelinated axons in the muscle nerve after 6 months (Badalamente et al., 1992, 1995). It has been suggested that these effects resulted from both muscle preservation and protection of the Schwann cell basal lamina, a site of normal CANP expression (Stracher, 1999). Although this approach to muscle and pathway preservation showed promise in primate experiments, it was never subjected to clinical trials because the pharmaceutical industry was not convinced of its profitability (Badalamente, personal communication).

Ectopic Motoneuron Transplantation

Temporary muscle reinnervation to provide trophic support and minimize atrophy is clinically feasible when sensory nerve is the axon source. Cutaneous nerves are relatively expendable, and a muscle and its adjacent skin are often served by different root levels, so that an axon source is often available. Although temporary reinnervation with motor axons would be preferable, motor nerves are less expendable, and potential donors may also be denervated. To overcome these difficulties, researchers at the Miami Project to Cure Paralysis implanted embryonic motoneurons into the distal stumps of transected rat tibial nerves. Many of these motoneurons survived in the intraneural environment, and their axons extended down the denervated tibial pathways and formed synapses in gastrocnemius muscle (Erb et al., 1993). Although few motor units were reestablished, gastrocnemius muscle contraction in response to stimulation of the motoneurons was strong enough to produce ankle movement in one-third of cases (Yohn et al., 2008). Subsequent experiments focused on enhancing the efficiency of the motoneuron transplant strategy revealed that a combination of GDNF, IGF-1 and HGF was particularly effective in enhancing motoneuron survival and muscle reinnervation (Grumbles et al., 2009). Although FGF-6 did not enhance overall reinnervation, it did influence the function of reinnervated muscle by changing the predominant fiber type to one that was stronger but more fatiguable (Grumbles et al., 2007). Recently, it was also shown that transplantation of embryonic stem cells into the nerve could produce similar results (Yohn et al., 2008).

Although the motoneuron transplant strategy was initially devised to facilitate electrical stimulation of muscle denervated by motoneuron death resulting from spinal cord trauma (Erb et al., 1993),

it might also be applied in some instances of peripheral nerve injury. After brachial plexus or proximal ulnar nerve transection, for instance, it might be possible to preserve the intrinsic muscles of the hand by injecting stem cells into the ulnar nerve at the wrist. The resulting ectopic motoneuron pool could then innervate and preserve these muscles until their native axons return 1–2 years later.

CONCLUSIONS

It is readily apparent that incremental improvements in the outcome of experimental nerve repair can be obtained by modifying a wide variety of regeneration components. Most of these improvements are in the 15–30% range; rarely has an experimental outcome measure been doubled or tripled. The majority of successful manipulations have been performed in rodents, but their effectiveness has not been confirmed in clinically relevant models. Although deficits resulting from nerve injury have been reduced dramatically by the advancement of specific techniques such as nerve transfer, the clinical outcomes of end-to-end nerve repair have improved little since the introduction of microsurgical techniques.

The void that separates frequent experimental success from rare clinical impact is a measure of the complexity of the regeneration process. It is likely that substantial inroads will require a program of multiple treatments that address two or more of the interdependent goals listed in the introduction: (1) Enhance and maintain the neuronal growth state to promote axons across the inhibitory milieu of the repair site and speed regeneration, (2) Create regeneration specificity by guiding axons to Schwann cell tubes in the distal stump that lead to functionally appropriate end organs, (3) Maintain the ability of chronically denervated Schwann cells to support regeneration, (4) Prolong the viability of denervated end organs, and (5) Maximize CNS compensation for peripheral miswiring.

Recently, the simultaneous use of two distinct treatments has been undertaken in an attempt to provide additive benefits for regeneration (English et al., 2005; Hetzler et al., 2008; Asensio-Pinilla et al., 2010; Udina et al., 2010). Two of these studies have addressed distinct aspects of nerve regeneration, neuronal regeneration state and pathway growth inhibition, in a model of nerve transection and repair. The effects of promoting regeneration with electrical stimulation and at the same time reducing pathway inhibition by breaking down proteoglycans were found to be additive, whereas the effects of proteoglycan breakdown were not additive with those of raising intracellular cAMP pharmacologically (English et al., 2005; Udina et al., 2010). Taken alone, the second set of results might suggest that once the neural regeneration state is enhanced, axons are able to proceed without interference from pathway inhibitors, so that their removal makes no difference. Together, however, these two sets of experiments suggest that either cAMP elevation is not as strong a stimulus as is electrical stimulation, or the two are signaling through overlapping but distinct pathways.

Most of the goals listed above involve accentuation or prolongation of an event that occurs naturally; neuronal regeneration state is elevated by axotomy, axons do cross the repair site, the distal stump does support regeneration, end organs are viable to begin with, and the CNS does compensate for miswiring to some degree. The one goal that remains, guiding axons to functionally appropriate Schwann cell tubes in the distal nerve stump, involves creating an entirely new activity. PMR generates partial sensory/motor specificity over time, but there is scant evidence to suggest that either PMR or other potential forms of specificity can be generated by initial recognition and selective reinnervation of Schwann cell tubes on a modality- or location-specific basis.

Potential reasons for the failure of pathway recognition can be found by comparing peripheral nerve development and regeneration in the context of evolution. As demonstrated by a series of elegant experiments in the frog, motoneuron regeneration is topographically specific up until the developmental stage when basal lamina is formed (Farel, Meeker, 1993; Meeker, Farel, 1993). Early in development axons navigate through an unconstrained environment in which they are free to respond to a variety of overlapping guidance cues. As they mature, axons become constrained within basal lamina tubes that are not part of the pathfinding process and thus have no reason to display specific pathway markers. Furthermore, it is unlikely that evolution has improved on this situation, as (1) animals that sustain nerve injury are unlikely to live long enough to reproduce, and (2) generation after generation of these animals would need to receive and survive nerve injuries in order to confer an evolutionary advantage to beneficial genes. Devising techniques to guide regenerating axons back to functionally appropriate Schwann cell tubes is thus likely to be a

substantial challenge. In view of the possible benefits, however, it is a challenge well worth undertaking.

REFERENCES

Aberg M, Ljungberg C, Edin E, Millqvist H, Nordh E, Theorin A, Terenghi G, Wiberg M (2009) Clinical evaluation of a resorbable wrap-around implant as an alternative to nerve repair: a prospective, assessor-blinded, randomised clinical study of sensory, motor and functional recovery after peripheral nerve repair. J Plast Reconstr Aesthet Surg 62: 1503–1509.

Al-Majed AA, Brushart TM, Gordon T (2000a) Electrical stimulation accelerates and increases expression of BDNF and TrkB rnRNA in regenerating rat femoral motoneurons. Eur J Neurosci 12: 4381–4390.

Al-Majed AA, Neumann CM, Brushart TM, Gordon T (2000b) Brief electrical stimulation promotes the speed and accuracy of motor axonal regeneration. J Neurosci 20: 2602–2608.

Al-Majed AA, Tam SL, Gordon T (2004) Electrical stimulation accelerates and enhances expression of regeneration-associated genes in regenerating rat femoral motoneurons. Cell Mol Neurobiol 24: 379–402.

Almquist EE, Nachemson A, Auth D, Almquist B, Hall S (1984) Evaluation of the use of the argon laser in repairing rat and primate nerves. J Hand Surg Am 9: 792–799.

Alto LT, Havton LA, Conner JM, Hollis ER, II, Blesch A, Tuszynski MH (2009) Chemotropic guidance facilitates axonal regeneration and synapse formation after spinal cord injury. Nat Neurosci 12: 1106–1113.

Anders GJ, Wierda J, Nienhaus AJ, Idenburg VJ (1978) Time and cell systems as variables in fusion experiments with polyethylene glycol. Hum Genet 42: 319–322.

Anders JJ, Borke RC, Woolery SK, Van de Merwe WP (1993) Low power laser irradiation alters the rate of regeneration of the rat facial nerve. Lasers Surg Med 13: 72–82.

Angelov DN, Ceynowa M, Guntinas-Lichius O, Streppel M, Grosheva M, Kiryakova SI, Skouras E, Maegele M, Irintchev A, Neiss WF, Sinis N, Alvanou A, Dunlop SA (2007) Mechanical stimulation of paralyzed vibrissal muscles following facial nerve injury in adult rat promotes full recovery of whisking. Neurobiol Dis 26: 229–242.

Asensio-Pinilla E, Udina E, Jaramillo J, Navarro X (2010) Electrical stimulation combined with exercise increase axonal regeneration after peripheral nerve injury. Exp Neurol 219: 258–265.

Ashley Z, Salmons S, Boncompagni S, Protasi F, Russold M, Lanmuller H, Mayr W, Sutherland H, Jarvis JC (2007) Effects of chronic electrical stimulation on long-term denervated muscles of the rabbit hind limb. J Muscle Res Cell Motil 28: 203–217.

Ashley Z, Sutherland H, Russold MF, Lanmuller H, Mayr W, Jarvis JC, Salmons S (2008) Therapeutic stimulation of denervated muscles: the influence of pattern. Muscle & Nerve 38: 875–886.

Aspalter M, Vyas A, Feiner J, Griffin J, Brushart T, Redett R (2008) Modification of Schwann cell gene expression by electroporation in vivo. J Neurosci Methods. 176: 96–103.

Atkins S, Loescher AR, Boissonade FM, Smith KG, Occleston N, O'Kane S, Ferguson MW, Robinson PP (2007) Interleukin-10 reduces scarring and enhances regeneration at a site of sciatic nerve repair. J Peripher Nerv Syst 12: 269–276.

Averill S, Michael GJ, Shortland PJ, Leavesley RC, King VR, Bradbury EJ, McMahon SB, Priestley JV (2004) NGF and GDNF ameliorate the increase in ATF3 expression which occurs in dorsal root ganglion cells in response to peripheral nerve injury. Eur J Neurosci 19: 1437–1445.

Badalamente MA, Hurst LC, Stracher A (1987) Localization and inhibition of calcium-activated neutral protease (CANP) in primate skeletal muscle and peripheral nerve. Exp Neurol 98: 357–369.

Badalamente MA, Hurst LC, Stracher A (1989) Neuromuscular recovery using calcium protease inhibition after median nerve repair in primates. Proc Natl Acad Sci USA 86: 5983–5987.

Badalamente MA, Hurst LC, Stracher A (1992) Recovery after delayed nerve repair: influence of a pharmacologic adjunct in a primate model. J Reconstr Microsurg 8: 391–397.

Badalamente MA, Hurst LC, Stracher A (1995) Neuromuscular recovery after peripheral nerve repair: effects of an orally-administered peptide in a primate model. J Reconstr Microsurg 11: 429–437.

Badke A, Irintchev AP, Wernig A (1989) Maturation of transmission in reinnervated mouse soleus muscle. Muscle & Nerve 12: 580–586.

Bailes JE, Cozzens JW, Hudson AR, Kline DG, Ciric I, Gianaris P, Bernstein LP, Hunter D (1989) Laser-assisted nerve repair in primates. J Neurosurg 71: 266–272.

Bain JR, Veltri KL, Chamberlain D, Fahnestock M (2001) Improved functional recovery of denervated skeletal muscle after temporary sensory nerve innervation. Neuroscience 103: 503–510.

Bain JR, Hason Y, Veltri K, Fahnestock M, Quartly C (2008) Clinical application of sensory protection of denervated muscle. J Neurosurg 109: 955–961.

Baptista AF, Goes BT, Menezes D, Gomes FC, Zugaib J, Stipursky J, Gomes JR, Oliveira JT, Vannier-Santos MA, Martinez AM (2009) PEMF fails to enhance nerve regeneration after sciatic nerve crush lesion. J Peripher Nerv Syst 14: 285–293.

Barakat-Walter I, Kraftsik R, Schenker M, Kuntzer T (2007) Thyroid hormone in biodegradable nerve guides stimulates sciatic nerve regeneration: a potential therapeutic approach for human peripheral nerve injuries. J Neurotrauma 24: 567–577.

Bassett CA, Campbell JB, Husby J (1959) Peripheral nerve and spinal cord regeneration: factors leading to success of a tubulation technique employing millipore. Exp Neurol 1: 386–406.

Bassett CA, Mitchell SN, Gaston SR (1981) Treatment of ununited tibial diaphyseal fractures with pulsing electromagnetic fields. J Bone Joint Surg Am 63: 511–523.

Bateman JE (1948) Plasma silk suture of nerves. Ann Surg 127: 456–463.

Berenberg RA, Forman DS, Wood DK, DeSilva A, Demaree J (1977) Recovery of peripheral nerve function after axotomy: effect of triiodothyronine. Exp Neurol 57: 349–363.

Birse SC, Bittner GD (1981) Regeneration of earthworm giant axons following transection or ablation. J Neurophysiol 45: 724–742.

Bittner GD, Ballinger ML, Raymond MA (1986) Reconnection of severed nerve axons with polyethylene glycol. Brain Res 367: 351–355.

Bjorkman A, Rosen B, Lundborg G (2004) Acute improvement of hand sensibility after selective ipsilateral cutaneous forearm anaesthesia. Eur J Neurosci 20: 2733–2736.

Bjorkman A, Rosen B, Lundborg G (2005) Anaesthesia of the axillary plexus induces rapid improvement of sensory function in the contralateral hand: an effect of interhemispheric plasticity. Scand J Plast Reconstr Surg Hand Surg 39: 234–237.

Blesch A, Tuszynski MH (2007) Transient growth factor delivery sustains regenerated axons after spinal cord injury. J Neurosci 27: 10535–10545.

Bouton MS, Bittner GD (1981) Regeneration of motor axons in crayfish limbs: distal stump activation followed by synaptic reformation. Cell Tissue Res 219: 379–392.

Boyd JG, Gordon T (2002) A dose-dependent facilitation and inhibition of peripheral nerve regeneration by brain-derived neurotrophic factor. Eur J Neurosci 15: 613–626.

Boyd JG, Gordon T (2003) Glial cell line-derived neurotrophic factor and brain-derived neurotrophic factor sustain the axonal regeneration of chronically axotomized motoneurons *in vivo*. Exp Neurol 183: 610–619.

Bozorg Grayeli A, Mosnier I, Julien N, El Garem H, Bouccara D, Sterkers O (2005) Long-term functional outcome in facial nerve graft by fibrin glue in the temporal bone and cerebellopontine angle. Eur Arch Otorhinolaryngol 262: 404–407.

Britt JM, Kane JR, Spaeth CS, Zuzek A, Robinson GL, Gbanaglo MY, Estler CJ, Boydston EA, Schallert T, Bittner GD (2010) Polyethylene glycol rapidly restores axonal integrity and improves the rate of motor behavior recovery after sciatic crush injury. J Neurophysiol 104: 695–703.

Broude E, McAtee M, Kelley MS, Bregman BS (1997) c-Jun expression in adult rat dorsal root ganglion neurons: differential response after central or peripheral axotomy. Exp Neurol 148: 367–377.

Brown TJ, Khan T, Jones KJ (1999) Androgen induced acceleration of functional recovery after rat sciatic nerve injury. Restor Neurol Neurosci 15: 289–295.

Brushart TM, Gerber J, Kessens P, Chen YG, Royal R (1998) Contributions of pathway and neuron to preferential motor reinnervation. J Neurosci 18: 8674–8681.

Brushart TM, Jari R, Verge V, Rohde C, Gordon T (2005) Electrical stimulation restores the specificity of sensory axon regeneration. Exp Neurol 194: 221–229.

Brushart TM, Hoffman PN, Royall RM, Murinson BB, Witzel C, Gordon T (2002) Electrical stimulation promotes motoneuron regeneration without increasing its speed or conditioning the neuron. J Neurosci 22: 6631–6638.

Bungner Ov (1891) Ueber die degeneratuins-und regenerationsvorgange am nerven nach verletzungen. Beitr Pathol Anat 10: 312–393.

Byers JM, Clark KF, Thompson GC (1998) Effect of pulsed electromagnetic stimulation on facial nerve regeneration. Arch Otolaryngol Head Neck Surg 124: 383–389.

Cafferty WB, Bradbury EJ, Lidierth M, Jones M, Duffy PJ, Pezet S, McMahon SB (2008) Chondroitinase ABC-mediated plasticity of spinal sensory function. J Neurosci 28: 11998–12009.

Campion ER, Bynum DK, Powers SK (1990) Repair of peripheral nerves with the argon laser: a functional and histological evaluation. J Bone Joint Surg Am 72: 715–723.

Cao X, Shoichet MS (2001) Defining the concentration gradient of nerve growth factor for guided neurite outgrowth. Neuroscience 103: 831–840.

Casellas P, Galiegue S, Basile AS (2002) Peripheral benzodiazepine receptors and mitochondrial function. Neurochem Int 40: 475–486.

Chen WZ, Qiao H, Zhou W, Wu J, Wang ZB (2010) Upgraded nerve growth factor expression induced by low-intensity continuous-wave ultrasound accelerates regeneration of neurotometicly injured sciatic nerve in rats. Ultrasound Med Biol 36: 1109–1117.

Cheng ASK, Hung LK, Wang JMW, Lau H, Chan J (2001) A prospective study of early tactile stimulation after digital nerve repair. Clin Orthop (no. 384): 169–175.

Cockett SA (1972) Rate of regeneration in peripheral nerves; a method for measuring. Exp Neurol 37: 635–638.

Cockett SA, Kiernan JA (1973) Acceleration of peripheral nervous regeneration in the rat by exogenous triiodothyronine. Exp Neurol 39: 389–394.

Cole BG, Gardiner PF (1984) Does electrical stimulation of denervated muscle, continued after reinnervation, influence recovery of contractile function? Exp Neurol 85: 52–62.

Condic ML (2001) Adult neuronal regeneration induced by transgenic integrin expression. J Neurosci 21: 4782–4788.

Crockett JL, Edgerton VR (1975) Exercise and restricted activity effects on reinnervated and cross-innervated skeletal muscles. J Neurol Sci 25: 1–9.

Danielsen N, Dahlin LB, Ericson LE, Crenshaw A, Lundborg G (1986) Experimental hyperthyroidism stimulates axonal growth in mesothelial chambers. Exp Neurol 94: 54–65.

Deepa SS, Carulli D, Galtrey C, Rhodes K, Fukuda J, Mikami T, Sugahara K, Fawcett JW (2006) Composition of perineuronal net extracellular matrix in rat brain: a different disaccharide composition for the net-associated proteoglycans. J Biol Chem 281: 17789–17800.

Dellon AL, Curtis RM, Edgerton MD (1974) Reeducation of sensation in the hand after nerve injury and repair. PRS 53: 297–305.

Dombrowski MA, Sasaki M, Lankford KL, Kocsis JD, Radtke C (2006) Myelination and nodal formation of regenerated peripheral nerve fibers following transplantation of acutely prepared olfactory ensheathing cells. Brain Res 1125: 1–8.

dos Reis FA, Belchior AC, de Carvalho Pde T, da Silva BA, Pereira DM, Silva IS, Nicolau RA (2009) Effect of laser therapy (660 nm) on recovery of the sciatic nerve in rats after injury through neurotmesis followed by epineural anastomosis. Lasers Med Sci 24: 741–747.

Dow DE, Cederna PS, Hassett CA, Kostrominova TY, Faulkner JA, Dennis RG (2004) Number of contractions to maintain mass and force of a denervated rat muscle. Muscle & Nerve 30: 77–86.

Dow DE, Cederna PS, Hassett CA, Dennis RG, Faulkner JA (2007) Electrical stimulation prior to delayed reinnervation does not enhance recovery in muscles of rats. Restor Neurol Neurosci 25: 601–610.

Duchenne G de Boulogne (1855) De l'electrisation localise, et de son application a la physiologie, a la pathologie et a la therapeutique. Paris: Bailliere.

Ducker TB, Hayes GJ (1968) Peripheral nerve injuries: a comparative study of the anatomical and functional results following primary nerve repair in chimpanzees. Mil Med 133: 298–302.

Eberhardt KA, Irintichev A, Al-Majed AA, Simova O, Brushart TM, Gordon T, Schachner M (2006) BDNF/TrkB signaling regulates HNK-1 carbohydrate expression in regenerating motor nerves and promotes functional recovery after peripheral nerve repair. Exp Neurol 198: 500–510.

Eggers R, Hendriks WT, Tannemaat MR, van Heerikhuize JJ, Pool CW, Carlstedt TP, Zaldumbide A, Hoeben RC, Boer GJ, Verhaagen J (2008) Neuroregenerative effects of lentiviral vector-mediated GDNF expression in reimplanted ventral roots. Mol Cell Neurosci 39: 105–117.

Egloff DV, Narakas A (1983) Nerve anastomoses with human fibrin: preliminary clinical report (56 cases). Ann Chir Main 2: 101–115.

Ekstrom PA, Mayer U, Panjwani A, Pountney D, Pizzey J, Tonge DA (2003) Involvement of alpha7beta1 integrin in the conditioning-lesion effect on sensory axon regeneration. Mol Cell Neurosci 22: 383–395.

English AW (2005) Enhancing axon regeneration in peripheral nerves also increases functionally inappropriate reinnervation of targets. J Comp Neurol 490: 427–441.

English AW, Meador W, Carrasco DI (2005) Neurotrophin-4/5 is required for the early growth of regenerating axons in peripheral nerves. Eur J Neurosci 21: 2624–2634.

English AW, Schwartz G, Meador W, Sabatier MJ, Mulligan A (2007) Electrical stimulation promotes peripheral axon regeneration by enhanced neuronal neurotrophin signaling. Dev Neurobiol 67: 158–172.

English AW, Cucoranu D, Mulligan A, Sabatier M (2009) Treadmill training enhances axon regeneration in injured mouse peripheral nerves without increased loss of topographic specificity. J Comp Neurol 517: 245–255.

Erb DE, Mora RJ, Bunge RP (1993) Reinnervation of adult rat gastrocnemius muscle by embryonic motoneurons transplanted into the axotomized tibial nerve. Exp Neurol 124: 372–376.

Fansa H, Schneider W, Wolf G, Keilhoff G (2002) Influence of insulin-like growth factor-I (IGF-I) on nerve autografts and tissue-engineered nerve grafts. Muscle & Nerve 26: 87–93.

Farel PB, Meeker ML (1993) Developmental regulation of regenerative specificity in the bullfrog. Brain Res Bull 30: 483–490.

Fischer DW, Beggs JL, Shetter AG, Waggener JD (1983) Comparative study of neuroma formation in the rat sciatic nerve after CO_2 laser and scalpel neurectomy. Neurosurgery 13: 287–294.

Franz CK, Rutishauser U, Rafuse VF (2008) Intrinsic neuronal properties control selective targeting of regenerating motoneurons. Brain 131: 1492–1505.

Fu Q, Hue J, Li S (2007) Nonsteroidal anti-inflammatory drugs promote axon regeneration via RhoA inhibition. J Neurosci 27: 4154–4164.

Fu SY, Gordon T (1995) Contributing factors to poor functional recovery after delayed nerve repair: prolonged axotomy. J Neurosci 15: 3876–3885.

Galtrey CM, Asher RA, Nothais F, Fawcett J (2007) Promoting plasticity in the spinal cord with chondroitinase improves functional recovery after peripheral nerve repair. Brain 130: 926–939.

Garcia-Alias G, Barkhuysen S, Buckle M, Fawcett JW (2009) Chondroitinase ABC treatment opens a window of opportunity for task-specific rehabilitation. Nat Neurosci 12: 1145–1151.

Gehlert DR, Stephenson DT, Schober DA, Rash K, Clemens JA (1997) Increased expression of peripheral benzodiazepine receptors in the facial nucleus following motor neuron axotomy. Neurochem Int 31: 705–713.

Geremia NM, Gordon T, Brushart TM, Al-Majed A, Verge V (2007) Electrical stimulation promotes sensory neuron regeneration and growth-associated gene expression. Exp Neurol 205: 347–359.

Gershenbaum M, Roisen F (1980) The effects of dibutyryl cyclic adenosine monophosphate on the degeneration and regeneration of crush-lesioned rat sciatic nerve. Neuroscience 5: 1565–1580.

Gibby WA, Koerber HR, Horch KW (1983) A quantitative evaluation of suture and tubulization nerve repair techniques. J Neurosurg 58: 574–579.

Gomez N, Schmidt CE (2007) Nerve growth factor-immobilized polypyrrole: bioactive electrically conducting polymer for enhanced neurite extension. J Biomed Mater Res A 81: 135–149.

Gómez-Pinilla F, Ying Z, Opazo P, Roy RR, Edgerton VR (2001) Differential regulation by exercise of BDNF and NT-3 in rat spinal cord and skeletal muscle. Eur J Neurosci 13: 1078–1084.

Gordon T, Amirjani N, Edwards DC, Chan KM (2010) Brief post-surgical electrical stimulation accelerates axon regeneration and muscle reinnervation without affecting the functional measures in carpal tunnel syndrome patients. Exp Neurol 223: 192–202.

Graham JB, Neubauer D, Xue QS, Muir D (2007) Chondroitinase applied to peripheral nerve repair averts retrograde axonal regeneration. Exp Neurol 203(1): 185-195.

Groves MJ, An SF, Giometto B, Scaravilli F (1999) Inhibition of sensory neuron apoptosis and prevention of loss by NT-3 administration following axotomy. Exp Neurol 155: 284–294.

Groves MJ, Schanzer A, Simpson AJ, An SF, Kuo LT, Scaravilli F (2003) Profile of adult rat sensory neuron loss, apoptosis and replacement after sciatic nerve crush. J Neurocytol 32: 113–122.

Groves ML, McKeon R, Werner E, Nagarsheth M, Meador W, English AW (2005) Axon regeneration in peripheral nerves is enhanced by proteoglycan degradation. Exp Neurol 195: 278–292.

Grumbles RM, Casella GT, Rudinsky MJ, Wood PM, Sesodia S, Bent M, Thomas CK (2007) Long-term delivery of FGF-6 changes the fiber type and fatigability of muscle reinnervated from embryonic neurons transplanted into adult rat peripheral nerve. J Neurosci Res 85: 1933–1942.

Grumbles RM, Sesodia S, Wood PM, Thomas CK (2009) Neurotrophic factors improve motoneuron survival and function of muscle reinnervated by embryonic neurons. J Neuropathol Exp Neurol 68: 736–746.

Gunderson RW, Barrett JN (1979) Neuronal chemotaxis: chick dorsal root axons turn toward high concentrations of nerve growth factor. Science 206: 1079–1080.

Guntinas-Lichius O, Wewetzer K, Tomov TL, Azzolin N, Kazemi S, Streppel M, Neiss WF, Angelov DN (2002) Transplantation of olfactory mucosa minimizes axonal branching and promotes the recovery of vibrissae motor performance after facial nerve repair in rats. J Neurosci 22: 7121–7131.

Guntinas-Lichius O, Hundeshagen G, Paling T, Streppel M, Grosheva M, Irintchev A, Skouras E, Alvanou A, Angelova SK, Kuerten S, Sinis N, Dunlop SA, Angelov DN (2007) Manual stimulation of facial muscles improves functional recovery after hypoglossal-facial anastomosis and interpositional nerve grafting of the facial nerve in adult rats. Neurobiol Dis 28: 101–112.

Gutmann E (1945) The reinnervation of muscle by sensory nerve fibers. J Anat 79: 1–8.

Guven M, Gunay I, Ozgunen K, Zorludemir S (2005) Effect of pulsed magnetic field on regenerating rat sciatic nerve: an in-vitro electrophysiologic study. Int J Neurosci 115: 881–892.

Haastert K, Grosheva M, Angelova SK, Guntinas-Lichius O, Skouras E, Michael J, Grothe C, Dunlop SA, Angelov DN (2009) Schwann cells overexpressing FGF-2 alone or combined with manual stimulation do not promote functional recovery after facial nerve injury. J Biomed Biotechnol 2009: 408794.

Hart AM, Wiberg M, Youle M, Terenghi G (2002) Systemic acetyl-L-carnitine eliminates sensory neuronal loss after peripheral axotomy: a new clinical approach in the management of peripheral nerve trauma. Exp Brain Res 145: 182–189.

Hart AM, Terenghi G, Kellerth JO, Wiberg M (2004) Sensory neuroprotection, mitochondrial preservation, and therapeutic potential of N-acetyl-cysteine after nerve injury. Neuroscience 125: 91–101.

Hazari A, Johansson-Rudén G, Junemo-Bostrom K, Ljungberg C, Terenghi G, Green C, Wiberg M (1999) A new resorbable wrap-around implant as an alternative nerve repair technique. J Hand Surg [Br Eur] 24B: 291–295.

Heine W, Conant K, Griffin JW, Hoke A (2004) Transplanted neural stem cells promote axonal regeneration through chronically denervated peripheral nerves. Exp Neurol 189: 231–240.

Henry FP, Goyal NA, David WS, Wes D, Bujold KE, Randolph MA, Winograd JM, Kochevar IE, Redmond RW (2009) Improving electrophysiologic and histologic outcomes by photochemically sealing amnion to the peripheral nerve repair site. Surgery 145: 313–321.

Hetzler LE, Sharma N, Tanzer L, Wurster RD, Leonetti J, Marzo SJ, Jones KJ, Foecking EM (2008) Accelerating functional recovery after rat facial nerve injury: effects of gonadal steroids and electrical stimulation. Otolaryngol Head Neck Surg 139: 62–67.

Hoke A, Redett R, Hameed H, Jari R, Li JB, Griffin JW, Brushart TM (2006) Schwann cells express motor and sensory phenotypes that regulate axon regeneration. J Neurosci 26: 9646–9655.

Hontanilla B, Auba C, Gorria O (2007) Nerve regeneration through nerve autografts after local administration of brain-derived neurotrophic factor with osmotic pumps. Neurosurgery 61: 1268–1274; discussion 1274–1265.

Hu X, Cai J, Yang J, Smith GM (2010) Sensory axon targeting is increased by NGF gene therapy within the lesioned adult femoral nerve. Exp Neurol 223: 153–165.

Huang TC, Blanks RH, Berns MW, Crumley RL (1992) Laser vs. suture nerve anastomosis. Otolaryngol Head Neck Surg 107: 14–20.

Hurst LC, Badalamente MA, Ellstein J, Stracher A (1984) Inhibition of neural and muscle degeneration after epineural neurorrhaphy. J Hand Surg Am 9: 564–572.

Hynes NM, Bain JR, Thoma A, Veltri K, Maguire JA (1997) Preservation of denervated muscle by sensory protection in rats. J Reconstr Microsurg 13: 337–343.

Ilha J, Araujo RT, Malysz T, Hermel EE, Rigon P, Xavier LL, Achaval M (2008) Endurance and resistance exercise training programs elicit specific effects on sciatic nerve regeneration after experimental traumatic lesion in rats. Neurorehabil Neural Repair 22: 355–366.

Imai H, Tajima T, Natsumi Y (1996) Successful reeducation of functional sensibility after median nerve repair at the wrist. J Hand Surg 16A: 60–65.

Ingvar S (1920) Reactions of cells to the electric current in tissue cultures. Proc Soc Exp Biol Med 17: 198–199.

Irintchev A, Simova O, Eberhardt KA, Morellini F, Schachner M (2005) Impacts of lesion severity and tyrosine kinase receptor B deficiency on functional outcome of femoral nerve injury assessed by a novel single-frame motion analysis in mice. Eur J Neurosci 22: 802–808.

Isaacs JE, McDaniel CO, Owen JR, Wayne JS (2008) Comparative analysis of biomechanical performance of available "nerve glues." J Hand Surg Am 33: 893–899.

Ito H, Bassett AL (1983) Effect of weak, pulsing electromagnetic fields on neural regeneration in the rat. Clin Orthop 181: 283–290.

Jaffe LF, Poo MM (1979) Neurites grow faster towards the cathode than the anode in a steady field. J Exp Zool 209: 115–128.

Jeans LA, Gilchrist T, Healy D (2007) Peripheral nerve repair by means of a flexible biodegradable glass fibre wrap: a comparison with microsurgical epineurial repair. J Plast Reconstr Aesthet Surg 60: 1302–1308.

Jubran M, Widenfalk J (2003) Repair of peripheral nerve transections with fibrin sealant containing neurotrophic factors. Exp Neurol 181: 204–212.

Kemp SW, Walsh SK, Zochodne DW, Midha R (2007) A novel method for establishing daily in vivo concentration gradients of soluble nerve growth factor (NGF). J Neurosci Methods 165: 83–88.

Kenney AM, Kocsis JD (1998) Peripheral axotomy induces long-term c-Jun amino-terminal kinase-1 activation and activator protein-1 binding activity by c-Jun and junD in adult rat dorsal root ganglia in vivo. J Neurosci 18: 1318–1328.

Kern H, Boncompagni S, Rossini K, Mayr W, Fano G, Zanin ME, Podhorska-Okolow M, Protasi F, Carraro U (2004) Long-term denervation in humans causes degeneration of both contractile and excitation-contraction coupling apparatus, which is reversible by functional electrical stimulation (FES): a role for myofiber regeneration? J Neuropathol Exp Neurol 63: 919–931.

Kerns JM, Fakhouri AJ, Weinrib HP, Freeman JA (1991) Electrical stimulation of nerve regeneration in the rat: the early effects evaluated by a vibrating probe and electron microscopy. Neuroscience 40: 93–107.

Kerns JM, Pavkovic IM, Fakhouri AJ, Gray GT (1994) Electrical stimulation of nerve regeneration in the rat: functional evaluation by a twitch tension method. Restor Neurol Neurosci 6: 175–180.

Kilmer S, Carlsen R (1984) Forskolin activation of adenylate cyclase in vivo stimulates nerve regeneration. Nature 307: 455–457.

Kilvington B (1912) An investigation on the regeneration of nerves, with regard to the surgical treatment of certain paralyses. Br Med J I:177–179.

Kim DH, Kline DG (1990) Peri-epineurial tissue to supplement laser welding of nerve. Neurosurgery 26: 211–216.

Kohmura E, Yuguchi T, Yoshimine T, Fujinaka T, Koseki N, Sano A, Kishino A, Nakayama C, Sakaki T, Nonaka M, Takemoto O, Hayakawa T (1999) BDNF atelocollagen mini-pellet accelerates facial nerve regeneration. Brain Res 849: 235–238.

Krekoski CA, Neubauer D, Zuo J, Muir D (2001) Axonal regeneration into acellular nerve grafts is enhanced by degradation of chondroitin sulfate proteoglycan. J Neurosci 21: 6206–6213.

Kuffler DP (1996) Chemotropic factors direct regenerating axons. News Physiol Sci 11: 219–222.

Kujawa KA, Kinderman NB, Jones KJ (1989) Testosterone-induced acceleration of recovery from facial paralysis following crush axotomy of the facial nerve in male hamsters. Exp Neurol 105: 80–85.

Kujawa KA, Jacob JM, Jones KJ (1993) Testosterone regulation of the regenerative properties of injured rat sciatic motor neurons. J Neurosci Res 35: 268–273.

Kuo LT, Simpson A, Schanzer A, Tse J, An SF, Scaravilli F, Groves MJ (2005) Effects of systemically administered NT-3 on sensory neuron loss and nestin expression following axotomy. J Comp Neurol 482: 320–332.

Kuo LT, Groves MJ, Scaravilli F, Sugden D, An SF (2007) Neurotrophin-3 administration alters neurotrophin, neurotrophin receptor and nestin mRNA expression in rat dorsal root ganglia following axotomy. Neuroscience 147: 491–507.

Li H, Wigley C, Hall SM (1998) Chronically denervated rat Schwann cells respond to GGF in vitro. Glia 24: 290–303.

Li Y, Yamamoto M, Raisman G, Choi D, Carlstedt T (2007) An experimental model of ventral root repair showing the beneficial effect of transplanting olfactory ensheathing cells. Neurosurgery 60: 734–741.

Lin JC, Schwentker-Colizza A, Curtis CG, Clarke HM (2009) Final results of grafting versus neurolysis in obstetrical brachial plexus palsy. Plast Reconstr Surg 123: 939–948.

Lindwall C, Dahlin L, Lundborg G, Kanje M (2004) Inhibition of c-Jun phosphorylation reduces axonal outgrowth of adult rat nodose ganglia and dorsal root ganglia sensory neurons. Mol Cell Neurosci 27: 267–279.

Ljungberg C, Novikov L, Kellerth JO, Ebendal T, Wiberg M (1999) The neurotrophins NGF and NT-3 reduce sensory neuronal loss in adult rat after peripheral nerve lesion. Neurosci Lett 262: 29–32.

Longo FM, Yang T, Hamilton S, Hyde JF, Walker J, Jennes L, Stach R, Sisken BF (1999) Electromagnetic fields influence NGF activity and levels following sciatic nerve transection. J Neurosci Res 55: 230–237.

Lore AB, Hubbell JA, Bobb DS, Ballinger ML, Loftin KL, Smith JW, Smyers ME, Garcia HD, Bittner GD (1999) Rapid induction of functional and morphological continuity between severed ends of mammalian or earthworm myelinated axons. J Neurosci 19: 2442–2454.

Lundborg G, Bjorkman A, Hansson T, Nylander L, Nyman T, Rosen B (2005) Artificial sensibility of the hand based on cortical audiotactile interaction: a study using functional magnetic resonance imaging. Scand J Plast Reconstr Surg Hand Surg 39: 370–372.

Lundborg G, Bjorkman A, Rosen B (2007) Enhanced sensory relearning after nerve repair by using repeated forearm anaesthesia: aspects on time dynamics of treatment. Acta Neurochir Suppl 100: 121–126.

Lutz BS, Wei FC, Ma SF, Chuang DC (1999) Effects of insulin-like growth factor-1 in motor nerve regeneration after nerve transection and repair vs. nerve crushing injury in the rat. Acta Neurochir (Wien) 141: 1101–1106.

Ma JJ, Novikov LN, Wiberg M, Kellerth JO (2001) Delayed loss of spinal motoneurons after peripheral nerve injury in adult rats: a quantitative morphological study. Exp Brain Res 139: 216–223.

MacInnis BL, Campenot RB (2002) Retrograde support of neuronal survival without retrograde transport of nerve growth factor. Science 295: 1536–1539.

Mai J, Fok L, Gao H, Zhang X, Poo MM (2009) Axon initiation and growth cone turning on bound protein gradients. J Neurosci 29: 7450–7458.

Malessy MJA, De Ruiter GCW, De Boer KS, Thomeer RTWM (2004) Evaluation of suprascapular nerve neurotization after nerve graft or transfer in the treatment of brachial plexus traction lesions. J Neurosurg 101: 377–389.

Maragh H, Hawn RS, Gould JD, Terzis JK (1988) Is laser nerve repair comparable to microsuture coaptation? J Reconstr Microsurg 4: 189–195.

Maragh H, Meyer BS, Davenport D, Gould JD, Terzis JK (1990) Morphofunctional evaluation of fibrin glue versus microsuture nerve repairs. J Reconstr Microsurg 6: 331–337.

Marinesco G (1910) Nouvelles recherches sur l'influence qu'exerce l'ablation du corps thyroide sur la degenerescence et la regenerescence des nerfs. Compte rendu de la Societe de biologie 68: 188–190.

Marqueste T, Alliez JR, Alluin O, Jammes Y, Decherchi P (2004) Neuromuscular rehabilitation by treadmill running or electrical stimulation after peripheral nerve injury and repair. J Appl Physiol 96: 1988–1995.

Marqueste T, Decherchi P, Desplanches D, Favier R, Grelot L, Jammes Y (2006) Chronic electrostimulation after nerve repair by self-anastomosis: effects on the size, the mechanical, histochemical and biochemical muscle properties. Acta Neuropathol (Berl) 111: 589–600.

Marsh G, Beams HW (1946) In vitro control of growing chick nerve fibers by applied electric currents. J Cell Comp Physiol 27: 139–157.

Marshall E (1999) Gene therapy death prompts review of adenovirus vector. Science 286: 2244–2245.

Martins RS, Siqueira MG, Silva CF, Godoy BO, Plese JP (2005) Electrophysiologic assessment of regeneration in rat sciatic nerve repair using suture, fibrin glue or a combination of both techniques. Arq Neuropsiquiatr 63: 601–604.

Massey JM, Hubscher CH, Wagoner MR, Decker JA, Amps J, Silver J, Onifer SM (2006) Chondroitinase ABC digestion of the perineuronal net promotes functional collateral sprouting in the cuneate nucleus after cervical spinal cord injury. J Neurosci 26: 4406–4414.

Matras H, Braun F, Lassmann H, Ammerer HP, Mamoli B (1973) Plasma clot welding of nerves. (Experimental report). J Maxillofac Surg 1: 236–247.

Mavrogenis AF, Spyridonos SG, Antonopoulos D, Soucacos PN, Papagelopoulos PJ (2009) Effect of sensory re-education after low median nerve complete transection and repair. J Hand Surg Am 34: 1210–1215.

McDevitt L, Fortner P, Pomeranz B (1987) Application of weak electric field to the hindpaw enhances sciatic motor nerve regeneration in the adult rat. Brain Res 416: 308–314.

McGinnis ME, Murphy DJ (1992) The lack of an effect of applied D.C. electric fields on peripheral nerve regeneration in the guinea pig. Neuroscience 51: 231–244.

McKenzie IA, Biernaskie J, Toma JG, Midha R, Miller FD (2006) Skin-derived precursors generate myelinating Schwann cells for the injured and dysmyelinated nervous system. J Neurosci 26: 6651–6660.

McQuarrie I, Grafstein B, Gershon M (1977) Axonal regeneration in the rat sciatic nerve: effect of a conditioning lesion and of dbcAMP. Brain Res 132: 442–453.

McQuarrie IG (1978) The effect of a conditioning lesion on the regeneration of motor axons. Brain Res 152: 597–602.

Mears S, Schachner M, Brushart TM (2003) Antibodies to myelin-associated glycoprotein accelerate preferential motor reinnervation. JPNS 8: 91–99.

Meeker ML, Farel PB (1993) Coincidence of Schwann cell-derived basal lamina development and loss of regenerative specificity of spinal motoneurons. J Comp Neurol 329: 257–268.

Menovsky T, van den Bergh Weerman M, Beek JF (1996) Effect of CO2 milliwatt laser on peripheral nerves: part I. A dose-response study. Microsurgery 17: 562–567.

Menovsky T, Van Den Bergh Weerman M, Beek JF (2000) Effect of CO(2)-Milliwatt laser on peripheral nerves: part II. A histological and functional study. Microsurgery 20: 150–155.

Menovsky T, Beek JF (2001) Laser, fibrin glue, or suture repair of peripheral nerves: a comparative functional, histological, and morphometric study in the rat sciatic nerve. J Neurosurg 95: 694–699.

Merzenich MM, Kaas JH, Wall J, Nelson RJ, Sur M, Felleman D (1983) Topographic reorganization of somatosensory cortical areas 3b and 1 in adult monkeys following restricted deafferentation. Neuroscience 8: 33–55.

Midha R, Munro CA, Chan S, Nitising A, Xu QG, Gordon T (2005) Regeneration into protected and chronically denervated peripheral nerve stumps. Neurosurgery 57: 1289–1298.

Mills CD, Bitler JL, Woolf CJ (2005) Role of the peripheral benzodiazepine receptor in sensory neuron regeneration. Mol Cell Neurosci 30: 228–237.

Mills C, Makwana M, Wallace A, Benn S, Schmidt H, Tegeder I, Costigan M, Brown RH, Jr., Raivich G, Woolf CJ (2008) Ro5-4864 promotes neonatal motor neuron survival and nerve regeneration in adult rats. Eur J Neurosci 27: 937–946.

Molteni R, Zheng JQ, Ying Z, Gomez-Pinilla F, Twiss JL (2004) Voluntary exercise increases axonal regeneration from sensory neurons. Proc Natl Acad Sci USA 101: 8473–8478.

Mourad PD, Lazar DA, Curra FP, Mohr BC, Andrus KC, Avellino AM, McNutt LD, Crum LA, Kliot M (2001) Ultrasound accelerates functional recovery after peripheral nerve damage. Neurosurgery 48: 1136–1140.

Murray GR (1891) Note on the treatment of myxedema by hypodermic injections of an extract of the thyroid gland of a sheep. Br Med J 2: 796–797.

Narakas A (1988) The use of fibrin glue in repair of peripheral nerves. Orthop Clin North Am 19: 187–199.

Neubauer D, Graham JB, Muir D (2007) Chondroitinase treatment increases the effective length of acellular nerve grafts. Exp Neurol 207: 163–170.

Nicolaidis SC, Williams HB (2001) Muscle preservation using an implantable electrical system after nerve injury and repair. Microsurgery 21: 241–247.

Nishimura MT, Mazzer N, Barbieri CH, Moro CA (2008) Mechanical resistance of peripheral nerve repair with biological glue and with conventional suture at different postoperative times. J Reconstr Microsurg 24: 327–332.

Nix W, Hopf H (1983) Electrical stimulation of regenerating nerve and its effect on motor recovery. Brain Res 272: 21–25.

O'Neill AC, Randolph MA, Bujold KE, Kochevar IE, Redmond RW, Winograd JM (2009) Photochemical sealing improves outcome following peripheral neurorrhaphy. J Surg Res 151: 33–39.

Ochi M, Kwong WH, Kimori K, Chow SP, Ikuta Y (1992) Reinnervation of denervated skeletal muscles by grafted dorsal root ganglion. Exp Neurol 118: 291–301.

Ochi M, Kwong WH, Kimori K, Takemoto S, Chow SP, Ikuta Y (1996) Delay of the denervation process in skeletal muscle by sensory ganglion graft and its clinical application. Plast Reconstr Surg 97: 577–586.

Orgel MG, O'Brien WJ, Murray HM (1984) Pulsing electromagnetic field therapy in nerve regeneration: an experimental study in the cat. Plast Reconstr Surg 73: 173–182.

Ornelas L, Padilla L, Di Silvio M, Schalch P, Esperante S, Infante PL, Bustamante JC, Avalos P, Varela D, Lopez M (2006a) Fibrin glue: an alternative technique for nerve coaptation—Part I. Wave amplitude, conduction velocity, and plantar-length factors. J Reconstr Microsurg 22: 119–122.

Ornelas L, Padilla L, Di Silvio M, Schalch P, Esperante S, Infante RL, Bustamante JC, Avalos P, Varela D, Lopez M (2006b) Fibrin glue: an alternative technique for nerve coaptation—Part II. Nerve regeneration and histomorphometric assessment. J Reconstr Microsurg 22: 123–128.

Otto D, Unsicker K, Grothe C (1987) Pharmacological effects of nerve growth factor and fibroblast growth factor applied to the transected sciatic nerve on neuron death in adult rat dorsal root ganglia. Neurosci Lett 83: 156–160.

Oud T, Beelen A, Eijffinger E, Nollet F (2007) Sensory re-education after nerve injury of the upper limb: a systematic review. Clin Rehabil 21: 483–494.

Papakonstantinou KC, Kamin E, Terzis JK (2002) Muscle preservation by prolonged sensory protection. J Reconstr Microsurg 18: 173–182; discussion 183–174.

Patel N, Poo MM (1982) Orientation of neurite growth by extracellular electric fields. J Neurosci 2: 483–496.

Paves H, Saarma M (1997) Neurotrophins as in vitro growth cone guidance molecules for embryonic sensory neurons. Cell Tissue Res 290: 285–297.

Pavlov SP, Grosheva M, Streppel M, Guntinas-Lichius O, Irintchev A, Skouras E, Angelova SK, Kuerten S, Sinis N, Dunlop SA, Angelov DN (2008) Manually-stimulated recovery of motor function after facial nerve injury requires intact sensory input. Exp Neurol 211: 292–300.

Peterson ER, Crain SM (1972) Regeneration and innervation in cultures of adult mammalian skeletal muscle coupled with fetal rodent spinal cord. Exp Neurol 36: 136–159.

Pichichero M, Beer B, Clody D (1973) Effects of dibutyryl cyclic AMP on restoration of function of damaged sciatic nerve in rats. Science 182: 724–725.

Pockett S, Gavin RM (1985) Acceleration of peripheral nerve regeneration after crush injury in the rat. Neurosci Lett 59: 221–224.

Podhajsky RJ, Sekiguchi Y, Kikuchi S, Myers RR (2005) The histologic effects of pulsed and continuous radiofrequency lesions at 42 C to rat dorsal root ganglion and sciatic nerve. Spine 30: 1008–1013.

Politis MJ, Zanakis MF, Albala BJ (1988) Facilitated regeneration in the rat peripheral nervous system using applied electric fields. J Trauma 28: 1375–1381.

Pomeranz B, Mullen M, Markus H (1984) Effect of applied electrical fields on sprouting of intact saphenous nerve in adult rat. Brain Res 303: 331–336.

Radtke C, Aizer AA, Agulian SK, Lankford KL, Vogt PM, Kocsis JD (2009) Transplantation of olfactory ensheathing cells enhances peripheral nerve regeneration after microsurgical nerve repair. Brain Res 1254: 10–17.

Raivich G, Bohatschek M, Da Costa C, Iwata O, Galiano M, Hristova M, Nateri AS, Makwana M, Riera-Sans L, Wolfer DP, Lipp HP, Aguzzi A, Wagner EF, Behrens A (2004) The AP-1 transcription factor c-jun is required for efficient axonal regeneration. Neuron 43: 57–67.

Raji AM (1984) An experimental study of the effects of pulsed electromagnetic field (diapulse) on nerve repair. J Hand Surg 9-B:105–112.

Ramon y Cajal, S. (1928) *Degeneration and Regeneration of the Nervous System*. London: Oxford University Press.

Ranson SW (1906) Retrograde degeneration in spinal nerves. J Comp Neuro 16: 265–293.

Raper SE, Chirmule N, Lee FS, Wivel NA, Bagg A, Gao GP, Wilson JM, Batshaw ML (2003) Fatal systemic inflammatory response syndrome in a ornithine transcarbamylase deficient patient following adenoviral gene transfer. Mol Gen Metab 80: 148–158.

Raso VVM, Barbieri CH, Mazzer N, Fasan VS (2005) Can therapeutic ultrasound influence the regeneration of peripheral nerves? J Neurosci Methods 142: 185–192.

Reid AJ, Welin D, Wiberg M, Terenghi G, Novikov LN (2010) Peripherin and ATF3 genes are differentially regulated in regenerating and non-regenerating primary sensory neurons. Brain Res 1310: 1–7.

Rich KM, Luszczynski JR, Osborne PA, Johnson EM, Jr. (1987) Nerve growth factor protects adult sensory neurons from cell death and atrophy caused by nerve injury. J Neurocytol 16: 261–268.

Robinson PP, Yates JM, Smith KG (2004) An electrophysiological study into the effect of neurotrophin-3 on functional recovery after lingual nerve repair. Arch Oral Biol 49: 763–775.

Rochkind S, Barrnea L, Razon N, Bartal A, Schwartz M (1987) Stimulatory effect of He-Ne low dose laser on injured sciatic nerves of rats. Neurosurgery 20: 843–847.

Rosen B, Lundborg G (2003) Early use of artificial sensibility to improve sensory recovery after repair of the median and ulnar nerve. Scand J Plast Reconstr Surg Hand Surg 37: 54–57.

Rosen B, Bjorkman A, Lundborg G (2006) Improved sensory relearning after nerve repair induced by selective temporary anaesthesia - a new concept in hand rehabilitation. J Hand Surg Br 31: 126–132.

Rosen B, Lundborg G (2007) Enhanced sensory recovery after median nerve repair using cortical audio-tactile interaction: a randomised multicentre study. J Hand Surg Eur 32: 31–37.

Rosoff WJ, Urbach JS, Esrick MA, McAllister RG, Richards LJ, Goodhill GJ (2004) A new chemotaxis assay shows the extreme sensitivity of axons to molecular gradients. Nat Neurosci 7: 678–682.

Rusovan A, Kanje M, Mild KH (1992) The stimulatory effect of magnetic fields on regeneration of the rat sciatic nerve is frequency dependent. Exp Neurol 117: 81–84.

Rydevik M, Bergstrom F, Mitts C, Danielsen N (2002) Locally-applied collagenase and regeneration of transsected and repaired rat sciatic nerves. Scand J Plast Reconstr Surg Hand Surg 36: 193–196.

Sabatier MJ, Redmon N, Schwartz G, English AW (2008) Treadmill training promotes axon regeneration in injured peripheral nerves. Exp Neurol 211: 489–493.

Salerno GM, Bleicher JN, Stromberg BV (1990) Blink reflex recovery after electrical stimulation of the reinnervated orbicularis oculi muscle in dogs. Ann Plast Surg 25: 360–371.

Sanchez EC (2007) Hyperbaric oxygenation in peripheral nerve repair and regeneration. Neurol Res 29: 184–198.

Santos X, Rodrigo J, Hontanilla B, Bilbao G (1998) Evaluation of peripheral nerve regeneration by nerve growth factor locally administered with a novel system. J Neurosci Methods 85: 119–127.

Schafer M, Fruttiger M, Montag D, Schachner M, Martini R (1996) Disruption of the gene for the myelin-associated glycoprotein improves axonal regrowth along myelin in C57BL/Wld mice. Neuron 16: 1107–1113.

Schenker M, Kraftsik R, Glauser L, Kuntzer T, Bogousslavsky J, Barakat-Walter I (2003) Thyroid hormone reduces the loss of axotomized sensory neurons in dorsal root ganglia after sciatic nerve transection in adult rat. Exp Neurol 184: 225–236.

Schober R, Ulrich F, Sander T, Durselen H, Hessel S (1986) Laser-induced alteration of collagen substructure allows microsurgical tissue welding. Science 232: 1421–1422.

Sebille A, Bondoux-Jahan M (1980) Effects of electric stimulation and previous nerve injury on motor function recovery in rats. Brain Res 193: 562–565.

Seijffers R, Allchorne AJ, Woolf CJ (2006) The transcription factor ATF-3 promotes neurite outgrowth. Mol Cell Neurosci 32: 143–154.

Shamir MH, Rochkind S, Sandbank J, Alon M (2001) Double-blind randomized study evaluating regeneration of the rat transected sciatic nerve after suturing and postoperative low-power laser treatment. J Reconstr Microsurg 17: 133–137; discussion 138.

Sisken BF, Smith SD (1975) The effects of minute direct electrical currents on cultured chick embryo trigeminal ganglia. J Embryol Exp Morphol 33: 29–41.

Sisken BF, Kanje M, Lundborg G, Herbst E, Kurtz W (1989) Stimulation of rat sciatic nerve regeneration with pulsed electromagnetic fields. Brain Res 485: 309–316.

Smahel J, Meyer VE, Bachem U (1987) Glueing of peripheral nerves with fibrin: experimental studies. J Reconstr Microsurg 3: 211–220.

Snyder SK, Byrnes KR, Borke RC, Sanchez A, Anders JJ (2002) Quantitation of calcitonin gene-related peptide mRNA and neuronal cell death in facial motor nuclei following axotomy and 633 nm low power laser treatment. Lasers Surg Med 31: 216–222.

Sretavan DW, Chang W, Hawkes E, Keller C, Kliot M (2005) Microscale surgery on single axons. Neurosurgery 57: 635–645.

Sterkers O, Badr el Dine M, Bagot d'Arc M, Tedaldi R, Sterkers JM (1990) [Anastomosis of the facial nerve using fibrin glue, apropos of 60 cases]. Rev Laryngol Otol Rhinol (Bord) 111: 433–435.

Stracher A, McGowan EB, Shafiq SA (1978) Muscular dystrophy: inhibition of degeneration in vivo with protease inhibitors. Science 200: 50–51.

Stracher A, McGowan EB, Hedrych A, Shafiq SA (1979) In vivo effect of protease inhibitors in denervation atrophy. Exp Neurol 66: 611–618.

Stracher A (1999) Calpain inhibitors as therapeutic agents in nerve and muscle degeneration. Ann N Y Acad Sci 884: 52–59.

Sulaiman OA, Gordon T (2002) Transforming growth factor-beta and forskolin attenuate the adverse effects of long-term Schwann cell denervation on peripheral nerve regeneration in vivo. Glia 37: 206–218.

Sulaiman OA, Voda J, Gold BG, Gordon T (2002a) FK506 increases peripheral nerve regeneration after chronic axotomy but not after chronic Schwann cell denervation. Exp Neurol 175: 127–137.

Sulaiman OAR, Midha R, Munro CA, Matsuyama T, Al-Majed A, Gordon T (2002b) Chronic Schwann cell denervation and the presence of a sensory nerve reduce motor axonal regeneration. Exp Neurol 176: 342–354.

Talman P (1979) Measurement of peripheral nerve regeneration in the rat and the effects of pyronin or hypothyroidism. Exp Neurol 65: 535–541.

Tandrup T, Woolf CJ, Coggeshall RE (2000) Delayed loss of small dorsal root ganglion cells after transection of the rat sciatic nerve. J Comp Neurol 422: 172–180.

Tannemaat MR, Eggers R, Hendriks WT, de Ruiter GC, van Heerikhuize JJ, Pool CW, Malessy MJ, Boer GJ, Verhaagen J (2008) Differential effects of lentiviral vector-mediated overexpression of nerve growth factor and glial cell line-derived neurotrophic factor on regenerating sensory and motor axons in the transected peripheral nerve. Eur J Neurosci 28: 1467–1479.

Tanzer L, Jones KJ (2004) Neurotherapeutic action of testosterone on hamster facial nerve regeneration: temporal window of effects. Horm Behav 45: 339–344.

Tarlov IM, Benjamin B (1942) Autologous plasma clot suture of nerves. Science 95: 258.

Tarlov IM, Benjamin B (1943) Plasma clot and silk suture of nerves. S G & O 76: 367–374.

Temple CL, Ross DC, Dunning CE, Johnson JA (2004) Resistance to disruption and gapping of peripheral nerve repairs: an in vitro biomechanical assessment of techniques. J Reconstr Microsurg 20: 645–650.

Terzis JK, Tzafetta K (2009) The "babysitter" procedure: minihypoglossal to facial nerve transfer and cross-facial nerve grafting. Plast Reconstr Surg 123: 865–876.

Tester NJ, Howland DR (2008) Chondroitinase ABC improves basic and skilled locomotion in spinal cord injured cats. Exp Neurol 209: 483–496.

Thanos PK, Okajima S, Tiangco DA, Terzis JK (1999) Insulin-like growth factor-I promotes nerve regeneration through a nerve graft in an experimental model of facial paralysis. Restor Neurol Neurosci 15: 57–71.

Thanos PK, Tiangco DA, Terzis JK (2001) Enhanced reinnervation of the paralyzed orbicularis oculi muscle after insulin-like growth factor-I (IGF-I) delivery to a nerve graft. J Reconstr Microsurg 17: 357–362.

Todorov AT, Yogev D, Qi P, Fendler JH, Rodziewicz GS (1992) Electric-field-induced reconnection of severed axons. Brain Res 582: 329–334.

Toma JG, Akhavan M, Fernandes KJ, Barnabe-Heider F, Sadikot A, Kaplan DR, Miller FD (2001) Isolation of multipotent adult stem cells from the dermis of mammalian skin. Nat Cell Biol 3: 778–784.

Tomita K, Kubo T, Matsuda K, Yano K, Tohyama M, Hosokawa K (2007) Myelin-associated glycoprotein reduces axonal branching and enhances functional recovery after sciatic nerve transection in rats. Glia 55: 1498–1507.

Tucker KL, Meyer M, Barde YA (2001) Neurotrophins are required for nerve growth during development. Nat Neurosci 4: 29–37.

Udina E, Furey M, Busch S, Silver J, Gordon T, Fouad K (2008) Electrical stimulation of intact peripheral sensory axons in rats promotes outgrowth of their central projections. Exp Neurol 210: 238–247.

Udina E, Ladak A, Furey M, Brushart T, Tyreman N, Gordon T (2010) Rolipram-induced elevation of cAMP or chondroitinase ABC breakdown of inhibitory proteoglycans in the extracellular matrix promotes peripheral nerve regeneration. Exp Neurol 223: 143–152.

Utley DS, Lewin SL, Cheng ET, Verity AN, Sierra D, Terris DJ (1996) Brain-derived neurotrophic factor and collagen tubulization enhance functional recovery after peripheral nerve transection and repair. Arch Otolaryngol Head Neck Surg 122: 407–413.

van Meeteren NL, Brakkee JH, Hamers FP, Helders PJ, Gispen WH (1997) Exercise training improves functional recovery and motor nerve conduction velocity after sciatic nerve crush lesion in the rat. Arch Phys Med Rehabil 78: 70–77.

Walker JL, Evans JM, Resig P, Guarnieri S, Meade P, Sisken BS (1994) Enhancement of functional recovery following a crush lesion to the rat sciatic nerve by exposure to pulsed electromagnetic fields. Exp Neurol 125: 302–305.

Walker JL, Kryscio R, Smith J, Pilla A, Sisken BF (2007) Electromagnetic field treatment of nerve crush injury in a rat model: effect of signal configuration on functional recovery. Bioelectromagnetics 28: 256–263.

Wallquist W, Zelano J, Plantman S, Kaufman SJ, Cullheim S, Hammarberg H (2004) Dorsal root ganglion neurons up-regulate the expression of laminin-associated integrins after peripheral but not central axotomy. J Comp Neurol 480: 162–169.

Walsh SK, Gordon T, Addas BM, Kemp SW, Midha R (2010) Skin-derived precursor cells enhance peripheral nerve regeneration following chronic denervation. Exp Neurol 223: 221–228.

Wang H, Gu YD, Xu JG, Shen LY, Li JF (2001) Comparative study of different surgical procedures using sensory nerves or neurons for delaying atrophy of denervated skeletal muscle. J Hand Surg 26A: 326–331.

Wang WJ, Zhu H, Li F, Wan LD, Li HC, Ding WL (2009) Electrical stimulation promotes motor nerve regeneration selectivity regardless of end-organ connection. J Neurotrauma 26: 641–649.

Webber CA, Xu Y, Vanneste KJ, Martinez JA, Verge VM, Zochodne DW (2008) Guiding adult mammalian sensory axons during regeneration. J Neuropathol Exp Neurol 67: 212–222.

Weiss P, Edds MV (1945) Sensory-motor nerve crosses in the rat. J Neurophysiol 30: 173–193.

Welin D, Novikova LN, Wiberg M, Kellerth JO, Novikov LN (2008) Survival and regeneration of cutaneous and muscular afferent neurons after peripheral nerve injury in adult rats. Exp Brain Res 186: 315–323.

Welin D, Novikova LN, Wiberg M, Kellerth JO, Novikov LN (2009) Effects of N-acetyl-cysteine on the survival and regeneration of sural sensory neurons in adult rats. Brain Res 1287: 58–66.

Williams HB (1996) The value of continuous electrical muscle stimulation using a completely implantable system in the preservation of muscle function following motor nerve injury and repair: an experimental study. Microsurgery 17: 589–596.

Wilson ADH, Hart A, Brannstrom T, Wiberg M, Terenghi G (2003) Primary sensory neuronal rescue with systemic acetyl-L-carnitine following peripheral axotomy: a dose-response analysis. Br J Plast Surg 56: 732–739.

Woodhall B, Beebe GW (1956) Peripheral nerve regeneration: a follow-up study of 3,650 World War II injuries. Washington, DC: US Government Printing Office.

Wynn Parry, C.B. (1966) Rehabilitation of the Hand, 2nd ed.. London: Butterworths.

Wynn Parry CB, Salter M (1976) Sensory re-education after median nerve lesions. Hand 8: 250–257.

Xu QG, Forden J, Walsh SK, Gordon T, Midha R (2009) Motoneuron survival after chronic and sequential peripheral nerve injuries in the rat. J Neurosurg 112: 890–899.

Yates JM, Smith KG, Robinson PP (2004) The effect of brain-derived neurotrophic factor on sensory and autonomic function after lingual nerve repair. Exp Neurol 190: 495–505.

Yin Q, Kemp GJ, Yu LG, Wagstaff SC, Frostick SP (2001) Neurotrophin-4 delivered by fibrin glue promotes peripheral nerve regeneration. Muscle & Nerve 24: 345–351.

Ying Z, Roy RR, Edgerton VR, Gómez-Pinilla F (2003) Voluntary exercise increases neurotrophin-3 and its receptor TrkC in the spinal cord. Brain Res 987: 93–99.

Yogev D, Todorov AT, Qi P, Fendler JH, Rodziewicz GS (1991) Laser-induced reconnection of severed axons. Biochem Biophys Res Commun 180: 874–880.

Yohn DC, Miles GB, Rafuse VF, Brownstone RM (2008) Transplanted mouse embryonic stem-cell-derived motoneurons form functional motor units and reduce muscle atrophy. J Neurosci 28: 12409–12418.

Young BL, Begovac P, Stuart DG, Goslow GE, Jr. (1984) An effective sleeving technique in nerve repair. J Neurosci Methods 10: 51–58.

Young C, Miller E, Nicklous DM, Hoffman JR (2001) Nerve growth factor and neurotrophin-3 affect functional recovery following peripheral nerve injury differently. Restor Neurol Neurosci 18: 167–175.

Young JZ, Medawar PB (1940) Fibrin suture of peripheral nerves. The Lancet: 126–130.

Yu LM, Wosnick JH, Shoichet MS (2008) Miniaturized system of neurotrophin patterning for guided regeneration. J Neurosci Methods 171: 253–263.

Yu WH, Srinivasan R (1981) Effect of testosterone and 5 alpha-dihydrotestosterone on regeneration of the hypoglossal nerve in rats. Exp Neurol 71: 431–435.

Yu WH (1982) Sex difference in the regeneration of the hypoglossal nerve in rats. Brain Res 238: 404–406.

Zhang JY, Luo XG, Xian CJ, Liu ZH, Zhou XF (2000) Endogenous BDNF is required for myelination and regeneration of injured sciatic nerve in rodents. Eur J Neurosci 12: 4171–4180.

Zuijdendorp HM, Tra WM, van Neck JW, Mollis L, Coert JH (2010) Delay of denervation atrophy by sensory protection in an end-to-side neurorrhaphy model: a pilot study. J Plast Reconstr Aesthet Surg. In press.

Zuo J, Neubauer D, Graham J, Krekoski CA, Ferguson TA, Muir D (2002) Regeneration of axons after nerve transection repair is enhanced by degradation of chondroitin sulfate proteoglycan. Exp.Neurol. 176: 221–228.

INDEX

Note: Page numbers followed by "*f*" and "*t*" indicate figures and tables, respectively.

electrical stimulation, brief, and, 411
  nerve regeneration and, 257–58, 298–99, 298f
  promoting regeneration at repair site/distal pathway, 424
brainstem nuclei, 393, 394f, 395–96, 395f
break test, 92
Brodmann areas, 43, 44f, 45
bundle regeneration, 291–92, 291f, 292f

cAMP. *See* cyclic adenosine monophosphate
cAMP response element-binding protein (CREB), 254–55, 256, 264
canonical programs, 59, 59f
cell counting, vituperous, 143
cellular augmentation, 422, 422f
central motor reorganization
  experimental, 381, 382f, 383f
  hand replantation/transplantation, 384
  intercostal nerve transfer, 384–85, 385f
  nerve transfer *vs.* repair, 385–87, 386f
central nervous system (CNS), plasticity promotion
  intraspinal chondroitinase injection and, 408–9, 410f
  sensory reeducation and, 407–8, 408f
  target muscle manual stimulation and, 408
central pattern generators, 69
chain fibers, 66, 67f
children
  digital nerve and, 112, 113f
  intercostal nerve transfers in, 226, 227–28
  median nerve repair and, 111–13, 112f, 113f
  2-PD and, 89, 112, 113f
  ulnar nerve repair and, 111–13, 112f
chondroitinase injection, 408–9, 410f
chondroitin sulfate proteoglycans (CSPGs), 255, 258, 275, 282–83, 295
  axon regeneration and, 312–13
chronic neuronal axotomy, 255f, 266
ciliary neuronotrophic factor (CNTF), 264–65, 265f
clinical outcomes, determining
  composite strength testing, 94–95, 94f, 95f
  electrodiagnostic testing, 95
  muscle testing, 92–94, 93t
  organization of sensory testing and, 85
  rationale of sensory testing and, 84–85
  reporting frameworks, 93t, 95–96, 97t, 98t
  sensory testing
    object recognition, 91–92, 92f
    organization of, 85
    rationale, 84–85
    spatial, 88–91, 91f
    threshold, 85, 86f, 86t, 87–88
CM. *See* direct cortico-motoneuronal projections
CMAP. *See* compound muscle action potential
CNS. *See* central nervous system
CNTF. *See* ciliary neuronotrophic factor
collagen, 4
collateral reinnervation, *vs.* terminal, 216–17, 218f, 219, 219f, 220f
collateral sprouting, 387–88
compartmentation, 201, 293–94, 293f
complement receptor-3 (CR3), 287
composite strength testing, 94–95, 94f, 95f
compound muscle action potential (CMAP), 136, 137f, 138
conditioning effect, 253–54
  cAMP and, 254, 255f
  conditioning in context and, 258
  electrical stimulation, brief, and, 414, 416f, 417f
conduction
  fraction, 138
  impulse, 8
  velocities in cat, 10, 11f

connective tissue layers
  endoneurium, 15f, 16–17, 17f
  epineurium, 13–14, 15f, 17f
  perineurium, 15f, 16, 17f
  vascular supply and, 18
contact recognition, specificity and, 364–65
convergence, 41
cortical changes, in response to experimental nerve injury/regeneration
  cortical plasticity mechanisms, 396
  false sensory localization, 390–91
  human cortical plasticity, 396
  thalamic/brainstem nuclei, 393, 394f, 395–96, 395f
  transection/crush/repair, 391–93, 392f
cortical column, cutaneous sensation and, 45–46
corticoneuronal receptive field, 46, 47f
CR3. *See* complement receptor-3
CREB. *See* cAMP response element-binding protein
crush
  cortical changes in response to experimental nerve injury/regeneration and, 391–93, 392f
  electrical stimulation, brief, and, 412, 415f
cutaneous end organ reinnervation, 171
cutaneous sensation
  central processing and
    cortical column, 45–46
    corticoneuronal receptive field, 46, 47f
    dorsal column/lemniscal system, 39–41, 41f
    dorsal horn, 41–43, 42f, 43f
    DRG, 38–39
    SI, 43, 44f, 45
  evaluation
    effectiveness, 87–88, 90
    monofilaments and, 85, 86f, 86t, 87
    of object recognition, 91–92, 92f
    organization, 85
    rationale, 84–85
    of spatial discrimination, 88–91, 91f
    statistics regarding, 87
    of threshold, 85, 86f, 86t, 87–88
    of vibration, 88
  general properties, 31–32
  mechanoreceptors
    Meissner corpuscle, 32t, 33f, 34f, 35–37, 36f
    Merkel cell-neurite complex, 32–35, 32t, 33f, 34f, 35f
    Pacinian corpuscle, 32, 32t, 33f, 34f, 36f, 37
    Ruffini organ, 32, 32t, 33f, 34f, 35f, 37–38
  proximo-distal lesion level and, 113–15, 114f
  secondary cortical projections, 48
cyclic adenosine monophosphate (cAMP), 250, 252, 258, 264, 271, 284, 287, 292, 313, 316, 317f. *See also* cAMP response element-binding protein
  conditioning and, 254, 255f
  neuropoietic cytokines and, 255, 256
  response element-binding protein, 254–55, 256, 264
  targeted modification of neuronal signaling and, 418
cyclosporin A, 200, 201

DASH. *See* disabilities of the arm, shoulder, and hand instrument
DCC. *See* deleted in colorectal cancer
deleted in colorectal cancer (DCC), 311, 316
de Medinaceli, L., 145
denervated Schwann cell, 284, 429–30
DGR neurons, 409
digital nerve
  grafting regarding, 122–23, 123f
  repair in children, 112, 113f
direct cortico-motoneuronal (CM) projections, 72

NGF, 424
NTs, 424
PEMFs, 423
VEGF, 198
GTP. *See* guanosine triphosphate
guanine nucleotide exchange factors (GEFs), 270
guanosine diphosphate (GDP), 270
guanosine triphosphate (GTP), 270
guanosine triphosphate hydrolase (GTPase), 255, 261, 264, 266, 269, 270, 271

hand
    replantation/transplantation, 384
    somatotopy and, 41*f*
heat shock protein-27 (Hsp-27), 257
heels-tail angle (HTA), 147–48, 149*f*
heparin sulfate proteoglycans (HSPGs), 6
hepatocyte growth factor (HGF), 303, 303*f*
HGF. *See* hepatocyte growth factor
HNK-1 carbohydrate, 361, 411–12
hormones, 426–27
horseradish peroxidase (HRP) labeling, 70–71
    retrograde labeling studies using, 139–41, 140*f*
    simultaneous double labeling and, 141, 142*f*, 143
host response, blunting, 199–201
House-Brackmann scale, 124
H reflex, 136
    after nerve repair/transfer, 380–81
HRP. *See* horseradish peroxidase labeling
Hsp-27. *See* heat shock protein-27
HSPGs. *See* heparin sulfate proteoglycans
HTA. *See* heels-tail angle
human cortical plasticity, 396
hyperbaric oxygen, 423–24
hyperpathic pain, 151–52

Ia
    afferent projections, 70–71, 70*f*, 71*f*
    inhibitory interneurons, 70*f*, 72–73
Ib interneurons, 73–74
IGF-1. *See* insulin-like growth factor 1
IGF-2. *See* insulin-like growth factor 2
IL-1β. *See* interleukin-1β
IL-6. *See* interleukin-6
IL-10. *See* interleukin-10
ILK. *See* integrin-linked kinase
impulse conduction, anatomy/function, 8
inhibition, overcoming, 255
inhibitory components removal, 427–29, 429*f*
innervation ratio, 59–60
inosculation, 197–98, 197*f*
insulin-like growth factor 1 (IGF-1)
    axon regeneration and, 305–7, 306*f*
    promoting regeneration at repair site/distal pathway, 425
insulin-like growth factor 2 (IGF-2), 305–6, 306*f*, 307
α7β1 integrin, 418–19
integrin-linked kinase (ILK), 293
integrins, 5–6, 293, 418–19
intercostal nerve transfers
    central motor reorganization and, 384–85, 385*f*
    in children, 226, 227–28
    for elbow flexion, 226–28, 227*f*
interleukin-1β (IL-1β), 286–87, 295
interleukin-6 (IL-6), 252, 257, 258, 264, 287
    neuropoietic cytokines and, 255–56
interleukin-10 (IL-10), 282
intraneural organization of axons

dissection, 18–19, 19*f*, 20*f*
    microneurography, 19*f*, 20, 20*f*
    retrograde tracing, 19, 21*f*, 22*f*
intraspinal chondroitinase injection, 408–9, 410*f*
inverted silicon "y" chamber, 355–56, 355*f*, 356*f*
isometric muscle strength, 169–70

JAK. *See* janus kinase
Jamar dynamometer, 94*f*
janus kinase (JAK), 264, 265
JNK. *See* c-Jun terminal kinase
c-Jun terminal kinase (JNK), 256, 261
c-Jun transcription factor, 419
juxtaparanode, 3, 4*f*
JVP grating dome, 90–91, 91*f*

kappa value, 87

L. *See* large light neurons
L1, 312
labeling techniques
    nerve repair/grafting experimental outcomes
        correlations in, 176, 177*f*
        sequential double labeling and, 144*f*, 175–76
        simultaneous double/triple labeling and, 142*f*, 173–75, 173*f*, 174*f*
        single labeling and, 171–73, 172*f*
    retrograde labeling studies
        HRP used in, 139–41, 140*f*
        TMB and, 139
        WGA and, 141
    sequential double labeling, 143–45, 144*f*
        nerve repair/grafting experimental outcomes and, 144*f*, 175–76
    simultaneous double labeling
        cell counting and, 143
        end-to-side nerve repair and, 216–17
        FG/FR and, 141, 142*f*
        HRP and, 141, 142*f*, 143
        nerve repair/grafting experimental outcomes and, 142*f*, 173–75, 173*f*, 174*f*
laminin, 4
    axon regeneration and, 309–10
    basement membrane grafts and, 202
large light neurons (L), 38–39
laser repair, 420
latency, 136
law of specific nerve energies, 31
lemniscal system, 39–41, 41*f*
leucine-rich repeat- and Ig domain-containing Nogo receptor-interacting protein (LINGO), 255, 261
leukemia inhibitory factor (LIF), 252, 255, 256, 257, 264, 287, 305, 307
LIF. *See* leukemia inhibitory factor
LINGO. *See* leucine-rich repeat- and Ig domain-containing Nogo receptor-interacting protein
local protein synthesis, 272–73, 273*f*
locognosia, 91
Louisiana State University (LSU) scale, 96
    radial nerve and, 127
    sciatic nerve and, 130
LSU. *See* Louisiana State University scale
lumbricals, 108*f*

M1. *See* primary motor cortex
MAG. *See* myelin-associated glycoprotein
magnetoneurography, 138
make test, 92

mammalian target of rapamycin (mTOR), 257
manual muscle testing (MMT), 92–94, 93t
manual stimulation of target muscles, 408
MAP1B. *See* microtubule-associated protein 1B
MAPK/ERK. *See* mitogen-activated protein kinase/extracellular
  signal-regulated kinase
matrix metalloproteinase-9 (MMP-9), 287
MBP. *See* myelin basic protein
MCP-1. *See* monocyte chemotactic protein-1
MCP-1α. *See* monocyte chemoattractant protein-1α
mechanical alignment, 366–67
mechanoreceptors
  cutaneous
    Meissner corpuscle, 32t, 33f, 34f, 35–37, 36f
    Merkel cell-neurite complex, 32–35, 32t, 33f, 34f, 35f
    Pacinian corpuscle, 32, 32t, 33f, 34f, 36f, 37
    Ruffini organ, 32, 32t, 33f, 34f, 35f, 37–38
  subcutaneous, 14t
median nerve
  anatomy, 106, 107f, 108, 108f
  axon loss and, 126–27
  fascicles, 228
  grafting, 120, 121f
    age and, 121
    analysis of variables, 120–23, 122f
    digital nerve and, 122–23, 123f
    end-to-end repair compared with, 111f, 120, 121f
    graft length regarding, 121–22
  repair, 108–11, 111f
    age regarding, 111–13, 112f, 113f
    faulty sensory localization and, 118–20, 119f
    grafting compared with, 111f, 120, 121f
    proximo-distal lesion level and, 113–15, 114f
    surgical technique and, 116, 117f, 118
    thalamic/brainstem nuclei regarding, 393, 394f, 395–96, 395f
    treatment delay and, 115
    violence of injury and, 115–16
Meissner corpuscles
  function of, 35–37
  location of, 34f, 35
  properties, 32t
  RA and, 32
  receptor density/fields and, 36f
  structure of, 33f, 36
Merkel cell-neurite complex
  function of, 33–34
  location of, 33, 34f
  NTs and, 34
  properties, 32t
  receptor density/fields and, 35f
  SA and, 32
  structure of, 32–33, 33f
  surround suppression and, 34–35
mesothelial tube, 207, 208f
microneurography, 19f, 20, 20f
microtubule-associated protein 1B (MAP1B), 279
microtubules, 270–71
Mitchell series, 95
mitogen-activated protein kinase/extracellular signal-regulated
  kinase (MAPK/ERK), 251
M-line, 57–58, 57f
MMP-9. *See* matrix metalloproteinase-9
MMT. *See* manual muscle testing
Moberg, E., 89, 91
molecules
  axon/myelin/Schwann cell interactions with, 5f
  CSPGs, 255, 258, 275, 282–83, 295, 312–13

electrical stimulation, brief, and, 411–12
FN, 4, 310
galectin-1, 311
L1, 312
laminin, 4, 202, 309–10
MAG, 5f, 7, 312
myosin, 57, 58–59, 58f
NCAM, 264, 283, 295, 308, 312
netrin-1, 311
neuropilins, 311–12
tenascin-C and, 310–11
monocyte chemoattractant protein-1α (MCP-1α), 287
monocyte chemotactic protein-1 (MCP-1), 286–87
monofilaments, 85, 86f, 86t, 87
Montoya staircase test, 149–50, 150f, 180
morphologic studies of skin/muscle, 139
motion
  age and, 112–13
  direct CM projections and, 72
  functional anatomy of, 68–69, 69f, 70f
  Golgi tendon organ and, 65–66, 65f
  Ia afferent projections and, 70–71, 70f, 71f
  Ia inhibitory interneurons and, 70f, 72–73
  Ib interneurons and, 73–74
  motoneuron-muscle interactions and, 62
  motoneuron pool and, 62, 63f
    inputs to, 69–70
  motor endplate and, 63–65, 64f
  motor unit
    distribution/innervation ratio, 59–60
    firing rate, 61–62
    physiologic classification, 59, 59f
    recruitment, 60–61, 61f
  muscle fiber types and, 58–59, 58f, 59f
  muscle receptors and, 65
  muscle spindle and, 66–68, 67f
  proximo-distal lesion level and, 113–15, 114f
  sarcomere and, 56–58, 57f
motoneuron
  death, 377
  direct CM projections and, 72
  ectopic transplantation, 433
  Ia afferent projections and, 70–71, 70f, 71f
  Ia inhibitory interneurons and, 70f, 72–73
  Ib interneurons and, 73–74
  muscle interactions with, 62
  neuronal rescue regarding, 409
  PMR and, 362
  pool, 62, 63f
    inputs, 69–70
  structure change, 377–78
motor-end organ specificity, 363–64
motor endplate, 63–65, 64f
motor system, after repair/transfer
  central motor reorganization
    experimental, 381, 382f, 383f
    hand replantation/transplantation, 384
    intercostal nerve transfer, 384–85, 385f
    nerve transfer *vs.* repair, 385–87, 386f
  experimental afferent fiber misdirection, 378–79
  Golgi tendon organs, 379–80, 380f
  H reflex, 380–81
  motoneuron death, 377
  motoneuron structure change, 377–78
  motor unit and, 375–77, 376f
  muscle afferents, 378, 379f
  stretch reflex, 380

nerve regeneration (*cont'd*)
    extracellular matrix/recognition molecules and (*cont'd*)
        galectin-1, 311
        L1, 312
        laminin, 309–10
        MAG, 312
        NCAM, 312
        netrin-1, 311
        neuropilins, 311–12
        tenascin-C, 310–11
    FGFS, 307–9
    GDNF and, 262, 263*f*, 264
    growth cone, 267
        actin bundles, 268–70
        form/function, 267–71, 269*f*, 270*f*
        guidance, 271–72, 271*f*
        manipulation with electric fields, 422–23
        microtubules, 270–71
    HGF, 303, 303*f*
    IGF-1, 305–7, 306*f*
    IGF-2, 305–6, 306*f*, 307
    local protein synthesis and, 272–73, 273*f*
    neuronal intrinsic growth state and, 253
    neuronal signaling and, 258–59
    neuron and, 252–53
    neuropoietic cytokines and, 255–56, 255*f*
    NTs
        BDNF, 298–99, 298*f*
        BMPs, 302–3
        GDNF, 300–302, 301*f*
        NGF, 295–98, 296*f*, 297*f*
        NT-3, 299–300
        NT-4/5, 300
        TGF-β, 302
        TGF-β superfamily, 300–303, 301*f*
    NTs/receptors and, 259–62, 260*f*, 262*f*, 263*f*
    overcoming inhibition regarding, 255
    overview, 250–51
    PMR and
        biological underpinnings of, 358, 358*f*, 359*f*
        described, 356
        femoral nerve and, 356–57
        mouse *vs.* rat and, 362–63
        potential mechanisms of, 359–62, 360*f*, 361*f*
        present/future of, 363
        pruning hypothesis and, 357–58
        retrograde tracing/electrophysiologic techniques and, 359
        simultaneous double labeling and, 357, 358*f*
    PTN, 304–5, 305*f*
    remyelination, 292–93
    repair site, 266–67
    signaling in adult mammalian neurons for, 272–73, 273*f*
    signaling in response to injury and, 255*f*, 264–66, 265*f*
    specificity regarding
        motor-end organ, 363–64
        motor-topographic, 363
        nerve trunk, 355–56, 356*f*, 357*f*
        organizational levels theoretically influencing, 354–55, 354*f*
        overview, 353
        PMR and, 356–63, 358*f*, 359*f*, 360*f*, 361*f*
        potential generation mechanisms, 364–68
        potential mechanisms of, 354, 354*f*, 359–62, 360*f*, 361*f*
        sensory-end organ, 364
        sensory-motor, 356–63, 358*f*, 359*f*, 360*f*, 361*f*
        sensory-topographic, 364, 365*f*
        tissue, 355, 355*f*
    speed, 289–91, 290*f*

transcription factors, additional, and, 255*f*, 256–57
transection/repair morphologic responses
    axon branching, 276, 277*f*, 278–79
    evolution of repair environment, 282–83
    retrograde regeneration, 268*f*, 283
    scar formation, 281–82
    staggered regeneration, 279, 280*f*, 281, 281*f*
    VEGF, 303–4, 304*f*
    Wallerian degeneration, 285
        axonal breakdown and, 285–86
        myelin breakdown/clearance and, 286–88, 286*f*, 288*f*
        terminating, 288–89
netrin-1, 311
NeuraGen©, 207–8
neural cell adhesion molecule (NCAM), 264, 283, 295, 308, 312
neural prostheses, enhancing regeneration across
    caveats regarding, 213
    growth factors for, 211–12
    Schwann/stem cells for, 212–13
Neuregulin-1 (NRG-1), 10
neurofilament proteins, 9
neuron. *See also* motoneuron; *specific subject*
    BDNF, role for, regarding, 257–58
    chronic neuronal axotomy and, 255*f*, 266
    conditioning effect and, 253–54
        cAMP and, 254, 255*f*
    conditioning in context and, 258
    GDNF and, 262, 263*f*, 264
    intrinsic growth state and, 253
    nerve regeneration and, 252–53
    neuronal signaling and, 258–59
    neuropoietic cytokines and, 255–56, 255*f*
    NTs/receptors and, 259–62, 260*f*, 262*f*, 263*f*
    overcoming inhibition and, 255
    signaling in adult mammalian, 272–73, 273*f*
    signaling in response to injury and, 255*f*, 264–66, 265*f*
    transcription factors, additional, and, 255*f*, 256–57
neuronal phenotype, DRG and, 38–39
neuronal rescue
    DRG neurons, 409
    motoneurons, 409
neuronal signaling, 258–59
neuropilins, 311–12
neuropoietic cytokines, 255–56, 255*f*
neurotization
    direct muscle, 215
    function restoration and, 214–15
    improvement of, 215
    muscle-nerve-muscle, 215
    nerve gap grafting and, 213–15, 214*f*
    polio and, 213
    process of, 214, 214*f*
neurotrophin (NT)
    BDNF, 298–99, 298*f*
    BMPs, 302–3
    CNTF, 264–65, 265*f*
    GDNF, 300–302, 301*f*
    Merkel cell-neurite complex and, 34
    NGF, 295–98, 296*f*, 297*f*
    NT-3, 68, 299–300, 424
    NT-4/5, 300, 424
    promoting regeneration at repair site/distal pathway, 424
    receptors and, 252, 255, 259–62, 260*f*, 262*f*, 263*f*, 289, 293, 295, 296
    TGF-β superfamily, 300–303, 301*f*
        BMPs, 302–3
        GDNF, 300–302, 301*f*